2000
YEAR BOOK OF
PEDIATRICS®

Statement of Purpose

The YEAR BOOK Service

The YEAR BOOK series was devised in 1901 by practicing health professionals who observed that the literature of medicine and related disciplines had become so voluminous that no one individual could read and place in perspective every potential advance in a major specialty. That has never been more true than it is today.

More than merely a series of books, YEAR BOOK volumes are the tangible results of a unique service designed to accomplish the following:

- to *survey* a wide range of journals of proven value
- to *select* from those journals papers representing significant advances and statements of important clinical principles
- to provide *abstracts* of those articles that are readable, convenient summaries of their key points
- to provide *commentary* about those articles to place them in perspective

These publications grow out of a unique process that calls on the talents of outstanding authorities in clinical and fundamental disciplines, trained literature specialists, and professional writers, all supported by the resources of Mosby, the world's preeminent publisher for the health professions.

The Literature Base

Mosby and its editors survey approximately 500 journals published worldwide, covering the full range of the health professions. On an annual basis, the publisher examines usage patterns and polls its expert authorities to add new journals to the literature base and to delete journals that are no longer useful as potential YEAR BOOK sources.

The Literature Survey

The publisher's team of literature specialists examines every original, peer-reviewed article in each journal issue. More than 250,000 articles per year are scanned systematically, including title, text, illustrations, tables, and references. Each scan is compared, article by article, to the search strategies that the publisher has developed in consultation with the 270 outside experts who form the pool of YEAR BOOK editors. A given article may be reviewed by any number of editors, from one to a dozen or more, regardless of the discipline for which the paper was originally published. In turn, each editor who receives the article reviews it to determine whether the article should be included in the YEAR BOOK. This decision is based on the article's inherent quality, its probable usefulness to readers of that YEAR BOOK, and the editor's goal to represent a balanced picture of a given field in each volume of the YEAR BOOK. In addition, the editor indicates when to include figures and tables from the article to help the YEAR BOOK reader better understand the information.

Of the quarter million articles scanned each year, only 5% are selected for detailed analysis within the YEAR BOOK series, thereby assuring readers of the high value of every selection.

The Abstract

The publisher's abstracting staff is headed by a seasoned medical professional and includes individuals with training in the life sciences, medicine, and other areas, plus extensive experience in writing for the health professions and related industries. Each selected article is assigned to a specific writer on this abstracting staff. The abstracter, guided in many cases by notations supplied by the physician editor, writes a structured, condensed summary designed so the reader can rapidly acquire the essential information contained in the article.

The Commentary

The YEAR BOOK editorial boards, sometimes assisted by guest commentators, write comments that place each article in perspective for the reader. This provides the reader with the equivalent of a personal consultation with a leading international authority—an opportunity to better understand the value of the article and to benefit from the authority's thought processes in assessing the article.

Additional Editorial Features

The editorial boards of each YEAR BOOK organize the abstracts and comments to provide a logical and satisfying sequence of information. To enhance the organization, editors also provide introductions to sections or individual chapters, comments linking a number of abstracts, citations to additional literature, and other features.

The published YEAR BOOK contains enhanced bibliographic citations for each selected article, including extended listings of multiple authors and identification of author affiliations. Each YEAR BOOK contains a Table of Contents specific to that year's volume. From year to year, the Table of Contents for a given YEAR BOOK will vary depending on developments within the field.

Every YEAR BOOK contains a list of the journals from which papers have been selected. This list represents a subset of approximately 500 journals surveyed by the publisher and occasionally reflects a particularly pertinent article from a journal that is not surveyed on a routine basis.

Finally, each volume contains a comprehensive subject index and an index to authors of each selected paper.

The 2000 Year Book Series

Year Book of Allergy, Asthma, and Clinical Immunology™: Drs Rosenwasser, Boguniewicz, Milgrom, Routes, Spahn, and Weber

Year Book of Anesthesiology and Pain Management®: Drs Tinker, Abram, Chestnut, Roizen, Rothenberg, and Wood

Year Book of Cardiology®: Drs Schlant, Collins, Gersh, Graham, Kaplan, and Waldo

Year Book of Chiropractic®: Dr Lawrence

Year Book of Critical Care Medicine®: Drs Parrillo, Balk, Calvin, Franklin, and Shapiro

Year Book of Dentistry®: Drs Zakariasen, Dederich, Boghosian, Horswell, McIntyre, and Hatcher

Year Book of Dermatology and Dermatologic Surgery™: Drs Thiers and Lang

Year Book of Diagnostic Radiology®: Drs Osborn, Birdwell, Dalinka, Groskin, Maynard, Oestreich, Pentecost, Ros, Smirniotopoulos, and Young

Year Book of Emergency Medicine®: Drs Burdick, Cydulka, Cone, Loiselle, Niemann, and Hamilton

Year Book of Endocrinology®: Drs Mazzaferri, Fitzpatrick, Horton, Kannan, Meikle, Molitch, Morley, Osei, Poehlman, and Rogol

Year Book of Family Practice®: Drs Berg, Bowman, Davidson, Dexter, Scherger, and Morrison

Year Book of Gastroenterology™: Dr Lichtenstein

Year Book of Hand Surgery®: Drs Amadio and Hentz

Year Book of Medicine®: Drs Mandell, Jett, Loehrer, Frishman, Barkin, Mazzaferri, Klahr, and Malawista

Year Book of Neonatal and Perinatal Medicine®: Drs Fanaroff, Maisels, and Stevenson

Year Book of Nephrology, Hypertension, and Mineral Metabolism: Drs Schwab, Bennett, Emmett, Moe, and Textor

Year Book of Neurology and Neurosurgery®: Drs Bradley and Gibbs

Year Book of Nuclear Medicine®: Drs Gottschalk, Blaufox, Coleman, Strauss, and Zubal

Year Book of Obstetrics, Gynecology, and Women's Health®: Drs Mishell, Herbst, and Kirschbaum

Year Book of Oncology®: Drs Loehrer, Glatstein, Gordon, Thigpen, Pratt, Eisenberg, and Johnson

Year Book of Ophthalmology®: Drs Wilson, Cohen, Eagle, Grossman, Laibson, Maguire, Nelson, Penne, Rapuano, Sergott, Shields, Spaeth, Tipperman, Ms Gosfield, and Ms Salmon

Year Book of Orthopedics®: Drs Morrey, Beauchamp, Currier, Tolo, Trigg, and Swiontkowski

Year Book of Otolaryngology–Head and Neck Surgery®: Drs Paparella, Holt, and Otto

Year Book of Pathology and Laboratory Medicine®: Drs Raab, Dabbs, Olson, Silverman, and Stanley

Year Book of Pediatrics®: Dr Stockman

Year Book of Plastic, Reconstructive, and Aesthetic Surgery®: Drs Miller, Bartlett, Garner, McKinney, Ruberg, Salisbury, and Smith

Year Book of Psychiatry and Applied Mental Health®: Drs Talbott, Ballenger, Frances, Jensen, Meltzer, Simpson, and Tasman

Year Book of Pulmonary Disease®: Drs Jett, Castro, Maurer, Peters, Phillips, and Ryu

Year Book of Rheumatology, Arthritis, and Musculoskeletal Disease™: Drs Panush, Hadler, Hellmann, LeRoy, Pisetsky, and Simon

Year Book of Sports Medicine®: Drs Shephard, Kohrt, Nieman, Torg, Alexander, and Mr George

Year Book of Surgery®: Drs Copeland, Bland, Deitch, Eberlein, Howard, Luce, Seeger, Souba, and Sugarbaker

Year Book of Urology®: Drs Andriole and Coplen

Year Book of Vascular Surgery®: Dr Porter

2000

The Year Book of PEDIATRICS®

Editor

James A. Stockman III, M.D.
President, The American Board of Pediatrics; Clinical Professor of Pediatrics, School of Medicine, University of North Carolina at Chapel Hill, Chapel Hill, North Carolina; Clinical Professor of Pediatrics, Duke University Medical Center, Durham, North Carolina

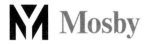 Mosby

St. Louis Baltimore Boston Carlsbad Naples New York Philadelphia Portland London
Madrid Mexico City Singapore Sydney Tokyo Toronto Wiesbaden

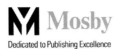

Dedicated to Publishing Excellence

Publisher: Susan Patterson
Developmental Editor: Colleen Cook
Manager, Periodical Editing: Kirk Swearingen
Production Editor: Stephanie M. Geels
Project Supervisor, Production: Joy Moore
Production Assistant: Karie House
Manager, Literature Services: Idelle L. Winer
Illustrations and Permissions Coordinator: Chidi C. Ukabam

2000 EDITION
Copyright © 2000 by Mosby, Inc.

Printed in the United States of America
Composition by Reed Technology and Information Services, Inc.
Printing/binding by Maple-Vail

Editorial Office:
Mosby, Inc.
11830 Westline Industrial Drive
St. Louis, MO 63146

International Standard Serial Number: 0084-3954
International Standard Book Number: 0-8151-9038-7

Contributing Editors

Mosby, Inc. and James A. Stockman III, M.D. would like to thank the following individuals for contributing their knowledge and expertise to this edition.

Alagappan Alagappan, M.D.
Benjamin S. Alexander, M.D.
Estella M. Alonso, M.D.
Yoshizo Asano, M.D.
Balu H. Athreya, M.D.
M. Douglas Baker, M.D.
Noosha Baqi, M.D.
Louis M. Bell, M.D.
Stephen Berman, M.D.
Paula A. Braveman, M.D., M.P.H.
Rebecca H. Buckley, M.D.
Mary T. Caserta, M.D.
Steven D. Chernausek, M.D.
Daniel I. Craven, M.D.
Barbara A. Dennison, M.D.
William H. Dietz, M.D., Ph.D*
Donna M. DiMichele, M.D.
David Driscoll, M.D.
Howard Dubowitz, M.D., M.S.
Andrea M. Dunk, M.D.
Michael S. Dunn, M.D., F.R.C.P.C.
Kai J. Eriksson, M.D., Ph.D.
Gary R. Fleisher, M.D.
Ilona J. Frieden, M.D.
Henry S. Friedman, M.D.
Herbert E. Fuchs, M.D., Ph.D.
Jeffrey B. Gould, M.D., M.P.H.
Michael Jellinek, M.D.
Joyce M. Koenig, M.D.
Nathan Kuppermann, M.D., M.P.H.
Edmund F. La Gamma, M.D.
Craig B. Langman, M.D.
Michael R. Lawless, M.D.
Christoph U. Lehmann, M.D.
Richard Liberthson, M.D.
M. Jeffrey Maisels, M.B., B.Ch.
David O. Matson, M.D., Ph.D.

---

*Dr. Dietz contributed to this book in his private capacity, and no official endorsement or support by the Centers for Disease Control and Prevention is intended or should be inferred.

Constantine Mavroudis, M.D.
John F. Modlin, M.D.
Paul W. Newacheck, Dr.P.H.
Michael E. Pichichero, M.D.
Charles G. Prober, M.D.
Richard A. Saunders, M.D.
Suzanne Schuh, M.D., F.R.C.P.C.
Peter G. Steinherz, M.D.
Meredith Stockman
Samantha Stockman, B.S.
Russell E. Ware, M.D., Ph.D.

Table of Contents

Journals Represented

Mosby and its editors survey approximately 500 journals for its abstract and commentary publications. From these journals, the editors select the articles to be abstracted. Journals represented in this YEAR BOOK are listed below.

American Journal of Cardiology
American Journal of Gastroenterology
Annals of Internal Medicine
Annals of Neurology
Annals of Surgery
Archives of Disease in Childhood
Archives of Ophthalmology
Archives of Otolaryngology-Head and Neck Surgery
Archives of Pediatrics and Adolescent Medicine
Blood
British Medical Journal
Child Development
Circulation
Clinical Pediatrics
Epilepsia
Journal of Adolescent Health
Journal of Allergy and Clinical Immunology
Journal of Clinical Microbiology
Journal of Clinical Oncology
Journal of Developmental and Behavioral Pediatrics
Journal of Infectious Diseases
Journal of Pediatric Gastroenterology and Nutrition
Journal of Pediatric Hematology/Oncology
Journal of Pediatric Orthopaedics
Journal of Pediatric Surgery
Journal of Pediatrics
Journal of Perinatology
Journal of Rheumatology
Journal of Urology
Journal of the American Academy of Child and Adolescent Psychiatry
Journal of the American Academy of Dermatology
Journal of the American College of Cardiology
Journal of the American Medical Association
Lancet
Medicine
New England Journal of Medicine
Ophthalmology
Pediatric Dentistry
Pediatric Dermatology
Pediatric Emergency Care
Pediatric Infectious Disease Journal
Pediatric Neurology
Pediatrics
Science

STANDARD ABBREVIATIONS

The following terms are abbreviated in this edition: acquired immunodeficiency syndrome (AIDS), cardiopulmonary resuscitation (CPR), central nervous system (CNS), cerebrospinal fluid (CSF), computed tomography (CT), deoxyribonucleic acid (DNA), electrocardiography (ECG), health maintenance organization (HMO), human immunodeficiency virus (HIV), intensive care unit (ICU), intramuscular (IM), intravenous (IV), magnetic resonance (MR) imaging (MRI), ribonucleic acid (RNA), and ultrasound (US).

NOTE

The YEAR BOOK OF PEDIATRICS® is a literature survey service providing abstracts of articles published in the professional literature. Every effort is made to ensure the accuracy of the information presented in these pages. Neither the editors nor the publisher of the YEAR BOOK OF PEDIATRICS® can be responsible for errors in the original materials. The editors' comments are their own opinions. Mention of specific products within this publication does not constitute endorsement.

To facilitate the use of the YEAR BOOK OF PEDIATRICS® as a reference tool, all illustrations and tables included in this publication are now identified as they appear in the original article. This change is meant to help the reader recognize that any illustration or table appearing in the YEAR BOOK OF PEDIATRICS® may be only one of many in the original article. For this reason, figure and table numbers will often appear to be out of sequence within the YEAR BOOK OF PEDIATRICS.®

Introduction

Given the infrequency with which we begin millenniums, it seems worthwhile to look back to see what those in their late 70s who might still be practicing pediatrics would have learned about the care of infants, children, and adolescents early in their careers. Chosen for this purpose was the 1953-1954 YEAR BOOK OF PEDIATRICS (the oldest in this editor's collection), with contents providing a snapshot of pediatrics a la the "Happy Days" era of the last millennium.

Through the articles selected for the YEAR BOOK OF PEDIATRICS, pediatricians of the 1950s learned to coat the ends of polyethylene feeding tubes with melted wax so as not to injure the esophagus of neonates. They were told to treat the anemia of prematurity with "molybdenized" ferrous sulfate and to give liver supplements and vitamin B_{12} to children with short stature. The continuing value of evaporated milk formulas was not yet a subject of concern or debate. There were only four vaccinations available: diptheria, tetanus, pertussis, and smallpox, although the 1953-1954 YEAR BOOK did include an abstract of an article from *JAMA* entitled: "Studies in human subjects on active immunization against poliomyelitis: 1. Preliminary report of experiments in progress" by Dr. Jonas E. Salk. The subject was not found to be sufficiently important to warrant a commentary.

The 1953-1954 YEAR BOOK OF PEDIATRICS was filled with talk of "saving" premature infants with oxygen, mist, and hyperbaric "locks," of retrolental fibroplasia, of neonatal staphylococcal pneumonia and *Pseudomonas* meningitis, and of irradiation of the nasopharynx to treat enlarged tonsils and "infectious" asthma. It was also 1953 that defined the treatment of otitis media as being 10 days of oral antibiotics (the drug of choice was Terramycin [Pfizer]). It was in 1953 that cat scratch encephalitis was first reported, along with the initial descriptions of idiopathic Heinz body anemia (later attributed to G6PD deficiency), and the association of a parasite, *Pneumocystis carinii*, in the lungs of newborns with "interstitial plasma cell pneumonia." Dr. Sydney Gellis, editor of the YEAR BOOK in those days, in commenting on that association, remarked that there was "no evidence...that [the parasite] is pathogenic, and its presence...may not bear an etiologic relationship to the pneumonitis,"[1] although he did recommend treatment with the standard antiprotozoals of the era: arasphen, quinine, and Atabrine. It was 1953 that saw the early reports of reduction of hydrostatic ileocecal intussusception. Dr. Gellis strongly opposed the technique ("We are still stubbornly opposed to the widespread use of reduction by barium enema)" and was supported by the famous surgeon of the time, Dr. Robert E. Gross, who remarked in a YEAR BOOK commentary: I distinctly fear that [babies undergoing this procedure] will have handling which...leaves the child in an exhausted state for the surgical procedure that must follow."[2] Similarly dismissed was the first description of the enuresis alarm that same year. Dr. Gellis noted that otherwise normal children with enuresis "...need no apparatus unless laundry problems are paramount."[3] On the other hand, support was provided for such interesting treatments such as infecting patients who had idiopathic nephrosis with malarial organisms. Some patients with ne-phrotic syndrome actually responded to this novel therapy, and besides, the infection itself was "...simple to transmit and to control."[4] It is obvious that those who are now our senior pediatricians learned much that was inaccurate as the science of child care evolved through the last century. Things aren't much different now, are they?

It should be mandatory for all those exiting residency training to take a look back at what was the basis of the teachings of the generation of pediatricians that preceded them. Old YEAR BOOKS are great for that purpose. One can see that easily half of the practice of medicine involves a continuous process of purging old, often wrong information, and that the only thing certain about change is that it will occur, usually sooner than expected. One wonders which part of the contents of the 2000 YEAR BOOK OF PEDIATRICS will quickly find itself in an information scrap yard. Read on and take a guess.

James A. Stockman III, M.D.

Editor

References

1. 1953-1954 YEAR BOOK OF PEDIATRICS, p 179.
2. 1953-1954 YEAR BOOK OF PEDIATRICS, p 207.
3. 1953-1954 YEAR BOOK OF PEDIATRICS, p 378.
4. 1953-1954 YEAR BOOK OF PEDIATRICS, p 229.

1 The Newborn

Reducing the Risk of Multiple Births by Transfer of Two Embryos After In Vitro Fertilization
Templeton A, Morris JK (Human Fertilisation and Embryology Authority, London; Wolfson Inst of Preventive Medicine, London)
N Engl J Med 339:573-577, 1998   1-1

Background.—The high risk of multiple births associated with in vitro fertilization is known to be a consequence of the number of embryos

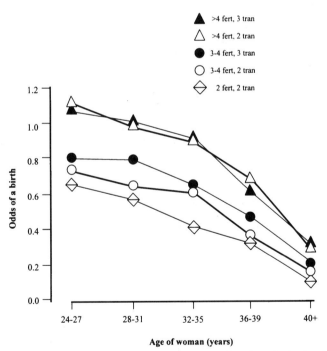

FIGURE 1.—Odds of a birth in relation to the woman's age, number of eggs fertilized, and number of embryos transferred. The odds of a birth were calculated as compared with those of a 30-year-old woman with more than 4 eggs fertilized and 2 embryos transferred (odds for this woman, 1.0). (Reprinted by permission of *The New England Journal of Medicine*, from Templeton A, Morris JK: Reducing the risk of multiple births by transfer of two embryos after in vitro fertilization. *N Engl J Med* 339:573-577. Copyright 1998, Massachusetts Medical Society. All rights reserved.)

transferred. Other factors that may contribute to this risk have not been delineated and were investigated.

Methods and Findings.—Data on 44,236 cycles in 25,240 women enrolled in the Human Fertilisation and Embryology Authority in the United Kingdom were analyzed. Factors associated with a significantly reduced chance of a birth and of multiple births were older age, tubal infertility, longer duration of infertility, and a greater number of previous in vitro fertilization attempts. A previous live birth was correlated with an increased chance of a birth but not of multiple births. The more eggs fertilized, the greater the likelihood of a live birth. More than 4 eggs fertilized was not associated with an increase in the birth rate for women receiving 3 transferred embryos compared with women receiving 2 embryos. However, the rate of multiple births was markedly increased when 3 were transferred (Fig 1).

Conclusions.—The chances of a live birth among women undergoing in vitro fertilization are correlated with the number of eggs fertilized, presumably because the selection of embryos for transfer is greater. When more than 4 eggs are fertilized and available for transfer, the transfer of only 2 embryos does not lessen a woman's chance of a birth, and transferring more embryos raises the risk of multiple births.

▶ This article created a fair amount of controversy. It was accompanied by an editorial.[1] The editorial points out that a decision to implant more than 2 embryos should be reserved to a couple and their physician. It is suggested that optimal pregnancy rates and simultaneous reduction of multiple gestation with the transfer of embryos cultured for 2 or 3 days can be achieved only with a flexible policy regarding the number of embryos transferred, which should be based on factors such as maternal age, the quality of the embryos, and the number of failed attempts previously.

Perhaps the day will come when it will be uniform policy, for good medical reasons, when only 2 embryos will be implanted. One might even look forward to the day when the transfer of a single embryo will be the usual and customary treatment for infertile couples. When that day comes, success will be also associated with a virtual elimination of the expense and tragic outcomes inherent in high-order multiple pregnancies and the painful decision that 1 or more fetuses in those circumstances should be selectively aborted. The concept of selective abortion is difficult to imagine, but it is occurring more and more frequently when many embryos are being implanted.

While we're on the topic of things related to pregnancy, have you ever heard the term "secondary spermatocytes"? A secondary spermatocyte is a spermatocyte obtained from a source other than an ejaculate. Men with non-obstructive azoospermia may be found to have foci of spermatids or spermatozoa in their testes. These can be injected into eggs, allowing fertilization and, subsequently, a viable pregnancy. Such sperm are known as secondary spermatocytes. Perhaps more interestingly, however, is the observation that one can take testicular tissue in which there are no definable spermatids or spermatozoa and use this material to inject in oocytes and achieve fertilization and pregnancy. Such biopsied material apparently contains enough haploid DNA to achieve its mark.[2]

You know you are in the 21st century when you hear about topics such as how to employ secondary spermatocytes. You also know you are in the 21st century when you've been to more than one shower that has 2 mothers and a sperm donor in attendance.

J.A. Stockman III, M.D.

References

1. Meldrum DR, Gardner DK: Two-embryo transfer: The future looks bright. *N Engl J Med* 339:624, 1998.
2. Sofikitis N, Mantzavinos T, Loutradis D, et al: Ooplasmic injections of secondary spermatocytes for non-obstructive azoospermia. *Lancet* 351:1177-1178, 1998.

An Optimality Score for the Neurologic Examination of the Term Newborn
Dubowitz L, Mercuri E, Dubowitz V (Royal Postgraduate Med School, London)
J Pediatr 133:406-416, 1998   1–2

Introduction.—To evaluate the neurologic state of the newborn infant, several methods have been developed. The Dubowitz neurologic examination was first developed in 1981 to assess preterm and term newborn infants. The method has been criticized, however, for not being quantitative in a research setting. A normal population of low-risk term newborns was assessed by using a modified version of the original assessment. The distribution of the findings for each item was evaluated in a normal population and the possible variability with gestational age was also determined. An age-specific optimality score was developed.

Methods.—Two hundred twenty-four low-risk, term newborn infants were assessed with a revised version of the Dubowitz neurologic examination (Figs 1 through 34). Less useful items were eliminated and new items were added that evaluated general movements and patterns of distribution of tone. To make the evaluation more quantitative, an optimality score was included. The distribution of the scores for each item in the population of low-risk term infants is the basis for the score. The variability of the findings was defined by using the tenth and fifth centiles.

Results.—Most of the items assessing tone and the Moro reflex varied with gestational age between 37 and 42 weeks, and these changes were incorporated into the new scoring system. The sum of the optimality scores of the individual items was the total optimality score. Deviant results on 1 or 2 single items could be observed in a third of this normal population, meaning that isolated deviant signs have little diagnostic value. In less than 10% of this population, the association of 4 or more deviant scores was found. This cohort did not have an abnormal distribution of tone patterns, which has been commonly observed in infants with brain lesions.

Tone (Figs 1-10)

	column 1	column 2	column 3	column 4	column 5
POSTURE Infant supine, look mainly at position of legs but also note arms. *score predominant posture*	arms & legs extended	legs slightly flexed	leg well-flexed but not adducted	leg well flexed & adducted near abdomen	abnormal posture: a) opistotonus b)

FIGURE 1.—Posture. Well-flexed and adducted legs (columns 3 and 4) were found in more than 90% of the infants assessed.

	column 1	column 2	column 3	column 4	column 5
ARM RECOIL Take both hands, quickly extend arms parallel to the body, Count to three. Let go. Repeat X 3	arms do not flex	arms flex slowly; not always; not completely	arms flex slowly; more complete	arms flex quickly and completely	arms difficult to extend; snap back forcefully

FIGURE 2.—Arm recoil. A complete recoil (columns 3 and 4) was found in more than 90% of the infants assessed.

	column 1	column 2	column 3	column 4	column 5
ARM TRACTION Hold wrist and pull arm upwards. Note flexion at elbow and resistance while shoulder lifts off table. *Test each side separately*	arms remain straight; no resistance	arms flex slightly or some resistance felt	arms flex well till shoulder lifts, then straighten	arms flex well approx 100° & mantained as shoulder lifts	flexion of arms <100°; mantained when body lifts up

FIGURE 3.—Arm traction. Good arm flexion (columns 3 and 4) was found in more than 90% of the infants assessed.

	column 1	column 2	column 3	column 4	column 5
LEG RECOIL Take both ankles in one hand, flex hips+knees. Quickly extend. Let go. Repeat X3	No flexion	incomplete flexion; not every time	complete but slow flexion	complete fast flexion	legs difficult to extend; snap back forcefully

FIGURE 4.—Leg recoil. A complete recoil (columns 3 and 4) was found in more than 90% of the infants assessed.

	column 1	column 2	column 3	column 4	column 5
LEG TRACTION Grasp ankle and slowly pull leg upwards. Note flexion at knees and resistance as buttocks lift. *Test each side separately*	legs straight - no resistance	legs flex slightly or some resistance felt	legs flex well till bottom lifts up	knee flexes -well ; remains flexed when bottom up	flexion stays when back+bottom up

FIGURE 5.—Leg traction. Good leg flexion (columns 3 and 4) was found in more than 90% of the infants assessed.

	column 1	column 2	column 3	column 4	column 5
POPLITEAL ANGLE Fix knee on abdomen, extend leg by gentle pressure with index finger behind the ankle. Note angle at knee. *Test each side separately*	180° R L	≈ 150° R L	≈110° R L	≈90° R L	<90° R L

FIGURE 6.—Popliteal angle. A popliteal angle between 90 and 110 degrees was found in more than 90% of the infants assessed.

	column 1	column 2	column 3	column 4	column 5
HEAD CONTROL (1) *(extensor tone)* Infant sitting upright; **Encircle chest with both hands holding shoulders** Let head drop forward.	no attempt to raise head	infant tries: effort better felt than seen	raises head but drops forward or back	raises head: remains vertical; it may wobble	

FIGURE 7.—Head control 1. Good head extensor tone (columns 3 and 4) was found in more than 90% of the infants assessed.

	column 1	column 2	column 3	column 4	column 5
HEAD CONTROL (2) *(flexor tone)* Infant sitting upright; **Encircle chest with both hands holding shoulders** Let head drop backward.	no attempt to raise head	infant tries: effort better felt than seen	raises head but drops forward or back	raises head: remains vertical; may wobble	head upright or extended; cannot be passively flexed

FIGURE 8.—Head control 2. Good head flexor tone (columns 3 and 4) was found in more than 90% of the infants assessed.

	column 1	column 2	column 3	column 4	column 5
HEAD LAG Pull infant to sit by wrists & support head slightly.	head drops & stays back	tries to lift head but it drops back	able to lift head slightly	lifts head in line with body	head in front of body

FIGURE 9.—Head lag. When pulled to sit, more than 90% of the infants assessed could fit their head slightly or maintain it in line with their body (columns 3 and 4).

	column 1	column 2	column 3	column 4	column 5
VENTRAL SUSPENSION Hold infant in ventral suspension; observe curvature of back, flexion of limbs and relation of head to trunk.	back curved, head & limbs hang straight	back curved, head ↓, limbs slightly flexed	back slightly curved, limbs flexed	back straight, head in line, limbs flexed	back straight, head above body

FIGURE 10.—Ventral suspension. A slightly curved or extended back (columns 3 and 4) was found in more than 90% of the infants assessed.

Tone Patterns (Figs 11-15)

	column 1	column 2	column 3	column 4	column 5
FLEXOR TONE (arm versus leg 1) compare scores of arm traction with leg traction		arm flexion less than leg flexion	arm flexion equal to leg flexion	arm flexion> leg flexion but difference 1 column or less	arm flexion > leg flexion but difference more than 1 column
incidence		25%	63%	12%	<1%

FIGURE 11.—Flexor tone (arm vs. leg 1). Arm flexion less than leg flexion (column 2) and arm flexion equal to leg flexion (column 3) r greater than leg flexion but with a difference of 1 column or less (column 4) were considered optimal. Arm flexion more than leg flexion but with a difference of more than 1 column was scored as suboptimal.

	column 1	col.2	column 3	column 4	column 5
FLEXOR TONE (arm versus leg 2) posture in supine			arms and legs flexed	strong arm flexion with strong leg extension *intermittent*	strong arm flexion with strong leg extension *continuous*
incidence			100%	<1%	<1%

FIGURE 12.—Flexor tone (arm vs. leg 2). Equal arm and leg flexion in the supine position (column 2) was considered optimal. All other patterns were scored as suboptimal.

	column 1	column 2	column 3	column 4	column 5
LEG EXTENSOR TONE compare scores of popliteal angle and leg traction		leg traction less than popliteal angle	leg traction equal to popliteal angle	leg traction > popliteal angle but difference 1 column or less	leg traction > popliteal angle but difference more than 1 column
incidence		4%	57%	35%	1%

FIGURE 13.—Leg extensor tone. Scores of leg traction equal to or greater than scores of popliteal angle but with a difference of less than 1 column were considered optimal. All other patterns were scored as suboptimal.

	column 1	column 2	column 3	column 4	column 5
NECK EXTENSOR TONE (SITTING) compare head control 1 and 2		head extension less than head flexion	head extension equal to head flexion	head extension > head flexion. but difference 1 column or less	head extension > head flexion but difference more than 1 column
incidence		3%	94%	3%	<1%

FIGURE 14.—Head control in flexion and extension. Head extension equal to head flexion was found in 94% and was considered optimal. All other patterns were scored as suboptimal.

	column 1	column 2	column 3	column 4	column 5
INCREASED EXTENSOR TONE (HORIZONTAL) compare scores of head lag and ventral suspension		ventral suspension less than head lag	ventral suspension equal to head lag	ventr suspension > head lag but difference 1 column or less	ventr suspension> head lag but difference more than 1 column
incidence		24%	55%	16%	<1%

FIGURE 15.—Head lag and ventral suspension. Ventral suspension less than head lag (column 2) and ventral suspension equal to head lag (column 3) or greater but with a difference of 1 column or less (column 4) were considered optimal. Ventral suspension greater than head lag but with a difference of more than 1 column was scored as suboptimal.

Reflexes (Figs 16-21)

	column 1	column 2	column 3	column 4	column 5
TENDON REFLEX test biceps, knee and ankle jerks.	absent	felt, not seen	seen	exaggerated	clonus
incidence	<1%	21%	78%	<1%	<1%

FIGURE 16.—Tendon reflexes. Reflexes that could be easily elicited (column 3) or that could be felt but not seen (column 2) were considered optimal. All other patterns were scored as suboptimal.

	column 1	column 2	column 3	column 4	column 5
SUCK / GAG Little finger into mouth with pulp of finger upwards.	no gag / no suck	weak suck only: • irregular • regular No stripping	strong suck: • irregular • regular Good stripping		no suck but strong clenching
incidence	1%	5%	92%		2%

FIGURE 17.—Sucking. A strong suck (column 3) was considered optimal. A weak suck was considered borderline, and all other patterns were scored as suboptimal.

	column 1	column 2	column 3	column 4	column 5
PALMAR GRASP Put index finger into the hand and gently press palmar surface. Do not touch dorsal surface. *Test each side separately*	no response — R L	short, weak flexion of fingers — R L	strong flexion of fingers — R L	strong finger flexion, shoulder ↑ — R L	very strong grasp; infant can be lifted off couch — R L
incidence	<1%	6%	85%	9%	<1%

FIGURE 18.—Palmar grasp. A strong flexion of fingers (column 3) was considered optimal. Short and weak flexion of fingers and strong flexion with lifting of the shoulder (columns 2 and 4) were considered borderline, and all other patterns were considered suboptimal.

	column 1	column 2	column 3	column 4	column 5
PLANTAR GRASP Press thumb on the sole below the toes. *Test each side separately*	no response — R L	partial plantar flexion of toes — R L	toes curve around the examiner's finger — R L		
incidence	<1%	2%	98%		

FIGURE 19.—Plantar grasp. A strong plantar grasp with toes curving around finger (column 3) was considered optimal. All other patterns were scored as suboptimal.

	column 1	column 2	column 3	column 4	column 5
MORO REFLEX One hand supports infant's head in midline, the other the back. Raise infant to 45° and when relaxed let his head fall through 10°. *Note if response is jerky.* *Repeat 3 times*	no response or opening of hands only	full abduction at shoulder and extension of the arms; no adduction	full abduction but only delayed or partial adduction	partial abduction at shoulder and extension of arms followed by smooth adduction	• no abduction or adduction; • only forward extension of arms from the shoulders • marked adduction only

FIGURE 20.—Moro reflex. Abduction with partial or full adduction (columns 3 and 4) was found in more than 90% of the infants assessed. This item was gestational age–dependent, with the number of infants showing full adduction increasing from 37 to 42 weeks.

	column 1	column 2	column 3	column 4	column 5
PLACING Lift infant in an upright position and stroke the dorsum of the foot against a protruding edge of a flat surface. *Test each side separately*	No response R L	dorsiflexion of ankle only R L	full placing response with flexion of hip, knee & placing sole on surface R L		
incidence	1%	18%	81%		

FIGURE 21.—Placing. A full placing response with flexion of hip, knees, and ankle (column 3) and a placing response with flexion of the ankle only (column 2) were considered optimal. The absence of response was scored as suboptimal.

Movements (Figs 22-24)

	column 1	column 2	column 3	column 4	column 5
SPONTANEOUS MOVEMENTS (quantity) Watch infant lying supine	no movement	sporadic and short isolated movements	frequent isolated movements	frequent generalised movements	continuous exaggerated movements
incidence	<1%	3%	5%	92%	<1%

FIGURE 22.—Spontaneous movements (quantity). Frequent generalized alternating movements (column 4) were considered optimal. Frequent isolated movements (column 3) were scored as borderline, and all other patterns were scored as suboptimal.

	column 1	column 2	column 3	column 4	column 5
SPONTANEOUS MOVEMENTS (quality) Watch infant lying supine	only stretches.	frequent stretches and abrupt movements; some smooth movements are also present	fluent movements but monotonous	fluent alternating movements of arms + legs; good variability	• cramped synchronised; • mouthing • jerky or other abn.mov.
incidence	2%	5%	<1%	93%	<1%

FIGURE 23.—Spontaneous movements (quality). Fluent alternating movements (column 3) with good variability were considered optimal. Frequent stretches alternated with fluent movements (column 2) were scored as borderline, and all other patterns were scored as suboptimal.

	column 1	column 2	column 3	column 4	column 5
HEAD RAISING PRONE Infant in prone, head in midline	no response	infant rolls head over, chin not raised	infant rolls head over raises chin	infant brings head and chin up	infant brings head up and keeps it up
incidence	<1%	10%	50%	40%	<1%

FIGURE 24.—Head raising (prone). When infants were put in the prone position, chin raising with the head rolling over (column 3) or with the whole head up (column 4) was considered optimal. Head rolling over without chin raised was scored as borderline, and all other patterns were scored as suboptimal.

Abnormal Signs (Figs 25-27)

	column 1	column 2	column 3	column 4	column 5
ABNORMAL HAND OR TOE POSTURES		hands open, toes straight most of the time	intermittent fisting or thumb adduction	continuous fisting or thumb adduction; index finger flexion, thumb opposition	continuous big toe extension or flexion of all toes .
incidence		85%	12%	3%	<1%

FIGURE 25.—Abnormal hand or toe posture. Hands open and normal posture of the toes (column 2) or intermittent hand fisting or adduction of thumb (column 3) was considered optimal. All other patterns were scored as suboptimal.

	column 1	column 2	column 3	column 4	column 5
TREMOR		no tremor or tremor only when crying	tremor only after Moro or occasionally when awake	frequent tremors when awake	continuous tremors
incidence		88%	12%	<1%	<1%

FIGURE 26.—Tremors. No tremor; tremors only when crying (column 2) or tremor only after Moro reflex, and occasional tremors when awake (column 3) were considered optimal. All other patterns were scored as suboptimal.

	column 1	column 2	column 3	column 4	column 5
STARTLE	no startle, even to sudden noise	no spontaneous startle but reacts to sudden noise	2-3 spontaneous startles	more than 3 spontaneous startles	continuous startles
incidence	<1%	94%	6%	<1%	<1%

FIGURE 27.—Startles. Absence of spontaneous startles (column 2) or 2 or 3 spontaneous startles (column 3) were considered optimal. All other patterns were scored as suboptimal.

Behavior (Figs 28-34)

	column 1	column 2	column 3	column 4	column 5
EYE MOVEMENTS	does not open eyes		full conjugated eye movements	*transient* • nystagmus • strabismus • roving eye movements • sunset sign	*persistent* • nystagmus • strabismus • roving eye movements • downward deviation
incidence	7		92%	1%	<1%

FIGURE 28.—Eye movements. Opening of the eyes (column 1) could not be elicited in 7%. Normal symmetrical eye movements (column 3) were considered optimal. All other patterns were scored as suboptimal.

	column 1	column 2	column 3	column 4	column 5
AUDITORY ORIENTATION Infant awake. Wrap infant. Hold rattle 10 - 15 cms from ear.	no reaction	auditory startle; brightens and stills; no true orientation	shifting of eyes, head might turn towards source	prolonged head turn to stimulus; search with eyes; smooth	turns head and eyes towards noise every time; jerky ,abrupt
incidence	<1%	30%	50%	20%	<1%

FIGURE 29.—Auditory orientation. Eye and head turning to the side of the noise (columns 3 and 4) or a weaker response (brightening or turning head with eyes closed) (column 2) was considered optimal. All other patterns were scored as suboptimal.

	column 1		column 2		column 3		column 4		column 5	
VISUAL ORIENTATION Wrap infant, wake up with rattle if needed or rock gently.Note if baby can see and follow red ball (B)or target (T)	does not follow or focus on stimuli		stills, focuses, follows briefly to the side but loses stimuli		follows horizontally and vertically; no head turn		follows horizontally and vertically; turns head		follows in a circle	
	B	T	B	T	B	T	B	T	B	T
incidence	<1%		7%		41%		51%		1%	

FIGURE 30.—Visual alertness. Seven percent of the infants had their eyes closed throughout the examination and could not be tested. The ability to track horizontally and vertically with and without head movements (columns 3 and 4) was considered optimal. Incomplete tracking was scored as borderline, and all other patterns as suboptimal.

	column 1	column 2	column 3	column 4	column 5
ALERTNESS Tested as response to visual stimuli (red ball or target)	will not respond to stimuli	when awake, looks only briefly	when awake, looks at stimuli but loses them	keeps interest in stimuli	does not tire (hyper- reactive)
incidence	1%	2%	38%	49%	<1%

FIGURE 31.—Alertness. Alertness was tested as the quality of the infant's response to track the stimulus presented (a red ball or a target). Looking at the stimulus with short interest (column 3) or long interest (column 4) was considered optimal. All other patterns were scored as suboptimal.

	column 1	column 2	column 3	column 4	column 5
IRRITABILITY in response to stimuli	quiet all the time, not irritable to any stimuli	awakes, cries sometimes when handled	cries often when handled	cries always when handled	cries even when not handled
incidence	<1%	93%	5%	2%	<1%

FIGURE 32.—Irritability. Occasional crying when handled (column 2) was considered optimal . Frequent crying when handled (column 3) was scored as borderline, and all other patterns as suboptimal.

	column 1	column 2	column 3	column 4	column 5
CRY	no cry at all	whimpering cry only	cries to stimuli but normal pitch		High pitched cry; often continuous
incidence	<1%	7%	92%		1%

FIGURE 33.—Cry. Normal cry in response to stimuli (column 3) was considered optimal. Whimpering cry was scored as borderline, and all other patterns as suboptimal.

	column 1	column 2	column 3	column 4	column 5
CONSOLABILITY Ease to quieten infant	asleep; awake, no crying; consoling not needed	awake; cries briefly; consoling not needed	awake; cries; becomes quiet when talked to	awake; cries ; needs picking up to console	awake; cries cannot be consoled
incidence	1%	41%	45%	12%	1%

FIGURE 34.—Consolability. Infants who were either not crying or cried briefly and did need consoling, could be consoled by talking, or needed to be picked up (columns 2, 3, and 4) were considered optimal. All other patterns were scored as suboptimal. (Figures 1-34 are courtesy of Dubowitz L, Mercuri E, Dubowitz V: An optimality score for the neurologic examination of the term newborn. *J Pediatr* 133: 406-416, 1998.)

Conclusion.—More quantitative and detailed information on the neurologic status of term infants is available with this new system. The original format of a pro forma scheme with diagrams is retained with the new format. The potential use of this system should be increased in longitudinal follow-up studies because it has an optimality score to allow comparison of clinical findings with neurophysiologic and imaging findings.

▶ It's not nice to fool with Mother Nature, or with the Dubowitz. The Dubowitz has held up well for the better part of 2 decades as being the standard neurologic examination of both preterm and term newborns. It has been the "Holy Grail" of such a neurologic examination and, as such, should not be tinkered with. However, when a Dubowitz does the tinkering (the first and last authors of this report are the authentic Dubowitzes), perhaps we will call such tinkering fine tuning of the Holy Grail.

No laboratory or radiologic test can yet supplant a high-quality neurologic examination as part of the assessment of the newborn who may have neurologic difficulties. With that as a fact, it is reasonable to expect that after 15 to 20 years of experience with the Dubowitz neurologic examination, some items will need to be updated and others eliminated. The Dubowitzes have eliminated habituation, arm release in the prone position, walking reflex, rooting reflex, and defensive reaction either because they were difficult to assess (they showed wide variability in otherwise normal babies) or because they simply did not distinguish between normal and abnormal responses. The new version of the Dubowitz examination is shown in the figures accompanying this abstract. The figures are well worth glancing through. There is much that we can all learn from the fine work of Dubowitz and Dubowitz.

J.A. Stockman III, M.D.

Increased Frequency of Genetic Thrombophilia in Women With Complications of Pregnancy

Kupferminc MJ, Eldor A, Steinman N, et al (Lis Maternity Hosp, Tel Aviv, Israel; Tel Aviv Univ, Israel)
N Engl J Med 340:9-13, 1999   1–3

Introduction.—Maternal and fetal morbidity and mortality are greatly affected by severe preeclampsia, abruptio placentae, fetal growth retardation, and stillbirth. Abnormal placental vasculature and disturbances of hemostasis, leading to inadequate maternal-fetal circulation, may be part of the causes. Important risk factors for obstetrical complications related to inadequate maternal-fetal circulation may be mutations predisposing patients to thrombosis. The relation between severe preeclampsia, abruptio placentae, fetal growth retardation, and stillbirth with several thrombophilic mutations were studied. Deficiencies of protein S, protein C, or antithrombin III were sought. The presence of anticardiolipin antibodies and lupus anticoagulant, which are also associated with thrombophilia, were examined.

Methods.—There were 110 women with an obstetrical complication compared with 110 control subjects, or women who had 1 or more normal pregnancies. Several days after delivery, the women were tested for the mutation of adenine to guanine at nucleotide 506 in the factor V gene (factor V Leiden), the mutation of cytosine to thymine at nucleotide 677 in the gene encoding methylenetetrahydrofolate reductase, and the mutation of guanine to adenine at nucleotide 20210 in the prothrombin gene. Tests for the deficiency of protein C, protein S, or antithrombin III, and for the presence of anticardiolipin antibodies were conducted between 2 and 3 months after delivery.

Results.—In 22 women with obstetrical complications and 7 with normal pregnancies, the mutation at nucleotide 506 in the factor V gene was detected (20% vs 6%) (Table 2). Homozygosity for the C677T mutation

TABLE 2.—Prevalence of Inherited and Acquired Thrombophilia in the Study Women*

Type of Thrombophilia	Thrombophilia Among Women With Complications (N=110)	Thrombophilia Among Women With Normal Pregnancies (N=110)	Odds Ratio (95% CI)	P Value
	No. (%)			
Inherited				
Factor V Leiden mutation, +/+ or +/−†	22 (20)	7 (6)	3.7 (1.5-9.0)	0.003
Methylenetetrahydrofolate reducease mutation, +/+	24 (22)	9 (8)	3.1 (1.4-7.1)	0.005
Prothrombin mutation, +/−	11 (10)	3 (3)	3.9 (1.1-14.6)	0.03
Total	57 (52)	19 (17)	5.2 (2.8-9.6)	<0.001
Acquired or inherited				
Deficiency of protein S, protein C, or antithrombin III	9 (8)	1 (1)	9.7 (1.2-78.0)	0.01
Presence of anticardiolipin antibodies	5 (5)	0	2.0 (1.7-2.3)	0.02
Deficiency of protein S, protein C, or antithrombin III or presence of anticardiolipin antibodies	14 (13)	1 (1)	15.9 (2.0-123.1)	<0.001
All types	71 (65)	20 (18)	8.2 (4.4-15.3)	<0.001

*CI denotes confidence interval, +/+ homozygous, and +/− heterozygous. Combined thrombophilias among the women with complications were as follows: factor V Leiden +/+ and the methylenetetrahydrofolate reductase mutation +/+ (1 patient), factor V Leiden +/− and the methylenetetrahydrofolate reductase mutation +/+ (4), factor V Leiden +/− and anticardiolipin antibodies (1), the methylenetetrahydrofolate reductase mutation +/+ and protein C deficiency (1), protein S deficiency and anticardiolipin antibodies (2), and anticardiolipin antibodies and lupus anticoagulant (1). Among the women with normal pregnancies, 1 had a combined prothrombin mutation +/− and factor V Leiden +/−.
†Among the women with complications, 2 were homozygous and 20 were heterozygous for factor V Leiden; all 7 with this mutation who had normal pregnancies were heterozygous.
(Reprinted by permission of *The New England Journal of Medicine*, from Kuperminc MJ, Eldor A, Steinman N, et al: Increased frequency of genetic thrombophilia in women with complications of pregnancy. *N Engl J Med* 340:9-13. Copyright 1999, Massachusetts Medical Society. All rights reserved.)

in the gene encoding methylenetetrahydrofolate reductase was found in 24 women with complications and 9 control subjects (22% vs 8%). The G20210A mutation in the prothrombin gene was discovered in 11 women with complications and 3 control subjects (10% vs 3%). A thrombophilic mutation was found in 57 women with complications compared with 19 control subjects (52% vs 17%). There were 14 women with complications and 1 control subject who had deficiency of protein S, protein C, or antithrombin III or anticardiolipin antibodies.

Conclusion.—An increased incidence of mutation was found in women with serious obstetrical complication, which predisposed them to thrombosis and other inherited and acquired forms of thrombophilia.

▶ Whoever said that having a baby is risk free? No one, actually. But now we know why some have the triad of preeclampsia, abruptio placentae, and fetal growth retardation (and, sometimes, fetal death). If the data from this report are believed, about half of women with this constellation of findings experience it on the basis of an inherited thrombophilia. We also see that the list of genetic causes of thrombophilia continues to grow. Just a few years ago that list consisted of antithrombin III deficiency, protein C deficiency, and protein S deficiency. Then along came resistence to activated protein C caused by an adenine-to-guanine mutation at nucleotide 506 in the factor V gene (the factor V Leiden mutation). Even more recently described is homozygosity for the mutation of cytosine-to-thymine at nucleotide 677 in the gene encoding methylenetetrahydrofolate reductase. The latter mutation results in decreased synthesis of 5-methylenetetrahydrofolate, the primary methyl-donor in the conversion of homocysteine to methionine. The resulting increase in plasma homocystine concentrations are a risk factor for venous and arterial thrombosis. A recently described guanine-to-adenine mutation at nucleotide 20210 in the prothrombin gene is associated with higher plasma concentrations of prothrombin and an increased risk of venous thromboembolism, myocardial infarction, and cerebral-vein thrombosis. Each and every 1 of these recently described problems is now a cause of potentially serious pregnancy-related complications.

So what do we do with this new information? First, we must put it into perspective. Most pregnant women (95%) have none of the obstetric complications in this report. Therefore, many women who have 1 or more types of inherited thrombophilia will never have difficulties with their pregnancy. The precise risk of serious complications in women with genetic or acquired thrombophilia remains unknown, even though we do know the prevalence of some of the inherited thrombophilias (for example, factor V Leiden mutation is seen in 5.2% of white women, 2% of Hispanic women, and 1.2% of black women). As of now, there is no reason to consider prescreening all pregnancies with complex coagulation studies that may yield results with no clinical implications. However, once a woman has a pregnancy complicated by severe preeclampsia, abruptio placentae, or unexplained fetal growth retardation or stillbirths, genetic testing for markers of thrombophilia is in order. Because these types of complications tend to recur in subsequent pregnancies, the identification of thrombophilia in women who have such problems offers an opportunity to reduce the risk of recurrence by prophylactic therapy with heparin and low-dose aspirin (for those with protein S deficiency, mutations in the factor V gene, or anticardiolipin antibodies), or prophylactic folic acid supplementation (for those with mutations in the gene for methylenetetrahydrofolate reductase causing high homocystine levels).

It is amazing, isn't it, how much we have learned about how blood disorders affect pregnancies in ways that no one would have believed 20 years ago.

J.A. Stockman III, M.D.

Declining Severity Adjusted Mortality: Evidence of Improving Neonatal Intensive Care

Richardson DK, Gray JE, Gortmaker SL, et al (Harvard Med School, Boston; Harvard School of Public Health, Boston; Children's Hosp, Boston)
Pediatrics 102:893-899, 1998　　　　　　　　　　　　　　　　　　　1–4

Introduction.—Improvements in neonatal intensive care are believed to be the cause of the rapid decline in neonatal mortality during the past 40 years. There has been continued improvement in birth weight–specific survival despite little change in birth weight distribution. This period has witnessed the introduction of surfactant replacement therapy, corticosteroid treatment of chronic lung injury and high-frequency ventilation, as well as improved infant formulas and nutritional supplements. It has also been postulated that very low birth weight infants have been delivered to the neonatal ICU less ill because of improving high-risk obstetric care. Better obstetric care is the result of better US imaging, more aggressive use of antenatal corticosteroid treatment, and delay of delivery with tocolytis, as well as more liberal use of cesarean section for preterm delivery. Evidence for the 2 competing hypotheses—better babies or better care—as the cause of improved survival of very low birth weight infants was examined.

Methods.—There were 739 infants born weighing less than 1500 g. One group was born between 1989 and 1990, and the other group was born between 1994 and 1995. Their mortality risk from birth weight and illness severity was estimated on admission. The therapeutic intensity was measured as well.

Results.—There was a decline in the neonatal ICU mortality rate from 17.1% to 9.5%. There was a total mortality decrease from 31.6% to 18.4%. "Better babies" was deemed the reason for one third of the decline and "better care" was deemed the reason for two thirds of the decline. There was more aggressive use of surfactant, mechanical ventilation, and pressors but decreases in transfusions procedures and monitoring resulted in little change in therapeutic intensity.

Conclusion.—For infants weighing less than 1500 g, the mortality rate decreased nearly 50% in 5 years. Improved condition on admission, reflecting improved obstetric and delivery room care, is the cause of one third of this decline. More effective newborn intensive care is responsible for two thirds of the decline, which was associated with more aggressive cardiovascular and respiratory treatments. The contribution of high-risk obstetric care in providing "better babies" may be underestimated as neonatal intensive care is overcredited as the sole reason for improved birth weight specific–mortality.

▶ Jeffrey B. Gould, M.D., M.P.H., professor of Maternal and Child Health, School of Public Health, University of California, Berkeley, and clinical professor of Pediatrics, Stanford University School of Medicine, Palo Alto, Calif, comments:

Historically, David and Siegel used a risk matrix approach in their 1983 article "Decline in neonatal mortality, 1968 to 1977: Better babies or better care?" which characterized a "better baby" in terms of birth weight, gestational age, and race.[1] They found that two thirds of the mortality decline was the result of better care and made a plea that, as a nation, we put more effort into increasing the percentage of healthy babies by reducing the incidence of low birth weight and prematurity. Although little progress has been made with respect to improving low birth weight, advances in perinatal care have been substantial, and declines in neonatal mortality continue to be impressive, even in the age of surfactant.

Richardson and colleagues have taken on the task of understanding the sources of the recent decline in neonatal mortality, using logistic modeling and objective scores for both neonatal condition and the intensity of therapeutic intervention. The authors are to be commended for providing an important analytic template. Their analysis of the 50% decline in neonatal mortality seen in 2 Boston nurseries between 1989 and 1995 extends risk adjustment to include physiologic condition immediately after birth (5-minute Apgar score) and during the first 12 hours of life (score for neonatal condition). In their paradigm, the temporal improvement in physiologic condition, after adjusting for birth weight and gestational age, is attributed to advances in maternal-fetal care. In 1995, the authors found a significant improvement in the risk profile of their population, and they demonstrate that one third of the decrease in neonatal mortality can be attributed to better babies.

The improved risk profile has several sources. The higher mean birth weight in infants weighing 750 to 1500 g and the increase in gestational age seen in the 1995 cohort could have been influenced by changes in the risk profile of mothers delivered (referral bias). However, the lower incidence of 5-minute Apgar scores and the lower neonatal condition scores for infants weighing 750 to 1000 g are suggestive of advances in the effectiveness of high-risk obstetric care—suggestive in that more effective resuscitation and early neonatal care could also result in improved 5-minute Apgar scores and 12-hour neonatal condition scores.

Two thirds of the decline in mortality was the result of better care. Changes in practice that may have contributed to better neonatal care include more extensive use of prenatal steroids and surfactant, significant increases in the therapeutic intensity sub scores for respiratory and cardiovascular support, and decreases in the sub scores for monitoring, procedures, and transfusions.

J.B. Gould, M.D., M.P.H.

Reference

1. David RJ, Siegel E: Decline in neonatal mortality, 1968 to 1977: Better babies or better care? *Pediatrics* 71:531-540, 1983.

First-Trimester Growth and the Risk of Low Birth Weight

Smith GCS, Smith MFS, McNay MB, et al (Cornell Univ, Ithaca, NY; Univ of Glasgow, Scotland)
N Engl J Med 339:1817-1822, 1998   1–5

Introduction.—Increased perinatal morbidity and mortality have been associated with a low birth weight of less than 2500 g and a birth weight that is low for gestational age. It was previously thought that variations in fetal size were largely determined in the second half of pregnancy; however, a more recent study showed a correlation between first-trimester crown-rump length and birth weight. A study was undertaken to determine whether a smaller-than-expected crown-rump length in the first trimester was associated with low birth weight and birth weight that was low for gestational age.

Methods.—Women who had no important medical problems, a normal menstrual history, and a first-trimester US scan in which the crown-rump length of the embryo or fetus had been measured were identified. The relationship between the outcome of 4220 pregnancies and the difference between the measured and the expected crown-rump lengths in the first trimester, expressed as equivalent days of growth, was examined.

Results.—An increased risk of birth weight below 2500 g was associated with a first-trimester crown-rump length that was 2 to 6 days smaller than expected, with a relative risk of 2.3. For a birth weight below the fifth percentile for gestational age, the relative risk was 3.0. For delivery between 24 and 32 weeks of gestation, the relative risk was 2.1. There was no increased risk associated with delivery between 33 and 36 weeks.

Conclusion.—Low birth weight, low–birth weight percentile, and premature delivery may be associated with suboptimal first-trimester growth. This is consistent with the hypothesis that the pathophysiology of extremely premature delivery may be different from that of moderately premature delivery. A possible causal relation between poor first-trimester growth and low birth weight may be a suboptimal environment or a disorder of placentation with suboptimal transfer of nutrients to the fetus.

▶ It's hard to imagine that this type of study had never been performed before, but it had not. The conclusions seem intuitively correct. Babies who are small in size during the first trimester do carry an excessive risk of being born with a low birth weight and of being born very prematurely. It may very well be that a suboptimal environment in the first trimester diminishes fetal growth potential throughout the entire pregnancy.

One can bet that the data from this report will be carefully scrutinized, repeated in further studies, and, if true, will form the basis for one more reason why all pregnancies might benefit from an early (first-trimester) fetal ultrasonogram. If nothing else, the parents will be happy with a copy of their new baby's picture.

Shifting gears a bit, were you aware that a baby's oxygen saturation might fall when flying on a commercial airline? There are data that suggest that babies who breath oxygen at less than normal atmospheric pressure may exhibit periodic respiration and occasional episodes of mild desaturation.[1] All aircraft used for medium and long flights are pressurized so that the pressure within a cabin is equivalent to that found at about 1700 m, as in a Boeing 747, and 2500 m, as in older DC-9s. At 2500 m, the atmospheric pressure is 75% of what it is at sea level. This is capable of reducing the arterial oxygen tension by about 35% in healthy adults. The oxygen saturation falls from 97% to about 89%. The issue is, however, whether this decrease in oxygen supply might or might not, in the first few weeks of life, cause babies on airplanes to have any difficulty. The answer to this question comes from British Airways. British Airways carries about 34 million passengers a year. Not a single case of sudden infant death syndrome has been recorded during flight. If one estimates that about 1 in 500 passengers is an infant, over a 10-year period British Airways has had experience with about three quarters of a million babies with zero incidents of sudden infant death syndrome in flight.[2] Babies can fly the friendly skies with confidence!

J.A. Stockman III, M.D.

References

1. Parkin KJ, Poets CF, O'Brien LM, et al: Effects of exposure to 15% oxygen on breathing patterns and oxygen saturation in infants: Intervention study. *BMJ* 316:887-894, 1998.
2. Milner AD: Effects of 15% oxygen on breathing patterns and oxygenation in infants: Infants are probably safe in aircraft. *BMJ* 316:873, 1998.

Recombinant Human Erythropoietin Therapy for Treatment of Anemia of Prematurity in Very Low Birth Weight Infants: A Randomized, Double-blind, Placebo-controlled Trial

Kumar P, Shankaran S, Krishnan RG (Wayne State Univ, Detroit)
J Perinatol 18:173-177, 1998   1–6

Background.—Research has shown that inadequate production of erythropoietin may be an important cause of anemia of prematurity. Recombinant human eythropoietin (rHuEpo) appears to stimulate endogenous erythropoiesis in affected infants. The safety and efficacy of rHuEpo in very low birth weight infants with anemia of prematurity were further investigated.

Methods.—By random assignment, 30 infants received rHuEpo, 300 U/kg per dose, or placebo twice a week. The infants were monitored for growth, caloric intake, hematologic factors, and transfusion requirements.

Findings.—Infants given rHuEpo had a significantly lower number and volume of erythrocyte transfusions. By the end of the study, serum ferritin concentrations declined and were significantly lower in the rHuEpo recipi-

TABLE 2.—Clinical and Laboratory Characteristics of Study
Infants at Exit From Study

	rHuEPO (n = 15)	Placebo (n = 15)
Entry to discharge duration (days)	28.3 ± 9.2	30.2 ± 10.7
Average caloric intake during study (calories/kg/day)	108.3 ± 6.8	109.0 ± 4.9
Rates of weight gain (gm/day/infant)	22.8 ± 3.2	22.0 ± 3.4
Volume of blood drawn during study (ml/infant)	8.8 ± 4.2	9.6 ± 4.3
Number of erythrocyte transfusions during study (per infant)*	0.07 ± 0.3	0.8 ± 0.8
Volume of erythrocyte transfusions during study (ml/infant)*	1.0 ± 3.9	11.7 ± 11.1
Hematocrit (%)	33.2 ± 4.1	30.2 ± 6.9
Reticulocyte count (%)*	7.5 ± 2.7	4.9 ± 3.8
TLC ($\times 10^9$/L)	8.4 ± 2.3	9.9 ± 2.4
ANC ($\times 10^9$/L)*	1.9 ± 0.9	3.2 ± 1.6
Platelet count ($\times 10^9$/L)	421.1 ± 137.5	378.2 ± 82.9
Serum ferritin (ng/ml)*	87.2 ± 55.2	173.6 ± 113.9

Note: Values represent mean ± 1 SD.
*$P < .05$.
(Courtesy of Kumar P, Shankaran S, Krishnan RG: Recombinant human erythropoietin therapy for treatment of anemia of prematurity in very low birth weight infants: A randomized, double-blind, placebo-controlled trial. J Perinatol 18:173-177, 1998.)

ents. Reticulocyte count was inversely correlated with absolute neutrophil count at study entry and completion (Table 2).

Conclusions.—Treatment with rHuEpo twice a week significantly decreases the need for erythrocyte transfusion in very low birth weight infants in stable condition. The significant decline in serum ferritin levels in infants given rHuEpo suggests the need to determine the best dose of iron supplementation in such patients.

▶ Dr. Alagappan Alagappan of Houston Neonatal Perinatal Associates, Houston, comments:

Despite several carefully conducted clinical trials, uncertainty still exists about the routine use of erythropoietin (EPO) in the treatment of anemia of prematurity.[1] Also unclear is whether all low birth weight infants would benefit, or whether low birth weight infants less than 1000 g benefit more than low birth weight infants in the 1000 to 1500 g range. Transfusion requirements tend to be higher in infants weighing less than 1000 g due to frequent phlebotomies. The majority of the transfusions are given in the first 3 to 4 weeks of life.[2] Studies testing the long-term effect of EPO by starting it early in the postnatal age in infants less than 1000 g are unavailable. However, Ohls et al.[3] recently tested the short-term effect by daily administration of EPO in the first 2 weeks of age and reported only modest benefit.

This may relate partly to the inability to prevent anemia due to phlebotomy loss. Also disappointing are reports that if EPO is started later, when these smallest infants are more stable, many infants have already had transfusions, thus exposure to a number of transfusion donors is not reduced.[4,5]

Kumar et al. enrolled infants weighing less than 1250 g at 5 to 6 weeks' postnatal age when the infants had received 80% of the total volume of transfusions they were to receive. Less than 1 transfusion per infant was prevented in the EPO group after study entry. Based on these studies, the use of EPO in the infants weighing less than 1000 g, either early or late, is of questionable value if the purpose is to lower donor exposure.

Though the risk for transfusion is less than the infants weighing 1000 to 1500 g, it is not negligible. Alagappan et al.[6,7] reported that even with adherence to strict transfusion guidelines, the majority of infants in this weight category required 1 or more transfusions. To test the efficacy of EPO in preventing transfusions in these larger infants, Alagappan et al. enrolled 28 infants in a randomized non–placebo-controlled clinical trial, starting EPO at 1 to 2 weeks of age at a dose of 300 U/kg, 3 times a week (SC) for 6 weeks. He reported a 90% reduction in the overall requirement of transfusion in the EPO-treated infants. Two transfusions were required in the EPO group compared with 18 transfusions in the control group.[7]

Based on currently available studies, a dose of 200 to 300 U/kg of EPO given 2 to 3 times a week subcutaneously along with enteral iron (6-12 mg/kg of elemental iron) or IV iron (500-1000 µg/kg of iron dextran in TPN solution) does appear relatively safe. The efficacy of EPO to reduce the overall requirement of transfusion in the smallest infants appears somewhat questionable; however, EPO does appear effective in reducing transfusion requirements among larger low birth weight infants (1000-1500 g).

A. Alagappan, M.D.

References

1. Strauss R: Recombinant erythropoietin for the anemia of prematurity: Still a promise, not a panacea. *J Pediatr* 131:653-655, 1997.
2. Widness J, Seward V, Kromer I, et al: Changing patterns of red blood cell transfusion in very low birth weight infants. *J Pediatr* 129:680-687, 1996.
3. Ohls R, Harcum J, Schibler K, et al: The effect of erythropoietin on the transfusion requirements of preterm infants weighing 750 grams or less: A randomized, double-blind, placebo-controlled study. *J Pediatr* 131:661-665, 1997.
4. Shannon K, Keith III J, Mentzer W, et al: Recombinant human erythropoietin stimulates erythropoiesis and reduces erythrocyte transfusions in VLBW preterm infants. *Pediatrics* 95:1-8, 1995.
5. Kumar P, Shankaran S, Krishnan R: Recombinant human erythropoietin therapy for treatment of anemia of prematurity in VLBW infants: A randomized, double-blind, placebo-controlled trail. *J Perinatol* 18:173-177, 1998.
6. Alagappan A, Shattuck K, Malloy M: Impact of transfusion guidelines on neonatal transfusions. *J Perinatol* 18:92-97, 1998.
7. Alagappan A, Alter B, Malloy M: Use of erythropoietin in stable preterm infants (1000-1500 grams) to reduce erythrocyte transfusions. *Pediatr Res* 43:235A, 1998.

Early Inhaled Glucocorticoid Therapy to Prevent Bronchopulmonary Dysplasia

Cole CH, Colton T, Shah BL, et al (Tufts Univ, Boston; Boston Univ; Pennsylvania Hosp, Philadelphia)
N Engl J Med 340:1005-1010, 1999   1–7

Background.—Inhaled glucocorticoid (GC) therapy is safe and effective in treating asthma in adults and children. This efficacy has led to its increasing use in the treatment of neonates with bronchopulmonary dysplasia (BPD). These authors examined whether early inhaled GC therapy indeed decreases the incidence of BPD.

Methods.—The patients were 253 infants 3 to 14 days of age who were born before 33 weeks' gestation, had a birth weight of 1250 g or less, and required mechanical ventilation. Patients were randomized to receive either placebo (n = 130) or beclomethasone dipropionate (n = 123) via a metered-dose inhaler delivering 42 µg of drug per actuation. Treatment continued for 4 weeks, during which time the dosage was reduced from 40 to 5 µg/kg/day. The number of infants who had BPD at 28 days of age was compared between the groups, as were the incidence of BPD at 36 weeks' gestational age, the requirement for systemic GC or bronchodilator therapy, the duration of respiratory support, the number of deaths, and the frequency of adverse clinical outcomes.

Findings.—The frequency of BPD was similar in the beclomethasone and placebo groups both at 28 days of age (43% and 45%, respectively) and at 36 weeks' gestational age (18% and 20%, respectively). However, significantly fewer patients receiving beclomethasone required systemic GCs both at 28 days of age (17% vs 29%) and at 36 weeks' gestational age (36% vs 48%). At 28 days of age, significantly fewer patients receiving beclomethasone required mechanical ventilation (48% vs 62%) and bronchodilator therapy. At 36 weeks' gestational age, however, the beclomethasone and placebo groups were similar in their requirement for ventilatory support (6% and 9%, respectively). The number of deaths (14 total) and other clinical outcomes—such as blood pressure, growth, retinopathy of prematurity, cataracts, intracranial hemorrhage, periventricular leukomalacia, necrotizing enterocolitis, or gastrointestinal bleeding—did not differ between the 2 groups.

Conclusion.—Early therapy with inhaled beclomethasone did not significantly affect the incidence of BPD at 28 days of age or at 36 weeks' gestational age. However, patients receiving beclomethasone required significantly less systemic GC and bronchodilator therapy. Furthermore, at 28 days of age, fewer patients receiving beclomethasone still required mechanical ventilation. Beclomethasone was not associated with any adverse effects.

▶ BPD has been with us going on 40 years now, according to the pediatric literature. Fortunately, the problem of respiratory distress syndrome has diminished with the widespread use of steroids to accelerate lung maturation, surfactant therapy, and improved methods of ventilation, with babies weighing between 500 and 750 g now surviving more than 50% of the time. With such survivorship comes a cost. Part of the cost involves the disease called BPD. We now know that BPD is hardly simply a matter of barotrauma or high oxygen concentration. Pathophysiologic factors that play into BPD likely include inflammatory mediators, cytokines, and proteolytic enzymes released by inflammatory cells whose influx into the lungs is the consequence of oxygen exposure and prenatal or postnatal sepsis.

Postnatal steroid therapy has been a major player in the treatment of BPD, even if its use remains controversial. Used systemically, typically beginning at 2 to 4 weeks of age, steroids have been successful in allowing weaning from mechanical ventilation to occur earlier. What they do not do, however, is change the overall outcome for these babies.

We see from this report that a randomized multicenter trial of inhaled steroids started in the first 2 weeks of life does not prevent BPD, but, like systemic steroids, does reduce the need for and duration of mechanical ventilation—a small plus, perhaps. By the way, inhaled nitric oxide has recently been reported to improve oxygenation in some patients with severe BPD.[1]

Babies in whom BPD develops are frequently the ones who require erythropoietin (EPO) administration. Kumar et al.'s article (Abstract 1–6) tells us how useful EPO can be. It is so readily available now that we are seeing more and more illicit use of it as a performance-enhancing device by some athletes. Physicians are frequently asked if they have any advice about how to detect the use of EPO by such athletes. You might suggest, under certain circumstances, that the criteria now used in western Europe to eliminate EPO users from cycling competitions is the way to go. There, the rule of the Union Cycliste Internationale is that blood samples for hematocrit must be taken. All athletes having a hematocrit level greater than 50% are excluded from competition. There is no assay available at this time to tell endogenous EPO from exogenous EPO, so the only test one can do is an assessment of packed-cell volume.[2]

Please note, however, before you recommend doing hematocrits to rule out EPO enhancement, that there are a number of factors that can affect an individual's hematocrit level, including the site of a sample, the time of the day, the posture of a subject, and whether that individual has recently eaten a meal. If a person has been standing for an extended length of time, fluid may pool in the extremities, artifactually raising the hematocrit level. If a tourniquet is left on a bit too long, the hematocrit level may be artificially elevated. Hematocrit levels tend to be lower after a meal in which liquids are given. Athletes hellbent on using EPO, particularly cyclists, are well aware of the factors that affect their hematocrits. Before having a venous sample drawn, some cyclists hang upside down to get as much fluid into their circulation as possible to dilute their hematocrits. Some will drink enormous quantities of fluids 30 to 45 minutes prior to the offering of a blood sample.

Sooner or later someone will figure out a way of placing a "tag" on recombinant human EPO so that we will be able to tell endogenous from exogenous EPO. But even tagging is not the answer. The reason is that EPO turnover is so quick, and the consequences (a raised hematocrit level) last so long. All an athlete has to do is to stop taking EPO several days before a planned blood drawing and it will be out of his or her system. So much for honest competition these days.

Four decades of BPD and no magic bullet as yet. One wonders what the next 4 decades will bring. Chances are that the key to success with BPD will be the prevention of prematurity, not the treatment of the disease after the fact.

J.A. Stockman III, M.D.

References

1. Banks BA, Seri I, Ischiropoulous H, et al: Changes in oxygenation with inhaled nitric oxide in severe bronchopulmonary dysplasia. *Pediatrics* 103:610-618, 1999.
2. Marx J, Vergouwen P: Packed-cell volume in elite athletes. *Lancet* 352:451, 1998.

Early Versus Late Surfactant Treatment in Preterm Infants of 27 to 32 Weeks' Gestational Age: A Multicenter Controlled Clinical Trial
Gortner L, Wauer RR, Hammer H, et al (Univ Children's Hosp, Lübeck, Germany; Univ Children's Hosp Charité, Berlin; Community Hosp, Dortmund, Germany; et al)
Pediatrics 102:1153-1160, 1998   1–8

Objective.—The timing of surfactant replacement therapy for infants of more than 27 weeks' gestational age with respiratory distress syndrome is controversial. Whether surfactant treatment with SF-RI1 (Alveofact) during hour 1 after birth is superior to treatment administered 2 to 6 hours after birth in infants of 27 to 32 weeks' gestational age requiring rescue was evaluated in a randomized, controlled, multicenter clinical trial.

Methods.—A total of 317 infants were randomly assigned to receive bovine surfactant SF-RI1 either during the first hour (n = 154) or 2 to 6 hours (n = 163) after birth. In case of unsatisfactory response, infants were retreated with surfactant at a dosage of 50 mg/kg to a maximum of 200 mg/kg at intervals of at least 8 hours. Pulmonary hemorrhage duration of mechanical ventilation, overall survival until discharge, survival without bronchopulmonary dysplasia, oxygen dependency at 36 weeks' gestational age, pulmonary interstitial emphysema, pneumothorax requiring chest tube drainage, and time receiving nasal continuous positive airway pressure were end points.

Results.—SF-RI1 was administered intratracheally at a dosage of 100 mg/kg to 59 infants within the first hour and to 60 infants 2 to 6 hours after birth. There were no significant differences between the early treatment and late treatment groups with respect to in-hospital deaths (5 vs 3), duration of mechanical ventilation (3 vs 2 days), death or bronchopulmonary dysplasia (40 vs 39), total time receiving nasal continuous positive airway pressure (1 vs 1 day), and duration of neonatal ICU treatment (19 vs 17 days). Gas exchange and ventilator settings for infants requiring mechanical ventilation were similar.

Conclusion.—Early surfactant treatment was not more beneficial than late surfactant treatment in infants 27 to 32 weeks' gestation with respiratory distress syndrome.

▶ Michael S. Dunn, M.D., F.R.C.P.C. Department of Newborn and Development Paediatrics, Women's College Hospital, Toronto, comments:

The study by Gortner and colleagues is the latest in a series of clinical trials examining the differences between early and delayed treatment of preterm neonates with surfactant. Most of the previous studies have compared prophylactic treatment at birth to treatment only if respiratory distress syndrome of a certain severity develops. A meta-analysis of these trials reveals an advantage to prophylaxis, especially in the smallest preterm infants.[1]

This study examines the timing issue in a slightly different way. Babies were randomized prior to birth, but none were given surfactant unless they required intubation and assisted ventilation. The results suggest that, if you need to intubate a baby of 27 to 32 weeks for respiratory distress, you do not need to rush in with surfactant right away.

This conclusion must be tempered by the possibility that the sample size used was too small to properly address the issue. Groups were analyzed according to "intention to treat," and both "early" and "late" groups contained a significant number of babies who were never given surfactant. The necessary inclusion of a large number of babies who would not be affected by the intervention "dilutes" any possible treatment effects that makes it necessary to boost up the sample size. The other 2 studies in the literature that most closely resemble this study enrolled 1400 and 2600 babies to examine similar questions.[2,3] Both studies concluded that earlier treatment is better.

Although this study suggests that it may not always be necessary to administer surfactant as soon as a decision is reached to intubate, complacency will almost certainly result in suboptimal outcomes for some babies. The bulk of the relevant data suggests that a baby who is surfactant-deficient will accrue the most benefit from exogenous surfactant if it is given as soon as possible after birth. In the developed world, surfactant is readily available, and one should not be stingy with it once a baby has demonstrated the need for intubation and supplemental oxygen.

M.S. Dunn, M.D., F.R.C.P.C.

References

1. Soll RF, Morley CJ: Prophylactic versus selective use of surfactant for preventing morbidity and mortality in preterm infants (Cochrane Review), in *The Cochrane Library*, issue 1, 1999: Update Software.
2. Kattwinkel J, Bloom BT, Delmore P, et al: Prophylactic administration of calf lung surfactant extract is more effective than early treatment of respiratory distress syndrome in neonates of 29 through 32 weeks' gestation. *Pediatrics* 92:90-98, 1993.

3. The OSIRIS Collaborative Group: Early versus delayed neonatal administration of a synthetic surfactant: The judgement of OSIRIS. *Lancet* 340:1363-1369, 1992.

Interleukin-1 Receptor Antagonist and Interleukin-6 for Early Diagnosis of Neonatal Sepsis 2 Days Before Clinical Manifestation

Küster H, Weiss M, Willeitner AE, et al (Univ of Munich; T Roosevelt Hosp, Banska Bystrica, Slovakia; Innsbruck Univ, Austria)
Lancet 352:1271-1277, 1998   1–9

Introduction.—Neonatal sepsis occurs with an incidence of up to 10 per 1000 live births—even higher for very low birth weight infants—and mortality of up to 50%. The nonspecific nature of the initial clinical signs and the absence of reliable laboratory tests often lead to delay in antibiotic therapy. The inflammatory markers interleukin 1 receptor antagonist (IL-1ra), interleukin 6 (IL-6), and circulating intercellular adhesion molecule-1 (cICAM-1) were studied for use in early diagnosis of neonatal sepsis.

Methods.—The prospective study included 182 very low birth weight infants at 6 neonatal ICUs. All were monitored for sepsis according to a

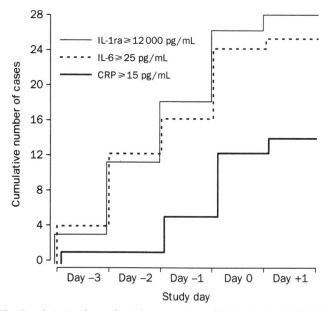

FIGURE.—Cumulative incidence of raised concentrations of IL-1ra, IL-6, and CRP in 28 cases of proven sepsis between day −3 and day +1. For practical reasons, the ROC-based cutoff values were rounded. cICAM-1 concentrations are not shown due to their inferior specificity of 64.1%. (Courtesy of Küster H, Weiss M, Willeitner AE, et al: Interleukin-1 receptor antagonist and interleukin-6 for early diagnosis of neonatal sepsis 2 days before clinical manifestation. *Lancet* 352[9136]:1271-1277, 1998. Copyright The Lancet Ltd.)

detailed protocol. Every time blood was taken, whether routinely or for clinical indications, IL-1ra, IL-6, cICAM-1, and C-reactive protein (CRP) were measured. The course of expression of these mediators was evaluated, along with their ability to make the diagnosis of sepsis before clinical diagnosis or CRP, the conventional laboratory marker.

Results.—The analysis included 101 infants; 21 had proven sepsis, 20 were free of infection, and 60 were unclassified. Fifty-seven patients were excluded because of missing data, and 24 because of early-onset sepsis. Levels of IL-1ra and IL-6 rose significantly 2 days before the diagnosis of sepsis (Figure). From 4 days before to 5 days after the diagnosis of sepsis, median peak increase was 15-fold for IL-1ra and 12-fold for IL-6 . Measured on the day of diagnosis, IL-1ra had a sensitivity of 93%, compared with 86% for IL-6 and 43% for CRP. Measured on the day before diagnosis, these values were 64%, 57%, and 18%, respectively. Specificity was 92% for IL-1ra, 83% for IL-6, and 93% for CRP, compared with 64% for cICAM-1.

Conclusions.—Measurement of the inflammatory markers IL-1ra and IL-6 in very low birth weight infants may permit earlier diagnosis of sepsis. Among those studied, using these markers would have led to earlier antibiotic therapy in nearly two thirds of proven sepsis cases. IL-6 measurements are available within 90 minutes, which should facilitate their routine clinical use.

▶ One of the several pots of gold at the end of the rainbow in the neonatal intensive care unit contains the perfect diagnostic test to tell when a neonate is infected. The early clinical signs of neonatal sepsis are often nonspecific as are laboratory indicators, including the CBC, the ratio of immature to total neutrophils, and CRP. The highly touted CRP is a very good example of how a commonly used tool proves not to be all that helpful. CRP concentrations have an initial sensitivity of only 50% when sepsis is first suspected. Sensitivity levels rise to 85% later when it is too late.

The examination of soluble immunologic mediators released within minutes to hours after invasion of pathogens could dramatically improve the early diagnosis of sepsis. A wide variety of cytokines have been described, including IL-1ra and IL-6. IL-1ra reaches its peak concentration 2 to 4 hours after the experimental administration of endotoxin and stays up for a day or so more. IL-6 also reaches its peak concentration very rapidly after the onset of a bacteremia and uses quite a bit ahead of the elevations in CRP.

What is neat about the study from Germany is that these investigators have documented rises in cytokine levels long before the clinical suspicion of onset of sepsis in newborns. Despite great variation in plasma concentrations, IL-1ra and IL-6 seem to clearly differentiate the proven sepsis group from the non-infection group, with specificities of 92% and 83%, respectively. Furthermore, the rises seem to occur in advance of the ability to unequivocally document clinical sepsis so that nearly two thirds of patients with subsequently proven sepsis would have qualified for earlier initiation of antibiotics than if you relied solely on clinical acumen.

We will definitely hear more about cytokines for the early triage of sepsis. Might it be that each morning in the neonatal ICU we will be ordering a CBC and cytokine profile . . . measuring cytokines perhaps as readily as taking a temperature?

J.A. Stockman III, M.D.

A Randomized, Controlled Trial of Prophylactic Granulocyte-Macrophage Colony-stimulating Factor in Human Newborns Less Than 32 Weeks Gestation

Carr R, Modi N, Doré CJ, et al (St Thomas' Hosp, London; Hammersmith Hosp, London)

Pediatrics 103:796-802, 1999   1–10

Background.—Morbidity from sepsis is high in preterm neonates receiving intensive care. When neutropenia develops in association with sepsis in such infants, mortality is high. The safety and efficacy of prophylactic granulocyte-macrophage colony-stimulating factor (GM-CSF) in producing a clinically relevant increase in neutrophil number in high-risk preterm neonates were investigated.

Methods.—Seventy-five neonates younger than 32 weeks' gestational age were enrolled in the open, randomized, controlled study. The infants were assigned to a control group or to treatment with GM-CSF, 10 µg/kg per day, by subcutaneous injection for 5 days beginning at less than 72 hours post partum. The main outcome measure was the neutrophil count during 14 days from study enrollment.

Findings.—During the study period, prophylactic GM-CSF completely eliminated neutropenia in both well and septic infants. By contrast, neutropenia developed in 16 of the 39 infants in the control group. Five control group infants had an acute decline in neutrophil count coinciding with sepsis onset. Treated infants showed no signs of hematologic, respiratory, or gastrointestinal toxicity. These infants also showed a trend toward fewer symptomatic, blood culture-positive septic episodes than did control group infants.

Conclusion.—Five-day prophylactic GM-CSF completely abolishes postpartum neutropenia and sepsis-induced neutropenia in preterm infants at high risk for sepsis. Thus, such prophylaxis eliminates an important risk factor for sepsis and sepsis-related mortality.

▶ This report has been a long time coming. In babies, particularly premature babies, neutrophil counts tend to drop under stress or in the presence of sepsis. The resulting neutropenia only makes a bad situation worse. Why the neutrophil count falls post partum is not totally known, but it appears to be caused by a reduced whole-body neutrophil cell mass, together with reduced numbers of committed neutrophil progenitors in the bone marrow at birth and an inability to increase granulopoiesis in response to sepsis. It takes more than a month for a newborn baby to begin to look like an adult in terms of neutrophil reserves. Thus, one might think that GM-CSF could be potentially helpful. If the conclusions of this report are true, indeed it is.

The issue with any relatively novel therapy is whether harm will be done with its use. The major concern over the use of CSFs in a newborn is that the neutrophils produced might cause a pulmonary sequestration and worsen pulmonary function. A similar concern exists about the mesenteric circulation and the possibility of an increased incidence of necrotizing enterocolitis. Neither of these complications was noted in this series. Also not found was any apparent increase in the risk of induction of a myeloid malignancy, although the study itself was perhaps too short in duration to perhaps detect this. The latter complication must be an extremely unusual one, if it occurs at all.

GM-CSF has not yet found its way into the routine management protocols of preterm infants. We will need to see more supportive data before this occurs, but preliminary insights into the possible benefits described suggest that we might just think about stocking up on GM-CSF in our neonatal ICUs.

Before leaving the topic of infections in newborns, try on the following case. Your diagnosis please: A 30-year-old gravida-4, para-3 woman who had immigrated to the United States from Mexico 8 years ago is having her fourth child here in the States and is living in Nashville. The pregnancy has had no abnormalities noted on the routinely scheduled prenatal visits to a Tennessee obstetrician. Labor and delivery are unremarkable and produce a male infant weighing 3340 g, with Apgar scores of 9 and 10. The newborn and mother are discharged, in good health, on the second hospital day. The infant does well until the third or fourth day of life, when the mother notes a foul-smelling discharge from the umbilical stump. The stump received routine hospital care and at home the mother had applied only isopropyl alcohol to it 2 or 3 times each day. On the sixth day of life, the infant becomes irritable, feeds poorly, and seems stiff. The next day the parents take the infant to a local pediatrician, who finds the child has no rash or fever, but the infant does appear irritable, stiff, and is experiencing difficulty swallowing with tight masseter muscles. Everyone else in this infant's home is healthy. The father works full-time as a laborer at a factory and also part-time on a farm feeding cattle and pigs. The home is adjacent to a pasture where cattle graze. Your diagnosis?

The Tennessee pediatrician who saw this infant made the correct diagnosis immediately based on the history and physical findings. The diagnosis was neonatal tetanus. Consistent with this history was the determination that this mother of Mexican background had never received appropriate tetanus immunization herself, and therefore the baby had no passive immunization protection. Although the infant's home was clean and tidy, it was located near a cattle pasture where tetanus spores would be commonly found in high concentrations in manure. It is likely that the infant's proximity to cattle manure may have increased his exposure to *Clostridium tetani*. This particular infant did especially well because of the prompt diagnosis by his pediatrician, who had experience as a volunteer in refugee camps on the Thai-Cambodian border and had seen several cases of neonatal tetanus. The baby required mechanical ventilation, muscle paralysis, and sedation for 1 month. He was treated with IV penicillin and multiple injections of human tetanus immunoglobulin, including shots subcutaneously administered around the umbilicus.[1]

The take-home message: Show me a home where the buffalo (cows) roam, and I'll show you a case of neonatal tetanus.

J.A. Stockman III, M.D.

Reference

1. Craig AS, Reed GW, Mohon RT, et al: Neonatal tetanus in the United States: A sentinel event in the foreign born. *Pediatr Infect Dis J* 16:955-959, 1997.

Length of Stay, Jaundice, and Hospital Readmission
Maisels MJ, Kring E (William Beaumont Hosp, Royal Oak, Mich; Wayne State Univ, Detroit)
Pediatrics 101:995-998, 1998   1–11

Background.—Early discharge from well-baby nurseries is now common practice in the United States. The association of early discharge with increased morbidity is unclear. The effect of infant age at discharge on the risk of readmission, especially for significant jaundice, was studied.

Methods and Findings.—A case-control design was used. Infants born between December 1, 1988, and November 30, 1994, at 1 hospital and readmitted within 14 days of discharge were compared with a randomly selected group of infants who were not readmitted. Of the total 29,934 infants discharged, 247 (0.8%) were readmitted by the age of 14 days. Fifty-one percent were rehospitalized because of hyperbilirubinemia, and 30% to rule out sepsis. Hospital readmission was associated with male sex, breastfeeding, diabetes in the mother, the presence of jaundice in the nursery, gestational age of 36 weeks or less and 37 to 38 weeks compared with 40 weeks or more, and a length of stay (LOS) of less than 48 hours or 48 to less than 72 hours compared with 72 hours or more. Readmission *for jaundice* was associated with male sex, breastfeeding, jaundice during nursery stay, gestational age of 36 weeks or less or 37 to 38 weeks compared with 40 weeks or more, and LOS of less than 48 hours or 48 to less than 72 hours compared with 72 hours or more. Infants discharged within 48 hours of birth were not at greater risk for rehospitalization for jaundice or other causes than were infants discharged 48 to less than 72 hours after birth.

Conclusions.—Compared with discharge 72 hours after birth, discharge at any time within the first 72 hours of life significantly increases the risk for readmission. Infants discharged within the first 72 hours of life should be seen by a health care professional within 2 to 3 days of discharge. Morbidity and readmission, especially for hyperbilirubinemia, may be reduced by helping mothers to nurse their babies more effectively from the time of birth.

▶ Dr. Paula Braveman, Family and Community Medicine, University of California at San Francisco, comments:

This well-designed case-control study examined risk factors for readmission among newborns discharged from a large community hospital's well-newborn nursery. One of the findings calls into serious question the current AAP guidelines for care of the normal neonate, that define "early discharge" as discharge in less than 48 hours, without specifying follow-up needs among infants staying from 48 to 72 hours.[1] In this study, babies with LOS from 48 to 71 hours were at similarly elevated risk as were babies staying less than 48 hours, compared with those staying 72 hours or more. The authors cite two other studies observing increased risks with newborn stays of less than 3 days.[2,3] The current guidelines should also be questioned on an *a priori* grounds, in light of the timing of peak bilirubin levels among many babies and of milk let-down and breastfeeding problems among many women.[4,5]

The authors acknowledge that their findings on LOS are confounded by delivery mode: almost all babies staying less than 72 hours, but few staying 72 hours or more, were delivered vaginally. This limitation would affect any nonrandomized study of the effects of different newborn LOS. However, even if a randomized study of LOS were feasible, it appears difficult to justify a 3-day LOS for apparently well newborns when a combination of better predischarge screening and early postdischarge follow-up for all newborns staying less than 72 hours (regardless of other risk factors) seems appropriate. I concur with the authors that well newborns should routinely be assessed within 2 to 3 days after discharge whenever initial LOS is less than 72 hours. I also believe these findings suggest that routine postdischarge newborn care should include early detection and intervention for breastfeeding problems, which would require significant changes in the content, not only the scheduling, of early pediatric care.

P.A. Braveman, M.D., M.P.H.

References

1. American Academy of Pediatrics, Committee on Fetus and Newborn: Hospital stay for healthy term newborns. *Pediatrics* 96:788-790, 1995.
2. Lee K-S, Perlman M, Ballantyne M: Association between duration of neonatal hospital stay and readmission rate. *J Pediatr* 127:758-766, 1995.
3. Soskolne EL, Schumacher R, Fyock C, et al: The effect of early discharge and other factors on readmission rates of newborns. *Arch Pediatr Adolesc Med* 150:373-379, 1996.
4. Braveman P, Egerter S, Pearl M, et al: Early discharge of newborns and mothers: A critical review of the literature. *Pediatrics* 96:716-726, 1995.
5. Braveman P, Kessel W, Ederter S, et al: Early discharge and evidence-based practice: Good science and good judgement. *JAMA* 278:334-336, 1997.

Control of Severe Hyperbilirubinemia in Full-term Newborns With the Inhibitor of Bilirubin Production Sn-mesoporphyrin

Martinez JC, Garcia HO, Otheguy LE, et al (Hosp Materno Infantil Ramon Sarda, Buenos Aires, Argentina; Rockefeller Univ Hosp, New York)
Pediatrics 103:1-5, 1999   1–12

Introduction.—The most frequent clinical problem that pediatricians must deal with during the newborn period is hyperbilirubinemia, which may cause severe brain damage. A new therapeutic approach to the treatment of newborn jaundice has been developed involving a synthetic heme analog that acts as a competitive inhibitor of heme oxygenase. The most potent and innocuous heme oxygenase inhibitor developed to date is Sn-mesoporphyrin (SnMP). It may seem more logical to suppress the production of bilirubin in the immediate postnatal period than to control elevated plasma bilirubin concentrations by phototherapy and exchange transfusion. The efficacy of SnMP was assessed in moderating the need for phototherapy.

Methods.—There were 84 healthy term breast-fed infants with plasma bilirubin concentrations of at least 256.5 µmol/L and no more than 307.8 µmol/L reached between 48 to 96 hours of age. Forty infants were randomized to receive SnMP at 6 µmol/kg birth weight, single dose, IM, and 44 were control subjects. The groups were similar in sex ratio, gestational age, birth weight, age at enrollment, and plasma bilirubin concentrations.

Results.—The need for supplemental phototherapy was entirely eliminated by SnMP to control hyperbilirubinemia. In the control group, 12 of 44 infants required phototherapy when their plasma bilirubin concentrations reached or exceeded the level of 333.5 µmol/dL (19.5 mg/dL). This level was not reached by any of the SnMP treated infants. The hours to case closure were also reduced with treatment to a median of 86.5 hours, whereas the control subjects had a median of 120 hours. The number of bilirubin determinations required for clinical monitoring of the infants was significantly reduced with the treatment patients having a median of 3 and the control subjects having a median of 5. There were no adverse effects with SnMP.

Conclusion.—In full-term breast-fed newborns with high bilirubin levels between 48 and 96 hours, a single dose of SnMP proved effective in controlling severe hyperbilirubinemia. The use of clinical medical resources was reduced, as well as the need for phototherapy and the emotional costs associated with the mothers and infants.

▶ M. Jeffrey Maisels, Department of Pediatrics, William Beaumont Hospital, Royal Oak, Mich, comments:

The management of jaundice in the term and near term infant is now an outpatient endeavor. This means, at the very least, visits by mothers to the pediatrician's office and the laboratory, and repeated heel sticks until the clinician is satisfied that the bilirubin level is declining. Phototherapy is a simple and safe intervention, but it requires blindfolding the infant's eyes, admission to hospital (sometimes), separation of mother and baby, and an increased likelihood that breastfeeding will be abandoned.[1] For all of these reasons, the possibility of turning off bilirubin production with a single shot of SnMP is extremely attractive, and there is no doubt that SnMP can both prevent and effectively treat hyperbilirubinemia in nonhemolyzing newborns. To date, several hundred newborns have received this drug in controlled clinical trials, and the only adverse effect has been a transient, nondose-dependent erythema that developed in a few infants who received photo-therapy after receiving SnMP.

So why are we not rushing to the drug store? First, although available for investigational use, the drug has not been released for general clinical use. Second, we need to have some idea of how many newborns would receive this drug and how many need to be treated to prevent a real or potential problem. A calculation of the "number needed to treat" depends on what you are trying to treat or, in this case, to prevent. The authors seem to suggest that we should attempt to interdict "the production of bilirubin for a short period immediately after birth. . . ." This approach would involve the treatment of almost 4 million newborns every year in the United States. If untreated with phototherapy, at least 2% of newborns will develop a bilirubin level of 20 mg/dL.[2] If SnMP reduced this to zero, the absolute risk reduction is $0.02 - 0 = 0.02$, and the number needed to treat is $1/0.02 = 50$. Thus, we would be treating 50 newborns to prevent 1 from developing a bilirubin of 20 mg/dL, a ratio that is more favorable than the use of vitamin K to prevent significant bleeding. We could restrict the administration of SnMP to those at significant risk for developing a high bilirubin level, and thus, reduce the number of newborns who received the drug by a half or more. Finally, we could substitute SnMP for phototherapy as done in this study. Assuming that about 5% of infants will require phototherapy, about 200,000 infants would receive SnMP each year in the United States.[3] The number needed to treat for this approach is $1/0.05$ or 20. If we chose a level of 20 mg/dL for treatment, rather than 17 mg/dL or 18 mg/dL to initiate therapy, the number needed to treat is higher, but the total number exposed to the drug would be reduced to about 80,000. The possibility of failure at higher bilirubin levels and the convenience of using SnMP, however, would likely persuade pediatricians to treat sooner (and, therefore, treat more infants). Earlier treatment would also get rid of the problem sooner, an attractive proposition for both physicians and parents. Whichever of these approaches is adopted, it is clear that there is the potential for treating a very large number of newborns in the United States and many more when the global population is included.

The issue, therefore, is safety. In spite of multiple clinical trials, and the criteria imposed by the FDA before drugs can be released for general use, there are numerous examples of very serious adverse effects, and even deaths, from drugs that initially appeared safe. An adverse event with the use of SnMP may be very uncommon, but when hundreds of thousands of newborns are exposed to the drug, it is possible (perhaps, likely) that some complications will emerge. There may be other reasons to be cautious. Although SnMP is cleared rapidly from the plasma, it may not be cleared so rapidly from the liver and other organs. SnMP affects hepatic heme levels, which in turn could influence levels of cytochrome P 450 enzymes and modify the baby's ability to metabolize drugs and endogenous compounds. And, while it is true that the dermal photosensitivity that has occurred is both mild and short lived, we do not have much data about the possibility of long-term phototoxicity. Nevertheless, to date, it does look as though the risk of significant toxicity following the small doses used is really quite small.

Martinez et al correctly point out that an intervention designed to inhibit bilirubin production would certainly eliminate many of the annoying and costly lengths to which we must now go to identify those few infants who might be at risk for bilirubin encephalopathy. On the other hand, phototherapy has been used throughout the world for more than 30 years and, with few exceptions, has been free of significant complications. In countries where phototherapy is not readily available, however, the use of SnMP is easily justified. But, closer to home, where it will find a niche in the management of neonatal jaundice, is yet to be defined.

M.J. Maisels, M.B., B.Ch.

References

1. James J, Williams SD, Osborn LM: Home phototherapy for treatment of exaggerated neonatal jaundice enhances breastfeeding. *Am J Dis Child* 144:431A-432A, 1990.
2. Newman TB, Escobar GJ, Branch PT, et al: Incidence of extreme hyperbilirubinemia in a large HMO. *Amb Child Health* 3:203A, 1997.
3. Bhutani VK, Johnson L, Sivieri EM: Predictive ability of a predischarge hour-specific serum bilirubin for subsequent significant hyperbilirubinemia in healthy-term and near-term newborns. *Pediatrics* 103:6-14, 1999.

Decreased Response to Phototherapy for Neonatal Jaundice in Breast-fed Infants
Tan KL (Natl Univ Hosp, Singapore)
Arch Pediatr Adolesc Med 152:1187-1190, 1998   1–13

Background.—Phototherapy has been found to be effective and safe in the treatment of neonatal hyperbilirubinemia. However, there have been no objective studies of the effect of breast-feeding on the efficacy of phototherapy in healthy, full-term infants with hyperbilirubinemia.

Methods.—One hundred sixty-three infants with nonhemolytic hyperbilirubinemia were studied. Seventy-nine infants were formula fed (group 1); 34 were breast fed (group 2); and 50 were fed both formula and breast milk (group 3). All feeding patterns were begun at birth. Conventional phototherapy with daylight fluorescent lamps was administered to all infants and was terminated only when bilirubin levels declined to less than 185 μmol/L.

Findings.—Mean weight loss as a percentage of birth weight was 2.8% in group 1, 6.1% in group 2, and 3.2% in group 3. Duration of phototherapy exposure was 54.1 hours in group 1, 64.6 hours in group 2, and 54.9 hours in group 3. The 24-hour rate of decline in the bilirubin concentration was 18.6%, 17.1%, and 22.9%, respectively. The overall hourly rate of reduction in bilirubin level for the duration of phototherapy exposure was 0.8%, 0.6%, and 0.8%, respectively. The 24-hour rate of reduction in the bilirubin concentration was significantly better in group 1 than in groups 2 or 3, with the latter 2 having similar rates. The overall rate of reduction in the bilirubin level during the duration of phototherapy exposure in group 2 was significantly lower than in groups 1 and 3, with the latter 2 having similar rates. The postexposure rebound bilirubin levels were similar in all groups in the first 2 days. However, the duration of moderate jaundice in group 2 was longer.

Conclusions.—In this series, exclusively breast-fed infants with hyperbilirubinemia responded significantly more slowly to phototherapy than infants fed formula only or a combination of formula and breast milk. Thus, adding formula to the diets of breast-fed infants with hyperbilirubinemia would enhance the efficacy of phototherapy and decrease phototherapy exposure time.

▶ It's nice to see a study that reinforces what most of us have seen over the years but have never bothered to document. In this case, the observation is that breast-fed jaundiced babies respond more slowly to phototherapy. That really is not too surprising, since the reason they are jaundiced is more complex than simple physiologic hyperbilirubinemia and so they might be expected to be more refractory to phototherapy. Fortunately, however, jaundiced breast-fed babies do respond to phototherapy, albeit a bit more slowly. The response to phototherapy is more than adequate to alleviate hyperbilirubinemia or to forestall thinking about more aggressive measures to reduce bilirubin levels. When the above article was published, there was an editor's note with it that read as follows: "For me, the take-home message from the study is that a clinician never (dangerous word!) needs to stop a mother from breast-feeding because of neonatal jaundice caused only by human milk. I just know someone will come up with a case that will force me to drink my words."[1] Actually, well before the article on phototherapy and breast feeding was published, Maisels et al.[2] did document that kernicterus can occur, albeit extremely infrequently, in otherwise healthy breast fed term infants with extreme hyperbilirubinemia. The latter report received a lot of attention, since it has been practically "bible" that nonhemolytic jaundice does not cause kernicterus. Journal editors aside, "never" means *sort of never*, or *almost never*, or *hardly ever*. Only "never, never" means *never*. When it comes to hyperbilirubinemia and kernicterus, "never" clearly means *well, sort of never*.

This is the last entry in the Newborn chapter, so we close with our habit of an ending query. What do Virginia Apgar and Soranus of Ephesus have in common? A little background on each of these luminaries is in order. Virginia Apgar was born here in the United States in 1909. She attended Mount Holyoke College and enrolled at the Columbia University College of Physicians and Surgeons. After graduation and a surgical residency, she elected to do anesthesiology and became the first woman in the United States to hold a full professorship at Columbia. She was also the first person to become a clinical professor in teratology in the United States. At the 27th annual Congress of Anesthetists in Virginia Beach in the fall of 1952, she presented a scoring system for the evaluation of the newborn infant after 1 minute of life. A year later, her scoring system was published and we now have, of course, the "Apgar score." By the time of her death in 1974, Apgar was already a legend.

Soranus, on the other hand, was born at Ephesus, a flourishing Ionian colony on the coast of Asia Minor, in the second half of the first century. He studied at the leading medical school of Alexandria, and he successfully practiced in Rome in the time of the emperors Trajan and Hadrian. He died in the same year that Galen was born (c 129 AD). Soranus, writing in Greek, prepared over 20 books related to medicine, philosophy, philology, and history. His book, *Gynaecia*, represents the most complete surviving account of gynecology, midwifery, and pediatrics of the Greco-Roman world.

So what do Virginia Apgar and Soranus of Ephesus have in common? Their descriptions of the health status of newborn infants. Within *Gynaecia*, Soranus prepared several chapters on the care of the newborn. The first chapter is strikingly called: "How to recognize the newborn that is worth rearing." In just 200 words, Soranus provides the midwife with a complete description of the healthy newborn ("worth rearing") and how to distinguish the healthy newborn from a handicapped infant. Four of the 5 criteria included in the Apgar score can be found more or less identically in Soranus' instructions on how to tell a healthy newborn from a "newborn not worth rearing." The only thing he missed was heart function. But this is not surprising, since the circulation had not been studied in the second century AD. By the way, Soranus, in addition to covering all of Virginia Apgar's assessments (except for heart rate), did recommend that a baby be inspected to determine if it was "perfect in all parts," "born at the due time," and "was delivered of a healthy pregnancy."

Soranus of Ephesus has long been the recipient of jokes of proctologists, but when it comes to pediatrics, he is a star.

Now you know your Soranus from your Apgar score.[3]

J.A. Stockman III, M.D.

References

1. DeAngelis CD: Editorial comment. *Arch Pediatr Adolesc Med* 152:1187, 1998.
2. Maisels MJ, Newman TB: Kernicterus in otherwise healthy, breast fed term infants. *Pediatrics* 96:30-33, 1995.
3. Galanakis E: Apgar score and Soranus of Ephesus. *Lancet* 352:2012-2013, 1998.

2 Infectious Disease and Immunology

Occupational Exposures to Body Fluids Among Medical Students: A Seven-Year Longitudinal Study

Osborn EHS, Papadakis MA, Gerberding JL (Palo Alto Med Found, Calif; Univ of California, San Francisco, Calif; Ctrs for Disease Control and Prevention, Atlanta, Ga)
Ann Intern Med 130:45-51, 1999
2–1

Background.—Because medical students lack experience and skill, they may be at high risk for occupational exposures to blood. The frequency of medical student exposure to infectious body substances and identified factors that affect the probability of such exposure were determined.

Methods and Findings.—All exposures reported by third- and fourth-year medical students in the classes of 1990 through 1996 at 1 center were reviewed. Of a total of 1022 medical students, 119 reported 129 exposures. Eighty-two percent of these exposures occurred on 4 services: ob-

TABLE 3.—Incidence of Exposure During Each Clerkship Rotation*

Rotation	Students Taking Rotation %	Exposures† n (%)	Exposure Incidence‡
Emergency department elective	52	25 (21)	4.7
Obstetrics-gynecology subinternship	6	2 (1.7)	3.3
Surgery subinternship	16	5 (4.2)	3.1
Medicine subinternship	95	17 (14.3)	1.8
Obstetrics-gynecology core clerkship	100	22 (18.5)	1.4
Surgery core clerkship	100	15 (12.6)	0.7
Neurology core clerkship	100	6 (5.0)	0.6
Medicine core clerkship	100	11 (9.2)	0.5
Pediatrics core clerkship	100	3 (2.5)	0.2
Psychiatry core clerkship	100	3 (2.5)	0.2
Family and community medicine core clerkship	100	2 (1.7)	0.1
Anesthesia core clerkship	100	2 (1.7)	0.1

*Six exposures were sustained on rotations taken by less than 2% of students and do not appear in this table.
†The percentages listed as percentages of the total number of exposures (n = 113).
‡Number of exposures per 100 student-months.
(Courtesy of Osborn EHS, Papadakis MA, Gerberding JL: Occupational exposures to body fluids among medical students: A seven-year longitudinal study. *Ann Intern Med* 130:45-51, 1999.)

stetrics-gynecology, surgery, medicine, and emergency medicine. Exposure probability was not correlated with graduation year, clerkship location, previous clerkship experience, or training site. Surveys of the first and last graduating classes in the 7 years of the study indicated that the percentage of exposures reported increased from 45% to 65%. Thus, the injury rates reported represent minimum estimates of actual occurrences. Although no cases of HIV infection or hepatitis were reported, follow-up was limited (Table 3).

Conclusions.—Instruction in universal precautions and clinical procedures is apparently not adequate for preventing exposure to blood during medical training. Medical schools must take more responsibility for ensuring that students are proficient in the safe performance of clinical procedures. Medical schools must also develop systems so that students can report and learn from their mistakes.

▶ This article makes you wonder how any of us made it out of medical school alive. While this statement is something of an exaggeration, there is still a problem these days. With 12% of medical students reporting 1 or more occupational exposures to needle stick hotlines, being educated these days is not without serious risk. This is especially true in a city such as San Francisco, where, at the San Francisco General Hospital, 34% of patients have antibodies to hepatitis C virus, 23% have HIV infection, and 2.3% have hepatitis B virus antigenemia. While San Francisco General Hospital is hardly typical of the rest of the country, no hospital is without similar type walking contagions. So what is the real risk to such medical students? The average risk for infection associated with a single parenteral exposure to HIV is approximately 0.3%. Fortunately, postexposure prophylaxis may reduce this risk somewhat. Transmission of hepatitis C virus carries a much higher risk of approximately 1.8% following needle puncture involving contaminated blood. The risk for hepatitis B virus transmission to those susceptible to infection exceeds 30% when the source patient has hepatitis B antigenemia. The risk is still substantial when this antigen is not present. Fortunately, medical students are now required to be immunized against hepatitis B virus. At the time of this report, a related article appeared in the *British Medical Journal.*[1] Being a medical student in Great Britain carries with it some interesting potential risks, since a large number of students will elect to spend time abroad, particularly in Africa. Given the high prevalence of HIV infection, particularly in sub-Saharan Africa, these students are not permitted to take an elective in obstetrics-gynecology or surgery. They are also told that they should take with them a 6-day course of zidovudine, which costs about £40. These precautionary measures make sense. Pregnant women in parts of Zimbabwe have recently been reported to have a prevalence of HIV infection of 32%. Imagine being splashed by amniotic fluid in such a country. Fortunately, despite these kinds of potential risks, very few medical students seem to get themselves into serious trouble. Indeed, insurance companies are very willing to write disability policies, since the actual risk of an untoward occurrence is small. If you're interested in an excellent review of the hepatitis viruses, see the update in hepatology that recently appeared in the *Annals of Internal Medicine.*[2]

J.A. Stockman III, M.D.

References

1. Gamester CF, Tilzey AJ, Banatvala JE: Medical students' risk of infection with bloodborne viruses at home and abroad: A questionnaire survey. *BMJ* 318:158-160, 1999.
2. Schiff ER: Update in hepatology. *Ann Intern Med* 130:52-57, 1999.

International Multicentre Pooled Analysis of Late Postnatal Mother-to-Child Transmission of HIV-1 Infection

Leroy V, for the Ghent International Working Group on Mother-to-Child Transmission of HIV (Université Segalen Bordeaux 2, France; et al)

Lancet 352:597-600, 1998   2–2

Introduction.—During pregnancy, in the intrapartum period or postnatally, mother-to-child transmission of HIV type 1 (HIV1) infection can occur. It is known that breastmilk has HIV1 DNA and that transmission can occur after birth through breastfeeding. If safe and affordable alternatives are available, the avoidance of breastfeeding by HIV1 infected women is recommended The risk of vertical transmission is doubled with breastfeeding; however, the exact risk and timing of transmission that can be attributed to breastfeeding is still not clear. To estimate the rate and timing of late postnatal transmission of HIV1, an international multicenter analysis was conducted.

Methods.—In 4 studies from the industrialized countries of the United States, Switzerland, France, and Europe 2807 children born to HIV-infected mothers were compared to 902 children born to HIV-infected mothers in the developing countries of Rwanda, Ivory Coast, and Kenya. The children were followed up from birth. If a child later became infected, late postnatal transmission was assumed. The analysis was stratified for breastfeeding.

Results.—Less than 5% of the children from the industrialized countries were breastfed, and no HIV1 infection was diagnosed. However, 5% of the children born in the developing countries where breastfeeding was the norm had postnatal transmission. There was an overall estimated risk of 3.2 per 100 child-years of breastfeeding follow-up. For 20 of the 49 children with late postnatal transmission, exact information on timing of infection and duration of breastfeeding was available. The transmission occurred between the last negative and first positive HIV1 tests. No infants would have been infected if breastfeeding had stopped at age 4 months, and if it had stopped at 6 months, only 3 children would have been infected (Figure).

Conclusion.—For breastfed children born to HIV1 positive mothers, the risk of late postnatal transmission is consistently shown to be substan-

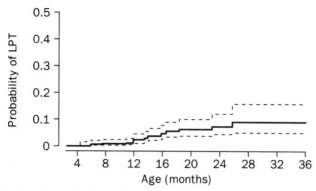

FIGURE.—Cumulative probability of late postnatal transmission (LPT) of HIV-1 among breastfed children with estimation of the timing of infection. Kaplan-Meier method with delayed entry (n = 20 of 429). *Dotted lines* represent 95% CI. (Courtesy of Leroy V, for the Ghent International Working Group on Mother-to-Child Transmission of HIV: International multicentre pooled analysis of late postnatal mother-to-child transmission of HIV-1 infection. *Lancet* 352[9128]:597-600, 1998. Copyright by The Lancet Ltd.)

tial. The effect of early weaning on infant mortality and morbidity and maternal fertility should be balanced against this risk. In the Ivory Coast, the stopping of breastfeeding at 6 months is being considered and, if put into effect, will need to be carefully monitored.

▶ It was only within this past decade that we have begun to understand that a mother who is HIV-positive could transmit the infective virus in her breast milk and that the breast milk itself could cause disease in an offspring. What we have not known is the exact risk and timing of transmission attributable to breast milk feeding. A rough estimate has been that breastfeeding approximately doubles the risk of vertical transmission. It would be easy to conclude that all one needed to do to eliminate this risk would be to insist that breastfeeding not take place. That indeed is the recommendation if safe and affordable alternatives are available. Unfortunately, in many developing countries, because of the expense associated with alternatives to breastfeeding and the problem of milk contamination, avoidance of breastfeeding causes more harm than good.

An alternative to recommending against breastfeeding would be to recommend a shortened period of such feeding if one were able to define when breastfeeding produced the greatest risk for a baby. Presumably, some babies become infected postnatally after they lose their passively-transferred maternal antibody. If this is so, one should be able to demonstrate that breastfeeding is safe initially, but carries risks beyond some specific period after birth. That is exactly what these investigators found. Before 4 months of age, no breastfed baby developed HIV-related disease. If you allow breastfeeding for the entire first year of life, you can expect an incidence of 3.2 cases of HIV infection per 100 babies (with the infection occurring only after 4 months of breastfeeding). The benefits of being able to breastfeed for the better part of the first half year of life should not be minimized. It is during that period that breast milk gives its greatest protection against other infections, as well as against malnutrition. Any period of breastfeeding, even if it is only for 4 months, is to be sought after in certain parts of the world. In such circumstances, despite maternal HIV infection, the breast still remains the best.

J.A. Stockman III, M.D.

The Mode of Delivery and the Risk of Vertical Transmission of Human Immunodeficiency Virus Type 1: A Meta-analysis of 15 Prospective Cohort Studies
Read JS, for the International Perinatal HIV Group (Natl Inst of Child Health and Human Development, Bethesda, Md)
N Engl J Med 340:977-987, 1999   2–3

Objective.—A reduction in vertical transmission of HIV type 1 (HIV1) with cesarean section has been suggested, but other studies have not shown an association, perhaps because the studies were small. Results of a meta-analysis using patient data from 15 prospective cohort studies were presented.

Methods.—Studies including at least 100 mother-child pairs enrolled on or before January 1, 1997 were analyzed for elective cesarean sections, nonelective cesarean sections, instrumental vaginal deliveries, and noninstrumental vaginal deliveries. Multiple regression analysis was performed.

Results.—Fifteen studies and 8533 mother-child pairs were selected. Compared with other modes of delivery, delivery by cesarean section reduced vertical transmission by approximately 50% after adjusting for confounding factors (odds ratio, 0.45) (Fig 2). After adjusting for receipt of retroviral therapy, advanced maternal disease, and low birth weight infants, elective cesarian section still reduced the risk of vertical transmission (odds ratio, 0.43). Vertical transmission rates after membrane rupture at less than 1 hour or at less than 4 hours before delivery were similar for patients having cesarean section. Without retroviral therapy, transmission rates were 10.4% for patients having cesarean section and 19.0% for patients not having cesarean section. With retroviral therapy, transmission rates were 2.0% for patients having cesarean section and 7.3% for patients not having cesarean section. Vertical transmission rates decreased by approximately 87% for patients with retroviral therapy having a cesarean section. Elective cesarean section was performed significantly more frequently in Europe than in North America (Fig 1).

Conclusion.—Cesarean section reduces vertical transmission of HIV1 independent of retroviral therapy.

▶ Whether mode of delivery makes any difference in terms of transmission of HIV to a baby during the process of labor and delivery has been an issue of quite some debate for the last 15 years or so. The ability to tease out

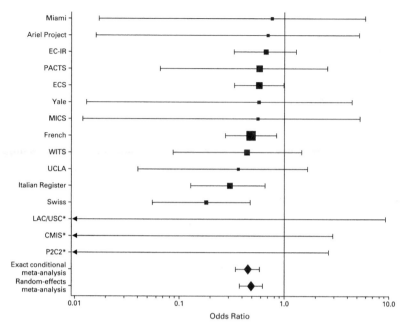

FIGURE 2.—Crude Odds ratios for the Association of Elective Cesarean Section with the Risk of Vertical Transmission of HIV-1 among 8533 Mother-Child Pairs in 15 Studies and in Meta-Analyses Based on the Exact Conditional Method and the DerSimonian-Laird Random-Effects model. Studies are listed in decreasing order of the odds ratios. *Bars* indicate 95 percent confidence intervals. The size of each square is proportional to the sample size of the corresponding study. *Asterisks* indicate that the lower limit of the confidence interval is less than 0.01; in these studies there were no cases of vertical transmission of HIV after elective cesarean section. *Abbreviations: Miami*, University of Miami Infants of HIV-1 Seropositive Mothers Study; *EC-IR*, mother-child pairs enrolled in both the European Collaborative Study and the Italian Register for HIV Infection in Children; *PACTS*, Perinatal AIDS Collaborative Transmission Studies; *ECS*, European Collaborative Study, with the Italian Collaborative Group on HIV and Pregnancy; *Yale*, Yale Prospective Longitudinal Cohort Study; *MICS*, Mothers and Infants Cohort Study; *French*, French Perinatal Cohort Study; *WITS*, Women and Infants Transmission Study; *UCLA*, UCLA–Los Angeles Maternal-Infant HIV Transmission Study; *Italian Register*, Italian Register for HIV Infection in Children; *Swiss*, Swiss Neonatal HIV Study–Swiss HIV and Pregnancy Study; *LAC/USC*, Los Angeles County–University of Southern California Perinatal Transmission Study; *CMIS*, Centre Maternel et Infantile sur le SIDA cohort; and *P2C2*, Pediatric Pulmonary and Cardiovascular Complications of Vertically Transmitted HIV Infection Study. (Reprinted by permission of *The New England Journal of Medicine*, from Read JS, for the International Perinatal HIV Group: The mode of delivery and the risk of vertical transmission of human immunodeficiency virus type 1: A meta-analysis of 15 prospective cohort studies. *N Engl J Med* 340:977-987. Copyright 1999, Massachusetts Medical Society. All rights reserved.)

differences in mode of delivery was made more difficult by the routine intrapartum use of zidovudine which, in and of itself, reduces the risk of transmission very significantly.

So what are the current understandings? The first is that mother-to-child transmission of HIV1 infection usually does occur around the time of delivery. In 1992, results from the European Collaborative Study suggested that infants of HIV1-infected women delivered by cesarean section did, indeed, have a lower risk of HIV1 infection than infants delivered vaginally, although the difference was hardly dramatic. A subsequent analysis of a larger data set from the European Collaborative Study—with allowance for other risk

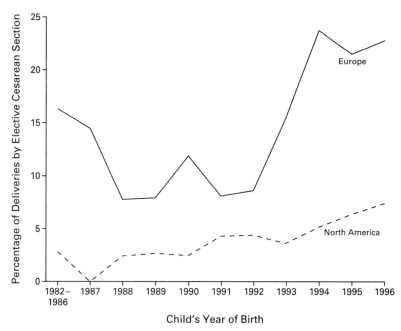

No. of Mother-Child Pairs										
Europe	435	408	439	507	565	583	596	591	565	373	189
North America	71	92	124	150	284	398	481	554	548	444	136

FIGURE 1.—Unadjusted proportions of elective cesarean sections among 8533 HIV type 1–infected women in Europe and North America, according to the child's year of birth. For each year, a significantly larger proportion of deliveries was performed by elective cesarean section in Europe than in North America (*P* < .05). (Reprinted by permission of *The New England Journal of Medicine*, from Read JS, for the International Perinatal HIV Group: The mode of delivery and the risk of vertical transmission of human immunodeficiency virus type 1: A meta-analysis of 15 prospective cohort studies. *N Engl J Med* 340:977-987. Copyright 1999, Massachusetts Medical Society. All rights reserved.)

factors such as prematurity and maternal clinical and immunological disease progression—suggested that elective cesarean section delivery significantly reduced the risk of vertical transmission by as much as 50%. Current data from the European Mode of Delivery Collaboration published just this past year indicated that only 1.8% of infants born to women who deliver by cesarean section became infected, compared with 10.5% of those delivering vaginally (all the pregnancies were appropriately treated with zidovudine).[1]

So, with several studies now pointing in the direction of recommending prophylactic cesarean section and the data from the above abstract, a meta-analysis of some 15 prospective studies also producing the same recommendation, will we see such a mode of delivery becoming the standard of future deliveries? The answer to this question is "maybe yes" and "maybe no." In a most interesting editorial on the topic of prophylactic cesarean section, Stringer et al admonish restraint, at least for now.[2] They suggest that in the absence of more complete morbidity data, a useful clinical measure for assessing the health consequences of prophylactic cesarean section is the number of operations required to avert a single case of pediatric HIV infection. For instance, if the rate of transmission among patients receiving zidovudine monotherapy is 4.3% and it could be reduced further with prophylactic cesarean section, the avoidance of a single case of mother-to-child transmission would require 29 prophylactic cesarean deliveries. However, if the rate of perinatal HIV transmission associated with monotherapy is 2% and could be reduced to 1% with prophylactic cesarean section, the avoidance of a single case of mother-to-child transmission would require approximately 100 prophylactic cesarean deliveries.

That's a lot of surgeries to relieve a single baby of infection, particularly when one takes into account the fact that there is some morbidity associated with cesarean delivery to the HIV-infected mother. In the latter regard, in a case-control study comparing 156 HIV-infected women with 156 uninfected women who had cesarean deliveries, Semprini et al reported 6 cases of major postoperative complications with cesarean section versus 1 major complication in those who did not have cesarean sections. There was also a threefold increased risk of minor complications with women with low CD4 lymphocyte counts who are at the highest risk of morbidity.[3]

A betting person would say that the "complete" package for prevention of perinatal (or subsequent) transmission of HIV infection includes the following: early detection of maternal HIV infection through universal screening, the use of antiretroviral therapy throughout pregnancy, neonatal antiretroviral therapy, selected intrapartum obstetrical interventions including elective cesarean section, and avoidance of breast feeding. The reason why decisions about cesarean sections should still be made on a case-by-case basis relates to the fact that unless everything else is being done to prevent HIV infection, cesarean section alone may make no difference, and it may not be appropriate to recommend cesarean section unless the "total package" can be delivered.

Sorry for the long-winded nature of this commentary, which recognizes that there is no absolute way to prevent perinatal transmission of HIV infection, only ways of reducing the risk. Life was simple when babies were delivered by storks, wasn't it?

J.A. Stockman III, M.D.

References

1. The European Delivery Collaboration: Elective C-section versus vaginal delivery in the prevention of HIV-1 transmission: A randomized clinical trial. *Lancet* 353:1035-1039, 1999.
2. Stringer JSA, Rouse DJ, Goldenberg RL: Prophylactic cesarean delivery for the prevention of perinatal human immunodeficiency virus transmission: The case for restraint. *JAMA* 281:1946-1949, 1999.
3. Semprini AE, Castagna C, Ravizza M, et al: The incidence of complications after cesarean section in 156 HIV-positive women. *AIDS* 9:913-917, 1995.

Lack of Long-term Effects of In Utero Exposure to Zidovudine Among Uninfected Children Born to HIV-infected Women
Culnane M, for the Pediatric AIDS Clinical Trials Group Protocol 219/076 Teams (NIH, Bethesda, Md; et al)
JAMA 281:151-157, 1999   2–4

Introduction.—The use of zidovudine for the prevention of mother-to-infant transmission of HIV has become widespread in the United States. Little is known about the late effects of perinatal exposure to antiretroviral drugs on the subsequent health of uninfected children. Zidovudine, a nucleoside analogue reverse transcriptase inhibitor, has had moderate antiviral effects for the treatment of persons with HIV infection at all stages of disease. The safety of perinatal zidovudine for the prevention of mother-to-child HIV transmission among HIV-uninfected children with in-utero zidovudine exposure was described.

Methods.—There were 234 uninfected children born to 230 HIV-infected women. Evaluations were made prospectively of the growth, immunologic, cognitive/developmental, cardiac, ophthalmologic, neoplasm, and mortality data. Children were assessed every 6 months when younger than 24 months and yearly thereafter. Before 36 months of age, they had a baseline echocardiogram and funduscopic evaluation. The children were randomized to receive zidovudine (122 children) or placebo prenatally (122), intrapartum, and during the immediate postnatal period. The children were studied for a median of 4.2 years and up to 5.6 years.

Results.—No significant differences were seen between the children exposed to zidovudine and those who received placebo in their weight, height, head circumference scores, cognitive/developmental function, and lymphocyte data. There were no deaths or malignancies. Two children exposed to zidovudine had abnormal, unexplained ophthalmic findings. A mild cardiomyopathy on echocardiogram at the age of 48 months was seen with 1 child exposed to zidovudine and the child is clinically asymptomatic.

Conclusion.—In-utero and neonatal exposure to zidovudine did not have any adverse effects on HIV-uninfected children. To assess the long-term safety of interventions that prevent perinatal HIV transmission, continued prospective evaluations of children born to HIV-infected women who are exposed to antiretroviral or immunotherapeutic agents are critical.

▶ It has been half a dozen years since the pediatric AIDS Clinical Trials Group first reported that zidovudine was effective in the prevention of mother-to-infant transmission of HIV if the drug was given prenatally to affected women and subsequently to their babies postpartum.[1] We have also had half a dozen years of experience with the offspring of such treated pregnancies and with any possible adverse effects following the administration of this potent nucleoside analogue reverse transcriptase inhibitor. If there are any untoward consequences, they haven't shown up yet. In particular, among the hundreds and hundreds of children followed, there was no short-term risk in terms of tumor formation. Carcinogenesis is of particular concern because female rats given zidovudine have developed vaginal epithelial neoplasms, a finding that may be explained by the presence of high concentrations of this agent in urine, which is capable of refluxing from the bladder into the vagina.[2]

For the second time, a health care worker has transmitted HIV infection and ultimately clinical AIDS to a patient or patients.[3] This case involved an orthopaedic surgeon who, in his early fifties, somehow transmitted the HIV virus during an operation to a woman who was undergoing a hip replacement. That surgeon in turn had developed his HIV infection from a needlestick injury involving blood from another patient he had operated upon. The orthopaedic surgeon had most likely been infected for about 10 years before he developed clinical AIDS. The more than 1200 patients he had operated on were then screened. Only 1 turned out to be HIV-positive related to a strain of virus virtually identical to his. The other health care worker was the well-known Florida dentist, who infected 6 of his patients, as reported 8 years ago.[4] Fortunately, transmission of the HIV virus from doctors to patients is extremely unusual, unlike transmission of hepatitis B or even hepatitis C. With improvement of instruments, use of reinforced gloves, and changes in surgical technique, as well as better education about transmission of infectious agents, I hope we will see even less of this problem in the future.

One final comment: even though HIV1-infected men who are receiving highly active antiretroviral therapy may have no detectable levels of viral RNA in plasma, the virus is still present in seminal cells and is therefore capable of being transmitted sexually.[5] Seminal cells harboring HIV1 can come in direct contact with leukocytes in the mucosa of sexual partners, resulting in transmission of the virus. Transmission of infection is not prevented by the low concentrations of antiviral drugs found in the semen.

Again, the rule is, condoms should be used on every conceivable occasion.

J.A. Stockman III, M.D.

References

1. Connor EM, Sperling RS, Gerber R, et al: Reduction of maternal-infant transmission of human immunodeficiency virus type 1 with zidovudine treatment. *N Engl J Med* 331:1173-1180, 1994.
2. Ayers KM, Clive D, Tucker WE Jr, et al: Nine clinical toxicology studies with zidovudine: Genetic toxicity and carcinogenicity bioassays in mice and rats. *Fundam Appl Toxicol* 32:148-158, 1996.
3. Lot F, Seguier J-C, Fegueux S, et al: Probable transmission of HIV from an orthopaedic surgeon to a patient in France. *Ann Intern Med* 130:1-6, 1999.
4. Ciesielski C, Marianos D, Ou ZY, et al: Transmission of human immunodeficiency virus in a dental practice. *Ann Intern Med* 116:798-805, 1992.
5. Zhang H, Dornadula G, Beaumont M, et al: Human immunodeficiency virus type 1 in the semen of men receiving highly active antiretroviral therapy. *N Engl J Med* 339:1803-1809, 1998.

Herpes Zoster in Children and Adolescents

Petursson G, Helgason S, Gudmundsson S, et al (Univ of Iceland, Reykjavik)
Pediatr Infect Dis J 17:905-908, 1998   2–5

Introduction.—Herpes zoster is caused by reactivation of latent varicella-zoster virus that had been acquired during a previous episode of chickenpox. There has been only one population-based study of zoster that involved children. All new cases of zoster in children and adolescents in a geographically well-defined primary care setting with a high quality of recording were prospectively collected. To determine the natural course of zoster, patients were followed for several years.

Methods.—All patients with acute zoster were enrolled by 61 general practitioners who had a computerized medical record system for registration of all patient contacts. The study population compassed 75,750 person years, and the patients were all younger than 20 years. At 1, 3, and 12 months from the start of the rash, a follow-up telephone interview was conducted, as well as another follow-up 3 to 7 years later. Questions concerned patient age and sex, discomfort or pain, and general health before and 3 to 6 years after the zoster episode.

Results.—There were 121 episodes of acute zoster that developed in 118 patients for a period of 75,750 person years, with an incidence of 1.6/1000 per year. After 554 person years of follow-up, end points were gained for all 118 patients. Postherpetic neuralgia, moderate or severe pain, or any pain lasting longer than 1 month from the start of the rash were not seen in any of the patients. The mean length of time for those having chickenpox before the age of 1 year until occurrence of zoster was 8.1 years and for those having chickenpox later, the mean length of time was 8.8 years. Within 3 months of contracting zoster, 3 patients were diagnosed with potential immunomodulating conditions (2.5%). A history of severe diseases was seen in only 5 patients (4%).

Conclusion.—There is an extremely low probability of postherpetic neuralgia in children and adolescents. In the primary care setting, zoster is seldom associated with undiagnosed malignancy.

▶ How many places can one capture an entire population in order to determine the incidence of any disease, much less the occurrence of acute zoster in children up to age 20? If you guessed Iceland, the country from which this report emanated, you would be right. The only reason that few, if any, cases might have been missed would be if a patient, for whatever reason, was never seen for the problem. This is unlikely with zoster. It is even more unlikely in Iceland where access to medical care by general practitioners is as readily available as popcorn in a movie theater.

It is clear that zoster during childhood in the nonimmunocompromised youngster has no real serious consequences. Virtually all children get better. They get better without a high likelihood of recurrence. Routine antiviral therapy has no place, despite pressures to the contrary by the pharmaceutical industry.

There is no reason to think that the information we have learned from Iceland cannot be used with reliability here in the United States. Doctors who hang out their shingles stateside can expect that the shingles of kids in Peoria are no different than the shingles of kids in Reykjavik.

J.A. Stockman III, M.D.

Prospective Study of Persistence and Excretion of Human Herpesvirus-6 in Patients With Exanthem Subitum and Their Parents
Suga S, Yoshikawa T, Kajita Y, et al (Fujita Health Univ, Toyoake, Japan; Showa Hosp, Kohnan, Japan)
Pediatrics 102:900-904, 1998   2–6

Introduction.—Human herpesvirus (HHV)-6 causes exanthem subitum which can be fatal. The etiologic role of HHV-6A is still not clear. It is not known whether patients with exanthem subitum transmit the virus to people around them and whether excretion of the virus occurs from various body sites during the course of exanthem subitum. Persistence and excretion of the virus were examined in 20 virologically confirmed infants with exanthem subitum. The HHV-6 status of the parents who were caring for the patients in the family setting was also examined.

Methods.—There were 20 infants from 20 families with primary HHV-6 infection and a typical clinical course of exanthem subitum and 15 parents from the 20 families. The infants had a mean age of 7.7 months and ranged in age from 4 to 11 months. The parents had a mean age of 28.2 years and ranged in age from 21 to 34 years. Isolation of the virus from peripheral blood mononuclear cells was conducted to confirm primary infection with HHV-6. By amplifying the viral deoxyribonucleic acid in serially collected peripheral blood mononuclear cells, plasma, saliva, stool, and urine samples, viral persistence or excretion was examined with a nested polymerase chain reaction (PCR) method.

Results.—During and after the disease, 20 infants with virologically confirmed exanthem subitum had HHV-6 DNA persistently in mononuclear cells. It was in plasma only in the first 5 days of exanthem subitum. During and after disease, the viral DNA was detected persistently or intermittently in saliva and stool, but rarely in urine. No HHV-6 viremia or viral DNA in peripheral blood mononuclear cells and plasma was seen in any of the parents, except for 1, but half of the parents excreted viral DNA in saliva during and after exanthem subitum. A fourfold increase in antibody titers to HHV-6 was seen in only 1 of the 15 parents after possible exposure from their children.

Conclusion.—It was found that HHV-6 is excreted into saliva and stool persistently or intermittently but rarely into urine, after systemic replication of HHV-6 in the blood of patients with exanthem subitum. Active infection with the virus was suggested by the presence of HHV-6 DNA in plasma. The source and transmission route of infection with HHV-6 is suggested by the excretion of the virus into the saliva of infants with exanthem subitum and their parents.

▶ Mary T. Caserta, M.D., Division of Pediatric Infectious Diseases, Children's Hospital at Strong, Rochester, NY, comments:

Our knowledge of the full scope of clinical and virologic consequences of infection with HHV-6 remains incomplete. Specifically, the connection between universal primary infection in infancy and diseases of normal or immunocompromised adults is unclear. The mode of transmission of HHV-6 is also undefined. Suga and colleagues have chosen a worthy goal in their attempt to more precisely define the virology of primary HHV-6 infection and to study adult caretakers of infected children to determine whether information regarding the transmission of HHV-6 could be obtained. Despite their efforts, however, the study is hampered by the small number of children enrolled, the short length of follow-up, and the ubiquity of infection with HHV-6 in adults.

Blood, saliva, urine, and stool were collected from 20 children with exanthem subitum and primary HHV-6 infection. Samples were also obtained once in the 2 weeks after the febrile illness, at 30 days, and again at between 60 and 90 days. The authors are to be commended for their rigorous definition of primary HHV-6 infection as requiring a combination of viral isolation and seroconversion. Additionally, they have extended the observation of Secchiero and colleagues that nested PCR on plasma as positive for cell-free HHV-6 DNA in a subset of children with primary infection concurrent with viremia.[1] Suga and colleagues also used nested PCR for HHV-6 on peripheral blood mononuclear cells and reported that all patients had HHV-6 DNA in the peripheral blood mononuclear cells during primary infection. Additionally, 90% of children had HHV-6 DNA detectable in peripheral blood mononuclear cells during follow-up, confirming previously published data by Hall and colleagues on 160 children in Rochester, New York, with primary HHV-6 infection.[2] In the larger study from Rochester, children were followed for up to 2 years with a 66% frequency of detection of HHV-6 DNA in peripheral blood mononuclear cells, demonstrating these cells as a site of long-term viral persistence or latency of HHV-6. The high frequency of detection of HHV-6 DNA in saliva and the low frequency of detection in urine reported by Suga and colleagues have also been previously reported.[3-5]

The majority of adult caretakers of children with primary infection had serologic evidence of past infection with HHV-6, with a large percentage harboring HHV-6 DNA in the saliva, similar to the matched adult controls. Therefore, it was impossible to draw any conclusions regarding the source or mode of transmission of infectious virus. Thus, the study by Suga and colleagues contributes no further data with regard to the transmission of HHV-6 and generally confirms previous studies demonstrating the persistence of viral DNA in several sites after primary infection.

M.T. Caserta, M.D.

References

1. Secchiero P, Carrigan DR, Asano Y, et al: Detection of human herpesvirus 6 in plasma of children with primary infection and immunosuppressed patients by polymerase chain reaction. *J Infect Dis* 171:273-280, 1995.
2. Hall CB, Long CE, Schnabel KC, et al: Human herpes virus-6 infection in children: A prospective study of complications and reactivation. *N Engl J Med* 331:432-438, 1994.
3. Cone RW, Huang MW, Ashley R, et al: Human herpesvirus 6 DNA in peripheral blood cells and saliva from immunocompetent individuals. *J Clin Microbiol* 31:1262-1267, 1993.
4. Jarrett RF, Clark DA, Josephs SF, et al: Detection of human herpesvirus-6 in peripheral blood and saliva. *J Med Virol* 32:73-76, 1990.
5. Gautheret-Dejean A, Aubin JT, Poierel L, et al: Detection of human *Betaherpesvirinae* in saliva and urine from immunocompromised and immunocompetent subjects. *J Clin Microbiol* 35:1600-1603, 1997.

Primary Human Herpesvirus 7 Infection: A Comparison of Human Herpesvirus 7 and Human Herpesvirus 6 Infections in Children
Caserta MT, Hall CB, Schnabel K, et al (Univ of Rochester, New York)
J Pediatr 133:386-389, 1998   2–7

Introduction.—There is widespread human infection with human herpesvirus (HHV)-6 and HHV-7; however, little is known about the latter. Hepatitis, upper respiratory tract infections, acute hemiplegia of childhood, and roseola infantum have been associated with primary HHV-7 infection. The clinical and virologic characteristics of primary HHV-7 infection in children was defined. These characteristics were compared with those of a group of children with primary HHV-6 infection identified during the same time period.

Methods.—A total of 496 children 3 years of age or younger were tested for HHV-6 and HHV-7 with polymerase chain reaction and serology. Medical records reviews and follow-up interviews were conducted to determine the clinical and laboratory characteristics of the patients.

Results.—There were 8 children with primary HHV-7 infection, compared with 29 children with HHV-6 infection. All children had a fever with a mean temperature of 39.8°C, and there was no difference in the degree of fever between the 2 groups, nor was there a difference in the frequency of rash or gastrointestinal complications. Children with primary HHV-6 infection had a median age of 9 months, compared with 26 months for those who had HHV-7 infection. Seizures associated with the illness were also more likely among the children with primary HHV-7 infection, compared with HHV-6.

Conclusion.—In childhood, a highly febrile illness can be caused by primary infection with HHV-7 and can be complicated by seizures. Cross-reacting antibodies may confound the serologic diagnosis of infection with primary HHV-6 and HHV-7.

▶ Yoshizo Asano, M.D., professor and chairman, Department of Pediatrics, Fujita Health University School of Medicine, Toyoake, Aichi, Japan, comments:

After the first isolation of HHV-7 by Frenkel et al. in 1990, a growing body of evidence has been produced regarding the causal relationship between the virus and several clinical features. HHV-7 is an ubiquitous virus, which is isolated from the saliva of most HHV-7 seropositive adults. However, from our experiences, the confirmation of primary HHV-7 infection is not easy in comparison with HHV-6 because of less intense fluorescence by indirect fluorescent antibody and indistinguishable cytopathic effects of infected mononuclear cells.

Although the sample size is small, this report suggested 2 important new findings: an equal severity of clinical manifestations by primary HHV-7 and HHV-6 infections and a more neuropathologic potential of HHV-7 than HHV-6. It is our clinical impression that the course of typical primary HHV-7 infection is milder than HHV-6 infection. HHV-6–associated exanthem subitum was characterized by high fever (mean, 39.4°C) lasting 4.1 days followed by an erythematous and macular or maculopapular rash of 3.8 days duration. In comparison, patients with HHV-7–associated febrile exanthem had a maximum fever of 38.7°C lasting 2.9 days followed by a skin rash of 2.9 days duration.[1,2] This may be explained by the fact that preexisting immunologic memory to HHV-6 would modify the clinical course of primary HHV-7 infection, as cross-reactions of antibodies and T-cell clones between HHV-6 and HHV-7 have been reported.

To confirm potential differences in the severity of clinical manifestations of primary infections with both viruses and in the neurotropic nature of these 2 viruses, a larger scale study will be required. I believe a consensus is needed on whether the term exanthem subitum (roseola infantum) should be used only for clinical features of primary infection with HHV-6 or for clinical syndromes featuring febrile exanthem by various infectious agents, including HHV-6, HHV-7, enteroviruses, etc.

Y. Asano, M.D.

References

1. Asano Y, Yoshikawa T, Suga S, et al: Clinical features of infants with primary human herpesvirus 6 infection (exanthem subitum, roseola infantum). *Pediatrics* 93:104-108, 1994.
2. Suga S, Yoshikawa T, Nagai T, et al: Clinical features and virological findings in children with primary human herpesvirus 7 infection. *Pediatrics* 99:4, 1997.

Transmission of Human Herpesvirus 8 Infection From Renal-Transplant Donors to Recipients

Regamey N, Tamm M, Wernli M, et al (Univ of Basel, Switzerland; Univ Hosp of Zurich, Switzerland)

N Engl J Med 339:1358-1363, 1998   2–8

Introduction.—Human herpesvirus (HHV)-8 has been observed in all forms of Kaposi's sarcoma, including transplantation-associated Kaposi's sarcoma. The route of HHV-8 transmission has not been clearly delineated; there is evidence that the virus cannot be transmitted sexually. The seroprevalence of HHV-8 in renal transplant recipients before and after transplantation was assessed to examine the possibility of transmission of HHV-8 through allografts.

Methods.—Serum samples from 220 renal transplant recipients were examined for the presence of antibodies to HHV-8 on the day of transplantation and 1 year later using an enzyme-linked immunosorbent assay with the recombinant HHV-8 protein orf 65.2. Positive results were determined by an indirect immunofluorescence assay that detects antibodies to latent antigen and by Western blotting. Patients were followed for 4 years.

Results.—The seroprevalence of HHV-8 in graft recipients rose from 6.4% on the day of transplantation to 17.7% 1 year after transplantation. Twenty-five patients seroconverted within the first year after transplantation. In 2 of these patients Kaposi's sarcoma developed within 26 months of transplantation. Ten of the patients who seroconverted had sequential serum samples taken. Of these, immunoglobulin M antibodies to HHV-8 were detected within 3 months after transplantation in 8 patients. Serum samples were available from donors of 6 patients who seroconverted. Five of these patients (83%) tested positive for HHV-8. Of 8 patients in a control group who were seronegative at the time of transplantation and received allografts from donors who were HHV-8 negative, none seroconverted within the year after transplantation.

Conclusion.—HHV-8 was able to be transmitted by donor organs. Patients who become seropositive after transplantation are at risk for Kaposi's sarcoma, particularly if they are severely immunosuppressed.

▶ HHV-8 is hardly the first virus to be transmitted through kidney transplantation. It is hardly likely to be the last virus either. Given the preciousness of donor organs, there is a strong inclination to letting "infected" organs be transplanted unless the infection is so potentially likely to cause problems that the organ must be excluded. A donor with HIV virus infection or with hepatitis B would fall into the latter category. When it comes to hepatitis C virus infection in a donor, the desirability of using transplanted organs is still being debated, although this editor would take a pass on being a recipient if he had his druthers.

HHV-8 is just one of a number of herpesviruses, some of which—if received via a donated organ—can cause problems. Other herpesviruses may not cause illness. The Epstein-Barr virus rarely causes illness, although there are isolated reports of complications post transplantation. Herpesvirus 3 (varicella-zoster virus) from donated organs is not a concern because the virus is largely latent in nervous tissue. The cytomegalovirus, also a herpesvirus, is a bad actor when transmitted via a transplant if the organ recipient has not already been exposed to this virus.

As this report tells us, the real risk with HHV-8 infection post transplantation is with its potential association with the development of Kaposi's sarcoma. It is most likely the immunosuppression that follows organ transplantation that allows the HHV-8 to emerge as an oncovirus triggering the Kaposi's sarcoma.

When something is as precious as a donated organ, you can bet that it will not be discarded without a very good reason. To date, there is not a clear and present danger from such donated organs when they harbor HHV-8. Some 5% to 10% of donors will be HHV-8–positive and although there *is* a possibility of posttransplantation complications, it is probably worth the risk of using such infected organs—at least for now—while we learn more about whether a real problem exists.

J.A. Stockman III, M.D.

Impact of a Large-scale Immunization Initiative in the Special Supplemental Nutrition Program for Women, Infants, and Children (WIC)
Hoekstra EJ, LeBaron CW, Megaloeconomou Y, et al (Ctrs for Disease Control and Prevention, Atlanta, Ga; Catholic Charities, Chicago; Chicago Dept of Public Health; et al)
JAMA 280:1143-1147, 1998   2–9

Introduction.—Nearly 80% of unvaccinated measles cases during the measles resurgence of 1989-1991 occurred among urban preschoolers. Immunization rates in inner cities frequently lag behind the rest of the country. High-risk urban children may lack the minimum level of population immunity needed to avoid outbreaks. The impact of an initiative linking immunization with distribution of food vouchers through the Special Supplemental Nutrition Program for Women, Infants, and Children (WIC) offices in the inner city of Chicago was assessed.

Methods.—A total of 16,581 children aged 24 months or younger were being served by 19 Special Supplemental Nutrition Program for WIC sites. During each WIC certification and recertification visit—which occurs every 6 months—the vaccination status was reviewed for each child age 24 months of age or younger. In Chicago, a 3-month supply of food vouchers is typically issued by WIC to enrolled families. With the immunization initiative (in which 14 of the 19 sites participated), children who were not age-appropriately vaccinated were issued a 1-month supply of vouchers. When the child was appropriately vaccinated, a 3-month supply was resumed. No voucher was withheld from a child because of immunization status. The impact of the immunization initiative was retrospectively evaluated for the period April 1996 through June 1997. Age-appropriate immunization rates and WIC enrollment rates were reviewed.

Results.—During the 15-month evaluation period, immunization rates rose from 56% to 89% at sites using the initiative program. The proportion of children needing voucher incentives decreased from 51% to 12%. The WIC sites not participating in the incentive program had no improvement in immunization coverage. Enrollment rates were similar for sites that did and did not use the voucher incentives.

Conclusion.—This large-scale initiative program demonstrates that voucher incentives at WIC can rapidly increase and sustain high childhood immunization rates in an urban population.

▶ If you aren't familiar with the national WIC initiative that links immunizations to this public health program, pilot studies have been underway now for several years. The concept here is similar to the United States policy that attempted to deal with the Saddam Hussein regime in Iraq and consists of carrots and sticks. The program allows WIC staff to review immunization records for each enrolled child and also to educate a parent concerning when immunizations are needed. Referrals are then made for immunizations as appropriate.

Parents of children found to be delayed in their immunizations or who will not bring in their infant's immunization card are provided only 1 month's supply of WIC food vouchers instead of the usual 3-month supply that is given if a child's immunizations are up to date. To say this differently, parents can avoid 2 "unnecessary" trips to a WIC center if they keep their child's immunization records up to date. In this report from Chicago, in just 15 months, immunization rates, which had been stubbornly low for more than a decade, increased dramatically from 56% to 89%, an absolutely stunning accomplishment! As importantly, there were no negative impacts on WIC participation rates.

The outstanding results linking the WIC program to immunization education has some interesting applications for other purposes. Children of poor, inner-city families are at risk not only for undernutrition and underimmunization, but also for many other problems that compromise their health, well being, and development. Is it possible that the higher rates of lead exposure, anemia, child abuse and neglect, growth and development problems, fatal and nonfatal injuries, premature birth, asthma, learning difficulties, etc., that are found in WIC populations might somehow be addressed by the WIC program as was done for immunizations? The possibilities are almost endless.

Some have criticized holding aspects of the WIC program hostage to other initiatives, but these initiatives are not "food for immunizations." They are avoidance of inconvenience for immunizations. No child is underfed because of these linkages, as far as anyone can tell. That having been said, why not go for it? Why not link more health initiatives to the WIC program?

J.A. Stockman III, M.D.

Reactions of Pediatricians to the Recommendation for Universal Varicella Vaccination
Newman RD, Taylor JA (Univ of Washington, Seattle)
Arch Pediatr Adolesc Med 152:792-796, 1998   2–10

Introduction.—Live attenuated varicella vaccine was licensed for use in children 12 months of age and older by the Food and Drug Administration. The recommendation of its use for this population has been endorsed by the American Academy of Pediatrics and the Centers for Disease Control and Prevention. This vaccine has been shown to be theoretically cost-effective, saving more than $5 for each dollar spent on immunization, and it reduces the morbidity and mortality associated with varicella infection. Nevertheless, the medical community has not unanimously endorsed routine immunization against varicella. A survey of pediatricians was conducted to determine the rate of adherence to the varicella immunization recommendation, to understand sources of concern, and to evaluate factors that might influence adherence.

Methods.—A survey was sent to 574 pediatricians in the state of Washington, and the response rate was 76%. The pediatricians were asked about demographic characteristics, attitudes about varicella vaccine, and previous experiences with the disease that were associated with self-reported adherence to universal varicella immunization recommendations.

Results.—Of those who completed the survey, 42% reported following a policy of universal varicella immunization. The recommendation was associated with pediatrician attitudes of agreement regarding the effectiveness of varicella vaccine in reducing rare but serious complications of the disease and in decreasing parental time lost from work. Those who universally recommended the vaccine disagreed with statements concerning the lack of the need for varicella immunization because complications are rare, that immunization is not required for school entry, or that it is not medically cost-effective. Adherence to the recommendations was also associated with experience with varicella encephalitis. Those who were less likely to report recommending universal vaccination were pediatricians who were concerned that varicella vaccine might not provide lifelong immunity.

Conclusion.—Universal varicella vaccination was recommended by fewer than 50% of the responding pediatricians. Personal experiences, perceptions about the potential seriousness of varicella, and beliefs about the societal and medical cost-effectiveness of varicella vaccine appear to influence adherence to the recommendation.

▶ If we pediatricians have difficulty recommending the use of the varicella vaccine, what are we going to do with the recent recommendations about the rotavirus vaccine? In all fairness, though, it is easy to see why there has been hesitancy on the part of some providers when it comes to immunizing against varicella. We don't know for sure whether vaccine-induced immunity will be truly lifelong. In children the disease is generally benign, whereas in adults it may not be. If protection fails over time, trying to play catch-up with the grown up will be an interesting challenge. Those who were cautious about the rotavirus vaccine were proven right in July of last year, when distribution of the vaccine was halted because of reports of postvaccination intusses option.

When all is said and done, the naysayers about varicella immunization should be setting their reservations aside and getting on with it fairly quickly. If many, but not all, are being vaccinated, the vaccine would have the potential to interrupt the natural cycle of varicella infection in ways that are not so good. Natural varicella would no longer flow freely through an entire community of children. A pool of unvaccinated children may emerge with a reduced likelihood of contracting infection in childhood, children who will grow up to adolescence or adulthood without any varicella immunity. That would be a worst-case, but nonetheless possible, scenario. The reason that such an occurrence is possible relates to a recent survey of pediatricians, which showed that 17% of the members of the American Academy of Pediatrics offered the varicella vaccine to "few or none" of their patients, whereas 14% give it to "some."[1] ...A pox on us if we make wrong decisions about this vaccine!

J.A. Stockman III, M.D.

Reference

1. Most fellows offer varicella vaccine, rates vary by location, payment system (editorial). *AAP News* 14:1, November 1998.

Deficiency of the Humoral Immune Response to Measles Vaccine in Infants Immunized at Age 6 Months

Gans HA, Arvin AM, Galinus J, et al (Stanford Univ, Calif; Palo Alto Med Found, Calif)
JAMA 280:527-532, 1998   2-11

Background.—Measles in infants can result in serious morbidity. In the United States, measles vaccine is typically given to children aged between 12 to 15 months. However, the infants of mothers with vaccine-induced immunity may lose antibodies acquired passively before 12 months, making them susceptible to measles. The immunogenicity of measles vaccine in children younger than 12 months was assessed.

Methods.—The cohort study included 27 infants aged 6 months, 26 aged 9 months, and 34 aged 12 months. Initial and follow-up samples, obtained before and after measles immunization, were available for 72 (83%) of the infants.

Findings.—Measles-neutralizing antibodies were detected before vaccination in 52% of the 6-month-old infants, in 35% of the 9-month-old infants, and in none of the 1-year-olds. In the absence of detectable passive antibodies, geometric mean titers after vaccination were significantly lower in the 6-month-old group than in the other age groups. The seroconversion rate (a 4-fold increase in antibody titer) in the 6-month-old infants was only 67%. Only 36% in this age group attained seroprotective neutralizing antibody titers of 120 or more after vaccination, compared with 100% of the 9- and 12-month-old infants without detectable passive antibody before vaccination. Age did not affect T-cell proliferation and cytokine responses.

Conclusions.—Even in the absence of detectable passively acquired neutralizing antibodies, vaccinated 6-month-old infants were deficient in humoral immunity. A developmental maturation of the immune response to measles, which affects the immunogenicity of measles vaccine, apparently occurs in the first year of life.

▶ The historical inability to immunize babies aged less than 12 months with the measles vaccine has been a plague upon pediatrics. Until recently, it really didn't matter. Most pregnant women who had natural measles as a child, had high titers of measles antibody that was reasonably protective, at least until about a year. That was the case during the first 3 decades or so after the measles vaccine was introduced. Now, in contrast, babies are born to mothers who have vaccine-induced immunity to measles. These mothers have significantly lower antibody levels. Such antibodies are lost before 12 months. One recent study showed that only 29% of 9-month-old infants and 5% of 12-month-old infants had persistent passive antibodies from their moms.[1] The consequence is fairly obvious. More infants now than ever, who are younger than 12 months, lack measles immunity, leaving them unprotected and in the highest age group for life-threatening complications.

It is well known that the younger one is in the first year of life, the more likely it is that one will have deficiencies in primary antigen presentation by dendritic cells, limited T-cell proliferation, impaired B-cell function, and reduced production of cytokines by helper T cells of the type 1 subset. These deficiencies are what cause a diminished antibody response to live virus vaccines. Whether these deficiencies, which could diminish the ability of a "take" of measles vaccine, are still present in a 6- to 9-month-old infant has not been determined. Because many infants now have early loss of passive antibodies, it should be feasible to distinguish the relative impact of age-related immune deficiencies attributed to maturation of the immune response from passive antibody inhibition of measles vaccine immunogenicity. The only way to find out what will happen is to give a group of 6-month-old infants the measles vaccine and see what occurs. That is exactly what these investigators did.

What they found was interesting, but probably predictable. A fair number, about 50% of 6-month-old infants already had nondetectable levels of passive antibodies in their blood (a result of the fact their mothers had low levels of antibodies, which was a consequence of their own vaccinations years ago). It was in these "zero" antibody babies that one could test the outcome of measles vaccination at 6 months. The results were mediocre, at best. Seroconversion was seen in only two thirds of these babies, and only one third had protective titers. By contrast, 100% of 9-month-old babies lacking passive antibody seroconverted and had protective titers. What does all this mean? It means that even if there were no interfering maternal antibody, the immune system of 6-month-old babies is not sufficiently and uniformly mature to allow them to be universally vaccinated. At the same time, the persistence of passive antibodies in half of 6-month-old infants and one third of 9-month-old infants makes measles immunization ineffective for these babies.

So where do we go from here? The twilight period for an at-risk state for babies getting measles seems to be between 6 and 12 months. Some babies are still protected by their moms, and others are not. Give the vaccine too early and it may not take because the baby's immune system is too immature to allow a take. Give it too early even if the baby's immune system is mature, and some babies' maternal antibody will block a take.

There is an increasing push to consider lowering the recommended age of measles immunization for infants whose mothers have vaccine-induced immunity. As this study suggests, there are many potholes in the path of such a consideration. What is a care provider to do?

J.A. Stockman III, M.D.

Reference

1. Meldonado YA, Lawrence EC, DeHovitz R, et al: Early loss of passive measles antibody in infants of mothers with vaccine-induced immunity. *Pediatrics* 96:447-450, 1995.

Etiology of Measles- and Rubella-like Illnesses in Measles, Mumps, and Rubella-Vaccinated Children
Davidkin I, Valle M, Peltola H, et al (Univ of Helsinki)
J Infect Dis 178:1567-1570, 1998   2–12

Background.—In Finland, a measles, mumps, and rubella (MMR) vaccination program was begun in 1982. Inaccuracy of clinical diagnoses was soon found to be a problem, as most suspected cases were not confirmed serologically as an MMR disease. The viral etiology of measles- or rubella-like illnesses after MMR vaccination was studied prospectively.

Methods.—Nine hundred ninety-three acutely ill children with fever and rash, seen from 1983 to 1995, were studied. Sera were analyzed for adenovirus, enterovirus, and parvovirus B19 antibodies. Previous antibody testing had excluded measles and rubella. The serologic diagnosis of adenovirus, enterovirus, or parvovirus infection was based on enzyme-linked immunosorbent assay. The diagnosis of human herpesvirus (HHV)-6 was based on indirect immunofluorescence.

Findings.—Viral etiology was verified in 368 children. Parvovirus was documented in 20%, enterovirus in 9%, and adenovirus in 4% (Fig 1). Twelve percent of young children had HHV-6 infection. Four percent of the children had double infections.

Conclusions.—Measles- or rubella-like illnesses in MMR-vaccinated children were frequently caused by other viruses. Infections in children

A

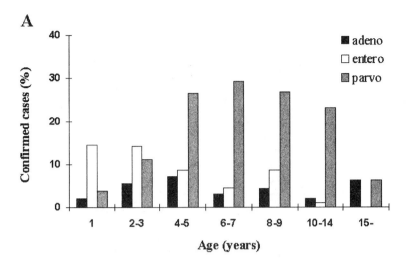

B

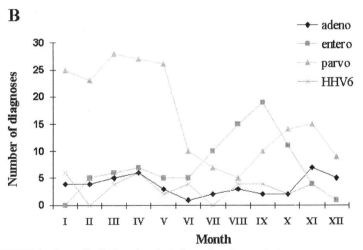

FIGURE 1.—**A**, age distribution of serologically confirmed cases of adeno-, entero-, and parvovirus infections (% of samples tested, by age group). **B**, seasonal variation in serologically confirmed acute cases of adeno-, entero-, and parvovirus and human herpesvirus 6 (HHV-6) infections. (Courtesy of University of Chicago, publisher, from Davidkin I, Valle M, Peltola H, et al: Etiology of measles and rubella-like illnesses in measles, mumps, and rubella-vaccinated children. *J Infect Dis* 178:1567-1570, © 1998 by the Infectious Diseases Society of America. All rights reserved.)

with suspected vaccine failure need laboratory confirmation to maintain reliable surveillance and control and to determine the cause of the illness.

▶ Dr. Ilona J. Frieden, clinical professor of Dermatology and Pediatrics, University of California, San Francisco, comments:

Exanthems are common. Some are so distinctive that they can be diagnosed on clinical grounds, but many have common morphologies and nonspecific accompanying signs and symptoms such as fever, cough, and rhinorrhea. Over the past few decades, a large number of laboratory methods have been introduced that allow specific diagnosis of exanthems, including viral serologies, cultures, and polymerase chain reaction. Despite the availability of these laboratory tests, most exanthems are still diagnosed clinically. Reasons for this include: (1) a reassuring clinical appearance of the patient; (2) the perception (often correct) that knowing which virus is causative will not change the patient management; and (3) expense and lack of cost-effectiveness, given the dozens of known infections that cause exanthems. There are certainly situations where precise knowledge of the etiology of an exanthem is very important, and can even be life-saving. These include those where a bacterial etiology (such as meningococcus) is suspected, signs of serious illness are present, or a potential public-health hazard such as rubella or measles is suspected. In these cases, cultures and/or serologies should always be obtained.

The article by Davidkin et al gives "exanthem watchers" new information about which infectious agents are relatively common causes of childhood exanthems in a highly immunized population.[1] Inclusion criteria apparently consisted of morbilliform or rubelliform rashes with or without fever. It is of note that even in this highly immunized population, 5.9% actually had either measles or rubella, a finding that hopefully will become less common with the addition of a booster MMR vaccine at age 5. The other infectious agents that were searched for included parvo-, entero-, and adenoviruses as well as HHV-6. The findings confirm existing epidemiologic information and are therefore not surprising.[1] Parvovirus was most common in school-aged children, occurring in epidemics, usually in the winter or spring. Enteroviruses were most common in the summer and fall, occurring in most age groups. Adenoviruses occurred in all age groups without seasonal trends. HHV-6 occurred mainly in 1- to 2-year-olds without seasonal trend.

Using serologies directed toward this set of etiologic agents, a verifiable viral cause for exanthem was found in only 37%. Since exanthems due to Epstein-Barr virus are fairly common in young children, evaluating for this agent might have increased the yield somewhat. The methodology used precludes other simple tests such as a bacterial throat culture which can confirm the presence of exanthem due to group A streptococcus. Nevertheless, this study gives us valuable information about the causes of exanthems in children and emphasizes the low probability of rubella and measles causing morbilliform and rubelliform rashes in a highly immunized population. Unfortunately, it also demonstrates that even when using many of the laboratory tests currently available, the etiology of exanthems still eludes us in many patients.

I.J. Frieden, M.D.

Reference

1. Goodyear HM, Laidler PW, Price EH, et al: Acute infectious erythemas in children: A clinico-microbiological study. *Br J Dermatol* 124:433-438, 1991.

Mother to Child Transmission of Hepatitis C Virus: Prospective Study of Risk Factors and Timing of Infection in Children Born to Women Sero-negative for HIV-1

Resti M, and Tuscany Study Group on Hepatitis C Virus Infection in Children (Univ of Florence, Italy)

BMJ 317:437-441, 1998   2–13

Introduction.—In mothers with HIV type 1 (HIV1) infection, mother-to-child transmission of hepatitis C virus (HCV) has been extensively studied, and transmission rates are as high as 36%. However, in women who are HIV1 seronegative, little is known about the risk of mother-to-child transmission of HCV or the correlates and timing of infection of their babies. In women who are not infected with HIV1, the risk factors for vertical transmission of HCV and the timing of such transmission to their children were determined.

Methods.—Four hundred forty-two mothers with HCV, but not HIV1, and their babies were included in the study. Of these, 403 (91%) completed the study. They were observed for a median of 28 months. The babies were tested for the presence of antibodies to hepatitis C, viral RNA, and alanine aminotransferase activity. The mothers and babies were also tested for the presence of viral RNA, and the method of infection with hepatitis C, the method of delivery, and type of infant feeding in the mothers were determined.

Results.—At the end of the follow-up period, 13 (3.2%) of the 403 children had acquired HCV infection. These children had mothers who were positive for HCV RNA. Of 128 RNA-negative mothers, none of their babies had the infection. Viral RNA was discovered immediately after birth in 6 children. IV drugs were used by 11 women, and blood transfusions were given to 20 women. These mothers had 11 of the infected children compared with 2 infected children born to the 144 mothers with no known risk factors.

Conclusion.—Only women with HCV RNA are at risk of infecting their babies among women not infected with HIV. It seems that transmission occurs in utero with the rate being higher in women who had blood transfusions or used IV drugs than in women who had no known risk factors for infection.

▶ At the start of this century, the HCV has yet to enter its teenage years. It was first described in the United States in 1989. Typical routes of transmission have included parenteral and sexual sources. This is an interesting virus in that, unlike hepatitis B where only 20% of those who become infected develop a chronic carrier state, some 80% of those infected with HCV do so. Transmission from mother to baby of these 2 viruses also differs. In mothers with hepatitis B virus, the vertical transmission rate is 90% or higher. The immaturity of the neonatal system may account for some of the inability to mount an immune response that clears hepatitis B. With hepatitis C, however, we see that vertical transmission occurs in only about 6% of pregnancies (somewhat higher if the mother is HIV positive). We can be fairly sure that the 6% figure is fairly accurate because several studies, including a recent report from the viral epidemiology branch of the National Cancer Institute, have shown the exact same frequency of vertical transmission.[1]

There are a few differences that are worthy of note regarding how vertical transmission statistics vary between HIV infection and hepatitis C infection. First, there appears to be no increase in the rate of hepatitis C transmission in children born by vaginal delivery, although given the relatively low probability of vertical transmission under any circumstance, it cannot be stated with assurance that a cesarean section might not reduce the risk of hepatitis C infection. Second, multiple studies have confirmed that breastfeeding does not represent a risk factor for vertical transmission of hepatitis C, unlike HIV infection.

Only time will tell what the natural history is of HCV-infected children. Some things are fairly clear even at this point. Persistent infection is to be expected. This is evidenced by intermittent transient elevations of liver enzymes, and in the few children who have had liver biopsies, persistent abnormalities are the norm.

While the likelihood of hepatitis C transmission from perinatal exposure isn't high, babies who are infected may be at long-term risk. Currently, there is no effective way to prevent vertical transmission, since unlike with HIV infection, effective antiviral therapies have not been identified.

J.A. Stockman III, M.D.

Reference

1. Granovisky MO, Minkoff HL, Tess PH, et al: Hepatitis C virus infection in mothers and infants cohort study. *Pediatrics* 102:355-359, 1998.

Interferon Alfa-2b Alone or in Combination With Ribavirin for the Treatment of Relapse of Chronic Hepatitis C
Davis GL, for the International Hepatitis Interventional Therapy Group (Univ of Florida, Gainesville; et al)
N Engl J Med 339:1493-1499, 1998   2–14

Background.—For patients with chronic hepatitis C virus (HCV) infection, interferon (IFN)-α is the only effective therapy. Nonetheless, relapse rates after the cessation of therapy are high. Some studies suggest that the combination of interferon plus ribavirin is associated with a longer sustained response than interferon therapy alone. This study compared interferon alone and in combination with ribavirin to determine the safety and efficacy of the combination in patients who relapsed after interferon therapy alone.

Methods.—The subjects were 345 patients with chronic HCV infection who relapsed after 1 or 2 courses of recombinant or lymphoblastic IFN-α treatment. Over a 24-week period, patients received either IFN–α-2b (3 ×

TABLE 4.—Rates of Symptoms During Treatment

Symptom	Interferon (N=172)	Interferon and Ribavirin (N=173)
	Percent	
Influenza-like symptoms		
Headache	54	55
Fatigue or asthenia	39	46
Myalgia	39	44
Arthralgia	23	21
Fever	33	32
Rigors	21	26
Gastrointestinal symptoms		
Anorexia	13	20
Nausea	20	35*
Diarrhea	18	12
Psychiatric symptoms		
Depression	11	16
Insomnia	23	20
Respiratory tract symptoms		
Cough	9	10
Dyspnea	6	14†
Pharyngitis	9	11
Dermatologic symptoms		
Alopecia	18	21
Rash	5	13†
Pruritus	6	13

Note: Only symptoms that occurred in 10% or more of all patients were included.
*$P = 0.002$ for the comparison with interferon alone.
†$P = 0.02$ for comparison with interferon alone.
(Reprinted by permission of *The New England Journal of Medicine* from Davis GL, for the International Hepatitis Interventional Therapy Group: Interferon alfa-2b alone or in combination with ribavirin for the treatment of relapse of chronic hepatitis C. *N Engl J Med* 339:1493-1499. Copyright 1998, Massachusetts Medical Society. All rights reserved.)

10^6 U 3 times a week) plus placebo (n = 172) or IFN–α-2b (same dosage) plus ribavirin (1000-1200 mg/day depending on the patient's weight) (n = 173). All patients were evaluated regularly to measure serum levels of HCV RNA and aminotransferases, and 24 weeks after the end of treatment a liver biopsy was performed in 277 patients (138 who had received IFN alone and 139 who had received the combination).

Findings.—Based on serum HCV RNA levels at the end of treatment, patients receiving combination therapy had a significantly better response than those receiving interferon alone (82% vs 47%). The difference between groups was still significant when assessed 24 weeks after the end of treatment (49% vs 5%). In both groups, patients whose baseline serum HCV RNA levels were 2 × 10^6/mL or less had a significantly better response to treatment. Based on biochemical responses, again, patients receiving the combination had a significantly better response than those receiving interferon alone, both at the end of treatment (89% vs 57%) and after follow-up (47% vs 5%). The same pattern was seen in histologic responses, with a significantly greater response in the combination group (63% vs 41%). Patients receiving combination therapy had a decrease in hemoglobin concentrations, with levels of less than 11 g/dL in 34% of patients. Other adverse events and symptoms between the 2 groups were similar (Table 4), although patients taking combination therapy did experience significantly more nausea (35% vs 20%), dyspnea (14% vs 6%), and rash (13% vs 5%).

Conclusion.—Based on virologic, biochemical, and histologic end points, combination therapy with IFN–α-2b and ribavirin provided a longer sustained response than interferon alone in patients with chronic HCV infection who had suffered a relapse. Although anemia was more common in the combination therapy group, the incidence of most adverse events was similar in the 2 groups.

Interferon Alfa-2b Alone or in Combination With Ribavirin as Initial Treatment for Chronic Hepatitis C

McHutchison JG, for the Hepatitis Interventional Therapy Group (Scripps Clinic and Research Found, La Jolla, Calif; et al)
N Engl J Med 339:1485-1492, 1998   2–15

Background.—Interferon therapy is often used to treat patients with chronic hepatitis C virus (HCV) infection, but in at least 15%, cirrhosis will develop. Thus, methods to improve the effectiveness of interferon therapy are needed, and some studies suggest that the combination of interferon (IFN) plus ribavirin is more effective than IFN therapy alone. This study compared interferon alone and in combination with ribavirin to determine the safety, efficacy, and optimal dosing scheme of the combined therapy.

Methods.—The subjects were 912 patients with chronic HCV infection who were randomized into 4 groups. In the IFN alone group (n = 456), patients received recombinant IFN–α-2b (3×10^6 U 3 times a week) plus placebo for either 24 weeks (n = 231) or 48 weeks (n = 225). In the combination groups (n = 456), patients received recombinant IFN–α-2b (same dosage) plus ribavirin (1000 or 1200 mg/day, depending on the patient's weight) for either 24 weeks (n = 228) or 48 weeks (n = 228). All 4 groups were similar in age, gender, weight, pretreatment serum HCV RNA levels, HCV genotype, and the incidence of cirrhosis. Patients were evaluated regularly to measure serum levels of HCV RNA and aminotransferases, and 24 weeks after the end of treatment, a liver biopsy was performed.

Findings.—Based on serum HCV RNA levels, patients receiving combination therapy for 48 weeks had a significantly better response than those receiving combination therapy for 24 weeks (38% vs 31%). Both of these groups had a significantly better response than patients receiving IFN alone for 48 weeks (13%), and all 3 groups had a significantly better response than patients receiving IFN alone for 24 weeks (6%). The same pattern was seen in biochemical responses, with significant differences between combination therapy for 48 weeks (34%), combination therapy

TABLE 5.—Rates of Discontinuation of Treatment, Dose Reductions, and
Other Adverse Events During Treatment

Adverse Event	Interferon		Interferon and Ribavirin	
	24 Wk (N=231)	48 Wk (N=225)	24 Wk (N=228)	48 Wk (N=228)
		Percent		
Discontinuation of treatment for any severe event	9	14	8	21
Dose reduction				
Due to anemia*	0	0	7	9
Due to other adverse events†	12	9	13	17
Influenza-like symptoms				
Headache	63	67	63	66
Fatigue	62	72	68	70
Malaise	7	5	4	11
Myalgia	57	63	61	64
Arthralgia	27	36	30	33
Musculoskeletal pain	26	32	20	28
Fever	35	40	37	41
Gastrointestinal symptoms				
Anorexia	16	19	27	25
Dyspepsia	6	9	14	16
Vomiting	10	13	11	9
Nausea	35	33	38	46
Diarrhea	22	26	18	22
Abdominal pain	17	20	15	14
Psychiatric symptoms				
Anxiety	9	13	10	18
Impaired concentration	14	14	11	14
Depression	25	37	32	36
Emotional liability	6	8	7	11
Insomnia	27	30	39	39
Irritability	19	27	23	32
Respiratory tract symptoms				
Cough	5	9	15	14
Dyspnea	9	10	19	18
Pharyngitis	9	10	11	20
Sinusitis	7	14	9	10
Dermatologic symptoms				
Alopecia	27	28	28	32
Pruritus	9	8	21	19
Rash	9	8	20	28
Dry skin	4	8	8	15
Inflammation at injection site	10	14	13	12

Note: Only events that occurred in 10% of patients or more are included.
*The daily dose of ribavirin was reduced to 600 mg for patients with hemoglobin values of less than 10 g/dL, and treatment with ribavirin was discontinued in patients with hemoglobin values of less than 8.5 g/dL.
†In the case of other severe events, the dose of interferon was decreased to 1.5×10^6 U 3 times a week, and the dose of ribavirin was decreased to 600 mg/day.
(Reprinted by permission of *The New England Journal of Medicine* from McHutchinson JG, for the Hepatitis Intervention Therapy Group: Interferon alfa-2b alone or in combination with ribavirin as initial treatment for chronic hepatitis C. *N Engl J Med* 339:1485-1492. Copyright 1998, Massachusetts Medical Society. All rights reserved.)

for 24 weeks (26%), IFN alone for 48 weeks (12%) and IFN alone for 24 weeks (5%).

Based on liver biopsy findings, patients taking combination therapy for 24 or 48 weeks had a significantly better response than those receiving IFN alone for 24 or 48 weeks (57% and 61% vs 44% and 41%, respectively).

In the 72% of patients with HCV genotype 1 infection, combination treatment for 48 weeks was 4 times as effective as IFN alone for 48 weeks (28% vs 7%). Adverse events, however, were more common with combination therapy (Table 5), and in 8% of patients, the dose of ribavarin was reduced because of the development of anemia. With either combination therapy or IFN alone, adverse events were higher after 48 weeks of treatment than after 24 weeks.

Conclusion.—Based on virologic, biochemical, and histologic end points, combination therapy with IFN–α-2b and ribavirin is more effective in treating chronic HCV infection than IFN alone. Treatment for 48 weeks was more effective than treatment for 24 weeks, but the incidence of adverse events was higher with longer dosing.

▶ This report (Abstract 2–15) and the one abstracted previously (Abstract 2–14) provide compelling evidence that the combination of IFN-α and ribavirin are significantly better than IFN-α alone as treatment for both the initial management and relapse of chronic hepatitis disease states. Currently, nearly 4 million Americans—or about 1.8% of the United States population—have been infected by HCV. Each year, this virus causes 8000 to 10,000 deaths. These are rough figures because HCV is something of a stealth disease, and tracking of it by public health officials is virtually impossible. Some 4 out of 5 newly infected patients do not have specific symptoms that would lead a care provider to do diagnostic anti-HCV antibody testing. This antibody, in any event, appears only months after initial exposure.

There are no firm guidelines for who should be receiving antiviral therapy when it comes to HCV infection. Usually, such a recommendation is made for patients in whom liver enzymes are persistently infected, liver biopsy shows evidence of inflamation and fibrosis, and HCV viremia is found. Even before we knew there was such a thing as HCV infection, we were treating it as non-A, non-B hepatitis with IFN-α. IFN therapy is hardly perfect. Only about 40% of patients respond, and of those who respond, only 10% to 15% have a sustained response once the antiviral agent is stopped. As we see from the reports abstracted here, the combination of IFN-α and ribavirin is remarkably more potent than IFN-α alone, both with respect to initial management and when such treatment is used for relapse. When it comes to the latter, response rates are 5 to 10 times greater than those achieved with IFN-α alone.

Please note that combination therapy for HCV infection is not without its side effects. Although the combination is relatively safe, a serious hemolytic anemia, albeit reversible, may occur and this is the result of ribavirin. This is made worse by the fact that such therapy commonly suppresses the bone marrow. Other nagging side effects have included cough, itching, rash, and insomnia.

Controversy surrounds the management of HCV infection, a controversy that relates to the manufacturer of IFN-α. *The Lancet* recently reported that the Schering Corporation had breeched the public trust with a United States newspaper campaign that appeared designed more to creating HCV hysteria than to creating public understanding. In its advertisements, the company gave the impression that anyone who has had their ears—or any other body part—pierced, has a tattoo, or has "shared a razor, toothbrush, or any item that could carry blood" is at risk for HCV infection and should be tested. "To put it bluntly," the company warned, "every living, breathing human being can get hepatitis C—even you." The *Lancet* commentary notes that in 1997, Schering sold $140 million worth of HCV treatment in the form of IFN-α in the United States alone, which helped make interferon its second biggest product worldwide.[1]

For more on the topic of HCV, see the excellent review by Liang.[2] You will see that, as is the case for the treatment of many viral infections, 2 antiviral drugs are better than 1. Although ribavirin hasn't found much success in the treatment of most children with bronchiolitis, it sure seems to have hit gold when it comes to chronic HCV infection. By the way, United States trials combining IFN-α with ribavirin have recently been reproduced with the same findings in Europe.[3]

J.A. Stockman III, M.D.

References

1. Making sense of hepatitis C (editorial). *Lancet* 352:1485, 1998.
2. Liang TJ: Combination therapy for hepatitis C infection. *N Engl J Med* 339:1549-1550, 1998.
3. Poynard T, Marcellin P, Lee SS, et al: Randomised trial of interferon α2b plus ribavirin for 48 weeks or for 24 weeks versus interferon α2b plus placebo for 48 weeks for treatment of chronic infection with hepatitis C virus. *Lancet* 532:1426-1432, 1998.

Intellectual Assessment of Children With Asymptomatic Congenital Cytomegalovirus Infection

Kashden J, Frison S, Fowler K, et al (Healthsouth Mountainview Regional Rehabilitation Hosp, Morgantown, WVa; Univ of Alabama, Birmingham)
J Dev Behav Pediatr 19:254-259, 1998   2–16

Background.—Many central nervous system sequelae of congenital cytomegalovirus (CMV) infection have been reported, including mental retardation, failure at school, sensorineural hearing loss, and other problems. This study evaluated whether children with congenital CMV infection are more likely than their uninfected siblings to be intellectually impaired.

Methods.—The subjects were 204 children (average age, 4 years; range, 5-200 months) with congenital asymptomatic CMV and 177 of their unaffected siblings (mean age, 6 years; range, 6-203 months). Each subject underwent a battery of tests to assess intellectual development. Tools included the Developmental Profile (in which the parent assesses the child's development) and standardized IQ tests: the Stanford Binet Intelligence

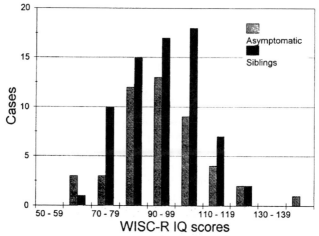

FIGURE 4.—Frequency distribution of the Wechsler Adult Intelligence Scale—Revised Full Scale IQ scores for children with asymptomatic congenital cytomegalovirus infection and for controls. (Courtesy of Kashden J, Frison S, Fowler K, et al: Intellectual assessment of children with asymptomatic congenital cytomegalovirus infection. *J Dev Behav Pediatr* 19[4]:254-259, 1998.)

Test LM Edition (for children 30 to 42 months old), the Wechsler Preschool and Primary Scale of Intelligence (for children 60- to 72-months-old), and the Wechsler Intelligence Scale for Children Revised (for children 72 or more months old).

Findings.—None of the 4 measures of intelligence differed significantly between patients with congenital CMV infection and controls (Fig 4). However, there was a tendency for parents to overestimate their children's intellectual functioning in both patients and controls; for example, for both groups, mean IQ scores were less than 100, but mean parent-assessed Developmental Profile IQ scores were 115 or more).

Conclusions.—Children with congenital asymptomatic CMV infection were not more likely than their unaffected siblings to have intellectual impairment. However, for both groups of children, parents tended to overestimate their children's level of neurocognitive functioning. The degree of overestimation was not insubstantial; thus, those who use studies that rely on a parent's assessment of the child's development must be aware of this response bias.

▶ Congenital CMV infection remains the most common congenital infection in the United States. At present it is found in 1% of live births. There is substantial evidence that congenital CMV infection is also the leading infectious cause of CNS damage in children. The curious thing about this virus, though, is its remarkable clinical variability, ranging from no evidence of sequelae to profound cognitive, motor, and sensory impairment. Some 90% of infected newborns have no signs of congenital infection at birth, and the disorder is uncovered only on screening for the virus. On the other hand, about 7% of infected newborns have serious clinical manifestations of congenital infection at birth, including microcephaly, splenomegaly, petechiae, jaundice, or retinitis. Such patients usually have CNS sequelae, including some degree of mental retardation, cerebral palsy, and hearing loss. Some studies have found that between 5% and 15% of the symptom-free patients will have sensorineural hearing loss. Whether or not children with asymptomatic congenital CMV infection are at increased risk of mental retardation has remained a point of controversy. This is the subject of the report abstracted here.

To determine whether asymptomatic congenital CMV is associated with intellectual impairment later in life, investigators from West Virginia and Alabama designed the study in which children known to have had asymptomatic congenital CMV infection were compared with uninfected siblings. Fortunately, the data show that asymptomatic congenital CMV infection is not associated with impairment of intellectual development.

Thank goodness for the outcome of this study. One percent of children in the United States represents a large number. Could you imagine that many children being intellectually impaired as a consequence of such a common perinatal infectious problem? Count our blessings.

J.A. Stockman III, M.D.

Clinical and Economic Impact of Enterovirus Illness in Private Pediatric Practice
Pichichero ME, McLinn S, Rotbart HA, et al (Univ of Rochester, NY; Scottsdale Pediatric Group, Ariz; Univ of Colorado, Denver; et al)
Pediatrics 102:1126-1134, 1998   2–17

Introduction.—Nonpolio enterovirus infections, such as coxsackievirus groups A and B, echoviruses, and the newer numbered enteroviruses, are common throughout late summer and early fall. The clinical course of signs and symptoms of nonpolio enterovirus disease in children were defined. The household spread of nonpolio enterovirus illness were determined. The rate of positive viral culture and polymerase chain reaction of nonpolio enterovirus in children with clinical presentations typical of the disease and in control, asymptomatic children were determined. The direct and indirect costs of care for children and adolescents with a clinical diagnosis of nonpolio enterovirus infection were assessed.

Methods.—Three hundred eighty children, aged 4 to 18 years, with systemic nonpolio enterovirus syndromes were compared with 73 asymptomatic controls. The presence of fever plus headache and stiff neck; myalgia and malaise; nonpuritic maculopapular rash; papulovesicular stomatitis; papular rash of the hands, feet, and mouth; or pleurodynia were the basis for a clinical diagnosis of nonpolio enterovirus. The frequency of health care contacts, the necessity for laboratory tests, medication use, and school/work absenteeism were recorded with a parent symptom diary card and twice weekly phone contacts by study nurses.

Results.—Of the patients, 33% were confirmed with nonpolio enterovirus infection. Rochester, NY had a greater frequency (58%) than Scottsdale, Ariz (14%). Meningitis resulted in 7 ill days and 2 missed days of school, summer camp, or work. Myalgia/malaise resulted in 9 ill days and 3 missed days. Rash resulted in 6 ill days and 4 missed days. Stomatitis resulted in 7 ill days and 2 missed days. Papular rash of the hands, feet and mouth resulted in 7 ill days and 1 missed day. Pleurodynia resulted in 8 ill days and 3 missed days. The direct medical costs varied from $69 for papular rash of the hands, feet, and mouth to $771 for meningitis per child. Indirect costs, which included parent missing work or sick-child care, varied from $63 for papular rash of the hands, feet, and mouth to $422 for meningitis per child. Papular rash of the hands, feet, and mouth spread to 50% of siblings and 25% of parents in households.

Conclusion.—Nonpolio enterovirus infection occurs more frequently in 4- to 12-year-olds than in adolescents; caused sufficient illness to prompt physician visits in summer and fall; varied in occurrence geographically; produced various clinical syndromes concurrently during the same months in the same season of a given year; produced a significant economic impact by generating direct and indirect costs; and was characterized by numerous symptoms of longer duration than previously recognized.

▶ John F. Modlin, M.D., Infectious Diseases Section, Dartmouth-Hitchcock Medical Center, Lebanon, NH, comments:

The stated objectives of this study were to assess the duration of symptoms, the secondary household transmission rate, and the economic impact of enterovirus infections among children who present to a private pediatrician. Readers will need to judge for themselves how close the authors have come to meeting these objectives, but they should consider that: (1) the study was conducted during a single enterovirus season; (2) children younger than 4 years old who experience the highest rates of enterovirus infection were excluded; (3) the case definition included non-specific illnesses (myalgia and malaise, or rash illness) often caused by other common pathogens, such as rhinoviruses, adenoviruses, and streptococci; (4) only one third of cases were confirmed to be caused by enteroviruses by a sensitive assay; and (5) costs were imputed by assigning estimated costs, rather than by calculating actual costs. Therefore, I suspect that the authors themselves (several of whom I consider friends), would admit that these data provide only a very rough estimate of direct and indirect costs associated with enterovirus infections.

An unstated objective of the study was to provide cost-benefit data to support the development of anti-enterovirus therapy by the sponsoring drug manufacturer. Drugs with potent activity against enteroviruses in vitro have shown promise in both animal studies and in early clinical trials. As 1 or more of these drugs come closer to market, we can anticipate seeing more data focusing on the monetary costs and other impacts of the lives of children with enterovirus infections and their families.

J.F. Modlin, M.D.

Prevalence of Astroviruses in a Children's Hospital

Shastri S, Doane AM, Gonzales J, et al (Stanford Univ, Calif)
J Clin Microbiol 36:2571-2574, 1998   2–18

Introduction.—Human infantile diarrhea may be caused by astroviruses, small, 28- to 34-nm, single-stranded RNA viruses which are part of the family Astroviridae. In infants, immunocompromised patients, and the elderly in nursing homes, and in the nosocomial diarrhea in children's hospitals, astroviruses have been increasingly identified as important diarrheal agents. A new, sensitive, monoclonal antibody–based enzyme-linked immunoassay that detects all 7 serotypes of human astrovirus was described, as was its application in surveying the astrovirus among symptomatic patients at a children's hospital.

Methods.—There were 278 symptomatic inpatients at a children's hospital who had an enzyme immunoassay performed for astrovirus. The assay screened 357 stool samples. The samples were analyzed for detection of astrovirus group antigen and for the presence of a serotype 1–specific epitope recognized by Mab 5B7.

Results.—Astrovirus antigen was found in 30 stool samples from 26 patients. In 34 samples, rotavirus was found. In 40 samples, *Clostridium difficile* was found. Half the astrovirus infections were nosocomial. In 6 of the astrovirus antigen–positive stool samples, additional pathogens were identified. Serotype 1 accounted for 80% of the astroviruses recovered.

Conclusion.—In very young infants and in those with surgical short-bowel syndrome, astrovirus infections were significantly more common than rotavirus or *C. difficile.* All 3 of these major pathogens may also be found in asymptomatic pediatric patients. To fully assess the role of each of these pathogens in diarrheal disease of hospitalized pediatric patients, further prospective case-control studies are warranted.

▶ Michael E. Pichichero, M.D., professor of Microbiology/Immunology, Pediatrics and Medicine, University of Rochester Medical Center, NY, comments:

Now that an effective rotavirus vaccine has been licensed and endorsed by the American Academy of Pediatrics and the Advisory Committee on Immunization Practices for universal administration to infants, we can expect to see an overall reduction in moderate-to-severe gastroenteritis in the winter. Several studies, including that of Shastri et al, suggest that astroviruses are likely to soon become the most common viral agent identified as causing gastroenteritis. Like rotavirus infections, astrovirus infections (1) occur mostly in the winter; (2) occur mostly in children aged 6 to 36 months; (3) cause diarrhea severe enough to warrant hospitalization; and (4) can produce infection without causing any symptoms. Because astroviruses are more frequently isolated in winter and in the same age group as those in whom rotavirus illness predominates, many rotavirus vaccine "failures" may, in fact, turn out to be caused by astrovirus. The majority of cases of astrovirus gastroenteritis occur in otherwise healthy children from the community. However, among the hospitalized children assessed in this current study, an overrepresentation of patients with short-bowel syndrome were included (reflecting the case mix at Stanford's Packard Children's Hospital).

M.E. Pichichero, M.D.

The Relationship Between Perceived Parental Expectations and Pediatrician Antimicrobial Prescribing Behavior
Mangione-Smith R, McGlynn EA, Elliott MN, et al (Univ of California, Los Angeles; RAND, Santa Monica, Calif)
Pediatrics 103:711-718, 1999   2–19

Background.—Despite increasing concern about antimicrobial resistance, physicians continue to prescribe such agents inappropriately. One important determinant of pediatricians' antimicrobial prescribing behavior may be parental expectations of prescriptions. The extent to which parental previsit expectations and physicians' perceptions of those expectations are related to inappropriate antimicrobial prescribing was investigated.

Methods.—Ten physicians and 306 consecutive parents seeking care for their children between October 1996, and March 1997 participated in the survey. Eligible parents were those seeking care for a child 2 to 10 years of age with ear pain, throat pain, cough, or congestion, who had not received antimicrobial treatment for the preceding 2 weeks and who was seeing one of the participating physicians.

Findings.—In a multivariate analysis, physicians' perceptions of parental expectations of antimicrobial agents was the only significant predictor of antimicrobial presciption for illnesses with presumed viral etiologies. When physicians thought a parent wanted such agents, they prescribed them 62% of the time, compared with 7% of the time when physicians did not think the parent wanted antimicrobials. However, physician antimicrobial prescribing behavior was uncorrelated with actual parental expectations. When physicians thought the parent wanted an antimicrobial agent, they were also significantly more likely to diagnose the child's condition as bacterial. Failure to meet parental expectations regarding communication events during the visit was the only factor significantly predicting parental satisfaction. Not prescribing expected antimicrobial agents did not affect parents' satisfaction with care.

Conclusion.—Physician perceptions of parents' desire for antimicrobial agents for viral infections in their children appear to be inaccurate. Further research to verify these findings and to explore interventions for changing physician perceptions is warranted.

▶ This report comes none too soon. Although containing no significant new information, it reinforces our current knowledge of the extent of antibiotic overprescription these days. The cost of therapeutic agents in the last 10 years has skyrocketed, far outpacing the cost of medical care (in general) in the United States. Within the pharmaceutical category, antibiotics represent one of the largest classes of medicinals. Imagine how dramatically health care cost in the United States would be reduced if we simply cut back on the use of antibiotics.

If you don't believe antibiotic use has increased, simply look at the number of prescriptions for amoxicillin written for adults and children in the United States. Between 1980 and 1992, amoxicillin use in children and adults attending outpatient clinics increased from 50 to 175 prescriptions per 1000 population. Cephalosporin use also increased significantly from about 25 to 90 prescriptions per 1000 population.[1] Take also the common cold. The average preschool child in the United States has 4 to 8 colds a year. Virtually all of these are self-limited illnesses. Despite this, as many as half of children still receive antibiotic prescriptions for this condition.[2] In this study from California, some 88% of children with a diagnoses of bronchitis were given prescriptions for antibiotics despite the fact that relatively few cases of bronchitis in children are caused by anything other than common viruses.

So why are we seeing such a wholesale over use of antibiotics? If there is one lesson to be learned it is that some care providers seem to want to make their patients, or their parents, satisfied. This has always been true in medicine, but is even more true these days given the pressures of managed care. When patient satisfaction becomes more important than good medicine, you know that managed care organizations, and their physician providers, have gone overboard to keep patients and their families happy. Also, it is sometimes easier to write a prescription than to sit down for 10 minutes to explain why it is not necessary to give antibiotics. It is strange medicine when productivity reins over quality.

In the long run, managed care organizations and care providers should recognize that the problems caused by antibiotic overuse will eventually—if they have not already—turn out to be far more expensive to society than good medicine practiced now. There is no new news here.

J.A. Stockman III, M.D.

References

1. McCraig LF, Hughes JM: Trends in antimicrobial drug prescribing among office-based physicians in the United States. *JAMA* 273:214-219, 1995.
2. Nyquist A, Gonzales R, Steiner JF: Antibiotic prescribing for children with colds, upper respiratory tract infections, and bronchitis. *JAMA* 279:875-877, 1998.

Self-reported Prescribing of Antibiotics for Children With Undifferentiated Acute Respiratory Tract Infections With Cough
Davy T, Dick PT, Munk P (Hosp for Sick Children, Toronto)
Pediatr Infect Dis J 17:457-462, 1998   2–20

Introduction.—About 13% of office visits in Canada account for patients with an acute respiratory tract infection, and the yearly cost in

Ontario is about $200 million. Tremendous implications are found in physicians' habits of prescribing antibiotics. A serious public health concern is the development of bacterial resistance, which is enhanced by unnecessary antibiotic use. It is important to contribute to evidence-based use of antibiotics and to delay the unnecessary development of bacterial resistance by formulating practice guidelines for physicians faced with undifferentiated acute respiratory tract infection with cough (UARTIC). Determining the current antibiotic-prescribing habits among pediatricians and family physicians is the first step. The variability of self-reported prescribing habits for antibiotics for children with UARTIC was assessed.

Methods.—The study included 181 primary care family physicians and pediatricians who were mailed a questionnaire that assessed their perceptions of their own antibiotic-prescribing habit. Of these, 136 (75%) completed the questionnaire, which consisted of 15 questions about the existence and prevalence of the problem, the physicians' self-reported prescribing of antibiotics, and factors that modified the treatment decision.

Results.—More than 10% of office visits were for UARTIC, in 32% of the physicians' offices. Antibiotics or antibiotics in reserve (a prescription to be filled if the patient's condition does not improve [AIR]) were prescribed for children with a 3-day history of UARTIC by 24% of physicians usually or always. When the UARTIC had worsened in the 24 hours before the office visit, this figure increased to 45%.

Conclusion.—Antibiotics or AIR was prescribed when a pediatric patient presented with UARTIC in the absence of clear indicators of bacterial infection. To support rational antibiotic use for UARTIC, research- and evidence-based guidelines are needed.

▶ Until someone figures out how to clearly distinguish an upper respiratory tract infection that may be due to a bacterial etiology from one that is viral, we will see more reports such as this. There isn't a single one among us who hasn't given a prescription for antibiotics on the "hunch" that something more was going on than a viral upper respiratory tract infection. That hunch may be based on a longer duration of fever than expected, a child who looks a little more ill than usual, or a runny nose with a bit more color to the secretions than not. There is not a single study which supports any of these as a legitimate criterion for antibiotic use.

This report also tells us that there is a difference between what family physicians do and what pediatricians do when faced with similar types of patients presenting with upper respiratory tract symptoms. Family physicians tend to prescribe antibiotics more frequently if there is a prior history of pneumonia or otitis media, or if a patient has persistent symptoms more than 3 days in duration and a fever greater than 38.5°C. Family physicians also tend to be more likely to prescribe antibiotics if parents seem anxious. Family physicians also tend to prescribe antibiotics "in reserve," asking parents to hold a prescription for use should symptoms worsen or fail to go away. Although there is a statistically higher probability that family practitioners would act in such a manner, a fair number of pediatricians prescribe antibiotics under similar circumstances.

This editor had not heard the term *antibiotics in reserve* (AIR) until he read this report. AIR apparently is becoming quite commonplace. With managed care, physicians are under a great deal of pressure to make patients (or their parents) happy. Patient satisfaction is critical these days. There is a great temptation to do whatever is necessary to forestall a repeat visit.

UARTIC and AIR now join the alphabet soup of our medical lexicon. Perhaps our patients would be better off without this part of our lexicon, maybe with a little chicken soup instead of AIR.

J.A. Stockman III, M.D.

An Epidemic of a Pertussis-like Illness Caused by *Chlamydia pneumoniae*
Hagiwara K, Ouchi K, Tashiro N, et al (Yamaguchi Univ, Ube, Japan; Saiseikai Shimonoseki Gen Hosp, Japan; Mito Hosp, Ooda, Japan; et al)
Pediatr Infect Dis J 18:271-275, 1999   2–21

Background.—An epidemic of a pertussis-like illness occurred in a rural Japanese junior high school in June and July 1994. The clinical manifestations and cause of this illness were reported.

Methods and Findings.—Of 230 adolescents, a severe cough illness developed in 136 (59%). One student had pneumonia, 9 had bronchitis, and 126 had upper respiratory tract infections (URIs). Patients with URIs had cough for a mean of 17.4 days. In patients with bronchitis and pneumonia, the mean duration of cough was 30.4 days. Serologic assessment or cultures were negative for *Bordetella pertussis, Bordetella parapertussis, Mycoplasma pneumoniae, Chlamydia trachomatis, Chlamydia psittai* and viruses. Infection with *Chlamydia pneumoniae* was documented in the patient with pneumonia, all 7 patients with bronchitis, and 84% of 38 patients with URIs.

Conclusion.—The causative agent in an epidemic of a pertussis-like illness at a junior high school in Japan was *C. pneumoniae* in most of the children tested.

▶ As residents, most of us learned that all that whoops is not pertussis, and all that is pertussis need not whoop. In the case of the epidemic described, the typical cough of pertussis sans whoop was not caused by pertussis, but rather was caused by *C. pneumoniae*. It has been recognized for a long time that *C. pneumoniae* does cause a pertussis-like illness, although the majority of cases to date have been in much younger children than are described in this outbreak in Japan. What is important about the outbreak in Japan is the observation that almost 60% of children in the school involved became clinically infected over the course of a 6-week period.

The next time you see a child with a pertussis-like cough, think *C. pneumoniae*, but do not forget that *B. pertussis* still might be a possibility. *B. parapertussis* and *M. pneumoniae* make up the remainder of the usual causes of a pertussis-like illness. All that has the bark of a pertussis-like illness is not true pertussis.

J.A. Stockman III, M.D.

A Serologic Study of Organisms Possibly Associated With Pertussis-like Coughing
Von König CHW, Rott H, Bogaerts H, et al (Univ of Kiel, Germany)
Pediatr Infect Dis J 17:645-649, 1998   2–22

Background.—Numerous reports have suggested causes other than infection with *Bordetella pertussis* in patients with pertussis-like coughing. Sera from patients with prolonged pertussis-like coughing were examined to determine the frequencies of infections with other microorganisms.

Methods.—During a field trial of an acellular pertussis vaccine, 1179 patients, aged 18 years or less, with prolonged (7 days or more) pertussis-like coughing were identified. Subjects provided acute- and convalescent-phase blood samples for microbiological analysis. Subjects who tested negative for *B. pertussis* were also tested for antibodies to 7 other microbes.

Findings.—Serologic tests for *B. pertussis* were negative in 149 children (12.6%). In 66 of these children (44%), none of the serologic tests performed revealed an infectious agent. The most commonly found agents in

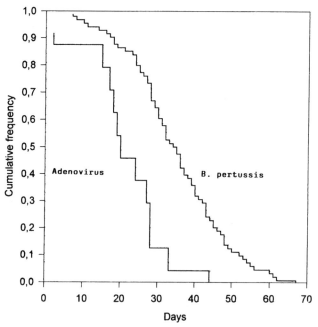

FIGURE 2.—Duration of paroxysmal cough in children with laboratory evidence for pertussis and for adenovirus infection. (Courtesy of Von König CHW, Rott H, Bogaerts H, et al: A serologic study of organisms possibly associated with pertussis-like cough. *Pediatr Infect Dis J* 17[7]:645-649, 1998.)

the remaining 83 children were adenovirus (33, or 22%), parainfluenza viruses 1, 2, and 3 (18, or 12%), *Mycoplasma pneumoniae* (11, or 7%), and respiratory syncytial virus (10, or 7%). These 83 children tended to have an age distribution similar to that of children with *B. pertussis*, except adenovirus infection was more common in children, aged 6 to 24 months. The duration of coughing differed between groups, with a significantly shorter period of paroxysms in the children with adenovirus (mean 18 days vs mean 35.1 days in children with *B. pertussis*)(Fig 2). Nonetheless, on the basis of a clinical criterion of paroxysmal coughing for more than 21 days, half the children with adenovirus infection would have been diagnosed as having pertussis. Children with *B. pertussis* infection were significantly more likely to experience whoops than children with adenovirus infection (79% vs 20%). However, vomiting was a common symptom in both groups (76% and 53%, respectively). Six percent of the children with *B. pertussis* had been vaccinated against pertussis, whereas 47% of the children with adenovirus infection had received the pertussis vaccine.

Conclusions.—Adenovirus, parainfluenza viruses, respiratory syncytial virus, and *M. pneumoniae* are significant causes of pertussis-like coughing in children. These infections should be part of the differential diagnosis for children with suspected pertussis, particularly for those who have been vaccinated against pertussis.

▶ Knowledge of the art of medicine seems to have a biphasic learning curve. When one is young in one's career, there is the rapid acquisition of all new information. When one is older in one's career, there is still new information to be learned, but a fair amount of time is expended on ridding ourselves of information that no longer is applicable, or may in fact be untrue. Take the story of pertussis-like coughing. When a child coughed for more than 2 weeks and had a whoop, that child had whooping cough. The etiology was *B. pertussis*. This is no longer so here in the United States. It may never have been so. It can be safely assumed that about 70% or more of pertussis-like coughs are not attributable to *B. pertussis*, but rather to other agents such as adenovirus, human parainfluenza virus, the respiratory syncytial virus, influenza virus A and B, and mycoplasma.

Of all the causes of pertussis-like cough, the adenovirus has now emerged to be the principle bad actor and imitator of clinical pertussis. This is particularly true of adenovirus type 9 infection. Although children with adenovirus will cough for a much shorter time than children who are infected with *B. pertussis*, the clinical severity of adenovirus infections is such that over 50% of children infected with this virus would fulfill the World Health Organization's clinical criteria for pertussis, and some 80% or more will have fulfilled the Center for Disease Control's clinical criteria that include 14 or more days of paroxysmal cough. It isn't just the length of the cough or its paroxysmal nature that mimics pertussis. About 20% of children with adenovirus infection will have whoops. More than 50% will have vomiting after a paroxysm of coughing.

This editor wishes the human mind were like a computer hard drive. Wouldn't it be nice if periodically we could simply push a button and delete all the disinformation that has accumulated over the years and then simply download the correct information that would replace it? There is an idea for Bill Gates.

J.A. Stockman III, M.D.

Tuberculin Skin Test Screening Practices Among US Colleges and Universities

Hennessey KA, Schulte JM, Cook L, et al (Ctrs for Disease Control and Prevention, Atlanta, Ga; Univ of Pennsylvania, Philadelphia)
JAMA 280:2008-2012, 1998   2-23

Introduction.—Six percent of all tuberculosis during a 4-year period occurred among persons aged 18 through 24, the age group most likely to be in college. Most came from 4 countries: Mexico (28%), Vietnam (14%), the Philippines (9%), and India (5%). Given the prolonged close contact students have with each other, a recent outbreak of tuberculosis at a university demonstrated how *Mycobacterium tuberculosis* can easily spread on college campuses. Some universities have instituted required tuberculin skin test screening. However, little is known about these screening practices. A survey of colleges and universities across the United States was conducted to determine the type and extent of required tuberculin skin testing and the number of students identified with positive skin test results or active tuberculosis.

Methods.—There were 796 of 3148 US colleges and universities who were sent a self-administered mail and telephone questionnaire. Of these, 624 (78%) responded. The survey investigated type of tuberculin screening required, types of schools requiring screening, and number and rate of students with positive skin test results and/or receiving a diagnosis of tuberculosis.

Results.—Tuberculin screening was required by 378 schools (61%). In 161 of 624 schools (26%), it was required of all new students, including US residents and international students. In 53 schools (8%), it was required of only new international students, but not new US residents. It was required in 294 (47%) of students in specific academic programs. Four-year schools were more likely than 2-year schools, American College Health Association members were more likely than nonmember schools, schools with immunization requirements were more likely than schools without, and schools with a student health clinic were more likely than schools without, to require screening. Tine or multiple puncture tests were accepted in 95 (25%) of schools. In 95 (25%), test results were recorded in millimeters of induration. Results were collected in a centralized registry or database in 100 (27%). Only 3.1% of students screened had positive skin test results in the 27% of schools accepting only Mantoux skin tests. A significantly higher case rate of active tuberculosis was found among international students than among US residents (35.2 vs 1.1 per 100,000 students screened).

Conclusion.—A low prevalence of skin test reactors and few tuberculosis cases were found with widespread tuberculin screening of students. Tuberculin screening should target students at high risk for infection, to optimize the use of limited public health resources.

▶ This editor was not aware that no medical screening for tuberculosis is required for international students entering the United States for the purposes of furthering their education. Screening for active tuberculosis is required of refugees and persons legally immigrating to this country—an interesting dichotomy, since foreigners who enter this country, and who ultimately develop tuberculosis, usually do so within a year or a year and a half of entry. By the middle of the 90s, approximately half a million foreign students came to the United States to study and made up about 3% of our college student population. Some 6% of all tuberculosis reported here in the last decade occurred in the age group that overlaps the college population. Of these cases, more than 60% were foreign-born individuals. Most were from 4 countries: Mexico (28%), Vietnam (14%), the Philippines (9%), and India (5%).[1] Despite the above comments, we see that for colleges and universities that do tuberculin screening (approximately 60% of all US colleges and universities have such programs in place), only about 3% of the general student population will be found to be positive. Most of these positives are in foreign students. The tuberculin screening actually identified few active cases of tuberculosis. Overall, the data indicate that slightly under 5 tuberculosis cases are being identified for every 100,000 students screened, with the rate of identification being 32 times higher in foreign-born students. The conclusion here is fairly obvious. Universal screening of college students with tuberculin skin testing will have low yields, except in high-risk foreign student populations. Even among foreign-born students, the value of screening exists only for those students coming from countries that have a significant problem with tuberculosis. It's time to save ourselves some public health dollars. Put away the PPD syringes on university campuses, except for use on high-risk students.

J.A. Stockman III, M.D.

Cerebrospinal Fluid Pleocytosis and Prognosis in Invasive Meningococcal Disease in Children
Malley R, Inkelis SH, Coelho P, et al (Harvard Med School, Boston; Harbor-UCLA Med Ctr, Lorrence, Calif; Univ of California, Davis)
Pediatr Infect Dis J 17:855-859, 1998   2–24

Introduction.—Invasive meningococcal disease (IMD) is typically categorized as either meningococcal meningitis or meningococcemia. Several reports have indicated that patients with CSF pleocytosis have a more favorable outcome than patients with meningococcemia without CSF pleocytosis. It has not been determined whether patients who lack a cellular response to CNS infection are at the same risk of untoward outcome as patients who lack CNS infection. A series of children with IMD was evaluated (1) to determine the frequency with which IMD occurs with bacteremia alone or with CNS infection without pleocytosis and (2) to compare the frequency of adverse outcome in either group with that of patients with CSF pleocytosis.

Methods.—Medical records of children at 4 pediatric referral hospitals were reviewed for the years 1985-1996. The 3 groups of children were compared regarding clinical and laboratory indices and severe adverse outcomes defined as death or limb loss. Multivariate logistic regression analysis was done to ascertain whether CNS infection without CSF pleocytosis was independently correlated with adverse outcome in IMD.

Results.—A total of 377 children with IMD were identified from the 4 participating hospitals. Of these, 86 children were excluded when it was determined that CSF analysis was either not done or was unevaluable. Of excluded patients, 22 (25.6%) had an adverse outcome. Of the 291 remaining patients, 204 (70.1%) had CSF pleocytosis, 52 (17.9%) had bacteremia alone, and 35 (12.0%) had CNS infection without CSF pleocytosis. Patients with CNS infection without CSF pleocytosis had significantly lower white blood cell and platelet counts and more coagulopathy, compared with patients with bacteremia alone or those with CSF pleocytosis. Frequencies of adverse outcome were 40%, 9.6%, and 3.4%, respectively, for patients with CNS infection without CSF pleocytosis, patients with bacteremia alone, and patients with CSF pleocytosis. The CNS infection without CSF pleocytosis was independently correlated with adverse outcome.

Conclusion.—Nearly 30% of all children with IMD do not have CSF pleocytosis. In patients with IMD, those with CNS infection without pleocytosis were at greater risk of adverse outcome than either patients with CSF pleocytosis or patients with bacteremia alone.

▶ One of the popular teachings when this editor was a resident was that it was far better for a patient to have meningococcal septicemia and meningitis than it was to have meningococcal septicemia alone. This made some sense because it implied that the patient had survived long enough with meningococcal septicemia for a meningitis to develop and, therefore, did not succumb early on to the consequences of fulminating meningococcal septicemia. Now we see that this rule applies only if the CSF has had a chance to develop some cells. If a patient has organisms in the CSF on culture, but a pleocytosis has not developed, the outcome is far worse than were that patient to have bacteremia alone. To say all this differently, meningococcal disease is one of the few conditions in which one wishes for overt meningitis to be present, cells and all.

On a related topic, a lot has been written about the polymerase chain reaction (PCR) detection of bacteria. It has been suggested that "molecular triage" might be performed, particularly in young patients suspected of having sepsis and meningitis. This presumably would be done on blood and spinal fluid testing for panels of various bacterial DNA. The question is, just how fast is it possible for PCR technology to detect bacteria? The answer comes from a recent technical review of the ability of PCR to detect bacteria using a relatively straightforward, tabletop piece of equipment known as the Advanced Nucleic Acid Analyzer (ANAA). Current versions of the portable ANAA measure about 16 × 24 × 8 in. Recent modifications made to the ANAA have sped up its ability to detect the DNA of bacteria using PCR technology. Using a sample organism, *Erwinia herbicola*, the ANAA turned out to be swifter than a well-trained athlete. The results demonstrate that the total time to perform complete DNA analysis on a sample containing realistic concentrations of bacteria can be as little as 7 minutes with this highly efficient instrument, which consists of inexpensive, low-power components.[1]

Maybe the time will be with us shortly when, in a 15-minute office visit, we can tell whether an 8-week-old febrile baby has a serious bacterial infection. How nice it would be to obviate hospital stays in such circumstances.

J.A. Stockman III, M.D.

Reference

1. Belgrader P, Benette W, Hadley D, et al: PCR detection of bacteria in seven minutes. *Science* 284:449-450, 1999.

Three-Year Multicenter Surveillance of Pneumococcal Meningitis in Children: Clinical Characterisitics, and Outcome Related to Penicillin Susceptibility and Dexamethasone Use

Arditi M, Mason EO Jr, Bradley JS, et al (Univ of Southern California, Los Angeles; Baylor College of Medicine, Houston; Univ of California–San Diego; et al)

Pediatrics 102:1087-1097, 1998   2–25

Introduction.—Despite effective antimicrobial therapy, meningitis caused by *Streptococcus pneumoniae* is associated with substantial morbidity and mortality. Few studies have investigated whether the antibiotic susceptibility of *S. pneumoniae* affects the severity or outcome of pneumococcal meningitis. The antibiotic susceptibility of *S. pneumoniae* isolates obtained from the CSF of children with meningitis was evaluated. The clinical presentation was described, as well as the current morbidity and mortality of pneumococcal meningitis among infants and children in relation to antibiotic susceptibility. The effect of the use of adjunctive dexamethasone on clinical outcome was assessed.

Methods.—There were 180 children with 181 episodes of pneumococcal meningitis identified in a 3-year period in this retrospective review. Determinations were made of pneumococcal isolates and their antibiotic susceptibilities for penicillin and ceftriaxone. Children infected with penicillin-susceptible isolates and those with nonsusceptible isolates and children treated with dexamethasone and those not treated with dexamethasone were compared for their clinical presentation, hospital course, and outcome parameters at discharge. Dexamethasone was given to 22% of the children at 8 or more doses before or within 1 hour after the first dose of antibiotics.

Results.—Fourteen children (7.7%) died; none of the deaths were the result of failure of treatment caused by a resistant strain. Neurologic sequelae, such as motor deficits, occurred in 25% of the 166 surviving children. Unilateral or bilateral moderate-to-severe hearing loss was found in 32% of children. Overall, 12.7% of pneumococcal isolates were intermediate and 6.6% were resistant to penicillin, whereas 4.4% were intermediate and 2.8% were resistant to ceftriaxone. Patients infected with penicillin- or ceftriaxone-susceptible or nonsusceptible organisms had no differences in clinical presentation, CSF indices on admission, hospital course, morbidity, or mortality. Nonsusceptible organisms do not seem to be more virulent intrinsically. The dexamethasone group had a higher incidence of severe hearing loss (46%) compared with those who did not receive dexamethasone (23%). The dexamethasone group also had a higher incidence of neurologic deficits, including hearing loss (55% vs 33%). Intubation and mechanical ventilation were required more frequently in the dexamethasone group. When the confounding factor of illness was controlled for, there were no longer any significant differences between the children who did or did not receive dexamethasone.

Conclusion.—Similar clinical presentations and outcomes were seen among children with pneumococcal meningitis caused by penicillin- or ceftriaxone-nonsusceptible organisms and those infected by susceptible strains. A beneficial effect was not associated with the use of dexamethasone.

▶ Charles G. Prober, M.D., Stanford University School of Medicine, Stanford, Calif, comments:

This article is loaded with valuable information regarding the clinical course, management, and outcome of pneumococcal meningitis in an era of increasing antibiotic resistance. The 11 authors prospectively collected and collated data on 181 episodes of pneumococcal meningitis cared for at 8 large children's hospitals over a recent 3-year period. The participating hospitals spanned the United States and cared for a racially diverse population of children. Clearly, pneumococcal meningitis remains a disease to be feared! The authors report a mortality rate of almost 8% and a frequency of motor deficits and hearing loss of 25% and 32%, respectively.

I suppose the good news is that resistance to penicillin and cephalosporins does not seem to adversely affect the clinical presentation, course, or outcome of infection. This observation needs to be tempered with 2 caveats. First, there were only 35 cases of meningitis caused by penicillin-nonsusceptible isolates, of which only 13 were also not susceptible to ceftriaxone. Second, empiric therapy for bacterial meningitis included vancomycin in more than half of the subjects. Therefore, a lack of difference in observed outcome, based upon antibiotic sensitivity pattern, should not engender complacency; antibiotic resistance is a problem of enormous magnitude.

In some areas of the United States, more than 80% of isolates of *S. pneumoniae* are resistant to penicillin, with many strains resistant to multiple antibiotics. This is especially troublesome considering that *S. pneumoniae* has become the most important bacterial pathogen of children. It is the most frequent cause of acute otitis media and sinusitis, bacterial pneumonia, walk-in bacteremia, and bacterial meningitis. Concern for this pathogen drives much of the use of vancomycin in children, and the consequences of increasing vancomycin use are now being felt nationally, especially in the form of vancomycin-resistant enterococci.

A final comment on the article relates to the use of steroids as adjuvant therapy for bacterial meningitis. The controversy lives! The authors compared the course and outcome of 37 children who receive dexamethasone before or within 1 hour of antibiotic receipt with those of 75 children not treated with dexamethasone. The frequency of hearing loss and other neurologic deficits actually was higher among the dexamethasone recipients. However, as pointed out by the authors, the steroid recipients were more ill at presentation and had lower concentrations of glucose in the CSF. Furthermore, therapeutic inferences should not be made on the basis of a nonrandomized, noncontrolled study. Therefore, although I am not a big fan of steroids, caution needs to be exercised in impugning their potential role in bacterial meningitis.

The authors should be congratulated for assembling this wealth of clinical information regarding pneumococcal meningitis. Hopefully, the new conjugate pneumococcal vaccines currently under investigation will be as successful as similar vaccines against *Haemophilus influenzae* type b, and a series of this size will never again appear in the literature!

C.G. Prober, M.D.

Clinical Characteristics and Outcome of Children With Pneumonia Attributable to Penicillin-susceptible and Penicillin-nonsusceptible *Streptococcus pneumoniae*

Tan TQ, Mason EO Jr, Barson WJ, et al (Northwestern Univ, Chicago; Baylor College of Medicine, Houston; Ohio State Univ, Columbus; et al)
Pediatrics 102:1369-1375, 1998   2–26

Background.—Although the typical clinical features and outcomes of pneumococcal pneumonia has been well documented in adults, little is known about the clinical characteristics of this illness in children. The clinical features, treatment, and outcomes of children with pneumonia attributed to isolates of *Streptococcus pneumoniae* susceptible or resistant to penicillin are reported.

Methods and Findings.—Two hundred fifty-four children with pneumococcal pneumonia seen in 8 US children's hospitals were included in the retrospective analysis. These children had a total of 257 episodes of pneumococcal pneumonia. Nine percent of the responsible isolates were intermediate, and 6% were resistant to penicillin. Three percent were intermediate to ceftriaxone, and 2% were resistant to ceftriaxone. The clinical presentation of patients with susceptible isolates did not differ from that of patients with nonsusceptible isolates. Pleural effusion occurred in 29% of the patients. Seventy-four percent of the children hospitalized were more likely than nonhospitalized children to have an underlying illness, multiple lung lobe involvement, and pleural effusion. A chest tube was placed in 52 of 72 inpatients, and 27 subsequently had a decortication drainage procedure. Eighty percent of the children treated as outpatients and 48% of those hospitalized were given a parenteral second or third generation cephalosporin, followed by a course of an oral antimicrobial agent. Treatment response was good in 97.6%. Although 6 children died, only 1 died from the pneumococcal infection.

Conclusions.—Children with penicillin-susceptible and those with nonsusceptible *S. pneumoniae* isolates have a similar clinical presentation and treatment outcome. Children who were hospitalized were more likely than outpatients to have underlying illnesses, multiple lobe involvement, and pleural effusions. Standard β-lactam therapy is effective in otherwise healthy children with pneumonia attributable to penicillin-resistant pneumococcal isolates.

▶ Dr, Louis M. Bell, associate professor of Pediatrics, University of Pennsylvania School of Medicine, and medical director of Infection Control, attending physician Infectious Diseases and Emergency Medicine, The Children's Hospital of Philadelphia, Pennsylvania, comments:

This study shows that the clinical characteristics, treatment, and outcome of pneumococcal pneumonia in children are the same whether the isolate is susceptible or resistant to penicillin. Standard therapy with β-lactam antibiotics seems to be effective for pneumonia and other invasive pneumococcal infections outside of the CNS.[1] While β-lactams are adequate, it would seem prudent to use doses at the higher end of those recommended for invasive infections caused by *S. pneumoniae*. If meningitis is suspected, presumptive therapy should be vancomycin (at a dose of 60 mg/kg/day) and a third generation cephalosporin until susceptibilities are known.

The results of this study are both reassuring and profoundly disturbing. It is reassuring that, although isolates of *S. pneumoniae* are increasingly resistant to antibiotics, the organisms don't appear to be more virulent as well. However, the frightening speed with which pneumococci have become resistant to antibiotics is disturbing. Less than 5% of isolates were penicillin-resistant at the beginning of the 1980s. Currently, rates of penicillin-resistance in the United States are estimated to be above 30%, with greater than 10% of isolates exhibiting multi-drug resistance.[2]

In a relatively short time, the resistance problem with pneumococci, a common cause of community-acquired infections, is affecting clinical decisions. Thanks to these authors, some questions about management and outcomes of infections with pneumococci in children have been answered.

However, important questions remain. What can be done to reverse this trend toward bacterial resistance? Is it too late?

Because the widespread use of antibiotics has caused resistance among pneumococci, it is important to examine antibiotic prescribing practices.[3-5] In a recent survey,[6] physicians have acknowledged that, without affecting patient health, antibiotic use in their practices could be reduced by 10% to 50%. The main diagnoses targeted for this reduction in children should be otitis media with effusion, nonstreptococcal pharyngitis, non-specific upper respiratory infection with purulent rhinitis, and cough illnesses or "bronchitis."[7] Once antibiotic use is reduced, it is hoped that pneumococcal resistance will decline. Experience in Japan showed that group A streptococcus resistance to erythromycin fell markedly after the use of this antibiotic was reduced.[8]

The discovery and routine use of antibiotics occurred a little over 50 years ago. Recent experience with antibiotic-resistant pneumococci over the last 10 years is alarming and reminds us that continued indiscriminate use of antibiotics could elicit the creation of a post-antibiotic era. As the holders of the prescription pad, it is within our power to reverse this trend toward antibiotic resistance.

L.M. Bell, M.D.

References

1. Deeks SL, Palacio R, Ruvinsky R, et al: Risk factors and course of illness among children with invasive penicillin-resistant *Streptococcus pneumoniae*. *Pediatrics* 103:409-413, 1999.
2. Mufson MA: Penicillin-resistant *Streptococcus pneumoniae* increasingly threatens the patient and challenges the physician. *Clin Inf Dis* 27:771-773, 1998.
3. Pallares R, Gudiol F, Linares J, et al: Risk factors and response to antibiotic therapy in adults with bacteremic pneumonia caused by penicillin-resistant pneumococci. *N Engl J Med* 317:18-22, 1987.
4. Ford KL, Mason EO Jr, Kaplan SL, et al: Factors associated with middle ear isolates of *S. pneumoniae* resistant to penicillin in a children's hospital. *J Pediatr* 119:941-944, 1991.
5. Tan TQ, Mason EO Jr, Kaplan SL, et al: Penicillin-resistant systemic pneumococcal infections in children: A retrospective case-control study. *Pediatrics* 92:761-767, 1993.
6. Barden LS, Dowell SF, Schwartz B, et al: Current attitudes regarding use of antimicrobial agents: Results from physicians' and parents' focus group discussions. *Clin Pediatr (Phila)* 37:665-671, 1998.
7. Schwartz B: Preventing the spread of antimicrobial resistance among bacterial respiratory pathogens in industrialized countries: The case for judicious antimicrobial use. *Clin Infect Dis* 28:211-213, 1999.
8. Fujita K, Murono K, Yoshikawa M, et al: Decline of erythromycin resistance of group A streptococcus in Japan. *Pediatr Infect Dis J* 13:1075-1078, 1994.

Effectiveness of Intramuscular Penicillin Versus Oral Amoxicillin in the Early Treatment of Outpatient Pediatric Pneumonia

Tsarouhas N, Shaw KN, Hodinka RL, et al (Univ of Pennsylvania, Philadelphia)
Pediatr Emerg Care 14:338-341, 1998   2–27

Background.—Traditional outpatient treatment of presumed bacterial pneumonia consists of oral amoxicillin for 10 days. IM injection of penicillin at the onset of illness may expedite recovery. The relative efficacy of IM and oral therapy in the early outpatient treatment of children with presumed bacterial pneumonia was investigated.

Methods.—One hundred seventy patients were enrolled in the prospective, randomized, blinded study. The patients were seen in the emergency department of an urban children's hospital. All had radiographically confirmed pneumonias and were managed as outpatients, receiving either 2 days of oral amoxicillin, 50 mg/kg per day divided into 3 separate doses, or an IM injection of procaine penicillin G, 50,000 units/kg. The children were re-examined 24 to 36 hours later.

Findings.—At initial and follow-up visits, the 2 groups did not differ in temperature, respiratory rate, accessory muscle use, pulse oximetry, or parental reports of activity level and oral intake. Three patients in the oral therapy group and 5 in the IM group did not respond to treatment. Four in the oral group and 5 in the IM group were admitted at the follow-up visit.

Conclusions.—The efficacies of oral amoxicillin and IM penicillin do not appear to differ in the early outpatient treatment of children with presumed bacterial pneumonia. The obvious advantage of oral administration is the avoidance of a painful injection. However, IM injection may be indicated for children with suboptimal oral intake or oral medication aversion or if parental compliance is a concern.

▶ Gary R. Fleisher, M.D., Children's Hospital, Boston, comments:

As they always do, these investigators from Emergency Medicine at Children's Hospital of Philadelphia have carefully designed and meticulously executed a study to answer an important question. I commend them, in particular, for their efforts to define a group of patients with bacterial pneumonia, rigorously determine the appropriate sample size, select objective and meaningful outcome measures, enroll a large portion of eligible patients, and appropriately analyze the data. Their conclusion, that IM procaine penicillin and oral amoxicillin offer equal therapeutic efficacy, offered physicians a well-substantiated basis for choosing between the two options for treatment of children with clinically diagnosed pneumonia caused by the spectrum of pathogens prevalent in 1994 and 1995.

This study has one significant limitation, as the authors acknowledge. Although most of the patients were highly febrile, young children with leukocytosis, a reasonably high proportion of those with negative viral cultures (153/170) likely had non-bacterial infections that would have improved with any regimen.

More relevant, as the new millennium dawns, is the continued emergence of *Streptococcus pneumoniae* not susceptible to penicillin. In many areas of the country, the incidence of intermediate and highly resistant organisms has climbed into the range of 25% to 50%. Given that procaine penicillin achieves a serum level of only 1 µg/mL, I would opt for "high dose" amoxicillin (80 mg/kg per day). Of course, keep in mind that changes in the bacteriologic landscape will date my comments in a short time, just as events of the past few years have altered the interpretation of these authors' conclusions. Most notably, we will need to reconsider our approach to the diagnosis and treatment of pneumonia following the introduction of a conjugated vaccine against *S. pneumoniae.*

G.R. Fleisher, M.D.

Once-Daily Therapy for Streptococcal Pharyngitis With Amoxicillin
Feder HM Jr, Gerber MA, Randolph MF, et al (Univ of Connecticut, Farmington; Univ of Connecticut, Hartford; Danbury, Conn; et al)
Pediatrics 103:47-51, 1999   2–28

Background.—Patients with group A β-hemolytic streptococcal (GABHS) pharyngitis may be better able to comply with once-daily oral amoxicillin therapy than with treatment taken several times a day. The efficacy of once-daily amoxicillin in the treatment of GABHS pharyngitis was investigated.

Methods.—One hundred fifty-two children, aged 4 to 18 years, seen in a private pediatric office during 16 months were enrolled in the study. All had GABHS pharyngitis. By random assignment, the children received oral

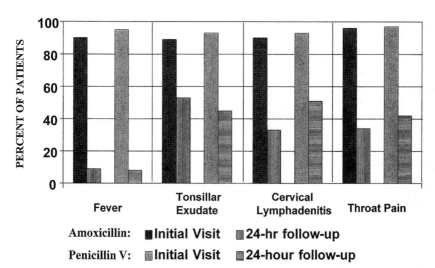

FIGURE 1.—Specific signs and symptoms before and after 18 to 24 hours of therapy. (Reproduced by permission of *Pediatrics*, from Feder HM Jr, Gerber MA, Randolph MF, et al: Once-daily therapy for streptococcal pharyngitis with amoxicillin. *Pediatrics* 103:47-51, 1999.)

amoxicillin, 750 mg once a day, or penicillin V, 250 mg 3 times a day, for 10 days. The 2 groups were comparable in age, illness duration before treatment initiation, and signs and symptoms at presentation. Urine antimicrobial activity was monitored to determine compliance.

Findings.—Compliance did not differ between groups. Clinical and bacteriologic responses did not differ at the 18- to 24-hour follow-up visit. Bacteriologic treatment failures occurred in 5% of the amoxicillin recipients and in 11% of the penicillin V recipients (Fig 1).

Conclusion.—Once-daily amoxicillin treatment is as effective as penicillin V therapy given 3 times daily in the treatment of GABHS pharyngitis. If these findings are verified by additional studies, once-daily amoxicillin treatment may become an alternative regimen for such patients.

▶ Michael E. Pichichero, M.D., professor of Microbiology/Immunology, Pediatrics and Medicine, University of Rochester Medical Center, Elmwood Pediatric Group, Rochester, NY, comments:

This is a well-written article by recognized, prominent researchers in the field of streptococcal pharyngitis treatment.[1] The study design, enrollment criteria, and bacteriology methods are well described and appropriate. The results suggest that once-daily amoxicillin for 10 days may be effective therapy for streptococcal pharyngitis. Unfortunately, only 79 evaluable children and adolescents were included in the amoxicillin group, and even combining the results with an earlier study by Shvartzman et al.[2] (who evaluated 75 children receiving once-daily amoxicillin), definitive conclusions cannot be reached. It would take 353 participants to reach a statistical conclusion with sufficient power plus Food and Drug Administration approval to make this treatment approach advisable in clinical practice.

An important feature of this study relates to the patient population age because older children and adolescents are more often successfully cured with penicillin and amoxicillin, compared with younger children.[3] The authors propose that once-daily amoxicillin therapy might work when once-daily penicillin therapy does not because a slightly longer half-life (1.1-1.8 hours for amoxicillin vs 0.95-01.2 hours for penicillin) and a higher peak concentration (3.86 µg/mL and 1.74 µg/mL, respectively) would allow for longer antibiotic time above the minimum concentration to kill GABHS pharyngitis.[1]

Last, Feder et al.[1] mention that 4 other agents already have Food and Drug Administration approval for once-daily administration (cefadroxil, cefixime, ceftibuten, and azithromycin). I would also note the important compliance-enhancing benefit of shortened duration of therapy and, in this regard, a 5-day regimen for GABHS pharyngitis has been approved by the Food and Drug Administration for azithromycin, cefuroxime axetil, and cefpodoxime proxetil.

M.E. Pichichero, M.D.

References

1. Feder M, Gerber MA, Randolph MF, et al: Once-daily therapy for streptococcal pharyngitis with amoxicillin. *Pediatrics* 103:47-51, 1999.
2. Shvartzman P, Tabenkin H, Rosentzwaig A, et al: Treatment of streptococcal pharyngitis with amoxycillin once a day. *BMJ* 306:1170-1172, 1993.
3. Pichichero ME, Hoeger W, Marsocci SM, et al: Variables influencing penicillin treatment outcome in streptococcal tonsillopharyngitis. *Arch Pediatr Adolesc Med* 153:1-6, 1999.

Vaccination Against Lyme Disease With Recombinant *Borrelia burgdorferi* Outer-Surface Lipoprotein A With Adjuvant
Steere AC, and the Lyme Disease Vaccine Study Group (Tufts Univ, Boston; et al)
N Engl J Med 339:209-215, 1998   2–29

Introduction.—Lyme disease is currently the most common vector-borne disease in the United States. The risk of acquiring this disease in areas in which it is endemic is high, making the development of a safe and effective vaccine a priority. The findings of a multicenter, double-blind, randomized trial involving individuals living in areas of the United States in which Lyme disease is endemic were reported. The efficacy, safety, and immunogenicity of the vaccine were examined.

Methods.—A total of 10,936 research subjects from 31 sites in 10 states in which Lyme disease is endemic were randomly assigned to receive either an injection of recombinant *Borrelia burgdorferi* outer-surface lipoprotein A (OspA) with adjuvant or placebo at baseline and 1 and 12 months later. In patients with suspected Lyme disease, culture of skin lesions, polymerase chain reaction testing, or serologic testing was performed. Individuals underwent serologic testing 12 and 20 months after baseline to detect asymptomatic infections.

Results.—In the first year after 2 injections, 1109 of 10,936 individuals (10%) were examined for suspected Lyme disease. Of these, 22 individuals in the vaccine group and 43 in the placebo group had definite Lyme disease. In the second year, after the third injection, 16 recipients of the vaccine contracted definite Lyme disease, compared with 66 recipients of placebo. Vaccine efficacy for the first and second years was 49% and 76%, respectively. The efficacy of the vaccine in preventing asymptomatic infection was 83% and 100% in the first and second years, respectively. Vaccine injection was associated with mild to moderate local or systemic reactions with a median duration of 3 days.

Conclusions.—A high level of protection from *B. burgdorferi* infection could be achieved with a series of 3 injections of L-OspA with adjuvant.

The rate of local and systemic side effects was acceptable. This vaccine provides an important new public health tool for preventing Lyme disease.

▶ Lyme disease has quickly emerged as the most common tick-borne disease in the United States. Somewhere between 15,000 and 20,000 cases are now reported annually, but the actual yearly incidence could be anywhere from 150,000 to 200,000 cases. Two recombinant vaccines are in the final stages of approval by the US Food and Drug Administration as of the writing of this commentary. One is being developed by SmithKline Beecham and contains an aluminum adjuvant, whereas the Pasteur Merieux Connaught product does not. Either one of these produces a 96% antibody response rate within 2 weeks after the second dose of the vaccine. Clinical trials suggest that a third dose is necessary to boost antibody levels and to provide a sustained protection efficacy of more than 80%. Older individuals do not seem to respond as well. The safety profile in the vaccine trials, which have included more than 10,000 persons to date, is highly reassuring, with participants having only mild local discomfort at the injection site. Although children are at the highest risk of Lyme disease, as of the end of 1998, no efficacy studies had been completed that have allowed FDA approval in children. This does not mean that the vaccine will not be given off-label.

So will pediatric care providers be using the Lyme vaccine? There are a number of rubs vis-à-vis routine administration. One is the uneven distribution of Lyme disease. More than 90% of cases occur in 10 states (Wisconsin, Minnesota, and states on the mid-Atlantic and New England seaboards). This uneven distribution confounds efforts to establish uniform recommendations for vaccine use. In regions where Lyme disease is highly endemic (incidence greater than 1% per year), the vaccines will likely be recommended for persons 15 to 65 years of age, excluding shut-ins and urban dwellers, who are at reduced risk of tick exposure. In regions of intermediate risk (incidence 0.1% to 1% per year), recommendations will target individuals whose activities increase their risk of tick exposure. The vaccine will not be recommended for individuals in regions of the United States with the lowest incidence of the disease. However, ours is a highly mobile society. What do you do with the person from Nevada who likes to spend 2 weeks in August on Cape Cod?

As with most newly introduced vaccines, the Lyme disease vaccine will see its fair share of naysayers. Of particular concern is whether the vaccine will alter the natural course of infection rather than preventing infection altogether, a possibility for which there may be a precedent with other infectious diseases. That circumstance could prove disastrous. For example, if vaccination prevented erythema migrans or other early (and more easily treated) manifestations of Lyme disease, vaccine recipients would probably have no signs or symptoms related to early infection and therefore there would be no tip-off that they had a problem that needed to be treated. Only with late manifestations, would the disease be recognized.

Finally, is the cost problem one that is true of all vaccines? It is estimated that this vaccine will be quite expensive in comparison to most commonly used vaccines.[1]

To read more on the topic of vaccines against Lyme disease, see the abstract which follows.

J.A. Stockman III, M.D.

Reference

1. Gardner P: Lyme disease vaccines. *Ann Intern Med* 129:583, 1998.

A Vaccine Consisting of Recombinant *Borrelia burgdorferi* Outer-Surface Protein A to Prevent Lyme Disease

Sigal LH, and the Recombinant Outer-Surface Protein A Lyme Disease Vaccine Study Consortium (Univ of Medicine and Dentistry of New Jersey, New Brunswick; et al)

N Engl J Med 339:216-222, 1998   2–30

Introduction.—Early clinical trials have shown that recombinant outer-surface protein A (OspA) is immunogenic and well tolerated, even in individuals with a history of Lyme disease. The protective efficacy of a 30-µg dose of vaccine without adjuvant in adults at risk of *Borrelia burgdorferi* infection was prospectively assessed in a multicenter, randomized, double-blind, placebo-controlled trial in areas of the United States in which Lyme disease is endemic.

Methods.—A total of 10,305 research subjects 18 years of age and older were recruited at 14 sites in Connecticut, Massachusetts, New York, and Wisconsin. Participants were randomized to receive either 30 µg of OspA vaccine (5156 research subjects) or placebo (5149). The second injection was administered 1 month after the first injection. A booster was administered at 12 months. Participants were observed for 2 seasons in which the risk of Lyme disease transmission was high. Patient groups were observed for the number of new clinically and serologically confirmed cases of Lyme disease.

Results.—Overall vaccine efficacy for the first year was 68%. Among the 3745 recipients of the third injection, efficacy was 92%. The vaccine was well tolerated, with mild, self-limited local and systemic reactions that lasted no longer than 7 days after injection. Recipients experienced no significant rise in the frequency of arthritis or neurologic events.

Conclusion.—The OspA vaccine was safe and effective in preventing Lyme disease in a large series of patients from areas in which the disease is endemic.

The Efficacy of Routine Outpatient Management Without Antibiotics of Fever in Selected Infants

Baker MD, Bell LM, Avner JR (Univ of Pennsylvania, Philadelphia)
Pediatrics 103:627-631, 1999   2–31

Background.—In a previous study of a new protocol for the outpatient treatment of febrile infants judged at low risk for serious bacterial illness (SBI), 40% of the patients were safely managed without antibiotic therapy at home. The emergency department staff established this protocol (the "Philadelphia protocol") as the standard of care at the authors' center. This study determined actual management practices 18 months after the establishment of the Philadelphia protocol as the standard of care as well as the continued efficacy of noninvasive outpatient management of fever in febrile infants identified as low risk for SBI based on this protocol.

Methods and Findings.—A cohort of 422 infants, aged 29 to 60 days, with rectal temperatures of 38°C or greater seen at 1 pediatric emergency department during 36 months was studied. Twenty-four percent of the febrile infants were identified prospectively as at low risk for SBI. Nearly 7% were managed in noncompliance with the Philadelphia protocol. Seven of these infants were admitted out of accordance, 10 were discharged out of accordance, and 11 inpatients initially received no antibiotics out of accordance with the protocol. Errors resulted from physician failure to consider the results of the complete blood count or urinalysis. None of the 43 febrile infants with SBI were erroneously classified as at low risk for SBI when the protocol was followed (Tables 2 and 3).

Conclusion.—The Philadelphia protocol for outpatient management of febrile infants at low risk for SBI without antibiotic therapy is practical, reliable, and safe. Physicians must be careful to comply with the protocol, especially in considering complete blood count and urinalysis.

▶ Nathan Kuppermann, M.D., M.P.H., divisions of pediatrics and emergency medicine, University of California, Davis Medical Center, Sacramento, comments:

The evaluation of the febrile infant continues to be a topic of considerable debate among clinicians. For ill-appearing febrile infants, few would disagree

TABLE 2.—Final Diagnoses of 422 Febrile Infants

Diagnostic Category	n (%)
Viral syndrome	228 (54.0)
Nonbacterial gastroenteritis	69 (16.4)
Aseptic meningitis	50 (11.8)
Serious bacterial illness	43 (10.2)
Bronchiolitis	20 (4.7)
Pneumonia (unidentified cause)	8 (1.9)
Otitis media	2 (0.5)
Varicella	1 (0.2)
Conjunctivitis	1 (0.2)

TABLE 3.—Serious Bacterial Illnesses Identified in 422 Febrile Infants

Disease	n (%)
Urinary tract infection	17 (4.0)
Esherichia coli	14
Enterococcus	1
Staphylococcus aureus	1
Citrobacter	1
Bacteremia	9 (2.1)*
Streptococcus pneumoniae	3
Group B streptococcus	3
Salmonella (untyped)	1
Staphylococcus aureus	1
Haemophilus influenzae type b	1
Meningitis	5 (1.2)
Streptococcus pneumoniae	2
Staphylococcus epidermidis	2
Haemophilus influenzae type b	1
Salmonella gastroenteritis	5 (1.2)†
Cellulitis (unidentified)	5 (1.2)‡
Chlamydia pneumonia	2 (0.5)
Necrotizing enterocolitis (unidentified)	1 (0.2)
Osteomyelitis (unidentified)	1 (0.2)
Septic arthritis (unidentified)	1 (0.2)

*Three infants with bacteremia had other concomitant bacterial diseases, including *Salmonella* gastroenteritis (n = 1), pneumonococcal meningitis (n = 1), and *Haemophilus* meningitis (n = 1).
†Three serogroup E, 1 serogroup G, and 1 untyped.
‡Three involved the periorbital region, 1 involved the neck, and 1 involved the toe.
(Reproduced by permission of *Pediatrics*, from Baker MD, Bell LM, Avner JR: The efficacy of routine outpatient management without antibiotics of fever in selected infants. *Pediatrics* 103:627-631, 1999.)

that a complete evaluation for sepsis and empirical administration of antibiotics is indicated. There is less agreement, however, regarding the evaluation of the well-appearing febrile infant. In infants younger than 3 months, it is unclear whether performance of a lumbar puncture and empirical administration of antibiotics are uniformly necessary. Clinical algorithms for the evaluation of febrile infants proposed by some authors have included both routine lumbar punctures and empirical administration of antibiotics, whereas others have recommended neither routine lumbar punctures nor empirical antibiotics for well-appearing infants[1-3].

Previously, Baker and colleagues developed and tested clinical and laboratory screening criteria for the evaluation of febrile infants 1 to 2 months of age with the goal of identifying infants with a low risk of SBI.[4] The screening evaluation includes an assessment of overall clinical appearance; analysis and culture of blood, urine and cerebrospinal fluid; and a chest radiograph. A stool specimen is also included when diarrhea is present. In the original study, this screening protocol had an excellent (100%) negative predicative value for SBI and allowed for the identification of a cohort of febrile infants who require neither hospitalization nor the empirical administration of antibiotics.[4] In the study abstracted here, Baker et al. further evaluated the use of these guidelines in the emergency department of the Children's Hospital of Philadelphia 18 months after the establishment of these criteria as the standard of care at their institution.[5] In reviewing a consecutive cohort of 422 febrile infants 1 to 2 months of age, the authors made several interesting and important observations: (1) had the protocol been universally employed, all 43 infants with SBI would have been correctly identified and (2) however, of the cohort, 6.6% of patients were not treated in accordance with the protocol, including 3 patients with SBI who were not treated with empirical antibiotics.[5]

Baker and colleagues have demonstrated that a subset of febrile infants 1 to 2 months of age can be managed as outpatients without empirical administration of antibiotics after a complete evaluation for sepsis. They have also shown, however, that physician adherence to these guidelines is not uniform, even within the institution where this protocol was developed. Several questions regarding the evaluation of febrile infants in this age group remain unanswered. Whether a lumbar puncture is an essential component of the evaluation of all febrile infants younger than 3 months remains to be determined. In addition, the lower age limit at which screening criteria can be applied safely is unclear. Baker et al. concluded that the Philadelphia protocol screening criteria were not sufficiently accurate in infants younger than 1 month of age.[5] Screening recommendations by other investigators, however, have included infants in this younger age group.[2,3]

N. Kuppermann, M.D., M.P.H.

References

1. Baskin MN, O'Rourke EJ, Fleisher GR: Outpatient treatment of febrile infants 28 to 89 days of age with intramuscular administration of ceftriaxone. *J Pediatr* 120:22-27, 1992.
2. Dagan R, Powell KR, Hall CB, et al: Identification of infants unlikely to have serious bacterial infection although hospitalized for suspected sepsis. *J Pediatr* 107:855-860, 1985.
3. Jaskiewicz JA, McCarthy CA, Richardson AC, et al: Febrile infants at low risk for serious bacterial infection: An appraisal of the Rochester criteria and implications for management. *Pediatrics* 94:390-396, 1994.
4. Baker MD, Bell LM, Avner JR: Outpatient management without antibiotics of fever in selected infants. *N Engl J Med* 329:1437-1441, 1993.
5. Baker MD, Bell LM: Unpredictability of serious bacterial illness in febrile infants from birth to 1 month of age. *Arch Pediatr Adolesc Med* 153:508-511, 1999.

Estimation of Direct and Indirect Costs Because of Common Infections in Toddlers Attending Day Care Centers

Carabin H, Gyorkos TW, Soto JC, et al (McGill Univ, Montreal; Montreal Gen Hosp; Régie Régionale de la Santé et des Services Sociaux de Laval, PQ; et al)

Pediatrics 103:556-564, 1999   2–32

Introduction.—Day care center services are increasingly needed as 2-wage earner families become the norm. It is well-known that children in day care become sick more often, and thus, additional costs on families and society are incurred. More than $14 billion has been spent per year to cover the cost of families for day care for children younger than 15 years of age, representing 6% of a family's income. The major cause of illness and absence of child care is respiratory illness, which often results in parental absenteeism from work. No comprehensive longitudinal study covering most actions taken by parents and their respective costs to help an ill child who attends day care has been conducted. The direct and indirect costs of illness were described in toddlers attending day care centers.

Methods.—This study involved 52 day care centers and 273 toddlers. Parents reported when their child had a cold, diarrhea, and vomiting, and they were called biweekly for their reports for 6 months. Costs measured included medication, visits to a physician, as well as alternative care provided by a family member, a babysitter, or an employed parent who missed work.

Results.—The adjusted average costs per child for medication was $47.47 and for a consultation was $49.10 during a 6-month period. The cost was $11.51 for a babysitter, $35.68 for care by a family member, and $117.12 for a parent missing work (when using opportunity cost). The total cost was $260.70 per child incurred to the parents and society.

Conclusion.—Future studies should determine economical ways to decrease illness frequency in toddlers attending day care centers and the associated costs.

▶ Dr. David O. Matson, professor of Pediatrics, head, Infectious Disease Section, and associate director, Center for Pediatric Research, Norfolk, Va, comments:

Estimation of costs for disease is complicated, and we are in our infancy with respect to methodology. This is a large study of the costs of common infections in the child care setting. For a 6-month winter period, the average cost of illness per toddler was $260.70. Adjusting for the increased incidence of disease during winter months, the annual cost might be on the order of $400 per toddler, which would represent a more than 20% increase in cost of care each year, over and above that of the usual tuition (if $100 per month), attributable only to these common infections. As expected for common infections usually of mild to moderate severity, indirect costs of illness exceeded direct costs. The number of purchases of medications, especially antibiotics (77% of prescription drugs), was huge. I believe the consensus of experts now is that such antibiotic prescribing for common infections in this age group is an abuse of powerful, and otherwise useful, medications.

The study has some limitations. First, the relative frequency of the common infections during the 6-month study period and during the other months of a calendar year is not known. Second, the average number of toddlers per center, 5.8, was small. Third, the recorded costs were the parents' declared costs, rather than costs documented at the source. Next, the influence of the toddler's time in the center is not known. We know that the highest incidence of common infections in the child care setting is in the first few months of attendance. If these toddlers had been present for more than 3 months, then the incidence of infection and associated costs would be reduced. A corollary of this point is that most toddlers in this study (median age, 24 months) would be experiencing their second or third infection with some common pathogens (such as rotavirus or respiratory syncytial virus) or experiencing comparatively mild episodes of otitis media, which would reduce severity and cost of care per episode of illness. Finally, there may be an observation bias. Simply asking parents about the study variable (costs) might have changed the parents' behavior and reporting.

The study confirms previous observations of the perhaps striking costs of infection among children receiving child care outside the home. The relative inflexibility of the work environment, often required by the content of the work, makes it harder for parents to adjust to episodic events like common illnesses in their child, and the costs measured in this study are a real burden to society.

D.O. Matson, M.D., Ph.D.

Immature Neutrophils in the Blood Smears of Young Febrile Children
Kuppermann N, Walton EA (Univ of Calif, Davis; Univ of Calif, San Diego)
Arch Pediatr Adolesc Med 153:261-266, 1999   2–33

Introduction.—A common symptom in children is fever, and it can be difficult to distinguish between viral and bacterial infections. There is controversy whether the presence of immature neutrophils (bands) in the peripheral blood smears of young febrile children helps to distinguish patients with bacterial infections from those with viral infections. Whether band count in the peripheral blood smear helps to distinguish young febrile children with bacterial or respiratory viral infections was determined.

Methods.—There were 100 febrile children, aged 2 years or younger. There were 31 with laboratory-documented bacterial infections, 24 with urinary tract infections, and 7 with bacteremia. There were 69 who had laboratory-documented respiratory viral infections. A clinical appearance score was given to each patient, using the Yale Observation Scale before the laboratory evaluation. All patients gave a complete blood cell count. Manual differential count of the peripheral blood smear was performed. Measurements were taken of band counts, represented as a percentage of white blood cells in the peripheral blood smear, the absolute band count, and band-neutrophil ratio. To determine whether the band count helps to distinguish bacterial infections from viral infections, logistic regression analysis was performed.

Results.—A higher mean absolute neutrophil count was seen in patients with bacterial infections than with respiratory viral infections (11.3 vs 5.9 $\times$ 10⁹/L). In percentage band count, however, there was no difference in patients with bacterial infections or respiratory viral infections (13.5% vs 13.3%). In band-neutrophil ratio, there was also no difference between the

2 groups. After adjusting for age, temperature, Yale Observation Scale score, and absolute neutrophil count in the regression analysis, the band count did not help to distinguish bacterial and viral infections.

Conclusion.—To distinguish bacterial infections from respiratory viral infections in young febrile children, the band count in the peripheral blood smear does not routinely help.

▶ M. Douglas Baker, M.D., chief, Pediatric Emergency Medicine, Yale–New Haven Children's Hospital, New Haven, Conn, comments:

Using sound scientific technique, the authors have added to our understanding of the issues surrounding the early identification of cause of fever in young children. Before globally embracing their conclusions, however, one must recognize the diversity of the study population, and consider the stated limitations of the study. The study population was comprised of children whose range of ages was, in this context, considerable. The current data clearly support the previous work of others who have investigated the issue of occult bacteremia in young children with fever beyond the newborn period. In previous reports, investigators have generally indicated that differential counts are of limited usefulness when evaluating fever in those children. In infants younger than 3 months, however, different observations have been made. The 2 largest studies of consecutively encountered febrile infants have indicated that band counts are useful components of clinical tools used to identify infants at low risk for bacterial disease.[1,2] Neither of those 2 studies used logistic regression in their analysis of data. As the authors of this study indicate, the number of patients that they studied was insufficient to stratify the analysis for patients younger than 3 months. I am hopeful that they will be able to continue their work to further address that issue. In the meantime, they should be acknowledged for a job well done.

M.D. Baker, M.D.

References

1. Baker MD, Bell LM, Avner JR: The efficacy of routine outpatient management without antibiotics of fever in selected infants. *Pediatrics* 103:627-631, 1999.
2. Baskin MN, O'Rourke EJ, Fleisher GR: Outpatient treatment of febrile infants 28 to 89 days of age with intramuscular administration of ceftriaxone. *J Pediatr* 120:22-27, 1992.

Hyper-IgE Syndrome With Recurrent Infections—An Autosomal Dominant Multisystem Disorder
Grimbacher B, Holland SM, Gallin JI, et al (NIH, Bethesda, Md)
N Engl J Med 340:692-702, 1999   2–34

Introduction.—Patients with the inherited disease of hyper–immunoglobulin (Ig) E syndrome have recurrent staphylococcal skin abscesses, pneumonia with pneumatocele formation, and very high serum IgE levels.

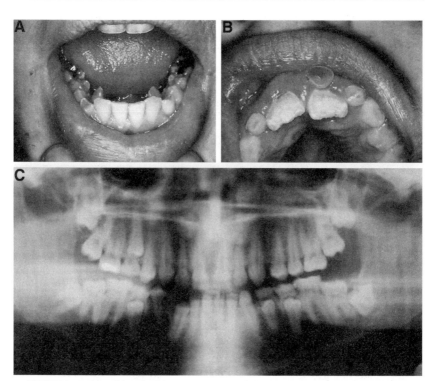

FIGURE 1.—Failure of dental exfoliation in patients with the Hyper-IgE syndrome. **Panel A** shows the lower canines of patient 8 (age, 11 years) and **Panel B** shows the upper central incisor of patient 4 (age, 8 years) and a high palate. Persistent deciduous teeth required extraction in both subjects. **Panel C** shows a panoramic radiograph of patient 11 (age, 23 years), revealing retention of 5 primary teeth with unresorbed roots. The eruption of 4 upper and lower premolars has been blocked by retained primary teeth, and a retained deciduous right lower canine can be seen behind and lateral to its erupted permanent counterpart. In contrast, timely removal of unshed primary teeth in the upper left quadrant of the patient's mouth (upper right) allowed normal eruption of the premolars. (Reprinted by permission of *The New England Journal of Medicine*, from Grimbacher B, Holland SM, Gallin JI, et al: Hyper-IgE syndrome with recurrent infections—An autosomal dominant multisystem disorder. *N Engl J Med* 340:692-702, 1999. Copyright 1999, Massachusetts Medical Society. All rights reserved.)

Nonimmunologic findings such as characteristic facial features, joint hyperextensibility, multiple bone fractures, and craniosynostosis have been reported as well, though their genetic basis is unclear. The genetic basis of the hyper-IgE syndrome is incompletely understood. These factors were addressed in a long-term follow-up study of 30 patients with the syndrome.

Methods.—The study included 30 patients with the hyper-IgE syndrome, with a total follow-up of 291 patient-years. There were 20 women and 10 men, mean age 26.5 years. The study included 5 families with more than 1 affected member. Seventy affected relatives were studied as well. The analysis addressed immunologic features and infections; nonimmunologic features, including dental, head and face, and skeletal abnormalities; and the genetic basis of the hyper-IgE syndrome.

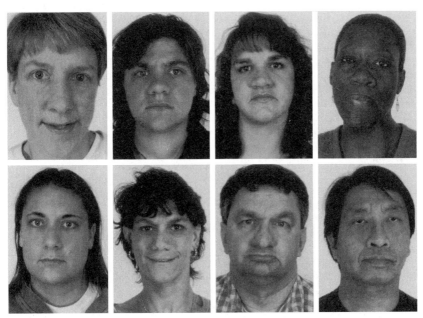

FIGURE 2.—Characteristic facial appearance of men and women of different races with the Hyper-IgE syndrome. (Reprinted by permission of *The New England Journal of Medicine*, from Grimbacher B, Holland SM, Gallin JI, et al: Hyper-IgE syndrome with recurrent infections—An autosomal dominant multisystem disorder. *N Engl J Med* 340:692-702. Copyright 1999, Massachusetts Medical Society. All rights reserved.)

Findings.—All affected patients older than 8 years had nonimmunologic features. Dental abnormalities were present in 72%, including retained primary teeth, noneruption of permanent teeth, or double rows of primary and permanent teeth (Fig 1). By age 16 years, all patients had distinctive facial features, consisting of facial asymmetry, a prominent forehead, deep-set eyes, a broad nose with a wide tip, and mild prognathism (Fig 2). Skeletal abnormalities included recurrent fractures in 57% of the patients, joint hyperextensibility in 68%, and scoliosis in 76% of those 16 years or older.

Seventy-seven percent of all patients, and 85% of those over age 8, had the classic triad of the hyper-IgE syndrome: abscesses, pneumonia, and elevated IgE levels. Twenty-six percent of adult patients had a decrease in their IgE levels over time, close to or within the range of normal. Twenty-seven relatives were identified as being at risk; 11 had the hyper-IgE syndrome, 11 were unaffected, and 6 had mild immunologic, dental, and skeletal manifestations.

Conclusions.—This study clarifies the nonimmunologic manifestations of the hyper-IgE syndrome, which affect the dentition, the skeleton, and the connective tissue. Failure to shed primary teeth because of lack of root resorption is a previously unreported characteristic. In a significant minority of patients, the elevated IgE level declines over time. The pattern of inheritance is autosomal dominant; expressivity is variable.

▶ Dr. Rebecca H. Buckley, professor of Pediatrics and Immunology and chief of Allergy and Immunology, Duke University Medical Center, comments:

This systematic study of patients who reportedly had the hyper-IgE syndrome, as determined by the National Genome Research Institute, confirms (1) that this is a distinct primary immunodeficiency disorder characterized by extremely elevated serum IgE, staphylococcal abscesses of the skin, lungs, and other sites, and eosinophilia; (2) that there are uniformly associated skeletal abnormalities that cause unusual facial features or that predispose to fractures (osteoporosis) or scoliosis; and (3) that the condition appears to have an autosomal dominant pattern of inheritance with incomplete penetrance.[1] While these features have been previously recognized, a new observation made by the authors is that these patients also have an apparent delay in the shedding of primary teeth. This was due to a reduced rate of resorption of the roots of the primary teeth. The authors also found that the mean nasal interalar distance in these patients was above the 98th percentile ($P < .001$). The limitations of the study were that only 77% of the patients had the necessary clinical diagnostic criteria of abscesses, pneumonias with pneumatoceles, and elevated IgE. Since there is no distinctive laboratory test for this condition, it is possible that not all of the patients in the study had the hyper-IgE syndrome. It is important to point out that, 27 years after the initial report of this syndrome, neither the precise host defect nor the fundamental biologic error underlying this condition has been found. The combination of elevated serum IgE and osteoporosis is also a feature of interleukin 4 transgenic mice, suggesting 1 possible mechanism for the coexistence of these 2 features.[2] Hopefully, the resources available to the National Genome Research Institute will eventually permit identification of the faulty gene causing this syndrome.

R.H. Buckley, M.D.

References

1. Buckley R, Wray B, Belmaker E: Extreme hyperimmunoglobulinemia E and undue susceptibility to infection. *Pediatrics* 49:59-70, 1972.
2. Lewis DB, Liggitt HD, Effmann EL, et al: Osteoporosis induced in mice by overproduction of interleukin 4. *Proc Natl Acad Sci U S A* 90:11618-11622, 1993.

Hematopoietic Stem-Cell Transplantation for the Treatment of Severe Combined Immunodeficiency

Buckley RH, Schiff SE, Schiff RI, et al (Duke Univ, Durham, NC)
N Engl J Med 340:508-516, 1999   2–35

Introduction.—Severe combined immunodeficiency is a rare, fatal syndrome that can be caused by a variety of genetic abnormalities and results in profound deficiency of lymphocytes. Immune function can be restored by techniques that deplete human marrow of T cells by marrow transplantation. In infants, successful marrow transplantation for the treatment of this disease does not require chemotherapeutic conditioning before transplantation because infants with severe combined immunodeficiency have an immunologic defect rather than a hematologic one. Data on the long-term efficacy of stem-cell transplantation in infants is lacking. Hematopoietic stem-cell transplantation was performed in infants with severe combined immunodeficiency.

Methods.—There were 89 infants with severe combined immunodeficiency who received hematopoietc stem-cell transplants. Their serum immunoglobulin levels and lymphocyte phenotypes and function were measured. Genetic analyses were also performed. Before transplantation, their bone marrow was depleted of T cells by agglutination with soybean lectin and by sheep-erythrocyte rosetting. T cell–depleted, HLA-haploidentical parental marrow was given to 77 infants. HLA-identical marrow from a related donor was given to 12 infants. Placental-blood transplants from unrelated donors were also given to 3 of the infants who received hap-

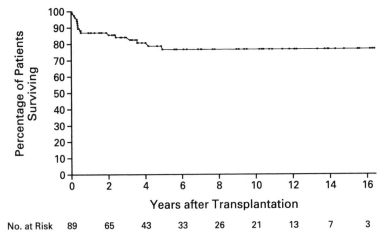

FIGURE 1.—Kaplan-Meier survival curve for 89 patients with severe combined immunodeficiency who received stem-cell transplants. Eight-one percent of the patients were alive at the most recent evaluation; only 12 received transplants from related identical donors. (Reprinted by permission of *The New England Journal of Medicine*, from Buckley RH, Schiff SE, Schiff RI, et al: Hematopoietic stem-cell transplantation for the treatment of severe combined immunodeficiency. *N Engl J Med* 340:508-516. Copyright 1999, Massachusetts Medical Society. All rights reserved.)

loidentical marrow. Chemotherapy before transplantation or prophylaxis against graft-versus-host disease was not given to any of the infants, except for 2 who received placental blood.

Results.—At 3 months to 16.5 years after transplantation, 72 of the 89 infants (81%) were still alive, including all 12 who received HLA-identical marrow, 60 of the 77 (78%) who received haploidentical marrow, and 2 of the 3 (67%) who received both haploidentical marrow and placental blood (Fig 1). In the infants who received unfractionated HLA-identical marrow, T-cell function became normal with 2 weeks after transplantation. In those who received T cell–depleted marrow, T-cell function became normal within 3 to 4 months after transplantation. Normal T-cell function was found in all but 4 of the 72 survivors at the time of the most recent evaluation, and all of the T cells in their blood were of donor origin. In many of the recipients of haploidentical marrow, B-cell function remained abnormal. Between 2% and 100% of B cells were of donor origin in 26 children (5 who received HLA-identical marrow and 21 who received haploidentical marrow). IV immune globulin was given to 45 of the 72 children.

Conclusion.—For patients with any type of severe combined immuno-deficiency, transplantation of marrow from a related donor is a life-saving and life-sustaining treatment, even when there is no HLA-identical donor.

▶ Everybody knows that bone marrow transplantation has been used for some time to treat severe combined immunodeficiency. In fact, it has been 30 years since the first patient with combined T-cell and B-cell immunode-ficiency was successfully treated with transplantation of bone marrow from an HLA-identical sibling. Over this 3 decades, hundreds of patients with this disorder have been treated and cured by transplantation of bone marrow from a brother or sister. One of the beauties of bone marrow transplantation in such patients is the absence of a need for preconditioning (myeloablative-conditioning) because the recipient of the transplant has no T cells and because graft-versus-host disease is uncommon in recipients of HLA-iden-tical bone marrow.

What is unique about the report above is that the results obtained by Buckley et al. are among the finest, if not the best, reported anywhere: survival rates were 100% for the 12 recipients of HLA-identical marrow and 78% (60 of 77 patients) for the recipients of haploincompatible marrow. The trick with the latter procedure was that the donor bone marrows were depleted of T cells by a methodology that reproducibly eliminates all mature T cells in the graft. The absence of T cells prevented graft-versus-host disease while still allowing immunologic reconstitution. Strikingly, virtually all (all, but one) patients transplanted younger than 3.5 months of age survived, showing that with early diagnosis and treatment, this condition can be licked in its infancy.

One important shortcoming of the treatment of severe combined immu-nodeficiency is the fact that most patients recover with somewhat impaired B-cell function. This means that most will require regular administrations of immunoglobulins just as one would do with hypogammaglobulinemia. The latter treatments are a small price to pay for a healthy, full life.

To read more about severe combined immunodeficiency and the results of bone marrow transplantation, see the superb review and commentary on this topic by Alain Fischer.[1]

The last entry in this YEAR BOOK'S chapter on Infectious Disease and Immunology closes with a query. In 1998, 362 Filipinos died of rabies, compared with 321 in 1997 and 337 in 1996. The question is, why is this happening? The answer is that it is not so much because "dog bites man," but rather vice versa. A little background is in order. The underlying problem of rabies in the Philippines is that public awareness of the disease remains poor, and dog owners are not taking advantage of the offer of subsidized rabies immunizations. Also, the government suspended the manufacturing of rabies vaccine for a lengthy period of time because of administrative snafus when its biological production service was relocated. By one estimate, there are only 42,000 doses of rabies vaccine in the entire country of the Philippines, hardly a drop in the bucket for the number of dogs. Most infections, 88% in fact, are caused by pet dogs, not by stray dogs. The real rub with rabies in the Philippines is the fact that folks still eat dogs there.

Please note that if you want to have your dog and eat it too, it must be thoroughly cooked; cooking will destroy the rabies virus. Recognize, however, that to cook a dog you have to prepare it, and that is how people have rabies transmitted to them in that part of the world. Traces of dog's fluid get on one's hands, which then come into contact with one's eyes or lips.

If you want to read all about this, see the excellent review of Wallerstein.[2] Whoever thought that an article entitled: "Man bites dog," would be the real McCoy?

J.A. Stockman III, M.D.

References

1. Fischer A: Thirty years of bone marrow transplantation for severe combined immunodeficiency. *N Engl J Med* 340:559-561, 1999.
2. Wallerstein C: Rabies cases increase in the Philippines. *BMJ* 318:1306, 1999.

3   Nutrition and Metabolism

Dietary Sources of Nutrients Among US Children, 1989-1991
Subar AF, Krebs-Smith SM, Cook A, et al (Natl Cancer Inst, Bethesda, Md; US
Dept of Agriculture, Riverdale, Md; Information Management Services, Inc,
Silver Spring, Md)
Pediatrics 102:913-923, 1998   3–1

Introduction.—Little is known about food consumption of children, particularly the quantities eaten of foods with the greatest concentration of a nutrient ("rich" sources) versus "important" sources of nutrients, those that contribute the most to a population's intake. The contributions of specific foods to nutrient, fiber, and cholesterol intakes of children were examined by using nationally representative data that account for the myriad of ways in which foods are consumed.

Methods.—There were 4008 children aged 2 to 18 years from whom 24-hour dietary recalls were collected. Calculations were made from each of 16 dietary constituents and 113 food groups by summing the amount provided by the food group for all individuals and dividing by total intake from all food groups for all individuals.

Results.—The top 10 sources of energy, fat, and protein are milk, yeast bread, cakes/cookies/quick breads/donuts, beef, and cheese. More than 2% of energy intake was contributed by many of the top 10 sources of carbohydrate such as yeast bread, soft drinks, sodas, milk, ready-to-eat cereal, cakes, cookies, quick breads, donuts, sugars, syrups, jams, fruit drinks, pasta, white potatoes; by protein such as poultry, ready-to-eat cereal, and pasta; and by fat such as potato chips, corn chips, and popcorn. Among the top contributors to folate, vitamin A, vitamin C, iron, and zinc is ready-to-eat cereal. About 14% of total vitamin C intake was contributed by fruit drinks containing little juice.

Conclusion.—Influential contributors of many vitamins and minerals are fortified foods. Major contributors to energy, fats, and carbohydrates are low nutrient–dense foods. Compliance with current dietary guidance may be impeded by the low nutrient–dense foods, which compromise intakes of more nutritious foods.

▶ William H. Dietz, M.D., Ph.D., director, Division of Nutrition and Physical Activity, Centers for Disease Control and Prevention, Atlanta, Ga, comments:

The Continuing Surveys of Food Intake of Individuals (CSFII), conducted periodically by the United States Department of Agriculture, characterize the principal food sources of major nutrients consumed by the United States population. Data from the 1989 to 1991 CSFII survey raise concerns that United States children increasingly rely on small numbers of foods as sources for micronutrients. In this survey, approximately 20% of energy intake for children aged 2 to 18 years was derived from milk and yeast bread, and an additional 20% was derived from cakes/cookies/quick breads/donuts, ready-to-eat cereals, soft drinks/soda, potato chips/corn chips/popcorn, or sugars/syrups/jams.

The foods that account for most of the intake of several specific nutrients constitute an even smaller number. For example, almost 50% of dietary folate intake for 2- to 18-year-olds derives from ready-to-eat cereals (30%), orange/grapefruit juice (10%), and yeast bread (8.5%). Because flour is now enriched with folic acid and because our own analysis of 1994 to 1996 CSFII data showed that only half of United States children consume cereal on a given day, for many children the relative contributions of cereals and yeast bread are likely to have increased even further. In the same age group, milk (51.5%) and cheese (14.3%) account for over 65% of calcium intake. The calcium now added to orange juice is likely to increase its rank contribution to calcium intakes.

The 1989 to 1991 data also emphasize the major contribution that milk and ready-to-eat cereals make to macronutrient and micronutrient intakes. Either milk or ready-to-eat cereals are among the top 5 food sources for 15 of the 16 nutrients examined in this studies (calories, carbohydrate, protein, fat, saturated fat, cholesterol, vitamin C, vitamin A, carotenes, fiber, folate, calcium, iron, zinc, and magnesium). Although both milk and cereals already contain a number of important nutrients, they are also fortified with micronutrients. Because they are so heavily consumed, they provide a disproportionate share of micronutrients.

Food fortification offers an attractive approach to the supply of micronutrients that may otherwise be limited in the United States diet. Enrichment of flour with folic acid or orange juice with calcium represents the most recent examples. However, before we rush to enrich additional foods, the following questions should be considered: What criteria justify fortification? How will we determine when fortification become excessive, particularly when fortification is combined with the use of over-the-counter dietary supplements? Finally, what unforeseen consequences will result from the reliance on enriched foods and supplements to provide micronutrients, rather than the use of a more varied food supply? The increase in lung cancer cases among beta carotene–supplemented Finnish smokers provides an important cautionary lesson.[1]

W.H. Dietz, M.D., Ph.D.

Reference

1. Alpha-Tocopherol, Beta Carotene Cancer Prevention Study Group: The effect of vitamin E and beta-carotene on the incidence of lung cancer and other cancers in male smokers. *N Engl J Med* 330:1029-1035, 1994.

Elimination Diet in Cow's Milk Allergy: Risk for Impaired Growth in Young Children
Isolauri E, Sütas Y, Salo MK, et al (Univ of Tampere, Finland)
J Pediatr 132:1004-1009, 1998   3–2

Background.—Therapeutic elimination diets in atopic patients with challenge-proven food allergy can alleviate symptoms, reduce allergen-specific immunoglobulin E concentrations, and decrease the proliferative response of peripheral blood mononuclear cells to food antigens. However, an increasing understanding of infant nutrition, suggesting a delicate balance between the benefits and risks of elimination diets, was investigated. The nutritional effect of therapeutic elimination diets was investigated along with risk factors predisposing infants with food allergy to poor growth.

Methods.—One hundred children, mean age 7 months, with atopic dermatitis and challenge-proven cow's milk allergy were studied. The children's growth was assessed during the symptomatic period before diagnosis and during the elimination diet.

Findings.—In all children, the elimination diet resulted in clinical control of symptoms. Compared with healthy, age-matched children, however, the patients' mean length standard deviation score and weight-for-length index were decreased. Six percent of the patients had low serum albumin; 24%, abnormal urea concentrations; and 8%, low serum phospholipid docosahexaenoic acid. A subgroup of patients with early symptom onset had a more pronounced growth delay than the patients with later symptom onset. Duration of breast-feeding correlated positively with the sum of n-3 polyunsaturated fatty acids and with the relative amount of docosahexaenoic acid.

Conclusions.—Although elimination diet resulted in clinical control of symptoms in these children, as well as a reduction in allergen-specific IgE and acquisition of clinical tolerance in 15%, it was also associated with a constant risk of nutritional inadequacy. The growth of the allergic children in this study differed from that expected and was reduced compared with that of a healthy control group.

▶ Wasn't it Roseanna Roseannadanna who said, "It's always something"? Here you have a child with cow's milk allergy. You decide to remove cow's milk from the diet. As a result, the allergic symptoms disappear, but the child now fails to grow. This world is full of unintended consequences. Please note the authors had no reasonable explanation for why removing such a nasty substance as cow's milk from the diet caused these youngsters to fail to grow. It could very well be that these youngsters had continual, subclinical, bowel inflammation that required an extensive period of time for healing. In any event, it would be illogical to conclude that the cow's milk had ever been good for them.

Did you ever stop to wonder when "man" first began to partake of cow's milk? Although sheep are thought to have been domesticated in the Near East around 9000 BC, and cattle and goats were domesticated around 7000 BC, there is no direct evidence that they were milked at that time. Pictorial and written records from the Sahara, Egypt, and Mesopotamia show that dairying likely began in that area somewhere between 4000 BC and 2900 BC.

As it turns out, milk obtained at that time may very well have been used for purposes other than ingestion. Recent archeological investigations show that milk was used to make pottery. Employing some fairly sophisticated stable carbon isotope methodologies, investigators have now shown that ancient pottery was not made with water, but rather with animal milk, presumably not human.

Given the known hazards of milk ingestion, it is entirely possible that the ancients knew more than we did about milk and the maladies it causes.

The lesson: calf's milk is for calves and cow's milk is for pots.[1]

J.A. Stockman III, M.D.

Reference

1. Dudd SN, Evershed RP: Direct demonstration of milk as an element of archeological economies. *Science* 282:1478-1480, 1998.

Trial on Timing of Introduction to Solids and Food Type on Infant Growth

Mehta KC, Specker BL, Bartholmey S, et al (Cincinnati Children's Hosp Med Ctr, Ohio; South Dakota State Univ, Brookings; Gerber Products Company, Fremont, Mich)
Pediatrics 102:569-573, 1998   3–3

Background.—When is the optimal time for introducing solid foods into an infant's diet? Does the timing of this introduction affect subsequent growth or body composition? And does the choice of food—commercially prepared food or food from the parents' table—affect growth or body composition? This randomized study addressed the effects of early versus late introduction of solid foods and of commercial versus prepared-at-home foods by assessing growth and body composition at 1 year of age.

Methods.—The 147 infants were randomized to 1 of 4 groups before they were 3 months of age. Before age 3 months, some of the infants were breast-fed; after enrollment in the study, however, all infants received formula. Infants received either an early introduction (at 3 months) to either commercial foods (n = 36) or the parents' choice of foods (n = 35), or a late introduction (at 6 months) to either commercial foods (n = 40) or the parents' choice of foods (n = 36). Infants were fed their assigned diet until they were 1 year of age. Anthropometric and body composition measurements (via dual energy x-ray absorptiometry) and 3-day diet diaries were collected at regular intervals until the infant was 1 year old.

Findings.—None of the 4 groups differed significantly in growth or body composition at 1 year of age. Total energy intake was similar in the early- and late-fed infants at all ages measured, indicating that the early introduction of solid foods did not add calories, but rather displaced calories the infant was receiving from formula. However, compared with the infants who were fed according to their parents' choice of food, infants who ate commercial food consumed fewer calories from protein at 9 months (80 vs 88 kcal/day) and at 12 months (101 vs 148 kcal/day), fewer calories from fat at 12 months (263 vs 343 kcal/day), and fewer total calories at 12 months (884 vs 1022 kcal/day).

Conclusion.—Anthropometric and body composition measurements did not differ whether infants were introduced to solid foods at 3 months or at 6 months. The introduction of solid foods at 3 months displaced energy intake from formula such that total energy intake was similar in the early versus late introduction groups. Beginning at 9 months, infants who consumed commercial foods (which have a relatively low caloric and protein content) were eating significantly fewer protein calories, and by 12 months they were eating significantly fewer protein, fat, and total calories, compared with infants fed from their parents' table. Despite these differences, anthropometric and body composition measurements did not differ between infants fed commercial foods and those fed their parents' choice of foods.

Fruit Juice Intake Is Not Related to Children's Growth
Skinner JD, Carruth BR, Moran J III, et al (Univ of Tennessee, Knoxville; Gerber Products Co, Fremont, Mich)
Pediatrics 103:58-64, 1999   3–4

Background.—Studies by Dennison et al. have reported that 2- and 5-year-old children who consume 12 or more oz/day of 100% fruit juice are at risk of short stature and obesity. These authors sought to confirm these findings in a group of children 24 to 36 months of age.

Methods.—The subjects were 105 children (55 boys and 50 girls) whose mothers were interviewed when the children were 24, 28, or 32 months of age, and again when the children were 28, 32, or 36 months of age. At each interview, 3 days of dietary data were collected (one 24-hour recall and a 2-day food record) and the children were weighed and had their height measured by a registered dietitian. Nutritionist IV software was used to analyze dietary data. Body mass index (BMI) (weight/height^2) and ponderal index (weight/height^3) were also measured at each interview.

These measurements were then compared between children drinking less than 12 or 12 or more oz/day of 100% fruit juice.

Findings.—There were no statistically significant correlations between fruit juice intake and height, BMI, or ponderal index. Compared with subjects in the Dennison et al. study, the subjects in this study by Skinner et al. consumed similar amounts of fruit juice (in interviews 1 and 2, respectively, 5.6 and 6.0 oz/day, vs 5.9 oz/day in the Dennison study). However, children in the current study consumed significantly more milk (12.5 and 12.2 oz/day, vs 9.8 oz/day in the Dennison study), soda pop (2.7 and 3.3 oz/day, vs 1.2 oz/day), and total beverages (64.7 and 63.2 mL/kg per day, vs 43.2 mL/kg per day). In the current study, BMI did not differ significantly between children with fruit juice intake less than 12 or 12 or more oz/day (BMI 75th percentile or greater, 29% vs 42%; BMI 90th percentile or greater, 13% vs 33%). Similarly, ponderal index did not differ significantly between children with fruit juice intake less than 12 or 12 or more oz/day (ponderal index 90th percentile or greater, 5% vs 17%). A greater intake of soda pop was related to less intake of milk and fruit juice. However, there was no correlations between the intakes of milk and fruit juice.

Conclusion.—Unlike the study of Dennison et al. the current data show no statistically significant correlations between obesity and stature in preschool infants based on daily intake of 100% fruit juice. Until more studies are available to characterize a relationship between growth and fruit juice intake, the previous recommendation to limit children's intake of 100% fruit juice to less than 12 oz/day seems unnecessary.

▶ Barbara A. Dennison, M.D., associate professor of Clinical Pediatrics, Columbia University College of Physicians and Surgeons, New York, comments:

This study attempts to replicate—or refute, given the negative tone of the paper—the findings of Dennison et al. that fruit juice is associated with childhood obesity and/or short stature.[1] Unfortunately, this paper lacks sufficient statistical power to detect differences in the prevalence of either obesity or short stature. This study included fewer children (n = 105) than the Dennison et al. study (n = 163). Less precise measures of height (a tape measure held against a doorway rather than a Harpenden stadiometer) and dietary intake (3 days rather than 7 days of records and a less sophisticated dietary software package) were also used compared with the study by Dennison et al.

In this study, the children who lived in warm Tennessee consumed more fluids than those living further north in colder upstate New York (the subjects of Dennison et al.). Surprisingly, the children's fruit juice intakes were the same, whereas the Tennessee children consumed more milk, soda pop, other drinks, and total beverages (64 vs 43 oz/kg per day) than the New York children.

The lack of statistical power is important because this study found, as did Dennison et al., that children who consumed 12 or more oz/day of fruit juice were more likely to be overweight than children who consumed less fruit juice. The findings, however, were not statistically significant. A comparison of the percentages of overweight children based on their fruit juice consumption is strikingly similar between the 2 studies. Dennison et al. found that 53% of children had a BMI in the 75th percentile or greater based on fruit juice intakes of 12 or more oz/day versus 32% of those drinking less than 12 oz/day. That compares with this study's 42% and 29%, respectively.

Dennison et al. found that 32% versus 9% of children had a BMI in the 90th percentile or greater based on fruit juice intakes of 12 or more oz/day and less than 12 oz/day, respectively, compared with this study's finding of 33% versus 13%. Although lack of statistical power is often a reason for not observing a statistically significant result, it is not a reason to negate the findings of a more powerful study, as the authors attempt to do in this paper. Whether they have an ax to the grind or really believe fruit juice is a wonder food is not clear.

To stem the current tide of obesity occurring in the United States, a multitude of interventions are needed. Specific recommendations to parents and caretakers should include limiting television watching, increasing physical activity, not encouraging overeating, not using foods as rewards, and limiting excessive intakes of all foods including fruit juice. Additional larger studies investigating the relationship of young children's growth to diet and other variables are, of course, always needed.

B.A. Dennison, M.D.

Reference

1. Dennison BA, Rockwell HL, Baker SL: Excess fruit juice consumption by preschool-aged children is associated with short stature and obesity. *Pediatrics* 99:15-22, 1997.

Florid Rickets Associated With Prolonged Breast Feeding Without Vitamin D Supplementation
Mughal MZ, Salama H, Greenaway T, et al (St Mary's Hosp, Manchester, England; Alexandra Practice, Manchester, England; Manchester Royal Infirmary, England)
BMJ 318:39-40, 1999   3–5

Background.—The incidence of rickets from vitamin D deficiency appears to be declining. The cases of 6 infants with florid rickets associated with prolonged breast feeding without vitamin D supplementation were reported.

Patients and Findings.—The infants were referred between 10 and 28 months of age. All had several of the clinical signs and symptoms of rickets, including bow legs, rickety rosary, swelling of the ends of long bones, frontal bossing of the skull, delayed dentition, poor growth, and slow motor development. In addition, all had the classic radiologic features of generalized osteopenia including growth plate widening and cupping of metaphyseal regions of long bones. Biochemical findings included increased serum alkaline phosphatase activity for their age, low serum levels of 25-hydroxycholecalciferol, and secondary hyperparathyroidism resulting in hypophosphatemia and normal or increased serum 1,25-dihydroxycholecalciferol concentrations. All children had been breast fed exclusively or for prolonged periods but had not received vitamin D supplements. None of the mothers had received vitamin D supplements during pregnancy or nursing. Four of the 5 mothers tested were deficient in vitamin D, with low serum 25-hydroxycholecalciferol levels. Oral cholecalciferol therapy effectively cured the rickets in all patients.

Conclusion.—Vitamin-D–deficiency rickets in these patients probably resulted from a combination of factors, including maternal vitamin D deficiency resulting in decreased maternal-fetal transfer of vitamin D during pregnancy, prolonged breast feeding by vitamin D–deficient mothers, and reduced sun exposure. These patients underscore the importance of providing vitamin D supplements for growing children and pregnant and lactating women with limited sunshine exposure.

▶ Chances are that it is not every day of the week that you will wind up seeing an infant with florid rickets as a consequence of being at the breast for too many months. It takes a combination of quite prolonged breast feeding, no vitamin supplementation, and little or no sun exposure to bring out the problem. In the reported infants, two thirds were born of mothers who were practicing Muslims who wore concealing clothing and who also wrapped their babies, thus inadvertently avoiding sunshine. As a result, the vitamin D deficiency rickets observed was caused by a combination of factors, including maternal vitamin D deficiency leading to reduced maternal-fetal transfer of vitamin D during pregnancy, prolonged breast feeding by mothers deficient in vitamin D, residence in Manchester, England (not the brightest spot on earth), and probably reduced overall exposure to the sun during summer months. As importantly, none of the reported infants was receiving vitamin D–containing vitamins.

Can prolonged breast feeding cause rickets? Yes, but it takes more than just that to produce the problem. Breast milk is still good for babies.

While we're on the topic of nutrition, please recognize that body size counts, particularly on airplanes. Everybody knows that there is a so-called "crash position" that should be assumed in case of an emergency or crash landing of an airplane. Some flight attendants still instruct passengers on such a technique, technically called the "brace-for-impact" position, in which the upper torso must be flexed totally forward to ensure a certain amount of protection in the case of an emergency. The question is, what is the likelihood that the average-sized individual can assume such an emergency position, given the way the airlines pack in customers these days? The answer to this question comes from an investigation that was undertaken by physicians, informed ahead of time of the nature of the study, who were traveling to New Orleans for the convention of the American Heart Association in March 1999. The aim of the study was to evaluate whether the suggested crash brace position could actually be achieved by passengers. Twenty-four doctors took part (22 men, 2 women; medium height, 1.80 m;

range, 1.7-1.93 m). No one who participated in the study was significantly overweight. Eighteen traveled in the "economy class" section, and six sat in first class. Only 2 of the 18 passengers in economy class could achieve a fully flexed brace position (both were women, the smallest participants), whereas this was possible for all 6 passengers in first-class. Failure to reach brace position was entirely due to the highly restricted space in economy class.[1]

Economy class is a second-class way to fly when it comes to airline safety. Wouldn't it be nice if airlines spaced their seats so that we could actually follow the recommendations that we are given to prevent injuries in emergency circumstances?

J.A. Stockman III, M.D.

Reference

1. Rodgia G, Moser B, Rodgia M: Seat space on airlines. *Lancet* 353:1532, 1999.

The Gluten-free Diet: A Nutritional Risk Factor for Adolescents With Celiac Disease?
Mariani P, Viti MG, Montuori M, et al (Istituto di Clinica Pediatrica Università "La Sapienza," Rome)
J Pediatr Gastroenterol Nutr 27:519-523, 1998   3–6

Background.—Patients with celiac disease are advised to follow a gluten-free diet. Compliance with this diet is less than ideal, particularly in adolescents. The nutritional choices of adolescents with celiac disease who were advised to stay on a gluten-free diet were investigated.

Methods.—The study included 47 patients (10 boys and 37 girls, aged 10-20 years) who had celiac disease and were prescribed a gluten-free diet, and 47 healthy, age-matched control subjects. All participants completed a 3-day alimentary record for analysis of their energy consumption, the distribution of their macronutrients, and their intakes of calcium, iron, and fiber. Additionally, blood samples of patients were tested to determine serum levels of immunoglobulin A antigliadin and antiendomysium antibodies to assess the compliance of patients with the gluten-free diet.

Findings.—Of the 47 patients, 25 (53%) were following the gluten-free diet, but 22 (47%) were eating foods containing gluten. On the basis of Recommended Daily Allowances, the patients and the control group did not differ significantly in their mean energy intake (110.4% vs 117%). Similarly, the macronutrient intakes of patients and the control group were similar, but weighted toward protein (129% and 140%) and lipids (106% and 104%) and a lower carbohydrate intake (71.5% and 73%). Patients were similar to control subjects in the inadequacy of their intakes of calcium (21% vs 17%), fiber (13% vs 22%), and iron (27% vs 21%), particularly in girls. Significant differences were noted between the patients who were adhering to a gluten-free diet and those who were not.

Patients not following the gluten-free diet consumed significantly more carbohydrates (284 vs 225 g) and significantly less protein (68.4 vs 82 g), iron (boys, 8.74 vs 10.8 mg; girls, 9.8 vs 13.2 mg), and calcium (600 vs 850 mg) than patients adhering to the diet. Compared with patients not following the diet, patients who avoided glutens had a greatly increased daily intake of meats, legumes, eggs, and snacks. Overweight and obesity were more common in patients following the gluten-free diet (72%) than in patients not following the gluten-free diet (51%) and in control subjects (47%).

Conclusions.—Only about half the adolescents in this study complied with the gluten-free diet. Their intakes of carbohydrates, protein, iron, and calcium were unbalanced and contributed to their greater rates of overweight and obesity. Thus, paradoxically, adhering to a gluten-free diet seems to be a nutritional risk factor in adolescents with celiac disease, because the diet leads these patients to make poor food choices.

▶ It really is not surprising that adolescents who strictly adhere to a gluten-free diet might get into trouble with eating a nutritionally balanced enough diet. It appears that patients with celiac disease who are on a strict gluten-free diet appropriately reduce their consumption of gluten-containing foods, such as bread, pizza, and pasta, but this diet is not counterbalanced by an increase in items from the same food groups, such as rice, corn, and potatoes. Instead you see a diet that is high in proteins (meat, eggs, and legumes) as well as a diet that is high in certain fats. On balance, this results in a greater percentage of celiac disease patients being overweight during the adolescent period. In recent years, there has been a great improvement in diagnostic tools for the detection of celiac disease. This progress is coming at a time when it would appear that the management of this disorder results in nutritional imbalances that can seriously adversely affect a youngster's cardiovascular risk factors, particularly during teenage years.

While on the topic of malabsorption states, one of the hottest things these days in the field of gastroenterology is a new hormonal entity called *oxyntomodulin-like immunoreactivity* (OLI). OLI is a group of proglucagon-derived intestinal peptides that may participate in gastrointestinal (GI) tract function. This hormone is secreted by ileal and colonic cells in response to nutrient stimulation within the gut. Lipids and carbohydrates are the primary stimuli. In adults, OLI plasma concentrations increase significantly within the first hour after a meal. In malabsorption states, OLI levels rise quite high, presumably because increased amounts of unabsorbed nutrients reach the distal gut mucosa and trigger transitory hyperactivation of the endocrine system of the GI tract, resulting in an exaggerated release of a number of hormonal peptides.

Recently, investigators from France examined circulating OLI in healthy children and in children with celiac disease. They found that children with celiac disease had seriously elevated OLI blood levels, although they were unable to use these levels as a diagnostic test for the disorder.[1]

If you're not familiar with the endocrinology of the GI tract, you soon will be. More and more is being written about GI hormones including OLI, motilin, enteroglucagon, neurotensin, peptide YY, secretin, vasoactive intestinal peptide, somatostatin, and gastric inhibitory peptide. These hormones may be the key to our understanding of many, if not most, GI tract disturbances.

J.A. Stockman III, M.D.

Reference

1. Le Quellec A, Clapie M, Callaamand P, et al: Circulating oxyntomodulin-like immunoreactivity in healthy children and children with celiac disease. *J Pediatr Gastroenterol Nutr* 27:513-518, 1998.

Growth of Hypercholesterolemic Children Completing Physician-initiated Low-Fat Dietary Intervention

Tershakovec AM, Jawad AF, Stallings VA, et al (The Children's Hosp of Philadelphia; Pennsylvania State Univ, University Park; Univ of Maryland, Baltimore)

J Pediatr 133:28-34, 1998   3–7

Background.—Although many groups have endorsed limitation of the fat intake of children over the age of 2 years, this idea remains controversial. The effect of reduced fat intake on growth is of particular concern. The Children's Health Project assessed the efficacy and safety of nutrition education programs that reduced fat intake in a group of hypercholesterolemic 4- to 10-year-old children.

Methods.—A cholesterol screening program was conducted in the offices of 9 suburban pediatricians to identify at-risk children. These children were randomly assigned to parent-child home-based nutrition education, standard nutrition counseling, or the at-risk control group. A non-at-risk control group was randomly selected from children without hypercholesterolemia. Groups were balanced by age, sex, and season of enrollment. Height, weight, skinfold thickness, total cholesterol, and blood pressure were evaluated at baseline and at 3, 6, and 12 months after intervention.

Results.—All intervention groups had significant decreases in fat and saturated fat intake after intervention. Weight z-score, height z-score, weight-for-height median, and skinfold sum did not vary among treatment groups over the year. At baseline, height z-score, weight z-score and weight-for-height median were positively associated with caloric intake, and weight z-score, weight-for-height median, and skinfold sum were positively associated with fat intake. When the children were grouped by average fat quintiles, there was no association between fat intake and changes in weight z-score, height z-score, or weight-for-height median.

Conclusions.—Hypercholesterolemic children, aged 4 to 10 years, can lower their fat intake through nutritional intervention and still maintain normal growth. These results support the safety of lower-fat diets for at-risk children.

▶ Thank goodness, you can lower cholesterol levels and not stunt growth. You can lower dietary fat intake and lower body fat at the same time without producing short kids. The ponderosity index here in the United States is moving along at a quite rapid pace. Today practically everyone is concerned about his or her weight—and seemingly for good reason, as it's clear that people have been getting fatter faster. By most stringent definitions, more than half of U.S. women and men 20 or more years of age are now considered overweight and nearly one quarter are clinically obese. The modern medical case against obesity began to build back in 1959, with the publication of the Metropolitan Life Insurance Company tables. Based on studies of hundreds of thousands of policy holders, these tables said that the risk of premature death increases steadily as weight increases above the so-called "desirable weight," corresponding to 126 pounds for a woman of 5 feet 4 inches and 154 pounds for a man of 5 feet 10 inches—remarkably lean standards that about 80% of men and women now exceed. Now, of course, we talk about body mass index instead of weight and height, but the story is still the same. It's not clear what is behind the increasing ponderosity index here in the United States, especially since the big leap seems to have occurred in the 1980s. Whether something happened in the 1980s to make food more available or us more sedentary is unclear.

The United States isn't the only place with a high ponderosity index. In Kuwait, the proportion of overweight children is rising quickly, as is the adult prevalence of coronary artery disease, hypertension, diabetes, and other weight-related illnesses.[1] The average Kuwaiti eats 3 hearty meals a day, with meat being the major constituent of all meals. The population of the country is only 2.2 million, yet 50,000 tons of red meat are consumed annually, mostly by the 80,000 indigenous Kuwaitis. This is in addition to large quantities of chicken and seafood. Breakfast can include fried liver and kidneys on top of dairy products such as cheese, clotted cream, and full-fat yogurt. Several meat dishes are usually prepared for lunch and in the evening. A household will often serve a whole roasted sheep on a bed of saffron rice if there is anything to celebrate. In addition, fast-food shops have sprung up all over Kuwait, offering snacks to assuage hunger between meals. Culturally, it is important to Kuwaitis to be generous in providing food to guests. To offer a meal that falls short in terms of richness of quantity is an insult. Similarly, the view that plump children must be healthy is still adhered to, even by parents who know that this is a fallacy. Relatives like nothing better than to playfully pinch the cheeks of young children, and the more rounded the face, the more satisfied the family members.

Obesity is not the only health-related problem in Kuwait. Smoking prevalence is as high there as just about anywhere. Statistics show that 62% of 10- to 18-year-olds smoke cigarettes, and the habit remains socially acceptable despite recent government provision of clinics to help those who wish to stop smoking. By law, stores that sell tobacco products now must donate 1% of their revenue to cancer-death-related projects.

One last comment: Apples do fare worse than pears. The data are now quite conclusive that individuals with mostly upper body fat (apple shapes) face more health risks than pear-shaped individuals. It's far better to have a big butt and fat thighs than to have skinny legs and a beer belly and a thick chest. The reasons are quite complex, but have to do with how abdominal fat cells, when overloaded, negatively interact with insulin, producing insulin resistance, which produces increased lipids in the blood and damage to the heart. If you want to read about more of this, see the editorial comment that recently appeared in *Science*.[2] It would seem that there is nothing wrong with a little Crisco fat in the can, when it comes to cardiovascular risk factors.

J.A. Stockman III, M.D.

References

1. Kandela P: The Kuwaiti passion for food cannot be shaken. *Lancet* 353:1249, 1999.
2. Wickelgren I: Do "apples" fare worse than "pears"? *Science* 280:1365-1367, 1998.

Body Composition Development of Adolescent White Females: The Penn State Young Women's Health Study
Lloyd T, Chinchilli VM, Eggli DF, et al (Pennsylvania State Univ, Hershey)
Arch Pediatr Adolesc Med 152:998-1002, 1998   3–8

Introduction.—Insight into the tempo of adolescent hormone changes and the likelihood of disease risk in adulthood may be obtained by studying body composition patterns acquired early in life. Managements of soft tissue and hard tissue development during growth, and changes in height and weight are possible with the advent of body composition assessment by dual-energy x-ray absorptiometry. The risk of osteoporotic fracture may depend on peak bone mass achieved by the end of the second decade of life and the rate or bone loss thereafter. A longitudinal analysis of soft and hard tissue measurements was conducted on women aged between 11 and 18½ years to determine and compare the ages for peak velocity and peak accumulation for hard and soft tissue components.

Methods.—The study included 82 premenarchal, healthy girls, aged 11 years, who completed the longitudinal, observational study during a 7-year period when they were aged 18 years. Dual-energy x-ray absorptiometry was used to obtain measurements of total body bone mineral content, total body bone mineral density, percentage of body fat, and lean body mass every 6 months for the first 4 years of study and yearly thereafter.

Results.—The mean age for peak velocity for height, weight, body mass index, and percentage of body fat was 11½ years; for lean body mass, 12 years; for total body bone mineral content and total body bone mineral density, 13½ years. The mean age for peak accumulation for height, weight, body mass index, lean body mass, total body bone mineral content, and total body bone mineral density was 17½ years; for percentage of body fat, 13½ years.

Conclusion.—The age of peak velocities for height, weight, body fat, and lean body mass occurs at 11½ to 12 years among a healthy population of white females. Peak accumulation of all tissue components is reached, on average, by age 17½ years, and peak soft tissue velocities precede hard tissue velocities by about 2 years. This study may help determine which women are most in need of hormone and calcium supplementation in postmenopausal years.

▶ Why would anyone go through the trouble of doing a study to determine the body composition development of adolescent females? All you have to do is to ask the average teenage male. The answer will come very quickly.

In all fairness to these investigators though, it is important to know precisely how young ladies mature. All the bone that a woman will ever have is acquired by age 18, and in most, well before that. Indeed, the age at which the peak growth is occurring, which includes the peak for laying down calcium in bone, is, on average, 11½ years in adolescent females. Between the start of puberty and its final terminus, mean tissue mass will approximately double and fat mass will increase threefold.

So what does all this mean? It means that good diet is especially important during such periods of rapid growth. If you want to form hard bones, that is the time to do it. Studies have shown that during periods of such growth, about 265 mg of calcium are incorporated into bone each day. That equates to a dietary intake of calcium of about 1000 mg, an amount not regularly consumed on a daily basis by the majority of adolescents here in the United States.[1]

Cow's milk is for calves. Perhaps it might also be for adolescent females, given the calcium requirements they have. Actually, given the fat accretion of young ladies at this age, perhaps a few milkshakes are in order.

J.A. Stockman III, M.D.

Reference

1. Martin AD, Bailey DA, McKay HA, et al: Bone mineral and calcium accretion during puberty. *Am J Clin Nutr* 66:611-615, 1997.

Reye's Syndrome in the United States From 1981 Through 1997
Belay ED, Bresee JS, Holman RC, et al (Ctrs for Disease Control and Prevention, Atlanta, Ga)
N Engl J Med 340:1377-1382, 1999   3–9

Background.—Although its cause is not known, Reye's syndrome is often preceded by a viral syndrome. In the early 1980s, many studies suggested a strong epidemiologic association between the ingestion of aspirin during a preceding viral syndrome and the subsequent develop-

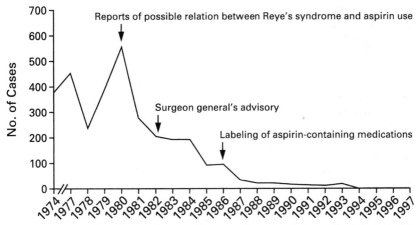

FIGURE 1.—Number of reported cases of Reye's syndrome in relation to the timing of public announcements of the epidemiologic association of Reye's syndrome with aspirin ingestion and the labeling of aspirin-containing medications. (Reprinted by permission of *The New England Journal of Medicine*, from Belay ED, Bresee JS, Holman RC, et al: Reye's syndrome in the United States from 1981 through 1997. *N Engl J Med* 340: 1377-1382. Copyright 1999, Massachusetts Medical Society. All rights reserved.)

ment of Reye's syndrome. Thus, in 1980 the Centers for Disease Control and Prevention issued an advisory against the use of salicylates in children with varicella or influenza-like illnesses. This was followed in 1982 by a warning from the Surgeon General of the United States and in 1986 by the requirement for aspirin-containing medications to carry a warning label. These authors reviewed the pattern of Reye's syndrome in the United States from 1980 through 1997.

Methods.—National surveillance data regarding Reye's syndrome were collected from December 1980 through November 1997. The number of cases of Reye's syndrome was determined, as were patient characteristics and risk factors for poor outcomes.

Findings.—During the period studied, 1207 children 18 years of age or younger sustained Reye's syndrome. The incidence peaked in 1980 (555 cases), right after the association of aspirin with Reye's syndrome was reported, and declined precipitously to the point that, since 1994, there have been 2 or less cases each year (Fig 1). The median age of the patients studied was 6 years; 52% were girls and 93% were white. The incidence peaked in January and February, coinciding with the respiratory virus season. Most of the patients (93%) reported an illness during the 3 weeks before the onset of Reye's syndrome. Additionally, most (82%) of those who underwent measurements of blood salicylate levels after hospital admission had detectable salicylate levels. The case fatality rate was 31% overall, with a significantly higher rate in children less than 5 years of age (relative risk [RR], 1.8) and in patients whose serum ammonia level was greater than 26 μmol/L (RR, 3.4). Serum ammonia levels greater than 26 μmol/L were also associated with significantly greater risk of neurologic complications (RR, 4.1).

Conclusion.—The number of infants and children with Reye's syndrome has decreased dramatically since 1980, when the epidemiologic association between aspirin ingestion during an antecedent varicella or influenza-like illness and the subsequent development of Reye's syndrome was announced. Since 1994, cases in the United States have been rare (2 or fewer per year). Thus, an extensive workup should be pursued in infants and children suspected of having Reye's syndrome to rule out treatable inborn metabolic disorders that can mimic Reye's syndrome.

▶ This is the last entry in the Nutrition and Metabolism chapter, and this important review of Reye's syndrome speaks for itself, so we close with a question. Supermodels have been criticized for being unrealistically thin and disproportionately shaped in comparison to "normal" women. They have also been compared, in their shapes, with teenagers and young adult women who have anorexia nervosa or bulimia. Are these purported comparisons appropriate? And, how would you make such a determination?

Leave it to investigators in the Department of Psychology of Newcastle University to answer these questions for us.[1] They compiled a biometric database of 300 fashion models, 300 glamour models, and 300 normal women. The fashion and glamour models' body data were obtained from model cards, displayed on the World Wide Web page of a large model agency. To check whether the model cards provided accurate biometric data (height, bust, waist, hip measurements), similar statistics for models were obtained from *Playboy*, a source which has apparently been judged reliable for this purpose.[1,2] "Normal" women in this study were undergraduate and graduate students, with no clinical history of eating disorders, who scored within the normal range on a battery of questionnaires related to eating disorders. Biometric data on dozens of anorectic and bulimic women were also used for comparison.

The Table below shows the biometric information for these groups of women. Believe it or not, there are behavioral studies suggesting that there is an optimum waist-hip ratio for female attractiveness; a waist-hip ratio of 0.7 is supposed to be the most attractive. This ratio corresponds to a fat distribution that gives optimum fertility.[1]

So what did these investigators find? They found that female fashion models were, as expected, taller than their peers, by an average of 11 cm.

TABLE.—Biometric Information

	Height (m)	Body-Mass Index	Waist-Hip Ratio	Waist-Bust Ratio	Bust-Hip Ratio
Fashion models	1.77 (0.00)	17.57 (0.26)	0.71 (0.02)	0.72 (0.02)	0.99 (0.00)
Glamour models	1.69 (0.00)	18.09 (0.07)	0.68 (0.00)	0.66 (0.00)	1.03 (0.00)
Anorexic women	1.65 (0.01)	14.72 (0.36)	0.76 (0.01)	0.78 (0.01)	0.96 (0.00)
Bulimic women	1.65 (0.01)	23.66 (1.05)	0.77 (0.01)	0.83 (0.01)	0.93 (0.01)
Normal women	1.66 (0.00)	21.86 (0.22)	0.74 (0.00)	0.80 (0.00)	0.92 (0.00)

Note: All values are mean (SE).
(Data from Singh D: Adaptive significance of female physical attractiveness. Role of waist to hip ratio. *J Pers Soc Psychol* 65:293-307, 1993.)

Both fashion models and glamour models were rated significantly under-weight on the basis of body mass index but were consistently heavier than anorexic women. Fashion models and glamour models did have a waist-hip ratio close to the "optimum" of 0.7 and tended to have an hourglass figure, as shown by the bust-hip ratio. Fashion and glamour models had similar measurements, although glamour models were regarded as more curvatious than fashion models, probably because they were shorter, allowing for the appearance of a "better" hourglass figure.

To learn what it takes to be a *Vogue* cover girl, see the article by Tovee et al.[3]

J.A. Stockman III, M.D.

References

1. Singh D: Adaptive significance of female physical attractiveness: Role of waist to hip ratio. *J Pers Soc Psychol* 65:293-307, 1993.
2. Bjorntorp P: Adipose tissue distribution and function. *Int J Obes* 15:67-81, 1991.
3. Tovee MJ, Mason SM, Emery JL, et al: Supermodels: Stick insects or hourglasses? *Lancet* 350:1474-1475, 1997.

4 Allergy and Dermatology

A Cost-saving Algorithm for Children Hospitalized for Status Asthmaticus
McDowell KM, Chatburn RL, Myers TR, et al (Univ Hosps of Cleveland, Ohio; Rainbow Babies and Childrens Hosp, Cleveland, Ohio; Case Western Reserve Univ, Cleveland, Ohio; et al)
Arch Pediatr Adolesc Med 152:977-984, 1998   4–1

Introduction.—The prevalence of asthma in children in the United States is rising. It is the most common discharge diagnosis for pediatric hospitals. Several attempts have been made to improve asthma management practices. It would be helpful if treatment that does not improve the quality of care could be eliminated. An effective predetermined algorithm may yield enormous economic effects by reducing treatment variation and improving patient outcomes. An assessment-driven algorithm for the treatment of pediatric status asthmaticus was evaluated for its ability to reduce length and cost of hospitalization in a nonrandomized, prospective, controlled trial in children aged 1 to 18 years.

Methods.—The asthma care algorithm (ACA) was used in 104 children hospitalized in a tertiary care children's hospital for treatment of status asthmaticus. Ninety-seven children receiving unstructured standard treatment acted as controls. The ACA group was treated with standard medications provided at a frequency driven by the patient's clinical condition. Specific criteria were used for decreasing or augmenting therapy, transferring to intensive care, and discharging to home. The patient records in the ACA group contained assessments, algorithm cues, and a record of treatment. Patients in the ACA group were interviewed by telephone 1 week after hospital discharge. Patients were followed for hosptial length of stay, cost per hospitalization, relapse rate, and protocol adherence.

Results.—The average hospital stay for patients in the ACA group was significantly shorter than for control patients (2.0 vs 2.9 days). Patients in the ACA group received fewer aerosolized albuterol doses, compared with controls, and there were no between-group differences in short-term relapse rate. A savings of $700 per patient was realized in the ACA group, compared with controls. Adherence to protocol was excellent; there were only 8 variances per patient stay out of more than 150 opportunities for variance.

Conclusion.—An intensive, assessment-driven algorithm for patients with pediatric status asthmaticus significantly decreased hospital length of stay and costs without increasing morbidity.

▶ Some have said that algorithms are for nonthinkers. That may or may not be true, but when it comes to asthma care, a consistent, logical approach to this disorder can only be helpful. If algorithms are about anything, they are about providing a logical and consistent framework for ones thinking. These investigators from Rainbow Babies and Children's Hospital in Cleveland have shown that one can seriously reduce hospital charges for the most common illness resulting in hospitalization to pediatric services.

While on the topic of asthma, have you wondered whether there might be a linkage between the increasing prevalence of childhood asthma and the decreased use of pediatric aspirin? Some investigators have considered that something as simple as a decline in aspirin use may be one cause of the increase in childhood allergic diseases and asthma seen in the last decade or two.[1] In the United States, the prevalence of childhood asthma has steadily increased over the last 30 years, but the rate of increase markedly accelerated beginning in the early 1980s when the use of aspirin decreased. Aspirin, but not acetaminophen, markedly inhibits cyclooxygenase-2, and the decreasing use of aspirin may be a factor in facilitating allergic sensitization and asthma by augmenting certain cytokine imbalances in genetically predisposed children. The theory here is that when a child gets a common respiratory infection with a little bit of fever, were that child treated with aspirin, wheezing might be prevented. This is an interesting theory, to say the least.

Before closing this commentary that started off with a discussion having to do with algorithms, do you know the origin of the word algorithm? The word itself relates to the term "algorism," referring to the Arabic system of numerals. "Algorism" comes from the proper name of an Arabic mathematician from the ninth century, a certain al-Khowarazmi. In fact, "arithmetic" and related words come from this native of Khawarazm.

J.A. Stockman III, M.D.

· *Reference*

1. Varner AE, Busse WW, Lemanske RF: Hypothesis: Decreased use of pediatric aspirin has contributed to the increasing prevalence of childhood asthma. *Ann Allergy Asthma Immunol* 81:347-351, 1998.

Montelukast, a Leukotriene-receptor Antagonist, for the Treatment of Mild Asthma and Exercise-induced Bronchoconstriction

Leff JA, Busse WW, Pearlman D, et al (Merck Research Labs, Rahway, NJ; Univ of Wisconsin, Madison; Colorado Allergy and Asthma Clinic, Aurora; et al)
N Engl J Med 339:147-152, 1998   4–2

Objective.—The release of inflammatory mediators such as leukotrienes is stimulated in exercise-induced bronchoconstriction. The effect of once-daily montelukast, a leukotriene-receptor antagonist, on airway hyperresponsiveness to exercise and methacholine challenges and on the overall clinical condition of patients with mild asthma was investigated in a 12-week, placebo-controlled, parallel-group study.

Methods.—After a 2-week washout/placebo period, either 10 mg montelukast (n = 54) or placebo (n = 56) was administered once daily at bedtime for 12 weeks to 110 asthma patients, aged 15 to 45 years, with exercise-induced bronchoconstriction. Exercise challenges were performed 20 to 24 hours after dosing at baseline; at weeks 4, 8, and 12, and after a 2-week washout period. Methacholine challenges were performed at baseline, at weeks 4 and 12 on nonexercise days, and after a 2-week washout period. The area under the curve for FEV_1 in the first 60 minutes after exercise was the primary end point.

Results.—Six patients in the montelukast group and 7 in the placebo group did not complete the study. Montelukast provided significantly more protection against bronchoconstriction during exercise than did placebo (Fig 2). Compared with placebo, montelukast significantly im-

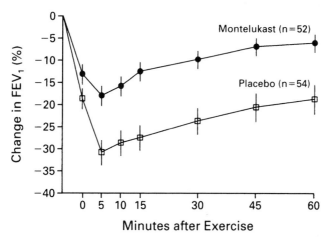

FIGURE 2.—Mean (±SEM) Changes in FEV_1 after Exercise Challenge after 12 Weeks of Treatment with Montelukast or Placebo. Treatment with montelukast was associated with a significant ($P = 0.002$) reduction in exercise-induced bronchoconstriction. (Reprinted by permission, from Leff JA, Busse WW, Pearlman D, et al: Montelukast, a leukotriene-receptor antagonist, for the treatment of mild asthma and exercise-induced bronchoconstriction. *N Engl J Med* 339:147-152. Copyright 1998, Massachusetts Medical Society. All rights reserved.)

proved the area under the curve (47.4%), and, after 12 weeks of therapy, significantly improved the maximal postexercise decrease in FEV_1 and significantly shortened the time for lung function to return to within 5% of preexercise FEV_1 at all time points. After 12 weeks of montelukast therapy, patients' global assessment of asthma control improved significantly. Montelukast patients were significantly less likely to require β-agonist rescue. Montelukast patients exhibited no rebound effect during the washout period. Methacholine challenges results were not significantly different between groups. The frequency of adverse effects was similar between groups.

Conclusion.—Montelukast provided significantly more protection than placebo against exercise-induced bronchoconstriction in asthma patients. There was no rebound effect during the washout period.

▶ In the 1999 YEAR BOOK OF PEDIATRICS, there was extensive commentary on the usefulness of montelukast as part of the treatment of asthma. Now we see even more convincing data that once-a-day treatment with montelukast provides significant protection against exercise-induced asthma. The terrific part about montelukast is that the degree of protection it affords does not seem to diminish after long-term therapy. On the other hand, tolerance is a particular problem with short-acting inhaled β-agonists, such as albuterol. Another nice aspect of montelukast is that while it provides no residual protective effect two or more weeks after treatment is stopped, neither is there any rebound worsening of exercise-induced bronchoconstriction.

Studies have shown that new therapies, such as using montelukast, tend to find their way into practice starting in areas with the largest concentrations of physician specialists in the population. If you have ever wondered which are the top cities that have more specialists per unit population, they are:

City	Specialists (Per 100,000)
1. Rochester, Minn	375
2. Boston, Mass	144
3. Iowa City, Ia	133
4. Charlottesville, Va	132
5. San Francisco, Calif	118
6. Columbia, Mo	107
7. Long Island, NY	104
8. Gainesville, Fla	104
9. Greenville, SC	101

(Data from the U.S. Department of Health and Human Services.)

Needless to say, for many of these towns, the main attraction is the medical center. What would Rochester, Minnesota be without its Mayo Clinic, or Charlottesville without its UVA? What about Long Island without its plastic surgeons?

J.A. Stockman III, M.D.

Effect of Long-term Salmeterol Treatment on Exercise-induced Asthma
Nelson JA, Strauss L, Skowronski M, et al (Univ Hosps of Cleveland, Ohio;
Case Western Reserve Univ, Cleveland, Ohio)
N Engl J Med 339:141-146, 1998   4–3

Background.—Selective β_2-adrenergic agonists such as salmeterol are
often used to treat acute exercise-induced asthma. Studies have shown that
salmeterol's protective effect decreases with long-term dosing, but these
studies have involved experimental precipitants of asthma (e.g., histamine,
methacholine, adenosine) that patients would not normally encounter.
This study evaluated the effectiveness of long-term salmeterol in response
to a clinically relevant stimulus of asthma: exercise.
Methods.—This randomized, double-blind, crossover trial included 20
nonsmoking patients (9 men and 11 women; mean age, 29 years) with
exercise-induced asthma. Patients took either 2 puffs (42 µg) of salmeterol
or placebo twice a day for 2 months, then after a 1-week washout period
they took the other study drug. Patients exercised on a cycle ergometer,
and their forced expiratory volume in 1 second (FEV_1) was measured while
they were breathing cold air. The FEV_1 was measured at baseline and on
days 1, 14, and 29 of each month, both before and after the dose of study
drug, and both in the morning and 9 hours later in the evening, (before the
next drug dose).
Findings.—At all times measured, FEV_1 decreased significantly in the
patients taking placebo (mean decrease from baseline, 19% ± 2% for
morning measurement and 18% ± 2% in the evening). Patients taking
salmeterol had significantly less airway narrowing after their morning dose
compared with baseline, with a decrease in morning FEV_1 values of 5% ±
2% on day 1, 10% ± 3% on day 14, and 9% ± 3% on day 29. With
prolonged use however, salmeterol gave significantly less protection
against exercise-induced asthma. At the evening measurement, FEV_1 values were 6% ± 2% on day 1, 15% ± 3% on day 14, and 14% ± 3% on
day 29. By the end of 1 month of dosing, 11 patients who were taking
salmeterol no longer gained any protective effect from this drug against
exercise-induced asthma (as determined by a greater than 10% decrease in
FEV_1).
Conclusions.—Although long-term use of salmeterol does protect
against exercise-induced asthma, its effectiveness decreases as dosing continues. Thus, patients with exercise-induced asthma who receive long-term
salmeterol therapy may have to have their dosing schedules altered, or they
may need to receive supplemental short-acting drugs to tide them over
until the next salmeterol dose.

▶ It's interesting to see how the therapies for asthma have expanded and
how quickly montelukast has been accepted here in the United States as
part of one of several mainstays for the treatment of chronic asthma. As a
potent, specific antagonist of leukotriene receptors, it can in fact be additionally effective against exercise-induced asthma. The latter problem is
thought to be mediated through the release of inflammatory substances,

including the leukotrienes. It isn't clear why exercise alone, through some cooling and drying effect on the airway, causes wheezing, but it does. For those who have to exercise and who have this problem, montelukast may be their cup of tea. Yes, it would be cheaper to stop running, but sometimes sensible approaches are not always preferred.

It is nice to have options when treating patients with significant symptoms. When it comes to exercise-induced asthma, albuterol may be just fine for the infrequent exerciser. For those who are physically active more than 30 to 60 minutes a day, inhaled salmeterol may be more appropriate because the duration of its clinical protection is likely to be longer than that achieved with albuterol if used regularly. Montelukast offers several practical advantages over both these drugs. It is taken once daily by mouth and has no known significant adverse effects or drug interactions. In those with a response, the protective effect lasts 20 to 24 hours, even during long-term administration. As of this past year, montelukast has been the only leukotriene modifier approved by the Food and Drug Administration for use by children 6 years of age and older. The National Collegiate Athletic Association, the US Olympic Committee, and the International Olympic Committee do allow competitors to use montelukast and other leukotriene modifiers without prior approval. Thus, for a variety of pragmatic reasons, many children and adults with mild, stable asthma manifested primarily by exercise-induced bronchoconstriction may wish to try montelukast for long-term control of symptoms. Three out of four patients will have a good response.

Montelukast: try it, you'll like it.

J.A. Stockman III, M.D.

Effect of Nebulized Ipratropium on the Hospitalization Rates of Children With Asthma

Qureshi F, Pestian J, Davis P, et al (Eastern Virginia Med School, Norfolk)
N Engl J Med 339:1030-1035, 1998   4–4

Introduction.—Several reports have indicated that the addition of the anticholinergic drug, ipratropium bromide (IB), to standard albuterol treatment significantly enhances pulmonary function, compared with albuterol alone. Other studies found that the addition of IB does not improve rates or durations of hospitalization. The addition of IB to standard emergency department therapy for asthma in children was assessed in a large, double-blind, randomized, prospective trial for its ability to decrease hospitalization rates.

Methods.—The study included 434 children, aged from 2 to 18 years. All patients had acute exacerbations of moderate or severe asthma treated in the emergency department. All children received 2 mg of oral prednisone or prednisolone per kilogram of body weight, and a nebulized solution of albuterol (2.5 or 5 mg per dose, depending on body weight) was administered every 20 minutes for 3 doses and then as needed. Children were randomized to treatment with 2.5 mL of saline placebo or 500 μg

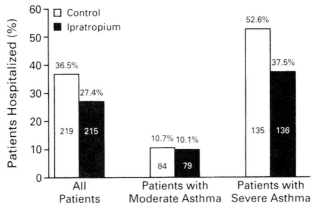

FIGURE 1.—Rates of hospitalization in the control and IB groups. When the 434 patients who completed the study were stratified according to the severity of the exacerbation of asthma at presentation, 163 were classified as having moderate asthma and 271 as having severe asthma. The number of children who received saline or IB in each group is shown within the bars. The overall rate of hospitalization was lower in the IB group ($P = .05$). In children with severe asthma, the rate of hospitalization was significantly lower in those receiving IB than in those receiving saline ($P = .02$). (Reprinted by permission, from Qureshi F, Pestian J, Davis P, et al: Effect of nebulized IB on the hospitalization rates of children with asthma. *N Engl J Med* 339:1030-1035, 1998. Copyright 1998, Massachusetts Medical Society. All rights reserved.)

(2.5 mL) of IB with the second and third doses of albuterol. Both treatment groups were observed for rates of hospitalization.

Results.—Children in the IB group had a significantly lower hospitalization rate than children in the placebo group (27.4% vs 36.5%). Hospitalization rates were similar for both groups in children with moderate asthma. For children with severe asthma, the addition of IB significantly diminished the need for hospitalization (37.5%, IB group; 52.6%, placebo) (Fig 1). The asthma score improved more often in patients treated with IB, than with saline treatment.

Conclusion.—The addition of IB to a nebulized β₂-adrenergic agonist has an additive effect of enhancing pulmonary function in children with severe asthma. The results suggest that treatment with IB could prevent approximately 14% of children with severe asthma from requiring hospitalization. This represents a substantial reduction in the national cost for this disease.

▶ Daniel I. Craven, M.D., Rainbow Babies and Children's Hospital, Cleveland, Ohio, comments:

Previous randomized, double-blind, placebo-controlled trials (RCTs) have provided less than overwhelming evidence that the laboratory and theoretical advantages of combined therapy with inhaled β-agonists and IB translates into improved lung function, or, more importantly, better clinical outcomes in the treatment of status asthmaticus. Some trials in adults have demonstrated nominal, but statistically significant, lung function benefits with combination therapy, while others detected no additional bronchodilation, and only 1 established a statistically significant reduction in hospitalization rate from the addition of anticholinergic therapy in the emergency room (ER) treatment of non-COPD asthmatics.[1] Even a pooled analysis of more than 900 adults from 3 ER trials showed only a trend of modest additional improvement in FEV_1 (.047L) and reduction in hospitalization rate (14% vs. 18%) for those patients treated with IB.[2]

The majority of RCTs studying children with acute asthma presenting to the ER demonstrate improved reduction in airway obstruction with the addition of inhaled anticholinergic therapy, although the detected effect size has been typically modest. Reduction in hospitalization rate from the addition of IB occurred in only 1 prior study, but the effect reached statistical significance only in the subgroup of children with FEV_1 less than 30% predicted.[3] However, the small size of this "ultra-severe" subgroup, and the fact that systemic corticosteroids were not administered during the study, detracts somewhat from the impact of the results.

The findings of Dr. Qureshi and colleagues, when considered in context with other published evidence, justify the addition of nebulized IB to adrenergic agents to enhance bronchodilation and reduce hospitalization rate for asthmatic children that present to the ER with acute severe airway obstruction. Their data also verify that the routine addition of IB in the ER treatment of children with less-than-severe exacerbations provides no additional clinically relevant benefit. These findings are complemented by another recent RCT that found no benefit in hospitalization rate or respiratory resistance from the addition of a single dose of IB to nebulized β-agonist therapy in children presenting with mild to moderate asthma exacerbations.[4] Although it may be tempting to do so, the results of this study cannot be reasonably extrapolated to justify the routine use of IB for hospitalized children with acute asthma as a means to hasten the resolution of symptoms and reduce length of stay. Nor should IB be routinely utilized for the management of chronic asthma. In these settings, the efficacy of IB remains inadequately supported by existing evidence, and its use should remain individualized until better data accumulate.

D.I. Craven, M.D.

References

1. Lin RY, Pesola GR, Bakalchuk L, et al: Superiority of ipratropium bromide over albuterol alone in the emergency department management of adult asthma: A randomized clinical trial. *Ann Emerg Med* 31:208-213, 1998.
2. Lanes SF, Garrett JE, Wentworth CD, et al: The effect of adding ipratropium bromide to salbutamol in the treatment of acute asthma: A pooled analysis of three trials. *Chest* 114:365-372, 1998.
3. Schuh S, Johnson DW, Callahan S, et al: Efficacy of frequent nebulized ipratropium bromide added to frequent high dose albuterol therapy in severe childhood asthma. *J Pediatr* 126:639-645, 1995.
4. Ducharme FM, Davis GM: Randomized controlled trial of ipratropium bromide and frequent low doses of salbutamol in the management of mild and moderate acute pediatric asthma. *J Pediatr* 133:479-485, 1998.

▶ The use of nebulized IB has received so much press this past year that we decided to continue the discussion of its pros and cons with another commentary. Suzanne Schuh, M.D., F.R.C.P.C., staff physician, Division of Emergency Pediatrics, associate scientist, Research Institute, The Children's Hospital for Sick Children, and associate professor of Pediatrics, University of Toronto, comments:

This paper is a timely one because it addresses the ongoing controversy about which children with acute asthma should be treated with nebulized IB. The best trial outcome to choose to convince the medical community about efficacy of a drug is the hospitalization rate. This is precisely what the authors did. To be able to analyze clinically meaningful differences in this outcome with a high degree of confidence requires a large sample size. The numbers need to be augmented even further to address the outcomes in subjects with a severe versus moderate degree of illness. Qureshi and her colleagues designed the study well to satisfy these tough requirements. The physicians making the decisions about disposition need to be blinded to the study results to avoid bias.

This landmark study very much strengthens the evidence that IB therapy is beneficial for children with severe acute asthma exacerbations, whereas those with moderate severity do not appear to derive significant benefit. Since most emergency attendings do not do pulmonary function testing, and because clinical scores largely represent a research tool, the decision to treat with IB is a clinical one.

Another controversial topic regarding IB is the optimum number of doses to administer. Although the existing literature supports using at least 2 to 3 consecutive doses, until further evidence arises, it may be advisable to titrate the number of doses to the clinical response.

S. Schuh, M.D., F.R.C.P.C.

A Comparison of Active and Simulated Chiropractic Manipulation as Adjunctive Treatment for Childhood Asthma
Balon J, Aker PD, Crowther ER, et al (Canadian Mem Chiropractic College, Toronto; Los Angeles Colleges of Chiropractic, Los Angeles; McMaster Univ, Hamilton, Ont; et al)
N Engl J Med 339:1013-1020, 1998   4–5

Introduction.—Several chiropractors and osteopaths report that chiropractic treatments are beneficial for nonmusculoskeletal conditions, including asthma. The beneficial effect in patients with asthma is based on 2 assumptions: (1) Reflex irritation of somatic and autonomic nerves at the spinal and nerve-root levels is the result of vertebral subluxation; and (2) this mechanical and neurologic disturbance influences chest wall function or alters airway tone or responsiveness directly or by means of neurogenic inflammation. Objective and subjective outcomes were assessed in children with asthma who were treated with active or simulated chiropractic manipulation in a randomized, controlled trial.

Methods.—Age range was 7 to 12 years in 91 children who required the use of a bronchodilator at least 3 times weekly for mild to moderate asthma. All children had continuing symptoms of asthma, despite usual medical treatment. Patients were randomized to 4 months of either active treatment or simulated chiropractic manipulation. No patients had received previous chiropractic care. Chiropractic visits were 3 times weekly for 4 weeks, twice weekly for 4 weeks, then weekly for 8 weeks. Research subjects were required to receive 20 to 36 treatments during the 4-month evaluation period. Patients were observed for change from baseline in peak expiratory flow before bronchodilator use. The frequency of morning peak expiratory flow falling below 85% of baseline value was compared in both groups.

Results.—Adequate data were available for 38 patients in the active treatment group and 42 patients in the control group. Patients in both groups experienced small increases of 7 to 12 L per minute peak expiratory flow in the morning and in the evening. The degree of change from baseline values was not significant in either group. Both groups experienced a decrease in symptoms of asthma and in use of β-agonists and an increase in quality of life; between-group differences were not significant. Most patients (63%) were not aware of whether they were in the active or simulated treatment group.

Conclusion.—Patients in the active treatment and simulated treatment groups had similar improvements in symptoms, quality of life, and reduced β-agonist use. Airway responsiveness did not change significantly in either group. The addition of chiropractic manipulation in the treatment of asthma in children offered no improvement in disease control. Earlier trials reporting the benefit of chiropractic treatment in children with asthma were not adequately controlled. Investigations of efficacy of treatment need to be adequately controlled, randomized, and blinded. The lack of airway responsiveness in this cohort suggests that improvements in the other parameters may be the result of a placebo or study effect. Other trials have reported that other alternative therapies, including hypnosis, acupuncture, and yoga, are effective in treating asthma.

▶ There is nothing wrong with alternative medicine except when it is unorthodox. You can be the judge whether acupuncture, homeopathy, yoga, hypnosis, chiropractic treatment, and herbal medicine are so unorthodox as to border on voodoo medicine. Clearly, some of each of these alternative therapies are meritorious and some are not. The trick is to figure out which is which. In some cases of asthma, hypnosis, acupuncture, and yoga may be of benefit. It is a stretch, though, to think that manipulating the spine would be of any benefit. Indeed, this form of chiropractic is about as useless as cracking one's knuckles in relieving reactive airway disease.

It was just in the last couple of years that the National Institutes of Health formed a specific working group dealing with alternative medicine. This was a reasonable decision. It will be a challenge to see whether this and other committed groups can separate the wheat from the chaff. Are you a conformist or a nonconformist when it comes to strict devotion to orthodox medicine?

One final reminder: The only thing a nonconformist hates worse than a conformist is another nonconformist who is failing to conform to the prevailing standards of nonconformity.

J.A. Stockman III, M.D.

Growth Hormone Treatment in Pediatric Burns: A Safe Therapeutic Approach

Ramirez RJ, Wolf SE, Barrow RE, et al (Univ of Texas, Galveston)
Ann Surg 228:439-448, 1998   4–6

Background.—For more than 10 years, these authors have been using recombinant human growth hormone (rhGH) to treat children with severe burns. However, a recent European report on adult ICU patients without burns indicates that adults given rhGH have twice the mortality rates of patients not given rhGH (42% vs 18%). Thus to reconfirm the safety of this protocol, these authors compared mortality and morbidity rates using rhGH with placebo in children with severe burns.

Methods.—The study included 263 patients aged between 1 and 18 years who had severe burns over more than 40% of their body surface area and more than 10% third-degree burns requiring skin grafting. In a randomized, prospective, double-blind study, 48 children received rhGH, 0.2 mg/kg/day subcutaneously, and 54 received placebo. Children in the randomized study were admitted within 3 days of the injury. An additional 82 younger and sicker children were given rhGH upon their transfer to the authors' institution, sometimes more than 8 days after injury (i.e., they were given rhGH for salvage). These patients were matched for age, sex, and burn size with 48 contiguous control patients. Finally, another 31 patients admitted after the European study was published and who received no rhGH were also studied as a control group. Exogenous albumin, insulin, calcium, and phosphorous were given as needed to maintain colloid osmotic pressures, euglycemia, normocalcemia, and normophosphatemia. Heart rates, rate-pressure products, complications, and deaths were compared between the 5 patient groups.

Findings.—Between all 5 groups, there were no significant differences in heart rate or rate-pressure product at any times measured. In the randomized study, the rhGH and placebo groups had similar rates of death (2% vs 2%), septic complications (23% vs 20%), renal failure (2% vs 2%), and cardiac arrest (6% vs 0%). Among the other 3 groups, mortality rates in the 82 children receiving rhGH were lower (10%) than in the other 2 groups of control subjects (17% and 13%). Overall, 22 of the 263 patients died; in no case was the use of rhGH implicated as a direct or associated cause of death. In the randomized study, patients receiving rhGH were significantly more likely to experience hyperglycemia (63% vs 41%) and to require exogenous insulin (46% vs 24%) than the patients receiving placebo. However, patients receiving rhGH also required significantly less exogenous albumin (75 vs 210 g) and calcium (69% vs 87%).

Conclusions.—In these children with severe burns, the use of rhGH was safe and efficacious. Mortality rates did not differ between patients receiving rhGH or placebo, nor did the rates of clinically significant complications or organ failure. However, patients receiving rhGH required much less exogenous albumin and calcium, and the higher rate of hyperglycemia in this group was effectively treated with insulin.

▶ You may not have been following the story that has suggested that children with burns may be benefitted by growth hormone therapy. This has been a quite controversial topic. The authors of this article are the ones who have previously noted and reported on the benefits of growth hormone treatment of children with burns. They have used this modality of therapy for more than a decade and their data have suggested that hospital stays are shorter (by 25%) and skin graft donor sites heal more quickly (up to 30% faster) when growth hormone is administered as part of the overall management of the burned child. The controversy relates to recent data from Europe that indicate that adults treated with growth hormone have more than a 2-fold greater probability of dying (42% vs 18% in untreated patients with serious burns).[1] Despite the adult data, further study of children seems to show little in the way for potential for deleterious side effects given the results from the Shriners Burns Hospital, Galveston, Texas.

The bottom line of any study examining growth hormone as part of the treatment of burns will have to look at risk-benefit ratios and cost effectiveness. The data regarding the latter are beginning to emerge. For example, the average 8-year-old with an 80% total body surface burn will consume about $12,000 in growth hormone therapy if the amount of growth hormone used is the same as in this article. The length of hospital stay for the same patient will decrease from 1 day per percent degree burn if given placebo to 0.66 days for each percent total body burn if growth hormone therapy is given. Even paying for the drug, the overall hospital cost for such a patient would be reduced by about $40,000.

Please note, rhGH has not been approved by the FDA for treating burns. There are still many unknowns. Centers that do use growth hormone therapy should keep very accurate records of what they are doing so that eventually we will know not only the benefits of such treatment, but also the potential harm. Only when bolstered with a "total" picture of what is going on can we adequately provide informed consent for our patients and their parents. In the meantime, 3 cheers for the Shriners Burns Hospital in Galveston for tossing the ball in the air when it comes to growth hormone and the treatment of burns. Hopefully it will land in the end zone for a touchdown some time in the near future.

J.A. Stockman III, M.D.

Reference

1. Public communications from Pharmacia & Upjohn Pharmaceuticals and Rolf Gunnarsson, M.D. to all industry and medical community involved with use or potential use of recombinant human growth hormone. October 31, 1997.

A Randomized, Vehicle-controlled Trial of Tacrolimus Ointment for Treatment of Atopic Dermatitis in Children

Boguniewicz M, Fiedler VC, Raimer S, et al (Univ of Colorado, Denver; Univ of Illinois, Chicago; Univ of Texas, Galveston; et al)

J Allergy Clin Immunol 102:637-644, 1998   4–7

Introduction.—The most common chronic skin disease in children is atopic dermatitis, which is characterized by chronic skin inflammation, cutaneous erythema, induration, severe pruritus, overexpression of inter-leukin 10, high immunoglobulin E levels, and eosinophilia. An immuno-suppressive agent with a spectrum of activity similar to that of cyclospo-rine is tacrolimus, which is currently used to prevent allograft rejection in liver and kidney transplantation. In a previous study of adults, it was found that treatment of atopic dermatitis with topical tacrolimus resulted in markedly diminished pruritus and skin inflammation. No previous studies have determined the effect of tacrolimus on children with atopic dermatitis. The efficacy and applicability of topically applied tacrolimus ointment in childhood atopic dermatitis were assessed.

Methods.—The study included 180 children aged from 7 to 16 years with moderate-to-severe atopic dermatitis covering 5% to 30% of their

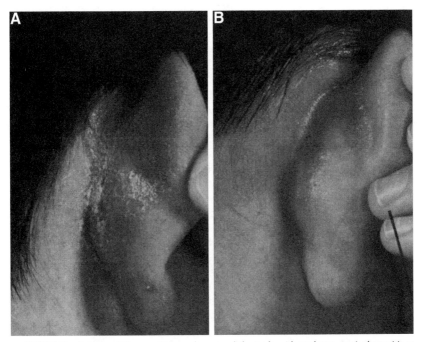

FIGURE 2.—Left ear of 12-year-old boy who entered the study with moderate atopic dermatitis at baseline (**A**) and day 15 (**B**). Improvement was noted by physician beginning on day 4 of treatment with 0.03% tacrolimus ointment. (Courtesy of Boguniewicz M, Fiedler VC, Raimer S, et al: A randomized, vehicle-controlled trial of tacrolimus ointment for treatment of atopic dermatitis in children. *J Allergy Clin Immunol* 102:637-644, 1998.)

body surface area. They received 1 of 4 treatments: 44 received vehicle; 43 received 0.03% tacrolimus ointment; 49 received 0.1% tacrolimus ointment; and 44 received 0.3% tacrolimus ointment.

Results.—A marked-to-excellent, (75% or more) improvement was found in 69% of children in the 0.03% tacrolimus ointment group, in 67% of the children in the 0.1% tacrolimus ointment group, and in 70% of the children in the 0.3% tacrolimus ointment group (Fig 2). These results were in comparison to only 38% in the vehicle group. For the 0.03% tacrolimus ointment group, the mean percent improvement for a modified Eczema Area and Severity Index at end of treatment was 72%; for the 0.1% group, it was 77%; and for the 0.3% group, it was 81%. This was significantly better than the 26% found in the vehicle group. A significantly greater median percent reduction in pruritus in the tacrolimus-treated patients (74%-89%) was found when compared to the vehicle-treated patients (51%). No serious systemic adverse events and minimal systemic absorption were noted.

Conclusion.—In children with atopic dermatitis, tacrolimus ointment is apparently safe and effective. Long-term studies are in progress to study the 1-year effects.

▶ It's interesting to see how quickly the discipline of immunodermatology has evolved. It is also fascinating to see how our understanding of atopic dermatitis has changed. It has become one of the most common immune disturbances of childhood. A decade or more ago, one would have never believed that the treatment of eczema would be based on an understanding of how skin inflammation relates to overexpression of certain cytokines, such as interleukin 10. Sure, we used topical steroids knowing that the skin was inflamed, but little did we know how or why steroids even worked. As importantly, we knew that steroids didn't always work, particularly in severe cases, and could result in growth retardation and adrenal problems on occasion.

Cyclosporine was the first "potent" alternative immunoregulatory agent to be used when steroids failed. It can be quite effective, but it must be given orally, and it is quite expensive. Additionally, it can have significant systemic toxicities. The latter has limited its use. Topical therapy is ineffective. This is where tacrolimus or FK506 comes in. This is an immunosuppressive agent isolated from an organism *Streptomyces tsukubaensis.* This drug has been found to be effective in preventing liver and kidney rejection following transplantation. It has a much smaller molecular weight and higher potency in comparison with cyclosporine, making it ideal as a topical agent. It does its job in the treatment of atopic dermatitis without producing blood levels that are known to be associated with toxicity. It is minimally absorbed through even inflamed skin. You can be guaranteed that you will be reading more about this interesting ointment. This editor has not yet seen any estimates about what it will cost.

A fast fact having to do with eczema. The first is that exposure to hard water in the home may increase the risk of eczema in children of primary school age.[1] McNally et al. have shown in a study of over 4000 randomly selected primary school-aged children, the more a home's water is like dilute cement, the more likely it is that children in that home will have eczema. This is true independently of whether or not there is a family history of allergy.

If you believe the linkage of atopic eczema with water hardness is a bunch of bologna, you won't think too much of the abstract that follows which suggests that when all else fails, you might try some massage therapy on your patients with refractory eczema.

J.A. Stockman III, M.D.

Reference

1. McNally NJ, Williams HC, Phillips DR, et al: Atopic eczema and domestic water hardness. *Lancet* 352:527-531, 1998.

Atopic Dermatitis Symptoms Decreased in Children Following Massage Therapy

Schachner L, Field T, Hernandez-Reif M, et al (Univ of Miami, Fla)
Pediatr Dermatol 15:390-395, 1998

4–8

Introduction.—Depression, stress, and anxiety have been correlated with the severity of atopic dermatitis, which may cause negative effects on the immune system via stress-increased cortisol levels. Described as a "shock organ" for emotional stress, the skin may manifest the stress in the form of a skin disease. A stress therapy may be a helpful adjunct to this disease, and massage therapy is a possibility because it requires less compliance from children, it may increase peripheral blood supply, and it may increase vagal activity. Massage therapy could also be provided by the child's parents. The effectiveness of stress therapy was assessed.

Methods.—The study included 20 children with atopic dermatitis who were massaged by their parents for 20 minutes daily for 1 month and treated with standard topical care. The effectiveness of their treatment was compared to a control group receiving standard topical care only.

Results.—Immediately after the massage therapy sessions, the children's affect and activity level significantly improved, and their parent's anxiety decreased. Lower anxiety levels in children were reported by parents of massaged children during the 1-month period. Significant improvements in all clinical measures were seen among the massaged children, including redness, scaling, lichenification, excoriation, and pruritus. A significant improvement was also seen in the control group in the scaling measure.

Conclusion.—For atopic dermatitis, massage therapy may be a cost-effective adjunct treatment, because there is only a one-time expense for the child to receive the massage and the parent to learn the technique. To explore residual or longer-term effects of massage therapy, futher research is required.

▶ Fascinating report. Now I know why I have never seen a boxer with eczema. Their "rub downs" are prophylactic.

So is stress reduction therapy some form of sorcery or is it truly a hopeful adjunct in the management of atopic dermatitis? The data suggest the latter. Indeed, when one thinks about it, relaxation therapy might be associated with a reduction in the tendency to itch and scratch. It could reduce stress and anxiety. It could increase peripheral blood supply. By reducing vagal activity (a known consequence of massage therapy), it could reduce peripheral vasoconstriction. If nothing else, a good massage just might make a child feel better.

This editor has never had a "proper" massage by a masseur. Given the prices involved, he is not likely to either. On a recent jaunt through the undergrounds at O'Hare Airport, there was a sign advertising massages at the Airport Hilton ($60.00 an hour). If the math is correct, the average masseur grosses $128,000 a year...not bad for someone who rubs you the right way. Please note, however, that if massage therapy ever does catch on as part of the treatment of atopic dermatitis, parents can learn this technique for about $30.00 (the published figure this report). If this form of therapy fails to work, at least the parents will have learned a new occupation.

By the way, in case you forgot, if the father does the massaging, the correct term is that he is a "masseur," if the mother does it, she is a masseuse. For the afficionados of the English language, the correct terminology for referring to one who gives a massage when one does not describe the gender of the massager is the word "massagist," not to be confused with a masochist...enough of Webster.

J.A. Stockman III, M.D.

Atopic Eczema and Domestic Water Hardness

McNally NJ, Williams HC, Phillips DR, et al (Univ of Nottingham, Univ Park, England; Queen's Med Centre, Nottingham, England; City Hosp, Nottingham, England)
Lancet 352:527–531, 1998   4–9

Purpose.—Although the causes of atopic eczema are unclear, many think environmental factors play an important role. One possible risk factor, which epidemiologic studies have not addressed, is domestic water supply, specifically exposure to hard water. This ecologic study examined the association between hard water exposure and prevalence of eczema in children.

Methods.—The analysis included questionnaire data on eczema and other atopic disorders collected from the parents of 4141 primary school children and 3499 secondary school children from 1 English district. Using information from the water company, domestic water hardness was classified into 4 categories. Water hardness was linked to eczema prevalence, with adjustment for sex, age, socioeconomic status, and access to health care.

Results.—Before and after adjustment, primary school children showed a significant and direct relationship between domestic water hardness and lifetime prevalence of eczema. Children in the highest water-hardness category had a 1-year period prevalence of 17%, compared with 12% for those in the lowest category (adjusted odds ratio 1:54). Lifetime prevalences of eczema for these groups were 25% and 21%, respectively (adjusted odds ratio 1:28). Water hardness did not significantly affect eczema prevalence for secondary school children. Primary school children exposed to higher water chlorine contents were also more likely to develop eczema. However, this trend was no longer significant after adjustment for confounding factors.

Conclusions.—Exposure to hard water at home is apparently a significant risk factor for eczema in primary school children. This effect appears age-related, because it does not appear in secondary school children. The findings await replication in other geographic locations, after studying the effects of water hardness in individual patients with eczema.

▶ This is the first article in a long time that has attempted to associate the hardness of home water with the prevalence of eczema. If the association between water hardness and eczema is real, what explains it? Water hardness may act more on existing eczema—exacerbating the disorder or prolonging its duration—than actually cause eczema. The stronger association with recent than with lifetime atopic eczema symptoms supports this argument. Calcium and magnesium (the minerals that make water hard) may act as a direct chemical irritant. I theorize that the association between water hardness and eczema, if real, may arise indirectly from the need for more soap and shampoo to obtain a lather when washing and bathing in hard water. It is known that increased exposure to soaps and their additives can have an irritant effect on the skin, which could exacerbate eczema in predisposed children.

On a slightly different topic, allergic disorders (particularly reactive airway disease) tend to occur more frequently in cities with high population concentrations per square mile. The following 5 cities have the greatest density of people, and might therefore be avoided if you get an allergic claustrophobia: New York (23,617 persons per square mile), San Francisco (15,609), Jersey City (15,341), Chicago (12,185), and Philadelphia (11,492). If it is elbow room you desire, there is always Anchorage, at 145 folks per square mile, or next to the least in line, Oklahoma City at 746.[1]

We'll need to wait to see if there are more scientific links described between water hardness and the prevalence of eczema. If such a link is unequivocally shown, some families will benefit from the help of a water treatment specialist...hey, Culligan man.

J.A. Stockman III, M.D.

Reference

1. United States Census Bureau: *City and County Data Book* 1994.

Side to Side Comparison of Topical Treatment in Atopic Dermatitis
Ainely-Walker PF, Patel L, David TJ (Univ of Manchester, England)
Arch Dis Child 79:149-152, 1998   4–10

Introduction.—Topical application of emollients and corticosteroids is the main treatment of atopic dermatitis. Much variation occurs with atopic dermatitis, making it difficult to evaluate the effectiveness of any treatment. In clinical trials of various topical treatments, side-to-side comparisons have been used. To determine the most effective topical treatment for children admitted to hospital for control of atopic dermatitis, the outcome of side-to-side comparisons of different corticosteroids were documented and assessed in a retrospective review.

Methods.—The records of 66 children with atopic dermatitis admitted to a children's hospital from June 1993 to October 1995 were reviewed. Applications of different topical corticosteroid ointments were given to the 2 sides of the body. A comparison between the 2 sides was conducted to determine which treatment was better.

Results.—On 25 occasions, more potent topical corticosteroid preparations appeared more effective than weaker preparations. On 20 occasions, there were no differences. A weaker preparation appeared more effective than a stronger one on 7 occasions. The efficacy of a preparation was not increased with the incorporation of an antimicrobial agent.

Conclusion.—Considerable spontaneous fluctuations in severity bedevil the management of atopic dermatitis, leading to uncertainty in determining whether new treatments are beneficial. A particular treatment may be wrongly implicated in a coincidental flare-up of the skin lesions. A feasible and rational way to determine the optimum treatment for an individual with atopic dermatitis is by comparing different topical treatments simultaneously on opposite sides of the body.

▶ This editor always thought that a side-to-side comparison of a treatment involved lining 2 people up who are otherwise perfectly matched and treating one 1 way and the other another way. Well, that apparently isn't needed with atopic dermatitis, since when it comes to dermatologic problems, you can treat your patient as if he or she had schizophrenia. Each side of the patient becomes an object of study. This allows 2 different topical agents to be given at the same time to opposite sides of the body in order to determine which one might work best. One can even use the same topical agent in differing concentrations. In the case of the report abstracted, the investigators used 2 levels of concentrations for the application of topical corticosteroid ointments. Interestingly, the weaker steroid fared as well as the more concentrated steroid, if not better, for most patients. Such a short trial has some practical implications in the sense that after a brief period of evaluation, one can quickly move to that topical agent which seems to work best rather than trying 1 therapy after another in sequence.

It is gratifying to learn the value of side-to-side comparisons of topical therapies. Next we'll be seeing "head-to-head" investigations of dandruff treatments (or is that "shoulder-to-shoulder"?). Or maybe sore "knee-to-knee" trials of Ben-Gay (Pfizer). Or perhaps eczematous "cheek-to-cheek" studies of tacrolimus.

Before you jump on the bandwagon of side-to-side comparisons of topical treatments, realize that your managed care organization may balk when seeing 2 prescriptions come through at the same time for treating the same problem. Whoever said that we live in a perfect world.

J.A. Stockman III, M.D.

Cutaneous Manifestations of Childhood Systemic Lupus Erythematosus

Wananukul S, Watana D, Pongprasit P (Chulalongkorn Univ, Bangkok, Thailand)
Pediatr Dermatol 15:342–346, 1998   4–11

Background.—Four of the 11 criteria for classifying systemic lupus erythematosus (SLE), according to the American College of Rheumatology, relate to cutaneous lesions. A detailed study of cutaneous lesions in childhood SLE was done.

TABLE 1.—Clinical Manifestations of 57 Children With SLE

Manifestations	Number of Patients	Percent
Renal	48	84
Skin lesion	44	77
Fever	23	40
Arthritis/arthralgia	22	39
Neurologic/psychiatric	12	21
Serositis	11	19
Pleural	5	9
Pericardial	7	12
Hematologic	33	58
Anemia	21	39
Leukopenia	10	19
Lymphopenia	9	18
Thrombocytopenia	10	18
Immunologic	25	45
LE	20	36
Anti-DNA	25	45
ANA	52	93
Depressed CH_{50}	50	88

TABLE 2.—Mucocutaneous Manifestations in 57 Patients

Manifestations	Number of Patients	Percent
Skin lesion; all types	44	77
Malar rash	42	74
Vasculitis	24	42
Raynaud's phenomenon	4	7
Periungual erythema	5	9
Bullous LE	1	2
Periungual gangrene	2	4
Nail involvement	2	4
Alopecia	18	32
Diffuse	15	26
Scarring	3	5
Subacute LE	2	4
Discoid LE	11	19
Photosensitivity	23	40
Oral ulcer	26	46

(Reprinted by permission of Blackwell Science, Inc., from Wananukul S, Watana D, Pongprasit P: Cutaneous manifestations of childhood systemic lupus erythematosus. *Pediatr Dermatol* 15[5]:342-346, 1998.)

Methods and Findings.—Fifty-seven children with classical SLE seen in a 6-year period were assessed. The children's ages at diagnosis ranged from 4 to 15 years, with a mean of 11.9 years. The ratio of females to males was 4.2:1. Seventy-seven percent of the children had cutaneous manifestations. Mucocutaneous signs were the second most common finding, next to renal involvement, which was present in 84%. Skin changes included malar rash, present in 74%; oral ulcer, in 46%; vasculitis, in 42%; photosensitivity, in 40%; alopecia, in 32%; and discoid lupus erythematosus (LE), in 19%. All of the patients with discoid LE were girls. Rarely seen manifestations were periungual erythema, Raynaud's phenomenon, periungual gangrene, nail involvement, and subacute LE. Antinuclear antibody reaction and anti-dsDNA were positive in 93% and 46%, respectively. Eight children died, 6 from severe infection and 2 from renal failure (Tables 1 and 2).

Conclusions.—The clinical manifestations of childhood SLE are similar to those of SLE in adulthood. Most children have multisystem involvement. In all age groups, females are affected predominantly. The presence of cutaneous lesions is important in the diagnosis of SLE. In this series, malar rash was the most common cutaneous manifestation, followed by oral ulcer, photosensitivity, and sensitivity. The incidence of skin manifestations in SLE may vary by age and among regions.

▶ This article is included in the 2000 YEAR BOOK OF PEDIATRICS to remind us of how commonly certain clinical manifestations show themselves in the presentation of SLE in children. In particular, the tip-off in most patients is the set of skin findings most patients present. Only 3 cutaneous presentations, however, are highly specific for lupus. These are malar rash, subacute cutaneous LE, and discoid LE.

The large majority of patients with lupus (some 74%) will have a malar rash. This can vary from a mild redness to a more severe erythematous, sharply demarcated eruption over the bridge of the nose and cheeks, with sparing of the nasolabial folds. The rash frequently follows sun exposure. Malar rash is clearly the hallmark of lupus, but it is not 100% sensitive nor 100% specific for this disease. Malar rash is more common in children than in adults, at least as noted in most reported series.

The subacute cutaneous findings of lupus are polycyclic erythema and psoriasiform lesions. These are relatively uncommon in children (perhaps about 5% will have these). They are usually widespread, symmetrical, and nonscarring on sun-exposed areas.

Chronic discoid lesions are seen in some 15% to 90% of children with lupus. Discoid lesions are much more common in girls. Interestingly, discoid lesions may be found in both light-exposed and light-protected areas of skin.

Children with lupus can have a variety of other less specific skin findings. For example, as many as half of children with lupus will have photosensitivity. As many as half of children will also show evidence of skin vasculitis in the form of petechiae, palpable purpura, urticaria, nodules, ulceration, and livido reticularis.

To say all this differently, while SLE is a multisystem disease, it is the skin findings that are critically important in its diagnosis. If you care for a child with lupus or merely want to know more about this disorder, this report should be on your "must" reading list.

The Allergy and Dermatology chapter is almost at a close, and this is one of the few YEAR BOOKS OF PEDIATRICS that has had nothing on the risks of sun exposure in it. So, here are a few fast facts about UV radiation, skin cancer, and how to protect yourself. First, stay out of the sun. One way of doing that is to stay in the shade, but recognize that not all shade is the same. For example, if you were under a shade tree, the mean UV protection is equivalent to a sunscreen with a sun protection factor (SPF) of 4.2 if you are flat on your back, but only 1.3 if you are standing up. The only shade that is sufficient to protect with the equivalent of an SPF greater than 15 would be the shade of a thickly wooded forest in which you could not see the sky.[1]

If you really want to protect yourself against UV radiation, please recognize that there is a very simple rule of thumb in this regard. The intensity of UV radiation is inversely proportional to the length of a person's shadow: when the shadow is shorter than you are, you should find shade. This rule applies whether you are a governor of Minnesota or Danny DeVito.[2]

Lastly, if you want to start a screening program for skin cancer, Sutton's Law would tell you where to start. Willie, as you will recall, when asked why he robbed banks, stated that it was because that was "where the money was." Most skin cancer screening programs unfortunately attract the "worried well," while those who are at greatest risk for skin cancer are less likely to attend. Take, for example, the skin cancer screening offered through the 1992 American Academy of Dermatology meeting, which sponsored a free cancer screening program on the beach (in this case the Texas Gulf Coast beach). This program showed that young surfers had a remarkably higher incidence of skin cancers, particularly basal cell carcinomas, in comparison with aged-matched populations.[3]

I can see it now: preventative cardiologists will hang out in restaurants to pick out those who have adverse risk factors for hypercholesterolemia and ischemic heart disease. Urologists will inhabit men's rooms to listen to the sounds to see who might have obstructive uropathies, and so on, and so on. Life does seem easier for the dermatologists, when it comes to screening programs, doesn't it?

J.A. Stockman III, M.D.

References

1. Parsons PJ, Neal R, Wolsk P, et al: Protection of UV exposure by shade. *Med J Aust* 168:327-330, 1998.
2. Keaveney J: Ultraviolet exposure. *South Med J* 91:619-623, 1998.
3. Dozier S, Wagner RF: Beachfront screening for skin cancer in Texas Gulf Coast surfers. *South Med J* 90:55-58, 1997.

The Natural History of Condyloma in Children
Allen AL, Siegfried EC (Saint Louis Univ, St Louis)
J Am Acad Dermatol 39:951-955, 1998   4–12

Introduction.—Since 1990, clinicians have reported increasing numbers of children with condyloma, also known as venereal warts. This increase in affected children probably reflects the prevalence of human papillomavirus in adults. Transmission can occur at birth, from warts on the hands of caregivers, or in the setting of sexual abuse. A cohort of children with condyloma was reviewed to determine the natural history of the warts in pediatric patients.

Methods.—Seventy-five cases were initially identified, and 41 (54%) had sufficient information to be included in the final analysis. Data recorded were age at onset, gender, duration of condyloma, distribution, and all treatments (Table 3). The parents or guardians of 38 children were successfully contacted by telephone; 15 agreed to follow-up examination. Three patients who were not contacted had sufficient chart information for inclusion. Outcome was defined as treatment-associated resolution (warts

TABLE 3.—Distribution by Age and Gender

	Perianal	Anogenital	Genital	Inguinal
Boys	5 (50%)	2 (18%)	2 (18%)	1 (9%)
Girls	15 (48%)	9 (29%)	6 (19%)	1 (3%)
Age (y)				
Average	3.6	2.8	3.2	5
(range)	(0.1-10)	(0.5-5.5)	(0.5-8)	(3-7)

(Courtesy of Allen AL, Siegfried EC: The natural history of condyloma in children. *J Am Acad Dermatol* 39:951-955, 1998.)

resolved within 1 month after completion of therapy) or as spontaneous resolution (condyloma resolved without therapy or more than 1 month after completion of unsuccessful therapy).

Results.—Thirty-three children (80%) received therapy and 31 (76%) had complete clinical resolution. Therapies included cimetidine, pulsed-dye laser, salicylic acid, cryotherapy, and acyclovir. Six of the 8 untreated children experienced spontaneous regression. Nine of the 33 treated children (27%) had resolution of the warts during treatment. There were 3 times as many girls as boys in the cohort, and resolution occurred comparatively more often in girls. Five of the 10 boys in the cohort had resolution of condyloma; 1 had resolution related to therapy.

Discussion.—In this group of children with condyloma, the rate of treatment-related resolution was no higher than the rate of spontaneous resolution. Active nonintervention for at least 1 year is a reasonable approach and nonpainful methods should be considered as first-line therapy.

▶ Thank goodness that not everything is like herpes—that is, not everything is forever. Human papilloma virus infection causing condyloma will self-resolve, at least in the majority of children and adolescents who become infected. In fact, venereal warts go away as quickly without treatment as with treatment, usually within a period of 1 to 2 years. Those in the pediatric population contract human papilloma virus by vertical transmission, by sexual contact, or by innocent contact. Perinatal transmission of oropharyngeal or genital sites occurs in as many as half of infants delivered vaginally of infected mothers. Pediatric condyloma can also be caused by human papillomavirus 2, typically found in common cutaneous warts. Children with such warts can autoinoculate their genital areas, causing condyloma. Lastly, condyloma can occur in the setting of sexual abuse; all children presenting with condyloma should be assessed for the possibility of such abuse.

This is the last commentary in the chapter on allergy and dermatology, so we'll close with some information about the skin. In the 1997 YEAR BOOK OF PEDIATRICS, we informed the reader that something having to do with the skin represented the longest word in the English language (15 letters) that uses no letter twice. It is the word "dermatoglyphics," the elegant version of the word for fingerprints. To expand on this topic, the word dermatoglyphics was invented in 1926 by Harold Cummings and Charles Midlo and was used for the first time in a paper on what they called "epidermal ridge configurations" when they restricted its use to ridges and their arrangements, including flexion creases and other secondary folds.[1] It derives from 2 Greek words loosely translated to derma (the skin) and gloupho (I sculpt).

"Fingerprints" have been around for centuries. They were used by the Greeks as signatures before the final firing of vases. In India, a fingerprint used as a signature was thought to be specific for an illiterate person and was known as "tipsahi," but fingerprints were first systematically described by Johannes Evangelista Purkinje in his thesis, *Commentatis de Examine Physiologico Rogani visus et Systematis Cutanei*, published in Breslau in 1823. Fingerprints were really put on the map by the astronomer William

Herschel (The Younger), who first devised a method for printing them in 1858, and by Francis Jolton, the geneticist, who in 1892 wrote a book, *Fingerprints*, about the differences in skin creases between individuals.

Finally, a question: which animal has fingerprints more closely resembling those of humans: the koala bear or the chimpanzee? It is the koala bear. As an aside, evolutionists believe that fingerprints developed over time in certain animal species as an aid to climbing.[2]

J.A. Stockman III, M.D.

References

1. Cummings H, Midlo C: Epidermal ridge configurations. *Am J Physiol Anthropol* 9:471-502, 1926.
2. Aronson J: Fingerprints. *BMJ* 315:930, 1997.

5 Miscellaneous

Would You Say You "Had Sex" If . . . ?
Sanders SA, Reinisch JM (Indiana Univ, Bloomington; Copenhagen Univ)
JAMA 281:275-277, 1999   5–1

Introduction.—There has been recent public discourse regarding whether oral-genital contact constitutes having "had sex." Using behaviors other than penile-vaginal intercourse can be viewed as a strategy to preserve "technical virginity." In a previous survey of college students it was found that almost 3 of 4 students reported that they would not consider someone with whom they had oral sex as a sexual partner. There has been a lack of empirical data on how Americans, as a population, define whether oral sex constitutes having "had sex" or sexual relations. Which interactions individuals would consider as having "had sex" were investigated.

Methods.—Among a random stratified sample of 599 students representative of the undergraduate population of a state university in the Midwest, such questions were included in a survey that explored sexual behaviors and attitudes. The students were from 29 states, and 79% classified themselves as politically moderate to conservative. They were asked to respond as to whether they believed the interaction described constituted having "had sex." The interactions included deep kissing, oral contact on the breast/nipples, person touching the breasts/nipples, touching other's genitals, oral contact with the genitals, penile-anal intercourse and penile-vaginal intercourse.

Results.—Regarding behaviors defined as having "had sex," individual attitudes varied, with 59% of the respondents indicating that oral-genital contact did not constitute having "had sex" with a partner. With regard to penile-anal intercourse, 19% responded that that did not constitute having "had sex."

Conclusion.—Americans hold widely divergent opinions about what behaviors do and do not constitute having "had sex." In this survey, most college students—of whom more were registered as Republicans than Democrats—did not define oral sex as having "had sex."

▶ At 8:15 AM Chicago time, January 15, 1999, George Lundberg was dismissed as editor-in-chief of the *Journal of the American Medical Association* during a brief telephone call to his home from the executive vice president of the AMA. The trigger for dismissal was the article (abstracted above) from the January 20, 1999 issue by Stephanie Sanders and June Reinisch from the Kinsey Institute for Research in Sex, Gender, and Reproduction at Indiana University. These authors submitted a paper to *JAMA* in November 1998 in which they reported data from a survey in 1991 of almost 600 college students. Asked, "Would you say you 'had sex' with someone if the most intimate behavior you engaged in was oral-genital contact?" 59% of students said they would not. The only type of behavior producing almost universal agreement about what constituted sex was penile-vaginal intercourse.

The authors argued that their findings had important implications for health care workers taking sexual histories of those involved in health education. Lundberg's firing was accompanied by the statement that he threatened the historic tradition and integrity of *JAMA* by inappropriately and inexcusably interjecting into a major political debate an article that had nothing to do with science or medicine.

As I think most of us know, Lundberg's dismissal created a firestorm of protest, protest mostly centered around the topic of editorial freedoms. The editor of the *British Medical Journal* remarked in an editorial: "Lundberg turned a journal that was an embarrassment into a respected major journal. Yet while *JAMA* has flourished, the AMA has withered. Its membership has fallen steadily to 38% of American doctors, and it is perceived as a reactionary organization concerned only with self interests."[1] Other journal editors followed suit. The Board of the Council of Biology editors said, "The firing marked a dark hour for scientific journals worldwide" and that the action "amounts to tacit support for suppression of scientific information that may be politically sensitive." *The New England Journal of Medicine* executive editor, Marsha Angell, was surprised by the firing of a "highly successful editor," although she called the Reinisch article "trivial and irrelevant."[2]

So what do we learn from this article, the hoopla occasioned by its publication, and the firing of a distinguished journal editor? We learn that adolescents think like adolescents and have their own definitions of sex. We learn that journal editors can easily be part of the collateral damage occasioned by impeachment mania. We also learn that some presidents (well, at least one) think like adolescents. If the last sentence offends, I've got my coat and hat ready.

Lastly, might there be a physical reason why some individuals cannot recall having had sexual activity? Well, it is just possible. There is a phenomenon known as transient global amnesia after sex. Two men have recently been described with this phenomenon, neither of whom had a reason to feign amnesia.[3] Both individuals experienced episodes of confusion and disorientation after sexual intercourse with their spouses. Both were taken to the hospital. Each had complete amnesia for what had happened to them in the preceding several hours. They misidentified the name of the current president of the United States when asked this question as part of a neurologic examination. The pathophysiology related to this has been recently hypothesized by Leuis.[4] The suspicion is that the trigger mechanism is Valsalva's maneuver. The sympathetic activation and Valsalva's maneuver occurring during sexual intercourse may lead to retrograde transmission of high venous pressure to the cerebral venous system, resulting in venous ischemia and transient global amnesia. The report of Dang et al.[3] describing this interesting entity concludes with the following comment: "As with our patients who did not recall the current U.S. president, a presidential Valsalva maneuver during each of his recent escapades may have legally allowed him to not recall specific events and may thereby help maintain international stability during the current transient global economic fluctuation."

Please note that the above words are those of Dang et al. not those of the editor, who would like to continue on preparing the YEAR BOOK OF PEDIATRICS without being dismissed from the position.

J.A. Stockman III, M.D.

References

1. Smith R: The fathering of brother George: The AMA has damaged itself. *BMJ* 318:210, 1999.
2. Holden C: Science Scope: JAMA editor gets the boot. *Science* 283:467, 1999.
3. Dang CV, Gardner LB: Transient global amnesia after sex. *Lancet* 352:1557-1558, 1998.
4. Leuis SL: Etiology of transient global amnesia. *Lancet* 352:397-399, 1998.

Health Outcomes in Offspring of Mothers With Breast Implants
Kjøller K, McLaughlin JK, Friis S, et al (Danish Cancer Society, Copenhagen; Internatl Epidemiology Inst, Rockville, Md)
Pediatrics 102:1112-1115, 1998   5–2

Introduction.—Case reports have suggested a relationship between a scleroderma-like esophageal disease and possible neonatal lupus in children breast-fed by mothers with silicone breast implants. The occurrence of esophageal malfunctions and disorders, connective tissue disease, and other rheumatic conditions was examined in a population-based cohort of children of mothers with cosmetic breast implants and was compared with the national childhood population and with children of mothers who underwent breast reduction surgery.

Methods.—The database of the central Danish National Registry of Patients was searched to identify all women who received breast implants for cosmetic reasons and all who underwent breast reduction surgery in public hospitals between 1977 and 1992. Offspring of these women were identified through the Central Population Register. Offspring were followed for occurrence of adverse health outcomes from date of birth to date of death, date of emigration, or December 31, 1993, whichever came first. Children were followed for esophageal disorders, definite connective tissue diseases, other rheumatic conditions, and congenital malformations.

Results.—There were 1135 and 7071 females who underwent breast implants or breast reduction surgery, respectively. Of 939 children of mothers with breast implants (660 before implants and 279 after), there were higher rates of hospitalization for esophageal disorders, but the excess was similar between children born before and after implant surgery. Higher than expected hospitalization rates were seen in 3906 children born of mothers who underwent breast reduction surgery. There was no significant rise in connective tissue diseases or congenital malformations in children of women who underwent breast implant or breast reduction.

Conclusion.—This first epidemiologic cohort investigation offers no evidence that silicone breast implants affect risks of esophageal or other disorders in children of these mothers. The observed risk pattern suggests a lower threshold exists among both groups of mothers who have undergone cosmetic breast surgery in seeking professional medical care for problems normally solved outside the hospital.

▶ The story relating a purported link between breast implants and a scleroderma-like esophageal disease in children breast-fed by mothers with silicone breast implants doesn't seem to want to die. The original report in 1994 received a lot of exposure.[1] This initial report based on just 8 children and subsequent reports seem to have waxed and waned, more waning than waxing, with respect to a true relationship between breast implants and scleroderma/rheumatologic problems in offspring. This report fails to show any evidence that silicone breast implants in any way increase the risk of esophageal or other disorders in children of women who have had implants. Interestingly, the report also suggests that children born of women who have not yet had transplants, but who will, have a higher prevalence of these types of problems, suggesting that the risk of these problems may be more related to a lower threshold on the part of the families for seeking professional medical care for infant feeding problems.

A few fast facts about silicon and breast implants. Silicon is the second most abundant element in the earth's crust, constituting about 28% by weight of our planet's veneer. By the way, oxygen is the most abundant element around us, constituting 48% (by weight) of the things that we touch. Because silicon is so ubiquitous, many foods and beverages, particularly those made from rice, grains (such as beer), etc., contain significant levels of silicon. All humans have silicon in their bodies. It's present in hair, bone, skin, and dental enamel. Silicon is considered an essential element in humans, although its physiology remains obscure. Silicone is a polymer, 40% silicon by weight, and is used in many prosthetics, medical devices, and pharmaceutical products.

Wouldn't it be nice to know whether the breast milk of women who have had silicone breast implants contains higher silicon levels than the breast milk of women who have never had a breast implant? Wouldn't it also be nice to know the blood silicon levels of these women as well? In fact, such a study has been recently reported by Semple et al.[2] The data are now clear. Whether you have had a silicone breast implant or not, your breast milk contains no more and no less silicon. Blood levels of silicon are a bit higher in those who have had breast implants, particularly if the breast implant has been placed under the pectoralis muscle. The differences, however, in comparison to women who have never had a breast implant, are at best marginally statistically significant.

So what would you say as a pediatrician the next time a prospective parent walks into your office and tells you that she has had a silicone breast implant and wants to know if it would be better to not breast-feed? Your answer should be fairly straightforward. It would be "go ahead and breast-feed." You would be on solid ground in recommending this. Cow's milk and cow's milk–related products, including cow's milk–based formulas, contain significantly higher levels of silicon than the breast milk of women who have had breast implants. The reason why is obvious. Cows feed on grass, grains, and other things found on or about the ground, and in the process, they eat a lot of silicon.

The long and the short of this is that in the final analysis, breast is always best, whether it's entirely your own or has had a bit of an augmentation.

J.A. Stockman III, M.D.

References

1. Levine JJ, Ilowite NT: Sclerodermalike esophageal disease in children breast fed by mothers with silicone breast implants. *JAMA* 271:213-216, 1994.
2. Semple JL, Lugowski SJ, Baines CJ, et al: Breast milk contamination and silicone implants: Preliminary results using silicon as a proxy measurement for silicone. *Plast Reconstr Surg* 102:528, 1998.

Correlation Between Down's Syndrome and Malformations of Pediatric Surgical Interest
Aquino A, Dòmini M, Rossi C, et al (Università "G. D'Annunzio" di Pescara, Italy)
J Pediatr Surg 33:1380-1382, 1998   5–3

Background.—Children born with Down's syndrome often have various congenital malformations. Surgical treatment of these malformations can improve and even save the lives of these children, about half of which

TABLE 1.—Down's Syndrome Patients With Associated Anomalies		
Total	69/127	54%
DS with no other anomalies	58	46%
DS and isolated cardiac malformations	16	
DS and isolated extracardiac malformations	36	
DS and both cardiac and extracardiac malformations	17	54%
DS patients with extracardiac malformations (isolated or not) operated on	17/53	32%

(Courtesy of Aquino A, Dòmini M, Rossi C, et al: Correlation between Down's syndrome and malformations of pediatric surgical interest. *J Pediatr Surg* 33:1380-1382, 1998.)

TABLE 3.—Malformations and Functional Diseases Associated With Down's Syndrome Observed in the Abruzzo Casuistry

	No. of Cases (%)	No. Operated On	No. Not Operated On
Gastroenteric apparatus			
Duodenal atresia or stenosis	3 (2.4)	3	
Hiatal hernia	2 (1.6)	2	
Esophageal atresia	1 (0.8)	1	
Anorectal malformations	1 (0.8)	1	
Hirschsprung's disease	1 (0.8)	1	
Hepatic neoplasm	1 (0.8)	1	
Cholelithiasis	1 (0.8)		1
Total	10	9	1
Genitourinary system			
Glanular groove	14 (17)		14
Retractil testis	11 (13.8)		11
Undescended testis	5 (6.2)	1	4
Phimosis	4 (5)	1	3
Hypospadias	3 (3.8)		3
VesicoUreteral reflux	1 (0.8)		1
Hypertrophic clitoris	1 (0.8)		1
Total	39	2	37
Abdominal wall and inguinal canal			
Umbilical hernia	15 (11.8)	1	14
Rectal diastasis	7 (5.5)		7
Hydrocele	2 (1.6)		2
Epigastric hernia	1 (0.8)		1
Inguinal hernia	1 (0.8)	1	
Total	26	2	24
Others			
Hemangiomas	5 (3.9)	2	3
Pectus excavatum	4 (3.1)		4
Palatoschisis	1 (0.8)		1
Syndactilia	1 (0.8)	1	
Hydrocephalus	1 (0.8)	1	
Total	12	4	8
Functional diseases			
Gastroesophageal reflux	17 (13.4)		17
Encopresis	17 (13.4)		17
Enuresis	1 (0.8)		1
Small left colon syndrome	1 (0.8)		1

Note: Seventeen patients underwent the surgery. Some of the others are waiting for it. The pathologies included in the functional diseases group were not surgical (i.e., functional gastroesophageal reflux, encopresis, enuresis, small left colon syndrome), once anatomical or organic disorders were excluded.

(Courtesy of Aquino A, Dòmini M, Rossi C, et al: Correlation between Down's syndrome and malformations of pediatric surgical interest. *J Pediatr Surg* 33:1380-1382, 1998.)

may live for 60 years. The incidences of congenital malformations associated with Down's syndrome were studied to determine which types of malformations pediatric surgeons could expect to treat.

Methods.—The study was performed over 10 years during which data from 127 patients (80 boys and 47 girls, aged from birth to 18 years) with Down's syndrome from the Abruzzo region of Italy were analyzed. The number and nature of cardiac and extracardiac malformations were determined, as were the associated surgical rates.

Findings.—Slightly more than half the patients (69, or 54%) had congenital malformations associated with Down's syndrome. The 33 patients with cardiac anomalies (either alone or in combination with other malformations)(26% of total sample) had 39 anomalies (Table 1). The most common cardiac malformations were interventricular defect (n = 19), interatrial defect (n = 8), and atrioventricular channel (n = 7). Surgery was performed for 9 cardiac anomalies. The 53 patients who had extracardiac anomalies (either alone or in combination) (42% of total sample) had 123 malformations, including 39 malformations of the genitourinary system, 26 of the abdominal wall and inguinal canal, and 10 of the gastroenteric apparatus (Table 3). Surgery was undertaken in 17 cases, mainly for gastrointestinal malformations. Thirty-six malformations were functional in nature (gastroesophageal reflux, encopresis, enuresis, and small left colon syndrome) and did not require surgery. When the patients with Down's syndrome were categorized according to the mother's age, most of the children (44%) had been born to mothers aged less than 30 years with mothers aged more than 38 years accounting for about 20% of these births. Children born of mothers aged more than 38 years had the lowest rates of associated congenital malformations (38% vs 50% or more for women of other age groups).

Conclusions.—Both cardiac and extracardiac congenital malformations are common in children with Down's syndrome. These malformations can be treated surgically, and operations to correct interventricular defect and gastrointestinal malformations were the most commonly performed. The pediatric surgeon can play a very important role in the treatment of associated congenital malformations in children with Down's syndrome. Finally, the higher percentage of children with Down's syndrome in women aged less than 30 years can be explained by the facts that this age group has the largest live-birth rate and receives the least Down's syndrome prevention.

▶ As we learn more about the natural and unnatural history of Down's syndrome, we see that with proper care, including surgery when needed, the mean age of survival has approached 60 years. As good as this statistic is, some 20% of affected children will die within the first decade of life, mostly of complications related to a variety of malformations, the most frequent of which appear to be cardiac in origin (some 40%-60% of cases). Other malformations in part include duodenal stenosis or atresia, esophageal atresia, anorectal malformations, umbilical hernias, rectal diastasis, genitourinary malformations, and pectus excavatum.

As we learn more about Down's syndrome, we recognize that it may be the most common human malformative syndrome with as many as 1 in 600 to 700 live births being affected. Each baby diagnosed must be very carefully examined to determine who does and who does not have a malformation. Given the high probability (slightly greater than 50%) of finding something, such infants will provide serious satisfaction to those who are appropriately curious.

A closing comment about Down's syndrome. It has been found that women who have children with Down's syndrome before age 36 have a higher risk of developing Alzheimer's disease at an early age. Why young women who have children with Down's syndrome seem to age more quickly is not known. It has been suggested that the mechanism for accelerated aging and the potential development of Alzheimer's disease in such young mothers relates to mutations in the presenilin gene.[1]

J.A. Stockman III, M.D.

Reference

1. Dorland M, van Montfrans JM, van Kooij RJ, et al: Normal telomere lengths in mothers of children with Down's syndrome. *Lancet* 352:961-962, 1998.

Impact of a Children's Health Insurance Program on Newly Enrolled Children
Lave JR, Keane CR, Lin CJ, et al (Univ of Pittsburgh, Pa; Western Pennsylvania Caring Found for Children, Pittsburgh)
JAMA 279:1820-1825, 1998   5–4

Introduction.—The State Children's Health Insurance Program (SCHIP), established in 1997, allocates $24 billion to states over a 5-year period to provide health insurance for children who would otherwise be uninsured. Few studies have examined the effect of extending health care coverage to uninsured children. Various effects of insurance designed to cover uninsured children were examined, including the impact of the programs on newly enrolled children and their families.

Methods.—A total of 887 families of newly enrolled children were interviewed by telephone; of the families who agreed to participate, 84% (659) responded to interviews at enrollment, at 6 months, and at 12 months to determine the program's effects on such factors as whether the children had a usual source of care, received health care service of different types, the number of physician visits, the number of dentist visits, whether they had experienced unmet need or delay in receiving services, and had restrictions on childhood activities. The baseline answers of the study families were compared with those of 330 other families of children who were newly enrolled into the program 12 months later to control for any underlying trends.

Results.—After enrollment in the program, access to health care services improved. A regular source of medical care was seen in 99% of children at 12 months after enrollment, up from 89% at baseline, whereas 85% had a regular dentist, up from 60% at baseline. At 12 months, only 165 of the children reported any unmet need or delayed care in the past 6 months, down from 57% at baseline. There was an increase from 59% to 64% in the proportion of children seeing a physician. Those visiting an emergency department decreased from 22% to 17%. The amount of family stress was reduced, family burdens were eased, and children were able to receive the care they needed as a result of having health insurance.

Conclusion.—There was a major positive impact on children and their families when health insurance was extended to uninsured children. Health insurance did not lead to excessive utilization in this sample but, instead, to more appropriate utilization.

▶ Paul W. Newacheck, Dr.P.H., professor of Health Policy and Pediatrics, Institute for Health Policy Studies, University of California, San Francisco, comments:

The report by Lave and associates on the impact of Pennsylvania's voluntary insurance program provides important insights into the role insurance plays as a determinant of access to and use of children's health services. This is a well-designed study that incorporates pretest and posttest measures as well as a comparison group. The results clearly demonstrate the powerful influence of insurance on increasing the likelihood that children will have a medical home and obtain medical and dental care when needed and on reducing parent's worries about their children's medical care.

The evidence presented bodes very positively for the new SCHIP. The results suggest that SCHIP could play a critical part in improving children's access to care nationally. However, when Congress set aside approximately $40 billion in federal funds for SCHIP, it provided no new funds for evaluation. This is unfortunate, because Congress gave states tremendous discretion in establishing their SCHIP plans. States have flexibility in setting eligibility thresholds, benefit levels, and outreach mechanisms. States were also given substantial leeway in the design of their delivery systems. They have the choice of using Medicaid or other insurance mechanisms and choosing between managed care approaches and traditional fee-for-service care. As a consequence, the great variety of state approaches now being implemented provides a natural experiment for identifying effective program designs. Without a strategy and funds to create a national evaluation of the SCHIP programs, this opportunity is forgone. Indeed, the opportunity for collecting pretest or baseline information in state SCHIP programs has already been lost in most cases. However, there is still time to meld an effective evaluation that would permit identification of more successful programs from those that are less successful in meeting children's needs. Doing so will require speedy and concerted action by the federal and state governments and other potential funders, such as foundations.

P.W. Newacheck, Dr.P.H.

Air Bags and Children: A Potentially Lethal Combination
McCaffrey M, German A, Lalonde F, et al (Univ of Ottawa, Ont)
J Pediatr Orthop 19:60-64, 1999   5–5

Introduction.—Since their introduction, the life-saving effects of air bags in high-speed collisions have been well documented; however, they

TABLE 1.—Summary of Case Studies

Case	Gender	Age	Seating/Restraint	Injuries Sustained	Accident
1	M	12	Front passenger, lap & torso belt	Ringing in ears, contusion to ear	Front of vehicle struck median; minor damage
2	M	8	Front passenger, lap & torso belt	Abrasion to left cheek	Vehicle in parking lot bumps wall; minor damage
3	F	12	Front passenger, lap & torso belt	Laceration to forehead, abrasion to right cheek	Case vehicle rear-ends truck; minor damage
4a	M	3	Front passenger, lap & torso belt	Contusions to forehead and right scalp	Vehicle sideswipes utility pole; minor damage
4b	F	2	Rear passenger, lap belt	Uninjured	As above
5	M	2	Front passenger, forward-facing child seat	Abrasion to left cheek	Vehicle impacts lamp standard; minor damage
6	M	4	Front passenger, lap belt only	Dislocation of spine (C1 & base of cranium), transection of spinal cord, hematoma from C1-C7, abrasion to right side of neck & face, right atrium bruised, died at accident scene	Case vehicle rear-ends another; minor damage
7	F	12	Front passenger, lap & torso belt	Burns to the face, posterior and right-sided neck pain, buckle fracture of the distal radial metaphysis	Vehicle struck head-on by oncoming vehicle; significant damage
8a	M	4	Front passenger, lap & torso belt	Minor facial abrasion	Left front fender/wheel struck light standard; moderate damage
8b	M	3	Right rear seat, lap & torso belt	Minor facial abrasion resulting from contact by the seat belt webbing	As above
9a	F	11	Front passenger, lap & torso belt	Minor facial contusions and abrasions	Frontal collision with side of another vehicle; moderate damage
9b	M	8	Left rear seat, lap & torso belt	Uninjured	As above
9c	M	9	Right rear seat, lap & torso belt	Uninjured	As above

(Courtesy of McCaffrey M, German A, Lalonde F, et al: Air bags and children: A potentially lethal combination. *J Pediatr Orthop* 19[1]:60-64, 1999.)

have been responsible for numerous injuries and fatalities, primarily in small women and children because of the explosive force with which they need to deploy. Children younger than 10 years have a 21% increased risk of fatality when an air bag is present. Experience with children who have sustained air bag injuries was reviewed because of increasing concern regarding pediatric air bag trauma sustained in minor collisions.

Case Review.—There were 13 children, aged 2 to 12 years, injured by air bags in cases in which seat belt wear was mandatory for all occupants (Table 1). Twelve children had relatively minor air bag trauma. Most injuries were of a superficial nature, consisting of lacerations, contusions, abrasions, or burns.

Fatality.—One of the children was killed by the air bag deployment. The child sustained an occipital-C1 dislocation. The child was 4 years old, weighed 40 pounds, and had the seat belt buckled with the torso portion of the belt behind his back. Just before the crash, the child was leaning forward, perhaps to play with the radio controls. When the right front air bag deployed, the boy received a large abrasion to the right side of the neck and face and a thermal burn to the right cheek. His cervical spine was dislocated with complete transection of the spinal cord, resulting in instant death. The father had only a minor contusion to his left hand when the air bag deployed.

Conclusion.—In these instances, had the car not been equipped with a passenger-side air bag, the children most likely would have been completely unharmed. As many parents continue to unwittingly place their children in the front seat, the pediatric population is at particular risk because they are in jeopardy of sustaining air bag–induced injuries should a collision occur. If the occupant is in the path of an air bag that is rapidly inflating, there is a greater chance of forceful contact occurring, resulting in more serious injuries.

▶ The authors of this report note that the pending "smart" air bag technology is expected to address the problem of air bags and injury to children. As you might have read, Ford recently announced the industry's first effort to produce an integrated smart air bag system, intending to feature this technology on redesigned cars and trucks beginning with this year's models. Smart technology does not deal just with children. Short adult drivers are at excess risk from air bag injuries as well. The technology that Ford uses is quite fascinating. The driver's seat position, the front passenger's weight (a surrogate for stature), seatbelt usage, and impact severity are all measured in the system's computer, which rapidly determines the most logical course of action. For instance, the passenger bag will not deploy if no weight is detected on its seat; it might not deploy in a low-speed collision if the seat belt is in use and the occupant is small; it might inflate slowly if the seatbelt isn't buckled; it will inflate quickly if the impact is severe.

What is key to any smart air bag system's judgment abilities is high-quality information, minimally, information as to the occupant's size and proximity to the air bag and impact violence. For instance, we know too well the dreadful consequences air bags have for children in the front passenger seat, but less publicized is the death rate among short drivers. According to a report in *Automobile Engineering*, of the 35 low-speed steering-wheel air bag–caused deaths recorded through October 1997, 25 were of women 5 ft 5 in or shorter. You guessed it; to reach the pedals, these drivers were too close to the steering wheel with a single-inflation–rate air bag. In many instances, these short drivers were properly buckled in. Ford's seat position sensor would know all this, and its 2-rate air bag would respond accordingly. Some Ford products also now have adjustable gas and brake pedals that allow short folks to sit further away from the steering wheel.

Stay tuned to the evolution of smart air bags. Even more sophisticated interior sensors are just over the horizon. Bosch, for example, is developing a system of infrared and ultrasonic sensing that can deduce the occupant's orientation on the seat (important for gauging whether it is even wise to fire a side air bag). Lastly, if you want to read more about smart air bags, read the review of this topic by Kim Reynolds.[1] (Yes, some editors of YEAR BOOKS are fast-car junkies and avid readers of *Road and Track*, *Motor Trend*, and *Car and Driver*).

One truly final comment. How would you respond if a parent, concerned about the possibility of air bag injury to a child, asked you whether they might simply remove the fuse for the air bag from the car's fuse box to deactivate the passenger-side air bag? The answer, here, also comes from *Road and Track* magazine. If the vehicle in question has separate fuses for the air bag, removing the fuse will indeed result in de-arming the air bag. However, industry experts note that air bag triggering systems are extremely sensitive and operate with minuscule electrical power. Thus, static electricity built up from an occupant's feet shuffling on the carpet of a car can be sufficient to trigger an air bag during an accident, even though a fuse is removed, assuming the bumper's sensor has been triggered. In this case, static electricity will bridge the fuse gap. Therefore, both removing the air bag fuse and grounding the trigger circuit are necessary to avoid air bag firing.

In the end, the only sure advice is to completely remove the air bag if absolute freedom from air bag deployment is desired. Good luck doing this yourself. It might be better to buy a Ford with a smart air bag system.[2] To read more about air bag–related deaths and serious injuries in children, their injury patterns, and related radiologic findings, see the superb review of this topic by Marshall.[3]

I drive a car that has a total of 8 airbags. If they all went off in a crash, I wouldn't have to worry about surviving a crash, I would be squashed on the spot like a bug. I hope to die peacefully in my sleep like my great grandfather did, not kicking and screaming like the other people in his car.

J.A. Stockman III, M.D.

References

1. Reynolds K: For safety technologies for the millennium: There is a strange new world of automotive safety coming—and sooner than you think. *Road and Track* 50:124, 1999.

2. Deflating concept (technical correspondence). *Road and Track* 50:146, 1999.
3. Marshall KW, Koch BL, Egelhoff CJ: Air bag–related deaths and injuries in children: Injury patterns and imaging findings. *Am J Neuroradiol* 19:1599-1607, 1998.

Prescription Drug Use and Self-prescription Among Resident Physicians

Christie JD, Rosen IM, Bellini LM, et al (Univ of Pennsylvania, Philadelphia; Veterans Affairs Med Ctr, Philadelphia; Johns Hopkins Univ, Baltimore, Md; et al)
JAMA 280:1253-1255, 1998   5–6

Introduction.—Physicians are able to prescribe medicines for themselves, yet many warn of the loss of objectivity that can accompany self-prescription. Little is known about self-prescription and self-care among resident physicians who have long and unpredictable work hours and who have easy access to prescription medications through on-site pharmacies and the presence of sample medications. Self-prescription and self-care practices among resident physicians were evaluated in internal medicine residency training programs.

Methods.—There were 381 residents who were mailed a survey to self-report their use of health care services and prescription medications and how the medications were obtained. The response was 316 residents (83%).

Results.—Among the responders, 244 residents (78%) reported using at least 1 prescription medicine and 52% reported self-prescribing the medications. A sample cabinet was the source of 25% of all medication and 42% of self-prescribed medication. A pharmaceutical company representative was the source of 7% of all medications and 11% of self-prescribed medications. There were 152 residents (49%) who indicated that they had no primary care physician or that they were their own primary care physician. The medications most often self-prescribed were antibiotics, followed by allergy and asthma medications.

Conclusion.—Among resident physicians, self-prescription is common. The source of these medications and the lack of oversight of medication use raise questions about the practice, although self-prescription is difficult to evaluate.

▶ Ben Alexander, M.D., and Andrea Dunk, M.D., chief residents, Department of Pediatrics, University of North Carolina School of Medicine, Chapel Hill, comment:

Congratulations are due the authors of this article for taking an interest in the health of house officers. They have identified an important and prevalent practice among training physicians. Their results are particularly striking given their self-report study design, which underestimates the true prevalence of self-prescription practices. This study surveyed internal medicine residents who should appreciate the importance of primary care. Only 27% of medications were prescribed by primary physicians and only 49% of residents had primary physicians. Interestingly , the rates of self-prescription were equal for residents with and without identified primary physicians. Although having available time to see a physician may be a factor in self-prescription, apparently having a primary physician is not. The overall results of the study are not surprising, given the previously demonstrated prevalence of self-prescription among practicing physicians.

For pediatricians, these questions and their corollaries take on another order of magnitude in complexity: Should pediatricians self-prescribe when they are trained to care for children? Should they prescribe for their children? Their spouse? The patterns of self-prescription and family prescription should be studied in pediatricians and pediatric residents to define practices within these groups. We suspect that they may differ significantly from those of physicians who care for adults only. Patterns of family prescription among nonpediatric physicians should also be studied. How often do internists prescribe for their children? How does the frequency relate to the child's age? Do these prescriptions generally fit the pediatric standard of care?

Obviously, these issues are important, existing at the crossroads of our professional and personal lives. They involve ethical boundaries and professional judgments that are not always black and white but involve a variety of gray areas which are nicely outlined by the authors of this study. Self-prescription clearly needs to be addressed by the medical profession as a whole, but the authors of this study have elegantly shown that it is rampant among resident physicians. As in most things pediatric, treatment (if not prevention) is best begun early and taught by example.

B.S. Alexander, M.D.
A.M. Dunk, M.D.

Trends in Clinical Education of Medical Students: Implications for Pediatrics
Hunt CE, Kallenberg GA, Whitcomb ME (Med College of Ohio, Toledo; George Washington Univ, Washington, DC; Assoc of American Med Colleges, Washington, DC)
Arch Pediatr Adolesc Med 153:297-302, 1999   5-7

Introduction.—There has been a call for more ambulatory care experience with the belief that ambulatory care settings provide clinical experience relevant to the future practice activities of most students. In response to these needs for curricular change, several national initiatives developed in the early 1990s. To determine how medical schools had responded to this imperative, the Association of American Medical Colleges conducted site visits at medical schools and collected clinical experiences that were implemented. The 3 major types of ambulatory care-based clinical experiences implemented by medical schools were described. The implications of these developments for the discipline of pediatrics were delineated.

Methods.—There were site visits to 26 medical schools and a review of detailed information from 12 other schools. The Council on Medical Student Education in Pediatrics developed the evaluation of the core curriculum within the context of the major curricular trends that were observed.

Results.—Community-based ambulatory experiences, continuity of care, integration, and population-based experiences were emphasized by the major observed curricular trends. Student-directed learning and performance-based assessments were the supporting educational principles. Early clinical experiences (longitudinal preceptorships), community-oriented/population-based experiences, and multispecialty clerkships were the 3 major curricular changes. The 3-year clerkship was the focus of the Council on Medical Student Education in Pediatrics objectives. The pediatric clerkship was primarily related to substantive participation by pediatric faculty in the overall curriculum.

Conclusion.—Clinical curricular opportunities for pediatrics will be extended beyond the traditional boundaries of the clerkship by revising the clerkship-based Council on Medical Student Education in Pediatrics guidelines according to the new educational trends. As a consequence, the discipline of pediatrics can achieve enhanced partnership in the planning, conduct, and evaluation of a clinical curriculum for medical students that is relevant to child health issues and that extends across all 4 years.

▶ Michael R. Lawless, M.D., chief, General Pediatrics and Adolescent Medicine, Department of Pediatrics and Adolescent Medicine, Wake Forest University School of Medicine, Winston-Salem, NC, and president, Council on Medical Student Education in Pediatrics, comments:

Medical education ranks high among systems resistant to change. Three important curricular trends in this article are among those making the 1990s a decade of remarkable change in medical student education. Clinical experience via a longitudinal preceptorship in the first year of medical school brings relevance and palpable enthusiasm to the study of basic sciences. Looking beyond the individual patient to consider the health needs of the population served broadens students' perspective, and for future pediatricians, identifies opportunities for child advocacy. Multispecialty (or interdisciplinary) clerkships are the greatest departure from the traditional block clerkship by discipline. Representing the integration of internal medicine, family medicine, and pediatrics, these clerkships vary greatly in format.

In each of the 3 curricular innovations, the community-based office of the generalist physician is partly or fully the site of the clinical encounter. With development of community-based preceptors as teachers and with clear educational goals for students, this can be a powerful site for students to learn from a physician who is an expert in office practice. The icing on this cake is the stimulus to continuing education of the preceptor that accompanies the teaching of students.

Of concern to pediatrics is that, of the 26 medical schools evaluated, only 20% to 25% of preceptors in the longitudinal preceptorships were pediatricians, even fewer in rural settings.

The milieu of academic medicine and of hospital and office-based practice has undergone dramatic change in this past decade. The challenge for pediatric educators in the midst of this change is to accurately predict the skills needed by the pediatrician of the future. Then we must be very deliberate in developing curriculum, developing performance-based assessment of pediatric clinical skills, and evaluating the outcome of pediatric education. Change always brings opportunity for improvement. The opportunities have never been greater.

M.R. Lawless, M.D.

Risk Factors for Infant Homicide in the United States
Overpeck MD, Brenner RA, Trumble AC, et al (Natl Inst of Child Health and Human Development, Bethesda, Md)
N Engl J Med 339:1211-1216, 1998   5–8

Introduction.—Almost one third of infant deaths are caused by homicide, most often occurring the first year of life. Fatal child abuse is the cause for more than 80% of documented homicides. Almost one fourth of infants discharged from acute care facilities with disabilities caused by injury are thought to have been intentionally injured, almost always as a result of child abuse. Birth certificates revealed that one third of the deaths were classified as caused by battering or other maltreatment (Table 1). To identify infants at high risk for homicide and to develop timely and effective interventions, risk factors that can be identified in the prenatal

TABLE 1.—Causes of Infant Deaths Classified as Intentional or of Undetermined Intent, 1983 to 1991

Cause*	ICD-9 e-Code†	Infant Deaths No. (%)
Total		2776 (100)
Battering or other maltreatment	967, 987	914 (32.9)
Assault by unspecified means	968.9, 988.9	779 (28.1)
Suffocation or strangulation	963, 983	282 (10.2)
Drowning	964, 984	120 (4.3)
Firearms	965, 985	84 (3.0)
Criminal neglect	968.4	81 (2.9)
Arson	968.0, 988.1	64 (2.3)
Cuts and stabbing	966, 986	58 (2.1)
Other		394 (14.2)

*Categories of battering or other maltreatment and criminal neglect include only deaths classified as intentional. An additional 52 deaths were classified as caused by unintentional neglect or abandonment (e-code 904).
†ICD-9, *International Classification of Diseases*, 9th revision.
(Reprinted by permission of *The New England Journal of Medicine*, from Overpeck MD, Brenner RA, Trumble AC, et al: Risk factors for infant homicide in the United States. *N Engl J Med* 339:1211-1216. Copyright 1998, Massachusetts Medical Society. All rights reserved.)

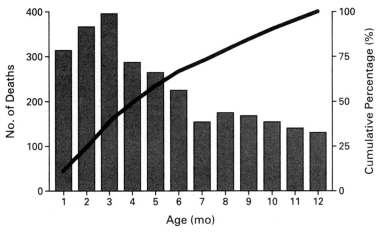

FIGURE 1.—Number and cumulative percentage of infant homicides, according to age at death, 1983 through 1991. *Bars*, numbers of deaths; *curve*, cumulative percentage. (Reprinted by permission of *The New England Journal of Medicine*, from Overpeck MD, Brenner RA, Trumble AC, et al: Risk factors for infant homicide in the United States. *N Engl J Med* 339:1211-1216. Copyright 1998, Massachusetts Medical Society. All rights reserved.)

period would be helpful. Deaths of infants born during an 8-year period were studied to establish estimates of risk factors for infant homicide.

Methods.—There were 2776 homicides, identified in an 8-year period, during the first year of life. Analyses were conducted of birth-certificate variables. Based on the increased relative risks among subcategories with adequate numbers for stable estimates, variables potentially predictive of homicide were selected.

Results.—By the fourth month of life, half of the homicides had occurred (Fig 1). A second or subsequent infant born to a mother younger than 17 years old (relative risk [RR], 10.9) or 17 to 19 years old (RR, 9.3), as compared with a first infant born to a mother 25 years old or older; a maternal age of less than 15 years, as compared with an age of at least 25 years (RR, 6.8); no prenatal care, as compared with early prenatal care (RR, 10.4); and less than 12 years of education among mothers who were at least 17 years old (RR, 8.0), as compared with 16 or more years of education, were the most important risk factors.

Conclusion.—Infant homicide is strongly associated with childbearing at an early age, particularly if the mother has given birth previously. These findings may have implications for prevention.

▶ The data from this article speak for themselves. Infant homicide is infanticide. Ours is not a society that should tolerate any such waste of our prodigy.

I have not seen any comparative data between infant homicide rates and overall homicide rates categorized by U.S. city data. The chart that follows shows the top 10 cities in this country based on total homicide rates in the mid-1990s. New Orleans led the list despite the fact that, between 1990 and 1995, its murder rate fell by approximately 25%.

City	Murders (Per 100,000, 1995)
1. New Orleans, La	32.7
2. Chicago	30.0
3. Philadelphia	28.2
4. Jackson, Miss	25.0
5. Oklahoma City, Okla	24.2
6. Memphis, Tenn	20.0
7. Pine Bluff, Ark	20.0
8. Shreveport-Bossier City, La	19.7
9. Los Angeles–Long Beach	18.3
10. Rocky Mount, NC	18.2

(Data from FBI Uniform Crime Reports, 1996.)

J.A. Stockman III, M.D.

Documentation of Child Physical Abuse: How Far Have We Come?
Limbos MAP, Berkowitz CD (Harbor–Univ of California Los Angeles, Torrance)
Pediatrics 102:53-58, 1998   5–9

Introduction.—Because the medical record is a legal document that is routinely used by public agencies, thorough documentation in cases of suspected child abuse is extremely important. An adequate medical record must include the history of the injury, a description of the injury, documentation of previous injuries or accidents, and compatibility or incompatibility between the history given and the injuries sustained. A 1980 study found that 60% of records had inadequate data to determine retrospectively whether child abuse had occurred. A study was undertaken to determine whether physician documentation of suspected child physical abuse has changed between 1980 and 1995.

Methods.—Emergency department records of children evaluated for physical abuse in 1980 and 1995 were reviewed to evaluate the completeness of medical documentation for each year, to determine whether an interval improvement in documentation had occurred, and to examine the effect of a structured form on the completeness of documentation. The review included documentation of 20 items, including history, physical examination, diagnostic procedures, and disposition.

Results.—There was better recording in 1995 concerning involvement of Child Protective Services and case disposition than in 1980. However, this was seen as the only improvement. Documentation of at least one item was missing in one half or more of the documents, and the missing items included witnesses to injury, past injuries, description of size and color of injuries, illustration, and a genital examination. A developmental history was not seen in any of the records, and fewer skeletal surveys were obtained in 1995 than in 1980. With the structured child abuse reporting form, there was improved documentation of 2 items: illustrations of injuries and time of arrival at the pediatric emergency department.

Conclusion.—Despite increased efforts to educate house staff in the evaluation of child abuse, little improvement in physician documentation of child physical abuse was seen between 1980 and 1995. A structured form did not significantly improve documentation of child abuse despite having prompts for physicians to document dates and times and to illustrate physical injuries on the diagram provided.

▶ Dr. Howard Dubowitz, director, Child Protection Program, and professor, Division of General Pediatrics, University of Maryland, comments:

This article on the documentation of child physical abuse asks: "How far have we come?" The findings suggest that the answer is, "not far." There were many gaps and little significant improvement between 1980 and 1995 in the documentation of physical abuse in the pediatric emergency department studied. Similarly, during both study years, the use of structured forms helped little, despite efforts to enhance knowledge and competency in the area of child abuse during the intervening years. The study design did not permit linkage between individual physicians and specific training efforts.

These are disappointing findings. However, it must be noted that the study involved a single emergency department and relatively few charts. It is possible that practice was better than the documentation. The study design did not permit this issue to be probed, and it is also possible that the poor documentation accurately reflected consistently poor practice. Others have found structured forms that include key issues to be useful. The lack of success here suggests the need to reconsider the form used as well as the accompanying training, before dispensing with this promising idea.

There are a few notable omissions in the data sought in the charts. Much attention has been given to separately interviewing children concerning sexual abuse; interestingly, this has not been true for physical abuse, and the authors make no mention of the child's history. Mention is made of the child's development but not of behavior; perhaps, the term *development* was used inclusively. In addition, it is clear that the family and social histories are often critical in evaluation of these cases, but they were not included.

The authors seek to draw constructive lessons from this study, offering several good ideas for future educational efforts. One challenge concerns the limited time often available for teaching residents and fellows about child maltreatment. And, given the time constraints, the not-so-scintillating topic of chart documentation is likely to be given short shrift. This remains an important issue, and this article is an impetus for us to reconsider our efforts and seek more effective approaches.

H. Dubowitz, M.D., M.S.

Changes in Sleep Position During Infancy: A Prospective Longitudinal Assessment

Lesko SM, Corwin MJ, Vezina RM, et al (Boston Univ School of Medicine, Brookline, Mass)

JAMA 280:336-340, 1998   5–10

Introduction.—Sudden infant death syndrome (SIDS) is defined as the sudden death of an infant that is not expected on the basis of history and is unexplained by a thorough postmortem examination, death scene investigation, and medical history review. The cause of SIDS is unknown, but its incidence is higher among blacks than whites, is increased by the mother's illicit drug use and smoking during pregnancy, is inversely proportional to birthweight, and may be decreased by breast-feeding. The American Academy of Pediatrics recommended in 1992 that infants be placed on their backs or sides to sleep, and in 1994 a campaign was launched to reduce the prevalence of prone sleeping among infants to 10% or less. The prevalence of the prone sleep position among infants born in 1995 and 1996 was described as these infants aged from 1 to 6 months. Factors that predict which infants will be placed on their stomachs at 3 months of age, the age at which SIDS has its peak incidence, were identified.

Methods.—A total of 7796 mothers whose infants weighed 2500 g or more at birth were enrolled in this prospective cohort study. The maternal and infant characteristics related to prone sleeping at 1 month and 3 months of age were recorded.

Results.—Prone sleeping increased from 18% at 1 month of age to 29% at 3 months of age. Non-Hispanic black or Hispanic race or ethnicity, younger age, less education, and higher parity were associated with prone sleeping at 1 month. Mother's non-Hispanic black or Hispanic race or ethnicity, younger maternal age (18-24 years), increasing parity (2 or more children), and infant gender were associated with switching from the nonprone to the prone position at 3 months.

Conclusion.—A substantial number of infants who slept nonprone at 1 month sleep prone at 3 months, if infant sleeping practices in the study communities are representative of practices throughout the United States.

▶ A few years ago, folks in Boston, Lowell, and Lawrence, Massachusetts, and Toledo, Ohio, got together to design a study to describe current newborn sleep practices, to document changes in sleep position with age, and to identify the health consequences of various sleep practices in the first 6 months of life. What they found was very interesting. At 1 month of age, prone sleeping was more common among non-Hispanic blacks and Hispanics than among other racial-ethnic groups. Male infants and infants born to unmarried women were more likely to sleep prone than female infants and infants born to married women. The prevalence of prone sleeping was inversely related to maternal age, education, and income and directly related to parity. Among Asian infants, the prevalence of prone sleeping was low and did not increase over time. What is important about these data is the comparison between the U.S. experience after the introduction of the "Back to Sleep" campaign begun in 1994 and data from other countries. Here, about 1 in 4 babies in the first few months of life still sleeps prone. In New Zealand, Australia, Norway, the United Kingdom, Hong Kong, and elsewhere, the prevalence of sleeping in the prone position is well under 10%.

We have a lot of work yet to do.

J.A. Stockman III, M.D.

Prevalence and Predictors of the Prone Sleep Position Among Inner-City Infants
Brenner RA, Simons-Morton BG, Bhaskar B, et al (Natl Inst of Child Health and Human Development, Bethesda, Md; Research Triangle Inst, Rockville, Md; Georgetown Univ, Washington, DC)
JAMA 280:341-346, 1998   5–11

Introduction.—An increased risk of sudden infant death syndrome (SIDS) has been associated with the prone sleep position, according to recent studies. Sudden infant death syndrome has declined by 50% in countries where the prevalence of the prone sleep position has been reduced to less than 10%. Research suggests that infants placed on their stomachs may rebreathe expired air, leading to increases in blood carbon dioxide levels, hypoxia, and asphyxia, or that the prone sleep position may cause infants to overheat through decreased dissipation of heat. However, the mechanism linking prone sleep position to SIDS has not been fully explained. The preferred sleep position, according to the American Academy of Pediatrics, is the supine position. Infant sleep position was examined in a low-income, inner-city population to identify predictors of the prone sleep position, particularly risk factors that may be amenable to interventions.

Methods.—There were 394 mothers and infants who were studied during a 1-year period. The mothers were interviewed shortly after delivery, and a follow-up interview was conducted at 3 to 7 months after delivery. The mothers were asked in which position the infants were placed for sleep on the night before the 3- to 7-month interview.

Results.—There were 157 infants (40%) who were placed for sleep in the prone position at 3 to 7 months. Poverty, black race, presence of the infant's grandmother in the home, and intent to place the infant in the prone position, as measured shortly after delivery, were independent predictors of prone sleep. Forty-three mothers saw their infants placed in the prone sleep position while in the hospital, and 40 (93%) of these intended to place their infants on their stomachs at home.

Conclusion.—In this predominantly low-income population, a substantial proportion of infants were placed in the prone sleep position. Initial intentions and reinforcement of the correct sleep position should be emphasized in education efforts. During the postpartum hospital stay, hospitals should ensure that healthy newborn infants are placed in the supine sleep position.

▶ This is the second report in this YEAR BOOK related to SIDS. The findings here reinforce the observations that race and young maternal age are factors affecting the probability that an infant will sleep in an undesirable position. We also see two more variables at play. It is not just the young mother who has a problem; it is also the mother who has had a number of prior pregnancies. Presumably, the latter circumstance is like trying to teach an old dog new tricks. Just as important, if there is a grandmother in the house, the risk that the infant willl sleep in the prone position increases markedly. In light of the discrepancy in the prevalence of prone sleeping positioning between the races, one logical conclusion is that the "Back to Sleep" message is not being adequately transmitted to certain populations here in the United States. There needs to be a more focused effort at directing the "Back to Sleep" campaign toward minority populations. This should start with the imprinting of new mothers that occurs in the nursery. In the report abstracted, the most important determinant of the early intentions of a mother to place her baby in the supine position is her observation of the position in which her infant was placed to sleep in the hospital shortly after delivery.

As this commentary closes, realize that the saga of SIDS and sleep positioning is both a bad news and a good news story. The bad news is that we still have a long way to go to match other countries' results in eliminating the prone sleep position. The good news is that we have at least gotten off to a good start. There has been a 66% reduction in the prevalence of prone sleeping in the last half dozen years and as much as a 40% decrease in the SIDS rate, presumably accounted for by the "Back to Sleep" campaign. However, there is a segment of our population that has not received or is not hearing this message. The message back to us is clear. We have to spread the word more widely.

To read an excellent commentary on effectively delivering the message on sleep position, see the review by Malloy.[1]

J.A. Stockman III, M.D.

Reference

1. Malloy MH: Effectively delivering the message on infant sleep position. *JAMA* 280:373-374,1998.

Comparison of Esophageal, Rectal, Axillary, Bladder, Tympanic, and Pulmonary Artery Temperatures in Children

Robinson JL, Seal RF, Spady DW, et al (Univ of Alberta, Edmonton)
J Pediatr 133:553-556, 1998   5–12

Background.—Where is the best site for measuring a child's body temperature? Temperature in the pulmonary artery in anesthetized children was measured and compared with temperatures measured at 5 other body sites.

Methods.—The subjects were 15 children, aged 6 months to 6 years, undergoing elective cardiac surgery. None had ear infection or drainage or incisions near the ear. Temperature probes were placed at the following 6 locations: (1) over the axillary artery; (2) 5 cm into the rectum; (3) in the esophagus behind the heart; (4) in the bladder; (5) in the right ear (2 probes, the Genius and the IVAC Core-Check); and (6) (in 5 children) in the pulmonary artery. Throughout the surgical procedure (including cooling and rewarming), an anesthetist measured temperature every 5 to 10 minutes from all sites. In total, 431 sets of readings from all sites except the pulmonary artery were made, and an additional 83 sets of readings included the pulmonary artery.

Findings.—In the 83 sets including the pulmonary artery, the readings closest to the temperature in the pulmonary artery were from the esophagus (mean difference 0.1°C). Mean differences for measurements at other sites were 0.6°C with the Genius tympanic thermometer, 0.7°C with the rectal thermometer, 0.8°C with the IVAC tympanic thermometer, 0.9°C with the bladder probe, and 1.3°C with the axillary thermometer. In the 431 sets excluding the pulmonary artery, esophageal readings were used as the reference standard. During cooling, both tympanic, bladder, and axillary temperatures differed by less than 0.20°C, and the rectal temperature differed by 0.53°C. During rewarming, the 2 tympanic thermometers were the closest to the esophageal readings (0.69°C and 0.78°C), whereas temperatures at the axillary artery, rectum, and bladder differed from the reference by 1.25°C or more. During both heating and cooling, differences between esophageal readings and both tympanic thermometers had the smallest standard deviations.

Conclusions.—Temperatures measured with the 2 tympanic thermometers were more accurate than temperatures measured at the axillary artery, bladder, and rectum. Furthermore, the performances of the tympanic thermometers were strikingly similar throughout the study, which suggests that their readings are precise. The rectal temperatures were the slowest to change during cooling and warming. The axillary temperatures varied greatly from the standard, particularly during rewarming.

▶ Bet you're a little tired about reading of the vagaries of taking a tympanic membrane temperature. If you are a believer in this technology, the results of this report will reinforce your beliefs. If you are a naysayer, the data from this report will not make you a convert, given the way in which this study was performed. The study itself was not intended to compare temperature readings in patients with elevated temperatures. It was intended to compare temperatures from various sites in the body at steady state temperature or as body temperature was decreasing during cardiovascular surgical cooling. The study itself was done extraordinarily elegantly. The investigators received permission to place temperature probes in the rectum, axilla, esophagus (immediately behind the heart), pulmonary artery, and in the bladder of patients undergoing elective cardiac surgery. This afforded an opportunity to compare temperatures at each of these sites with temperatures taken by tympanic thermometry.

So what were the results? The results were pretty straightforward. Pulmonary artery temperature most closely represents core body temperature. That is not unexpected. Under ideal conditions, tympanic thermometry does seem to be very accurate. In the real world, not in the operating room however, there are many pitfalls that create non-ideal conditions. A narrow external canal that is a little crooked will reek havoc with the accuracy of a tympanic thermometry instrument.

The aural infrared thermometer has been around now for a good decade or more. A parent can buy 1 over-the-counter at any pharmacy or your local corner Wal-Mart. Serious concern still exists about how accurate this type of thermometer is in comparison to other ways to take a temperature.

The real rub is that in the practical world, there is no gold standard for taking a temperature. A rectal temperature is accurate in the sense that it takes the temperature within the rectum. Please realize, though, that the rectal temperature rises somewhat more slowly than will the temperature elsewhere in the body during the evolution of a fever. It would appear that stool is a fairly good insulator against rapid ups and downs in temperature if that's what the end of a rectal thermometer happens to be sitting in. Other areas where temperature is taken (oral, axillary, etc.) are areas where children frequently do not allow the probe to sit for any length of time. Because of this, some have suggested that in younger children, you might attempt using a pacifier thermometer (a technology which this editor calls a "thermometer in a binky").[1]

When all is said and done, it may be that the touch of the back of a mother's hand is as good as anything to screen for a significant fever. Whybrew et al tell us that as a screening procedure, touch, while seriously overestimating the incidence of fever, rarely misses a fever.[2] In a sense, this is ideal since screening tests are allowed to have some false-positives, but few false-negatives.

It's time for a moratorium on more of this fever and how to detect it nonsense. All any of us can do is our best at telling who is and who is not febrile. Who was it that said: "When you're hot, you're hot, when you're not, you're not"? Bet they didn't have an aural infrared thermometer in mind.

For more on this topic, see a practitioner's prospective.[3]

J.A. Stockman III, M.D.

References

1. Press S, Quinn J: The pacifier thermometer, comparison of supralingual with rectal temperatures in infants and young children. *Arch Pediatr Adolesc Med* 151:550-554, 1997.
2. Whybrew K, Murray M, Morley C: Diagnosing fever by touch: Observational study. *BMJ* 317:321, 1998.
3. Prazar GE: The aural infrared thermometer: A practitioner's prospective. *J Pediatr* 133:471-472, 1998.

Diagnosing Fever by Touch: Observational Study

Whybrew K, Murray M, Morley C (Univ of Cambridge, England)
BMJ 317:321, 1998   5–13

Background.—Fever, a useful indicator of whether a child is seriously ill, is often estimated by touch. Whether mothers and medical students could reliably use touch to determine the presence of fever was investigated.

Methods.—One thousand ninety children, aged 1 month to 16 years, were included in the study. Two medical students and the child's mother felt the child's abdomen, forehead, and neck and independently recorded whether the child felt hot. At the same time, a mercury thermometer was used to determine axillary temperature.

Findings.—Twenty-seven percent of the children had fever, defined as 37.8°C or higher. By touch, the mothers determined that 67% of the children were warm or hot. The sensitivity and specificity of the mother's touch were 94% and 44%, respectively, with positive and negative predictive values of 39% and 95%. The medical students judged 48% of the children as being warm or hot. The students' sensitivity and specificity were 94% and 67%, respectively, with positive and negative predictive values of 49% and 97%.

Conclusions.—Using touch, mothers and medical students rarely missed a child with a fever, though they overestimated the number who had a fever. Thus, a child who does not feel hot is unlikely to have a fever. A child who feels hot should have his or her temperature taken before fever is diagnosed.

▶ Who can deny that a mother's touch is as good as a thermometer, at least in some respects, when it comes to detecting a baby's temperature? Few, if any, fevers will be missed. So what if half the time mothers tend to over-diagnose a fever? It is better to be more sensitive than specific in this regard.

So what does all this mean? It means that if a parent is concerned about a fever, it's okay to take a temperature by touch because fever will rarely be missed. Before calling the doctor at 3 AM, however, it would be wise to verify the finding with a thermometer.

J.A. Stockman III, M.D.

Use of Topical Lidocaine in Pediatric Laceration Repair: A Review of Topical Anesthetics

Stewart GM, Simpson P, Rosenberg NM (Wayne State Univ, Detroit)
Pediatr Emerg Care 14:419-423, 1998   5–14

Introduction.—As medical personnel acknowledge prior insensitivity to pediatric pain management, they are now increasing their attention to this issue. Up to 55% of total pediatric emergency department visits are accounted for by lacerations. For suture repair, lidocaine injection is traditionally used. To eliminate the pain of the injection, topical anesthetics have been used; however, no pediatric study has tested the anesthetic effect of topical aqueous lidocaine alone in laceration repair. Whether the application of topical lidocaine to a laceration decreased pain from the lidocaine injection in children was studied.

Methods.—In this prospective, double-blind study were 100 children, aged 5 to 16 years, who had simple lacerations during a 6-month period. A Telfa pad was soaked with an unlabeled 3-mL solution of either 1% lidocaine or placebo (saline) and then was placed onto the laceration for 10 minutes. An injection of 1% lidocaine was performed into the wound, which was then irrigated and sutured. The patient and parent were asked to record pain response 4 times: before any intervention, after the soak, after the injection, and at the end of the procedure. At the same intervals, blood pressure and heart rates were recorded. The 2 groups had similar age, sex, race, laceration length, and physiologic parameters.

Results.—The groups did not differ in the 4 pain ratings in the categories of age, sex, race, laceration length, or location. In relieving pain from the injection, topical lidocaine was ineffective. A significant negative correlation was noted for age versus injection pain when the groups were combined, with older children reporting less pain from injection than younger children.

Conclusion.—Pain from subsequent lidocaine injection was not decreased by soaking a simple laceration with 1% lidocaine in children. Development of a new effective, safe, and cost-efficient topical anesthetic may provide a viable alternative to the lidocaine injection.

▶ There is nothing like a simple study with a simple conclusion: Soaking a Telfa pad with 1% lidocaine and then placing it on a laceration for 10 minutes adds nothing to the normal routine of infiltrating a wound with 1% lidocaine before suturing.

So are there other good options when sutures are required? EMLA is a fine topical anesthetic but has to be left on for as long as an hour to be effective. It may prolong wound healing and is not recommended for laceration repair. Refrigerant topical anesthetics, including ethyl chloride, work by producing a noxious cold stimulus which is thought to alter transmission of the pain impulse. Most data suggest that such agents are no better than nothing in reducing pain related to suturing.

In summary, soaking a cut with lidocaine will do nothing for either you or your patient. If you insist on using a topical agent, try lidocaine combined with adrenalin or with adrenalin and tetracaine. The rub is that such combinations are somewhat more expensive and can be associated with some morbidity. All in all, a syringe of 1% lidocaine remains the safest and quickest way to close a wound.

This commentary is written as the Special Olympics are being held just a few miles from my home. Such events bring about the need to close a few lacerations. Take the last "big" Summer Olympics, for example. The 1996 Olympic Games in Atlanta attracted an estimated 5 million people, making it the largest peace-time gathering in history. Over 10,000 of this 5 million needed help from the Games' medical services. Those seeking help included 890 officials, 480 Olympic dignitaries, and some 2000 athletes. In addition to the usual cuts and bruises, the subtropical weather contributed over 1000 consultations for heat-related illness, and heat stations handed out some 645,000 cups of water, 600,000 hats, nearly 400,000 packets of sunscreen, and 162,000 hand fans.[1]

J.A. Stockman III, M.D.

Reference

1. Health care delivery and olympic games (editorial). *BMJ* 316:1684, 1998.

Frozen Oral Hydration as an Alternative to Conventional Enteral Fluids
Santucci KA, Anderson AC, Lewander WJ, et al (Rhode Island Hosp, Providence)
Arch Pediatr Adolesc Med 152:142-146, 1998   5–15

Introduction.—For mild-to-severe acute diarrheal disease of various causes, the efficacy of oral rehydration therapy has been proven. Mild dehydration is associated with infant diarrhea and oral hydration is the treatment; however, 400 deaths per year still occur. In the United States, the practice is to commonly administer clear liquids such as fruit juices, carbonated beverages, and sports drinks; however, because of their high osmolality and inappropriate ratio of sodium to carbohydrate content, they are inappropriate for rehydration. Pedialyte and Infalyte are best suited for use as maintenance solutions; however, at times there is resistance associated with their use. A frozen product may facilitate the initiation of oral rehydration or maintenance hydration without the use of IV fluids in children with ongoing losses. The tolerability of the frozen solution was compared with that of the conventional solution.

Methods.—There were 91 children with enteritis ranging in age from 6 months to 13 years who had mild-to-moderate dehydration. They were offered either the frozen solution (Revital) or the conventional solution (glucose electrolyte solution). During a 90-minute trial period, the patients were offered 10 mL/kg of either product in 3 equal aliquots, and they were monitored for the quantities consumed and vomited. The alternate product was offered with complete treatment failures, or absolute refusal, and the intake was recorded.

Results.—Fifty-five percent tolerated the full amount offered of the frozen solution in comparison with 11% of those offered the conventional solution. Fifty-seven percent completely refused the conventional solution. After they crossed over to the frozen solution, 20% tolerated the full amount and 33% tolerated between 5 and 9 mL/kg. For the frozen solution, the treatment failures were 12%, and after those patients were crossed over the conventional solution, none could tolerate more than 5 mL/kg.

Conclusion.—The frozen solution was more easily tolerated by the children with mild or moderate dehydration in comparison to the conventional solution. A greater tolerance rate was seen in the conventional solution failures who crossed over to the frozen solution compared with the reverse.

▶ Oral rehydration fluids have been around for a long time. Although they were first introduced in 1946, it was not for another 20 years or so that early controlled trials documented their effectiveness in managing acute diarrheal disease in children.[1,2] Now, balanced electrolyte solutions for such purposes are big market items and include solutions such as Pedialyte and Infalyte. The rub with these is that many children—particularly those who have nausea and vomiting—just will not take oral rehydration solutions.

So why are frozen rehydration solutions, the "medicinal popsicles," more acceptable and potentially effective? The answer is obvious. Humans are oral creatures. In this sense, swallowing odorous fluids does not produce much in the way of satisfaction. Sucking on a popsicle, on the other hand, does. That is why babies like binkies, adults like ice cream cones, and some men like cigars. Add to this a better taste, a cool and soothing object to suck on, and you can see why a child with nausea, vomiting, and diarrhea might prefer an ice pop's appeal.

There is only 1 rub to all this and that rub is pretty obvious: Among the world's populations, those at greatest risk from dying of dehydration from diarrheal illness are those who have no freezer at home. Unless the Good Humor man is willing to stock balanced electrolyte solution–flavored popsicles and unless he is willing to drive over hill and dale in third world countries, oral rehydration via the popsicle will have only limited benefits, if one is talking about mankind as a whole. This disclaimer is no reason not to join the bandwagon here in the United States where most homes, even in impoverished areas, have a reasonable likelihood of having a freezer or access to one.

J.A. Stockman III, M.D.

References

1. Finberg L, Kravath RE, Hellerstein S: *Water and Electrolytes in Pediatrics: Physiology, Pathophysiology and Treatment.* Philadelphia, WB Saunders, 1993.
2. Pierce NF, Sack RB, Mitra R, et al: Replacement of electrolyte and water losses in cholera by oral glucose-electrolyte solution. *Ann Intern Med* 70:1173-1181, 1969.

Bacteriologic Analysis of Infected Dog and Cat Bites
Talan DA, for the Emergency Medicine Animal Bite Infection Study Group (Univ of California, Los Angeles; et al)
N Engl J Med 340:85-92, 1999   5–16

Objective.—Dog and cat bites are a very common problem that can lead to serious sequelae if they become infected. Past microbiologic studies of

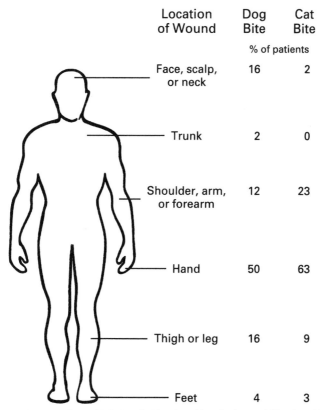

Location of Wound	Dog Bite	Cat Bite
	% of patients	
Face, scalp, or neck	16	2
Trunk	2	0
Shoulder, arm, or forearm	12	23
Hand	50	63
Thigh or leg	16	9
Feet	4	3

FIGURE 1.—Location of wound infections in 50 patients bitten by dogs and 57 patients bitten by cats. (Reprinted by permission of *The New England Journal of Medicine*, from Talan DA, for the Emergency Medicine Animal Bite Infection Study Group: Bacteriologic analysis of infected dog and cat bites. *N Engl J Med* 340:85-92. Copyright 1999, Massachusetts Medical Society. All rights reserved.)

animal bites have included small numbers of patients, vague definitions of infection, and variable specimen collection and pathogen isolation techniques. A prospective, multicenter bacteriologic study of dog and cat bites was designed to avoid these shortcomings.

Methods.—To be included in the 21-month, 18-center study, patients had to have a dog or cat bite resulting in a cutaneous wound large enough for at least a miniswab to be inserted for deep culture. Patients had to meet at least 1 of 3 specified major criteria for infection—fever of greater than 38°C, abscess, and lymphangitis; or 4 of 5 minor criteria—wound-associated erythema, wound site tenderness, wound site swelling, purulent drainage, and leukocytosis. Specimens for microbiologic analysis were taken by needle aspiration from abscesses, cotton swabs for open wounds, and miniswabs for puncture wounds. Aerobic and anaerobic cultures were performed at a research laboratory and sometimes at local hospital laboratories. Various methods were used to isolate the infecting strains. Outcomes were assessed by medical records review and telephone follow-up.

TABLE 3.—Aerobic and Anaerobic Bacteria Isolated From 50 Dog Bites and 57 Cat Bites

Bacteria	Dog Bite No. of Patients (%)	Cat Bite No. of Patients (%)
Aerobes		
Pasteurella		
Past. canis	25 (50)	43 (75)
Past. multocida spp. multocida	13 (26)	1 (2)
Past. stomatis	6 (12)	31 (54)
Past. multocida ssp. septica	5 (10)	2 (4)
Past. dagmatis	2 (4)	4 (7)
Past. multocida ssp. gallicida	1 (2)	0
Other†	1 (2)	0
Streptococcus		
Strep. mitis	23 (46)	26 (46)
Strep. mutans	11 (22)	13 (23)
Strep. pyogenes	6 (12)	6 (11)
Strep. sanguis II	6 (12)	0
Strep. intermedius	4 (8)	7 (12)
Strep. constellatus	3 (6)	2 (4)
Strep. equinus	2 (4)	2 (4)
Strep. sanguis I	1 (2)	3 (5)
Strep. agalactiae	1 (2)	1 (2)
Strep. sanguis	1 (2)	1 (2)
β-Hemolytic, group G	1 (2)	0
Strep. dysgalactiae	1 (2)	1 (2)
β-Hemolytic, group F	0	0
Staphylococcus	23 (46)	20 (35)
Staph. aureus	10 (20)	2 (4)
Staph. epidermidis	9 (18)	10 (18)
Staph. warneri	3 (6)	6 (11)
Other†	3 (6)	0
Staph. intermedius	1 (2)	1 (2)
Staph. hominis	1 (2)	1 (2)
Aerobes (cont.)		
Moraxella	5 (10)	20 (35)
Other†	5 (10)	18 (32)
Morax. catarrhalis	1 (2)	6 (11)
EF-4b	5 (10)	9 (16)
Enterococcus	5 (10)	7 (12)
Ent. faecalis	3 (6)	2 (4)
Ent. avium	1 (2)	0
Ent. malodoratus	1 (2)	0
Ent. durans	0	
Bacillus	4 (8)	5 (9)
Bac. firmus	2 (4)	6 (11)
Bac. circulans	1 (2)	1 (2)
Bac. subtilis	1 (2)	0
Other†	0	3 (5)
Pseudomonas	3 (6)	3 (5)
Pseud. aeruginosa	1 (2)	0
Pseud. vesicularis	1 (2)	1 (2)
Pseud. diminuta	1 (2)	0
Pseud. putida	0	1 (2)
Pseud. stutzeri	0	1 (2)
Actinomyces	3 (6)	2 (4)
Act. viscosus	2 (4)	1 (2)
Act. neuii ssp. anitratus	1 (2)	0
Other†	0	1 (2)
Brevibacterium†	3 (6)	2 (4)
Gemella morbillorum	3 (6)	2 (4)
EF-4a	3 (6)	0
Escherichia coli	1 (2)	1 (2)
Weeksella	1 (2)	4 (7)
Aerobes (cont.)		
Actinobacillus†	0	2 (4)
Alcaligenes	0	2 (4)
Alcal. faecalis	0	1 (2)
Alcal. odorans	0	1 (2)
Enterobacter cloacae	0	2 (4)
Erysipelothrix rhusiopathiae	0	2 (4)
Reimerella anatipestifer	0	2 (4)
Rothia dentocariosa	0	2 (4)
Aeromonas hydrophila	0	1 (2)
Pantoea agglomerans	0	1 (2)
Rhodococcus†	0	1 (2)
Streptomyces†	0	1 (2)
Anaerobes		
Fusobacterium	16 (32)	19 (33)
Fuso. nucleatum	8 (16)	14 (25)
Other†	6 (12)	4 (7)
Fuso. russii	1 (2)	8 (14)
Fuso. gonidiaformans	1 (2)	1 (2)
Fuso. alocis	1 (2)	0
Bacteroides	15 (30)	16 (28)
Bact. tectum	7 (14)	16 (28)
Bact. forsythus	2 (4)	0
Bact. gracilis	2 (4)	0
Bact. ureolyticus	2 (4)	0
Bact. tectum group E	1 (2)	2 (4)
Bact. fragilis	1 (2)	1 (2)
Bact. ovatus	1 (2)	0
Porphyromonas	14 (28)	17 (30)

Organism	Dog	Cat
Staph. auricularis	1 (2)	0
Staph. cohnii	1 (2)	0
Staph. xylosus	1 (2)	0
Staph. sciuri-lentus	0	2 (4)
Staph. capitis	0	1 (2)
Staph. haemolyticus	0	1 (2)
Staph. hyicus	0	1 (2)
Staph. saprophyticus	0	1 (2)
Staph. simulans	0	1 (2)
Neisseria	8 (16)	11 (19)
N. weaverii	7 (14)	8 (14)
N. subflava	1 (2)	1 (2)
Other†	1 (2)	0
N. cinerea-flavescens	0	1 (2)
N. mucosa	0	1 (2)
Corynebacterium	6 (12)	16 (28)
Group G	3 (6)	3 (5)
Coryne. minutissimum	2 (4)	4 (7)
Coryne. aquaticum	1 (2)	8 (14)
Coryne. jeikeium	1 (2)	1 (2)
Coryne. afermentans	1 (2)	0
Group E	1 (2)	0
Coryne. pseudodiphtheriticum	1 (2)	0
Other†	0	0
Group B	0	1 (2)
Group F-1	1 (2)	1 (2)
Coryne. kutscheri	0	1 (2)
Coryne. propinquum	0	1 (2)
Coryne. striatum	0	1 (2)
W. virosa	0	0
W. zoobelcum	0	2 (4)
Klebsiella	2 (4)	2 (4)
K. oxytoca	1 (2)	1 (2)
K. pneumoniae	0	1 (2)
Lactobacillus	1 (2)	2 (4)
L. lactis	0	1 (2)
Other†	1 (2)	2 (4)
Citrobacter	0	1 (2)
Citro. amalonaticus	0	1 (2)
Citro. koseri	0	2 (4)
Flavobacterium	0	1 (2)
Group IIa	0	1 (2)
Flavo. brevis	0	2 (4)
Micrococcus	0	1 (2)
Micro. lylae	0	1 (2)
Other†	0	2 (4)
Proteus mirabilis	0	2 (4)
Stenotrophomonas maltophilia	4 (7)	1 (2)
Capnocytophaga	2 (4)	1 (2)
Cap. ochracea	3 (5)	1 (2)
Other†	1 (2)	1 (2)
Eikenella corrodens	1 (2)	1 (2)
Flavimonas oryzihabitans	0	1 (2)
Dermabacter hominis	0	1 (2)
Oerskovia†	0	1 (2)
Pediococcus damnosus	0	1 (2)
Stomatococcus mucilaginosus	0	1 (2)
Acinetobacter	4 (7)	1 (2)
Acine. baumannii	2 (4)	1 (2)
Acine. luoffii	2 (4)	1 (2)
Porph. macacae	4 (7)	3 (6)
Porph. cansulci	1 (2)	3 (6)
Porph. gingivalis	6 (11)	2 (4)
Porph. canoris	5 (9)	2 (4)
Porph. cangingivalis	2 (4)	2 (4)
Other†	0	1 (2)
Porph. circumdentaria	3 (5)	1 (2)
Porph. levii-like	0	0
Prevotella	11 (19)	14 (28)
Prev. heparinolytica	5 (9)	7 (14)
Prev. intermedia	0	4 (8)
Other†	4 (7)	1 (2)
Prev. zoogleoformans	1 (2)	2 (4)
Prev. melaninogenica	1 (2)	1 (2)
Prev. denticola	0	1 (2)
Propionibacterium	10 (18)	10 (20)
Prop. acnes	9 (16)	7 (14)
Prop. acidi-propionicus	0	1 (2)
Prop. freudenreichii	0	1 (2)
Other†	0	0
Prop. avidum	1 (2)	1 (2)
Prop. lymphophilium	1 (2)	0
Peptostreptococcus	3 (5)	8 (16)
Pept. anaerobius	3 (5)	4 (8)
Other†	0	3 (6)
Pept. asaccharolyticus	1 (2)	1 (2)
Eubacterium†	0	2 (4)
Lactobacillus jensenii	1 (2)	1 (2)
Filifactor villosus	3 (5)	0
Clostridium sordellii	1 (2)	0
Veillonella†	1 (2)	0

*Some patients were infected with more than 1 type or species of bacteria.

†The isolate could not be identified beyond the genus level.

Results.—The analysis included 107 patients with infected bite wounds—50 patients with dog bites and 57 with cat bites (Fig 1). Median age was 28 years for patients with dog bites versus 39 years for those with cat bites; 22% of patients were less than 18 years old. Most dog bite victims were male, whereas most cat bite victims were female. Sixty percent of dog bite wounds and 85% of cat bite wounds were puncture wounds.

The median number of isolates per culture at the research laboratory was 5, compared with a median of 1 isolate per culture at the local laboratories. Fifty-six percent of wounds yielded both aerobes and anaerobes, 36% aerobes only, and 1% anaerobes only; 7% of cultures yielded no isolate (Table 3). One half of dog bites and three fourths of cat bites yielded *Pasteurella* species, especially *Pasteurella canis* in dog bites and *Pasteurella multicoda*, species *multicoda* and *septica* in cat bites. Other commonly isolated organisms included aerobic organisms of the genera *Streptococcus, Staphylococcus, Moraxella,* and *Neisseria* and anaerobic species of the genera *Fusobacterium, Bacteroides, Porphyromonas,* and *Prevotella*. Several organisms not previously identified as pathogenic in humans were isolated, including *Reimerella anatipestifer, Bacteroides tectum, Prevotella heparinolytica,* and various *Porphyromonas* species. The microbiologic results supported the use of a β-lactam antibiotic and a β-lactamase inhibitor, which was the most frequent treatment.

Conclusions.—The findings highlight the complex microbiologic characteristics of infected dog and cat bite wounds. *Pasteurella* species are the most common isolates, but other less common organisms are identified as well. The results suggest that empiric therapy for infected dog and cat bites wounds should consist of a β-lactam antibiotic and a β-lactamase inhibitor, a second-generation cephalosporin with anaerobic activity, or combination therapy with either penicillin and a first-generation cephalosporin or clindamycin and a fluoroquinolone.

▶ Most cat and dog bites are ones administered to their owners by their own pets. Apparently, such domestic animals do not believe in the philosophy of never biting the hand that feeds them. Be it an animal bite from the patient's own Rover or Felix or not, when you see a patient with an animal bite, a whole series of decisions have to be entertained by you as the care provider. How do you clean the wound? Can the wound be closed with sutures? Are there areas of the body that differ from other areas? Does the use of a prophylactic antibiotic make any difference? Do you need to give tetanus toxoid? Do you need to give tetanus immune globulin? Are the considerations different if the bite is from a human? The answer to the above questions can at times be somewhat complex. Bites occasionally do not look serious when they are. A puncture wound over a joint, a tendon, a blood vessel, or a nerve, or even certain facial areas, can seed parts of the body that quickly get into trouble, even though the initial wound may look quite benign. In general, wounds should be left open unless they are at risk of a cosmetic problem. This is certainly true if the wound is more of a puncture than a laceration, particularly if it involves the legs, arms, and hands as opposed to the face. The longer the time after a bite has occurred, the less inclined you should be to close a wound. Please note, however, that a dog bite causing a laceration on the face, or one caused by a cat in the same area, can almost always be closed without getting into too much trouble. If you do decide to close a laceration caused by an animal bite, avoid any use of subcutaneous sutures if at all possible, since such foreign material drives up the risk of infection fairly significantly. The article abstracted above merely tells us what the infectious agents are that cause problems after an animal bite delivered by a dog or cat. The report does not tell us whether we should use antibiotics. Antibiotics use is somewhat controversial, but most people do employ them if faced with a high-risk wound (a deep puncture, particularly if from a cat bite, wounds requiring suturing, and those involving the hands). In the absence of these kinds of risk conditions, routine use of antibiotics is probably not warranted. When antibiotics are used, the most commonly employed one is amoxicillin combined with a β-lactamase inhibitor. Don't forget the risk of tetanus. Those who are bitten who have had 2 or fewer primary immunizations probably should receive both tetanus toxoid and tetanus immune globulin. Tetanus toxoid alone is fine for those whose primary immunizations have been completed, but who have not received a booster in the last 5 years. Two final precautions: always worry about rabies. If in doubt, see your Red Book. Also, remember that human bites represent an entirely different kettle of fish. Human bites can transmit HIV, hepatitis B, hepatitis C, and other odds and ends, including syphilis. You would be better off being bitten by a horse than by another human.

This commentary closes with a few fast facts about animals and animal bites. In 1995 and 1996, at least 25 persons died as a result of dog attacks. Of these deaths, 20 occurred among children (3 were under the age of 30 days, 1 was 5 months old, 10 were aged 1-4 years, and 6 were aged 5-11 years). Five deaths occurred among adults. The oldest was an 86-year-old woman in Tennessee who went outside her home simply to check the weather and was fatally mauled by 2 rottweilers owned by a neighbor. The dogs had also attacked and injured the woman 1 month before the final attack. Of the 25 deaths reported with sufficient information to understand exactly what happened, 30% involved an unrestrained dog off the owner's property. One in 5 involved a restrained dog on the owner's property, and approximately half involved an unrestrained dog on the owner's property. Of the 25 deaths, 36% involved 1 dog, 36% involved 2 dogs, and 8% involved 3 dogs. Some 20% involved between 6 and 11 dogs. All of the attacks by unrestrained dogs off an owner's property involved more than 1 dog. Of the 3 deaths among neonates, all occurred on the dog owner's property and involved 1 dog and a sleeping child. Rottweilers were the most commonly involved dog.[1]

By the way, a study of the intelligence of dogs suggests that the smartest breed of dog is the Border collie. The least intelligent breed of dog is the basset hound. There is no overall general correlation between the intelligence of a dog and the likelihood that it will or will not bite.

J.A. Stockman III, M.D.

Reference

1. Dog-bite–related fatalities: United States, 1995-1996 (editorial). *MMWR* 46:467-470, 1997.

Course and Outcome of Chronic Fatigue in Children and Adolescents

Krilov LR, Fisher M, Friedman SB, et al (New York Univ, Manhasset; Albert Einstein College of Medicine, Bronx, NY)
Pediatrics 102:360-366, 1998   5–17

Background.—Chronic fatigue syndrome is a recognized disorder that occurs in people of all ages. These authors characterized the course of chronic fatigue syndrome in children and adolescents.

Methods.—Fifty-eight children (29% male, 71% female; 94% white) who were evaluated for chronic fatigue between 1990 and 1994. Half the patients were children 7 to 14 years of age, and half were 15 to 21 years of age. In summer 1994, all records were reviewed to standardize demographic and psychosocial data, signs, symptoms, results of laboratory tests, and data obtained at follow-up. Additionally, 42 of the families were interviewed by telephone to discuss how the patient was getting along.

Findings.—When initially seen, 50% of patients had experienced fatigue for 6 months or less, and 50% had experienced fatigue for 7 to 36 months. In most cases, the fatigue was brought on by acute illness (60%), and most patients had a history of allergies (60%). The most common symptoms

TABLE 2.—Symptoms Most Commonly Reported by Young Patients Seen for Evaluation of Chronic Fatigue

	(*n*)	(%)
Fatigue	58	100
Headache	43	74
Sore throat	34	59
Abdominal pain	28	48
Fever	21	36
Impaired cognition	19	33
Myalgia	18	31
Diarrhea	17	29
Adenopathy	17	29
Anorexia	16	28
Nausea/vomiting	15	26
Congestion	13	22
Dizziness	10	17
Arthralgia	10	17
Otitis	6	10
Cough	6	10
Rash	5	9
Sweats	5	9
Chills	4	7
Depression	4	7

reported were fatigue (100%), headache (74%), and sore throat (59%) (Table 2), although abdominal symptoms, fever, impaired cognition, and myalgia were also frequent (reported by more than 31% of patients). Evidence of earlier Epstein-Barr virus infection was seen in 32 patients, and 9 had antibodies to cytomegalovirus, 2 had antibodies to toxoplasma, and 2 had antibodies to *Borrelia burgdorferi*. However, none of the patients had significantly abnormal immunoglobulin levels. Most students reported that their school performance and social activities had suffered due to their fatigue. At follow-up, many patients' symptoms had improved significantly by the first year after treatment (41% of patients were "at their best most of the time," vs 12% of patients when initially seen), as did their participation in activities (56% vs 20%). By the second year of follow-up, 70% of symptoms and 75% of activities were "at their best most of the time." By the fourth year, almost all of the patients were doing well almost all of the time. Telephone interviews indicated that families considered the child to be "cured" or "improved" in 43% and 52% of cases, respectively, and in only 5% of cases did the family consider the child to be "the same." None of the demographic or clinical factors examined correlated with the patients' performance during follow-up.

Conclusions.—The types of symptoms reported by children and adolescents with chronic fatigue syndrome are similar to those reported by adults. However, children and adolescents with chronic fatigue syndrome are often seen earlier than adults (within 6 months of syndrome onset), and the vast majority (95%) can expect improvement, if not total resolution, of symptoms with appropriate medical and psychosocial care.

▶ Thank goodness the Centers for Disease Control and Prevention (CDC) have provided us with uniform criteria for making a diagnosis of the chronic fatigue syndrome. The CDC tells us we can make this diagnosis if a patient has persistent or relapsing fatigue of greater than 6 months' duration in association with at least 4 minor criteria including impaired cognition, sore throat, adenopathy, muscle pain, joint pain, headache, unrefreshing sleep, and/or postexertional malaise.[1]

Please recognize that the chronic fatigue syndrome is not a new entity. In the middle of the 19th century, the term neurasthenia was used to describe it. People with neurasthenia were thought to have a form of nervous exhaustion. One of the reasons for thanking the CDC for codifying the diagnosis is that we now can use 1 term to describe the illness. "Chronic fatigue syndrome" is a far better term than others used in the past—terms such as "skiver's sickness" and "yuppie flu," as well as more conventional terms such as "postviral fatigue syndrome," "myalgic encephalomyelitis," "neuromyasthenia," "fibromyalgia," "myasthenia," "myalgic syndrome," and "Iceland disease."

So is long-term, low-dose hydrocortisone treatment the magic bullet for the chronic fatigue syndrome? Supplementation with small daily doses of hydrocortisone (that is, 20-30 mg for young adults at about 8:00 AM, and 5 mg at about 2:00 PM, for 12 weeks) results in slight, but consistent improvements compared with placebo-treated controls. These low doses of steroids will still suppress the adrenal glands and probably should not be used for prolonged treatment courses.

In a review of the management of chronic fatigue syndrome, Franklin makes some very appropriate comments about the disorder.[2] He states: "Chronic fatigue syndrome is a real illness and currently affects a large number of children whose education is interrupted for prolonged periods due to sickness. This illness is a genuine disability whether it is thought to be of biological, psychological, or mixed origin. The doctor may be called upon to advocate for the patient with chronic fatigue syndrome, and I believe the families need more empathy rather than criticism from the medical profession. Those young people who have recovered, gradually feel more secure in their own ability than those who have been forced to submit to a regimen which they resent for years afterwards."

Even though many of us are tired of hearing about this enigmatic disorder, it is well worth reading Dr. Franklin's review if you have time.

Lastly, patients with the chronic fatigue disorder often use smelling salts at times of faintness. Smelling salts can be dangerous to young children if the salts are bitten into. Several cases involving children biting into these pellets have recently been reported. Smelling salts are ammonia pellets. They are produced and manufactured by numerous companies. An example of the ingredients of a typical capsule includes 15% ammonia hydroxide, 35% denatured alcohol, 4% ammonium carbonate, and 46% water. The contents are usually packaged within a 0.33-mL glass ampule and covered with a tough filter paper. When broken, the capsule or ampule releases a solution having an aromatic and pungent odor of ammonia, which immediately colors the filter paper pink from rubine dye. If a child bites into such a capsule, the ammonia that is released will be extremely caustic and can easily damage the throat, esophagus, and other areas of the gastrointestinal tract.

If you should ever run across this problem, the cardinal rules are as follows: (1) do not induce vomiting; (2) give water or milk in large volumes (no more than 15 mL/kg body weight); (3) wash skin and eyes with large amounts of running water; and (4) call an otolaryngologist. It would be wise for the latter specialist to inspect the upper airway and possibly the esophagus for burns.[3]

J.A. Stockman III, M.D.

References

1. Fukuda K, Straus SE, Peterson P, et al: The International Chronic Fatigue Syndrome Study Group. The chronic fatigue syndrome: A comprehensive approach to its definition and study. *Ann Intern Med* 121:953-959, 1994.
2. Franklin A: How I manage chronic fatigue syndrome. *Arch Dis Child* 79:375-378, 1998.
3. Rosenbaum AM, Walner DL, Dunham ME, et al: Ammonia capsule ingestion causing upper aerodigestive tract injury. *Otolaryngol Head Neck Surg* 119:678-680, 1998.

In Which Journals Will Pediatricians Find the Best Evidence for Clinical Practice?

Birken CS, Parkin PC (Univ of Toronto; Hosp for Sick Children, Toronto)
Pediatrics 103:941-947, 1999   5–18

Background.—A knowledge of which medical journals contain the best evidence relating to clinical pediatric practice would allow the clinician to make the most efficient use of journal reading time. These authors applied 3 different strategies to identify which journals contain the best evidence pertaining to clinical pediatric practice.

Methods.—Three strategies of analysis were developed, based on the assumption that the medical literature itself would identify the highest quality journal articles. All 3 strategies were based on systematic reviews covering the topics of pediatrics, children, infants, newborns, neonates, neonatology, and adolescents. The first strategy involved a review of the Cochrane Database of Systematic Reviews (CDSR), Issue 4, 1997, published by the Cochrane Collaboration, which is a network that prepares, maintains, and disseminates systematic reviews on the effects of health care. The second strategy involved policy statements of the American Academy of Pediatrics (AAP) from 1994 to 1996, as found in the AAP policy reference guide. The third strategy involved policy statements of the Canadian Paediatric Society (CPS) from 1990 to 1997, as found in *Pediatrics and Child Health*.

Stringent criteria were applied to exclude topics related to tertiary neonatology, health care professionals other than physicians, public health policy, and ethics; also excluded were nonjournal citation sources, statements with no references, CDSR journal citations with no pediatric subjects, citations of AAP policy statements cited in AAP policy statements, and non-English articles. Then, under the 3 different strategies, the citations from the 10 most frequently cited journals were tallied and expressed as a percentage of the total citations identified.

TABLE 2.—Top 10 Journals Cited: American Academy of Pediatrics Strategy

Journal Title	Number of Citations	Percent of Total Citations (n = 960)
Pediatrics	106	11.4% (95% CI: 9.4, 13.4)
Journal of Pediatrics	63	6.8%
New England Journal of Medicine	45	4.8%
Journal of the American Medical Association	42	4.5%
Journal of Infectious Diseases	35	3.8%
American Journal of Diseases in Childhood	30	3.2%
Pediatric Infectious Diseases Journal	21	2.3%
Lancet	20	2.3%
British Medical Journal	18	1.9%
Archives of Diseases in Childhood	13	1.4%
Total citations of top 10 journals cited	393	42.3% (95% CI: 39.3, 45.3)

Abbreviation: CI, confidence interval.
(Reproduced by permission of *Pediatrics*, from Birken CS, Parkin PC: In which journals will pediatricians find the best evidence for clinical practice? *Pediatrics* 103:941-947, 1999.)

Findings.—All 3 strategies identified 7 journals as being among the 10 most frequently cited journals. They are (in alphabetic order): *Archives of Diseases in Childhood, British Medical Journal, Journal of the American Medical Association, Journal of Pediatrics, Lancet, New England Journal of Medicine,* and *Pediatrics* (Table 2). *Pediatrics* was the journal cited most frequently, according to all 3 strategies, and represented 6.0%, 11.4%, and 11.9% of the total citations identified by the CDSR (n = 234), AAP (n = 960), and CPS (n = 873) strategies. Furthermore, citations from the top 10 journals in the CDSR, AAP, and CPS strategies accounted for 38.9%, 42.3%, and 60.6% of the total citations with that strategy.

Conclusion.—A handful of medical journals serve as the best sources for medical evidence pertaining to clinical pediatric practice. Nonetheless, high-quality evidence relevant to pediatric practice can be found in many medical journals. It is hoped that these results help clinicians to develop a strategy for making efficient use of evidence-based medicine as reported in the current medical literature.

Size and Age-Sex Distribution of Pediatric Practice: A Study From Pediatric Research in Office Settings
Bocian AB, Wasserman RC, Slora EJ, et al (American Academy of Pediatrics, Elk Grove Village, Ill; Univ of Vermont, Burlington; Arvada Pediatrics Assoc, Colo; et al)
Arch Pediatr Adolesc Med 153:9-14, 1999   5–19

Introduction.—Little is known about the size of pediatricians' practices or the number of children cared for by an individual pediatrician. HMO sources estimated the number of patients per pediatrician to be 885:1 to a high of 1750:1. Their estimates may be artificially low because children seen in HMOs have higher visit rates than children seen in fee-for-service settings. Recent data on age distribution of patients seen by office-based pediatricians are also lacking. The average number of patients per practitioner was estimated. The total number of active patients cared for was determined. The age and sex distribution of patients seen in pediatric practice was estimated.

Methods.—There were 89 practices in 31 states with 373 practitioners. The practices were asked to reveal how many patients visited the practice during the prior 2 years. Patients visiting more than once were counted only once. Computer billing records or medical-record sampling were used to determine age-sex registers.

Results.—There were 529,513 active patients among the practitioners, of which 50.75% were male. An average of 1546 patients was cared for by each practitioner. In less-populated areas and in solo practices, the number of patients per practitioner was significantly higher. Eighty-one percent of the patients were 12 years and younger, and more than half of the children were 6 years or younger. Before age 5 a slightly, but significantly, higher number of patients were accounted for by boys; however, after age 14, girls comprised a significantly larger proportion of patients.

Conclusion.—HMO-based estimates were in line with the average number of 1546 patients per practitioner derived from these private-practice data. Younger children are predominantly served by pediatric practitioners. This was the only current national estimate of the size and age-sex distribution of independent pediatric practices. This data can help health service researchers and pediatricians plan for the future provision of health care to children.

▶ Everyone, pediatricians included, likes to know the score. This is the same whether one is talking about the Bulls, the Packers, or the comparisons among us in terms of the number of patients for whom care is provided in a primary care practice. The Pediatric Research in Office Settings (PROS) provides us with the answer. The average pediatrician cares for 1546 patients. If you're caring for significantly more than that (many of you are), you either live in a rural area (rural primary care providers have more patients), your managed care organizations have squeezed you too tightly, or you're just in over your head.

Three cheers for PROS. The American Academy of Pediatrics organized the PROS network a good decade and a half ago to address the shortage of research being done in primary care settings. This network and others like it (such as the Pediatric Practice Research Group out of Illinois and Indiana) contribute valuable information on how we provide care and how we should provide care.

One last comment. The 1500 or so patients per pediatrician found in this report is very similar to the recommendations that have emerged from the Future of Pediatric Education II Task Force. The task force suggests that the ratio of pediatricians to patients 0 to 17 should be approximately 1:1300. If one enlarges the circle to patients 0 to 21, you have to add an additional 6.6%, which brings us pretty close to the 1 in 1500 number found in the PROS report. The task force report also suggests, however, that we need more pediatricians. The reason why is that as of now, just a bit over 50% of children in the United States are cared for by pediatricians. There really is no reason why that percentage should not be higher. Raising the percent of visits cared for by pediatricians to 65%, for example, would require an increase in our current pediatric workforce.

This chapter of the YEAR BOOK closes with a question that any pediatric care provider should be able to answer. Just how good are continuing medical education (CME) speakers these days? Investigators from Minnesota and Illinois recently analyzed the results of the evaluation forms for 9 speakers who participated in a CME symposium.[1] There were 245 attendees, 94 of whom submitted evaluation forms. One speaker had to withdraw abruptly because of an unforeseen event before the scheduled presentation. The remaining 8 speakers were graded very high—80% of the attendees gave them "excellent" or "good" mean scores for quality at presentation. The missing speaker was actually graded by a large number of responders.

The evaluations of his canceled presentation, never given, ran higher than the mean.

Indeed, less is more, more or less.

J.A. Stockman III, M.D.

Reference

1. Christian TF, Bonow RO: Evaluating CME speakers. *N Engl J Med* 338:1163, 1998.

6 Neurology and Psychiatry

National Distribution of Child and Adolescent Psychiatrists
Thomas CR, Holzer CE III (Univ of Texas, Galveston)
J Am Acad Child Adolesc Psychiatry 38:9-16, 1999   6–1

Background.—Earlier reports on the relative number of child and adolescent psychiatrists (CAPs) in the United States suggested a serious shortage of such specialists. However, the advent of managed care and its reduction in psychotherapy by psychiatrists raises the possibility that there is now a surplus of CAPs. The national distribution of CAPs was described by state, community, and youth population.

Methods.—Data on such psychiatrists were compiled for states and counties, then compared by state, county characteristics, number of youth, percentage of youths living in poverty, and child and adolescent psychiatry residents.

Findings.—The number of CAPs per 100,000 youths varied substantially among states and counties (Table 2). These psychiatrists were significantly more likely to live in metropolitan areas and counties with a low percentage of children living in poverty. Distribution was not significantly associated with the distribution of residency training programs in child and adolescent psychiatry.

Conclusions.—The current pattern of CAPs indicates that the shortage of these physicians is most severe in nonmetropolitan areas and in areas where youths are at the greatest risk for mental disorders. These patterns are similar to but more pronounced than those among general psychiatrists.

▶ Dr. Michael Jellinek, professor of Psychiatry and Pediatrics, Harvard Medical School, Boston, comments:

These authors ask two critical questions related to mental health services for children: How many CAPs are needed and what is their geographic availability? Before answering how many CAPs are needed, they appropriately ask how many children need psychiatric services and what is the role of the CAP in their care. Most epidemiologic studies defining prevalence use criteria of impairment in major developmental areas to define which children

TABLE 2.—Youth Aged 0 to 17 Years and Child and Adolescent Psychiatrists by State

State	Youth 0-17 1990 Census	% of Youth 0-17 in Poverty 1990 Census	No. of Child Psychiatrists 1990	Rate of Child Psychiatrists Per 100,000 Youth
Alabama	1,048,610	24.19	23	2.19
Alaska	168,473	11.45	7	4.15
Arizona	962,146	22.03	43	4.47
Arkansas	613,946	25.31	12	1.95
California	7,563,329	18.25	539	7.13
Colorado	847,298	15.29	80	9.44
Connecticut	739,346	10.69	121	16.37
Delaware	160,601	11.99	8	4.98
District of Columbia	112,247	25.49	39	34.74
Florida	2,810,959	18.69	150	5.34
Georgia	1,705,808	20.11	66	3.87
Hawaii	275,518	11.59	34	12.34
Idaho	303,969	16.17	9	2.96
Illinois	2,907,761	17.04	144	4.95
Indiana	1,435,285	14.20	44	3.07
Iowa	709,017	14.34	29	4.09
Kansas	652,636	14.26	65	9.96
Kentucky	943,858	24.79	46	4.87
Louisiana	1,212,904	31.41	49	4.04
Maine	303,858	13.79	20	6.58
Maryland	1,142,102	11.25	180	15.76
Massachusetts	1,333,396	13.22	252	18.90
Michigan	2,424,941	18.57	165	6.80
Minnesota	1,152,575	12.70	53	4.60
Mississippi	739,268	33.64	6	0.81
Missouri	1,296,368	17.75	63	4.86
Montana	218,523	20.46	4	1.83
Nebraska	424,287	13.78	10	2.36
Nevada	287,456	13.30	7	2.44
New Hampshire	274,702	7.44	24	8.74
New Jersey	1,775,286	11.31	121	6.82
New Mexico	440,038	27.78	25	5.68
New York	4,181,056	19.12	626	14.97
North Carolina	1,586,601	17.20	75	4.73
North Dakota	173,549	17.13	5	2.88
Ohio	2,766,663	17.83	121	4.37
Oklahoma	825,896	21.71	22	2.66
Oregon	708,631	15.75	33	4.66
Pennsylvania	2,755,035	15.69	243	8.82
Rhode Island	223,365	13.81	21	9.40
South Carolina	909,732	20.98	43	4.73
South Dakota	195,966	20.36	3	1.53
Tennessee	1,198,879	20.98	45	3.75
Texas	4,774,027	24.29	249	5.22
Utah	622,104	12.54	23	3.70
Vermont	141,350	12.04	15	10.61
Virginia	1,480,087	13.34	114	7.70
Washington	1,232,559	14.54	57	4.62
West Virginia	439,107	26.21	12	2.73
Wisconsin	1,271,165	14.86	65	5.11
Wyoming	133,236	14.40	2	1.50
Total	62,605,519	18.26	4,212	6.73

(Courtesy of Thomas CR, Holzer CE III: National distribution of child and adolescent psychiatrists. *J Am Acad Child Adolesc Psychiatry* 38[1]:9-16, 1999.)

need psychiatric services. Using mild to moderate impairment (a level most pediatricians would find clinically relevant), the prevalence rate of children needing mental health services would be 10% to 13%. Using criteria of moderate to severe impairment leads to an estimate of 5% to 7%. These prevalence figures double in populations of poor or at-risk children.

What is the CAP's role in the care of these children? Before managed care, CAPs often completed comprehensive evaluations, coordinated treatment, and prescribed medication in the context of providing psychotherapy. With the advances in psychopharmacology and with managed care directing treatment, the CAP's role has been narrowed to diagnosis and medication management. Comprehensive evaluations, implementation of treatment plans, and psychotherapy are diffused over a number of other clinicians including the pediatrician, social worker, psychologist, school guidance personnel, and the managed care company's case manager. Based on current data, 3 million to 10 million children need services, which is an overwhelming number given the 5000 CAPs in the United States, many of whom also have teaching, supervisory, administrative, and research responsibilities. The practical access to CAPs is further reduced since most children are not readily available during school hours. Finally, as these authors describe in detail, there is a serious distribution problem both state-to-state and in rural versus urban settings.

Children's mental health needs and CAP distribution issues should negate any turf struggles between primary care pediatricians, behavioral/developmental subspecialists, and CAPs. The central issue is not who should help these children; that answer is easy—everyone working together would still be insufficient. The core issue is the lack of resources in pediatric and psychiatric settings, in schools, and in the tattered social "safety net." Our society has pressured and constrained resources for children's mental health services. Less than one quarter of children get the care they need. The poor get less, those who can afford to pay out-of-pocket get more, and providers are encouraged to compete and cost-shift rather than coordinate and collaborate.

M. Jellinek, M.D.

A Comparison of Rectal Diazepam Gel and Placebo for Acute Repetitive Seizures
Dreifuss FE, Rosman NP, Cloyd JC, et al (Univ of Virginia, Charlottesville; New England Med Ctr, Boston; Univ of Minnesota, Minneapolis)
N Engl J Med 338:1869-1875, 1998   6–2

Introduction.—About 2 million individuals in the United States are affected by epilepsy. Repetitive seizures are those that last minutes or hours and whose pattern is different from the usual seizure pattern. If left untreated, these seizures can turn into a serious problem, such as status epilepticus. The treatment of choice involves administration of benzodiazepines, which have a rapid onset of action and are safe. When the patient

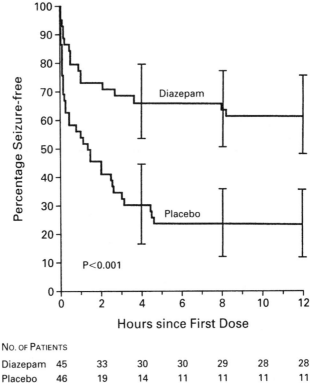

No. of Patients

Diazepam	45	33	30	30	29	28	28
Placebo	46	19	14	11	11	11	11

FIGURE 3.—Kaplan-Meier estimate of the time to a first recurrence of seizures. Data from all patients were censored at 12 hours, the observation period for children. Only 2 patients, both in the placebo group, had their first seizure recurrence between 12 and 24 hours after the initial treatment. The vertical bars show 95% confidence intervals. (Reprinted by permission of *The New England Journal of Medicine*, from Dreifuss FE, Rosman NP, Cloyd JC, et al: A comparison of rectal diazepam gel and placebo for acute repetitive seizures. *N Engl J Med* 338:1869-1875. Copyright 1998, Massachusetts Medical Society. All rights reserved.)

is actively convulsing, oral and sublingual administration is frequently difficult and hazardous, and rectal administration results in slower absorption. Rectal diazepam has been used to treat acute repetitive, prolonged, and febrile seizures. A clinical trial was conducted to assess the safety and efficacy of diazepam rectal gel for acute repetitive seizures.

Methods.—In this randomized, double-blind, parallel-group, placebo-controlled study, 125 patients were randomly assigned to receive placebo or rectal diazepam gel at doses ranging from 0.2 to 0.5 mg/kg of body weight on the basis of age. There were 47 children and 44 adults. The first dose was given to children at the onset of acute repetitive seizures, and the second dose was given 4 hours later. Three doses were given to adults, with the first at onset, the second at 4 hours, and the third at 12 hours after onset. A caregiver, such as a parent, who received special training, administered the treatment in the home. In children, the seizures after the first dose were counted; in adults, the seizures were counted for 24 hours.

Results.—In reducing frequency of seizures and improving global assessment of treatment outcome by the caregiver (frequency and severity of seizures and drug toxicity), diazepam treatment was superior to placebo. Post hoc analysis showed diazepam to be superior to placebo in reducing frequency of seizures in children and adults. In improvement in global outcome, post hoc analysis showed that diazepam was superior to placebo only in children. In the patients receiving diazepam, it took longer for the first recurrence of seizure to occur after initial treatment than in those receiving placebo (Fig 3). At least one adverse effect of treatment was reported by 35 patients, with somnolence being the most frequent. There were no reports of respiratory depression.

Conclusion.—An effective and well-tolerated agent for treatment of acute repetitive seizures is rectal diazepam gel, administered at home by trained caregivers.

▶ This is an important study. It could well be one of the most important studies on the management of neurologic disorders in children in the last several years. The study shows us that diazepam given rectally as a gel is quite effective in the control of repetitive seizures. This is true in both children and adults. Earlier studies using diazepam suppositories have been less impressive. Such suppositories have slow, erratic absorption, which limits their usefulness as part of the management of an acute seizure. On the other hand, rectal diazepam solutions have many characteristics that are ideal in treating acute repetitive seizures. Their high lipid solubility permits both prompt absorption and rapid penetration into the central nervous system. Peak serum plasma concentrations are reached within 5 to 45 minutes, with bioavailability ranging from 80% to 100%. That is almost as good as an IV administration.

There is probably little reason to use diazepam gel rectally in an emergency room. Its real benefit is in the home. The benefits of a safe and effective treatment for acute repetitive seizures were highlighted recently by Alldredge et al. who reviewed 45 episodes of convulsive status epilepticus in 38 children given prehospital treatment with rectal or intravenous diazepam.[2] Rectal diazepam shortened the duration of status epilepticus by one half and reduced by one third the likelihood that seizures would recur in the emergency department. In the study abstracted, no patients given rectal diazepam and 13% of patients in the placebo group required emergency medical care. The cost savings could be profound if parents were given the freedom of administering rectal diazepam gel as noted in a study of Kriel et al.[1] who found a 67% decrease in emergency room visits and a cost savings in excess of $1000 per family in the year after the families began using rectal diazepam. There was also reduced family disruption and improved quality of life.

If you decide to use diazepam rectal gel, the dose reported in this study is 0.5 mg/kg of body weight for children 2 to 5 years of age, 0.3 mg/kg for children 6 to 11 years of age, and 0.2 mg/kg for patients 12 and older.

J.A. Stockman III, M.D.

References

1. Kriel RL, Lloyd JC, Hadsall RS, et al: Home use of rectal diazepam for cluster and prolonged seizures: Efficacy, adverse reactions, quality of life, and cost analysis. *Pediatr Neurol* 7:13-17, 1991.
2. Alldredge BK, Wall DB, Ferriero DM: Effect of prehospital treatment on the outcome of status epilepticus in children. *Pediatr Neurol* 12:213-216, 1995.

Emergency Brain Computed Tomography in Children With Seizures: Who Is Most Likely to Benefit?
Garvey MA, Gaillard WD, Rusin JA, et al (Children's Natl Med Ctr, Washington, DC)
J Pediatr 133:664-669, 1998   6–3

Background.—Guidelines on the use of neuroimaging in adults seeking emergent care for new-onset seizures have recently been published. The applicability of these guidelines to children was investigated.

Methods.—One hundred seven neurologically normal children undergoing neuroimaging after being brought to an emergency department with a possible first seizure were included in the retrospective analysis. Children with simple febrile seizures were excluded.

Findings.—Eight children were found to have nonepileptic events, with final diagnoses of gastroesophageal reflux, syncopal event, or rigor. Forty-nine of the remaining 99 children had provoked seizures, including complicated febrile seizure, meningoencephalitis, and toxic or metabolic abnormalities, and 50 children had unprovoked seizures. Brain abnormalities were identified by CT in 19 children. Seven children underwent further examination or intervention based on CT findings. CT scan abnormalities requiring treatment or monitoring occurred more often in children with their first unprovoked seizure, in those whose seizure onset had been focal, and in those with focal abnormalities on postictal neurologic assessment.

Conclusion.—With some modifications, the recently published guidelines on neuroimaging for new-onset seizures in adults are useful in the care of children with first seizures. Seizure associated with fever in children rarely indicates the presence of an unexpected CT scan lesion requiring intervention.

▶ Guidelines as to which child who has experienced a first seizure should have an emergent CT scan are virtually nonexistent. We tend to rely on the "adult" recommendations. The published guidelines for adults identify certain factors that point to an increased risk for a CT scan abnormality that might require intervention. These factors can be found in the history (age older than 40 years, persistent headache, or seizures with focal onset); results of physical examination (new focal deficits, persistently altered mental status, fever); and initial laboratory results (no identified metabolic or toxic cause for seizure). In some pediatric emergency rooms, it is customary to perform a CT scan on each and every child with a first seizure. Nonetheless, in such settings the high cost of emergency CT scanning, its relatively low yield of new-onset seizures, and perhaps the more appropriate use of MRI in the investigation of seizures call into question whether routine CT scanning in such circumstances really makes sense. This is the dilemma that these investigators from the National Children's Medical Center in Washington attempted to sort out.

It was found that about 1 in 5 children seen in the emergency department with a first seizure did have a CT scan abnormality, although fewer than half of these children required anything to be done about that abnormality. As importantly, if the first seizure was associated with a fever, the likelihood of a CT scan showing anything (assuming there were no other findings other than the fever on physical examination) was negligible.

So who should have an emergent scan and who should not? A simple febrile seizure, even if it is a first seizure, should not alone demand an emergency CT scan. An emergency scan can be reserved for those first seizures associated with focality on neurologic examination or cases in which focal postictal deficits are present. As the authors note, if an accurate history is difficult to obtain or if the neurologic examination is compromised in some way, or, lastly, if follow up cannot be assured, you have every excuse, indeed every reason, for going ahead and ordering a CT scan while the child is still in the emergency room.

Lastly, see if you would do a CT scan in the following situation. This is a whodunit. A 15-year-old boy with normal development milestones and intelligence was transferred to an emergency room because of a generalized tonic convulsion lasting for 4 minutes. He had been watching TV and experienced his seizure at 6:51 PM. There is no personal or family history of epilepsy. The date of this occurrence was December 16, 1997. The location was Japan. The question is, What caused this youngster to come to the emergency room, the same cause that resulted in 685 other children also being taken to hospitals in Japan because of convulsions, headache, nausea, general malaise, and eye irritation with blurred vision beginning also precisely at 6:51 PM that same day?

If you guessed that this is the largest ever occurrence in history of seizures evoked by watching a particular television program, you would be correct. What was going on here is fairly straightforward. Approximately half of all Japanese children aged 6 to 12 years watched a half-hour program titled: "Pocket Monsters," a made-for-television animation program. A segment of that program, called "Computer Warrior Porygon" featured characters fighting each other inside a computer. Almost all the children who wound up with problems developed symptoms at 6:51 PM, just after a scene depicting exploding vaccine missiles launched to destroy a computer virus. This scene was followed by several seconds of deep red and bright blue colors, occupying the entire screen, colors alternating at a frequency of 12 Hz. This particular scene was determined to be the critical one, because most of the children with seizures—including 4 recently described patients—developed the problem at or immediately after the scene.[1]

In case you weren't aware, many countries have very specific broadcast guidelines to prevent the production and showing of cartoons, other animation, etc., that might induce seizures. Remember the phenomenon "Pocket Monsters–induced seizures." Kids like these sort of things. They are literally glued or tied to their seats. If there are reruns of "Pocket Monsters," in Japan or elsewhere, such kids may be "fit" to be tied . . . literally.

J.A. Stockman III, M.D.

Reference

1. Ishida S, Yamashita Y, Matsuishi T, et al: Photosensitive seizures provoked while watching "Pocket Monsters" a made for television animation program in Japan. *Epilepsia* 39:1340-1344, 1998.

Epidemiology of Epilepsy in Childhood: A Cohort of 440 Consecutive Patients

Kramer U, Nevo Y, Neufeld MY, et al (Tel Aviv Sourasky Med Ctr, Israel; Tel Aviv Univ, Israel)
Pediatr Neurol 18:46-50, 1998   6–4

Introduction.—During the first 20 years of life, the onset of seizures occurs in about one third of all new epileptic patients. Broad categories of seizure types are used in most population-based studies of childhood epilepsy, and the incidence of relatively rare epileptic syndromes is not known. Epileptic patients in a 20-year period were analyzed to verify the relative frequency of all seizure types and to delineate the age of onset of the different seizure types.

Methods.—The study included 440 patients with 2 or more unprovoked seizures with neonatal seizures excluded. Records were studied for clinical description of the epileptic event, age at the time of the first seizure, EEG abnormalities, and findings of neurologic and radiologic examinations.

Results.—In order of frequency, the different types of seizures recorded were as follows: partial seizures secondarily generalized (20.6%), complex partial seizures (12.5%), unclassified seizures (12%), West syndrome (9%), simple partial seizures (8.6%), benign rolandic epilepsy of childhood (8%), absence seizures (7%), generalized tonic-clonic seizures (6.6%), generalized tonic seizures (5%), myoclonic seizures (2.2%), benign occipital epilepsy of childhood (2%), mixed type seizures (1.8%), Lennox-Gastaut syndrome (1.5%), juvenile myoclonic epilepsy (0.9%), and atypical absence (0.6%). The following seizures each had a frequency of 0.2%: Landau-Kleffner syndrome, Ohtahara syndrome, myoclonic astatic epilepsy, electrical status epilepticus in sleep, and startle epilepsy (Table 1). The first seizure occurred when aged between 1 month and 1 year for 18%, between 2 and 5 years for 33%, between 6 and 10 years for 31%, and between 11 and 15 years for 18%.

Conclusion.—More pediatric patients with partial seizures (52%) were observed than with primary generalized seizures (33%). In this age group, the most frequent seizure type was partial seizures secondarily generalized.

TABLE 1.—Relative Frequencies of Seizures in the 440 Study Patients

Seizure Type	n	% of Total
Partial with secondary generalization	91	20.7
Complex partial	55	12.5
West syndrome	40	9.0
Simple partial	38	8.6
BREC	36	8.0
Absence	31	7.0
Generalized tonic-clonic	29	6.6
Generalized tonic	21	5.0
Myoclonic seizures	10	2.2
BOEC	8	2.0
Mixed type	8	1.8
Lennox-Gastaut	7	1.5
Juvenile myoclonic	4	0.9
Atypical absence	3	0.6
Landau-Kleffner	1	0.2
Ohtahara syndrome	1	0.2
Myoclonic astatic	1	0.2
ESES	1	0.2
Startle epilepsy	1	0.2
Unclassified	54	12.3

Abbreviations: BOEC, benign occipital epilepsy of childhood; *BREC*, benign rolandic epilepsy of childhood; ESES, electrical status epilepticus during slow-wave sleep.
(Reprinted by permission of the publisher, from Kramer U, Nevo Y, Neufeld MY, et al: Epidemiology of epilepsy in childhood: A cohort of 440 consecutive patients. *Pediatr Neurol* 18:46-50, 1998. Copyright 1998 by Elsevier Science Inc.)

▶ Kai J. Eriksson, M.D., Ph.D., pediatric neurologist, Tampere University Hospital, Finland, comments:

The authors describe results of a noteworthy study on a difficult but important subject: distribution of seizure and epilepsy types in a pediatric patient population. Even though the authors are not able to give any epidemiologic data on the incidence or prevalence of epilepsy in childhood, the results clearly add to our knowledge about the age at onset of various seizures and certain epilepsy types as well as the overall distribution of various seizure types in pediatric patients.

The method of retrospectively analyzing and classifying such brief and transient clinical symptoms—as epileptic seizures many times are—must have posed a real challenge for the authors. The most interesting results and greatest contribution of this study are clearly the identification of the age at onset of major seizure categories: in partial onset seizures (excluding rolandic seizures), the peak age is under 6 years and in primarily generalized seizures, a bimodal distribution results (peak ages 4-6 years and 9-11 years). This result is consistent with the research data and clinical experience we have on the age at onset of many clinically distinct epileptic syndromes in childhood and may also be regarded as reflecting the more prevalent symptomatic etiologies of epilepsy in younger age groups as well as aspects related to the maturation of central nervous system in childhood.

One of the most controversial results of this study was the rather high number (20.6%) of partial onset seizures with secondary generalization. The identification of secondary generalization, for example, in tonic-clonic seizures is difficult, especially in retrospective studies. This may also account for the rather low percentage (6.6%) of primarily generalized tonic-clonic seizures compared to earlier studies. However, this same problem of differentiating primary from secondary generalization in epileptic seizures is a very crucial one also in clinical practice (e.g., for the selection of effective antiepileptic drug) and may sometimes need extensive diagnostic efforts, including for example, video EEG monitoring. The true percentages in this respect do still remain obscure and provide therefore an interesting subject for further studies.

K.J. Eriksson, M.D., Ph.D.

Staring Spells in Children: Descriptive Features Distinguishing Epileptic and Nonepileptic Events
Rosenow F, Wyllie E, Kotagal P, et al (Cleveland Clinic Found, Ohio)
J Pediatr 133:660-663, 1998   6–5

Background.—Staring spells in children, a common presenting symptom, may or may not be epileptic. The sensitivity and specificity of certain questions asked during history taking to distinguish between epileptic staring (absence seizures) and nonepileptic staring (NES) spells were investigated.

Methods.—The parents of 40 children with staring spells completed a questionnaire. Data on 17 children with absence seizures were compared with data on 23 with NES. All children had normal interictal electroencephalographic findings and no neurologic disease.

Findings.—Preserved responsiveness to touch, lack of interruption of playing, and initial identification by a teacher or health professional had sensitivities of 43% to 56% for NES, but their specificities were 87% to 88%. These features were more frequent in children with NES than in those with absence seizures. Although body rocking occurred only in NES, its sensitivity was only 13%. Limb twitches, upward eye movements, and

TABLE 3.—Epileptic Staring Spells: Specificity and Sensitivity of Reported Clinical Features

Clinical Features	n	Specificity (95% CI)	n	Sensitivity (95% CI)
1. Twitching of arms or legs	23	1.0 (0.85-1.00)	17	0.23 (0.07-0.50)
2. Urine loss	22	1.0 (0.85-1.00)	16	0.13 (0.02-0.38)
3 Upward eye movements	23	0.91 (0.72-0.99)	17	0.35 (0.14-0.62)
4. Occurrence when tired	23	0.74 (0.52-0.90)	17	0.58 (0.33-0.82)
1 or 2	22	1.0 (0.85-1.00)	16	0.35 (0.15-0.65)
3 and 4	23	0.96 (0.78-1.00)	17	0.29 (0.07-0.50)

Abbreviation: CI, confidence interval.
(Courtesy of Rosenow F, Wyllie E, Kotagal P, et al: Staring spells in children: Descriptive features distinguishing epileptic and nonepileptic events. *J Pediatr* 133:660-663, 1998.)

urinary incontinence had specificities of 91% to 100% for absence seizures, but their sensitivities were only 13% to 35% (Table 3).

Conclusion.—Staring spells in children are probably nonepileptic when parents report preserved responsiveness to touch, body rocking, or initial identification by a teacher or health professional but report no limb twitches, upward eye movement, interruption of play, or urinary incontinence. In such children, physicians may confidently diagnose NES, with confirmation based on long-term follow-up.

▶ One of the most common things that pediatricians scratch their heads about is the dilemma presented to them when a teacher or a parent is concerned that their child's staring spells might represent a seizure disorder. Even though the physical examination may be entirely normal, such children, depending on the history, will usually wind up having an EEG performed. Recognize, however, that a normal EEG does not rule out an epileptic event. Indeed, the only sure way of ruling out the latter is a video EEG performed to correlate the EEG findings with the clinical spells. As we all know, a video EEG is a fairly expensive endeavor. What would be ideal would be to avoid the EEG with some degree of confidence that no seizures are occurring, based on clinical and historical findings. That is what this report is all about.

It would appear that in children with staring spells, these spells are unlikely to represent a seizure disorder if the child is responsive to touch during the episodes; experiences no interruption of playing; and has no limb twitches, upward eye movements, or urinary incontinence. Also, interestingly, if the stares are identified by a teacher or a health professional, the likelihood of the stares being caused by epilepsy actually diminishes. At first glance, this would seem to be counterintuitive as one might expect that a teacher or speech therapist or nurse would be more accurate than a parent in the identification of a true epileptic seizure. This, however, does not appear to be the case according to this report. Is it possible that what the teachers had to teach was boring to children and "spaced them out"?

In any event, it is probably not necessary to go the video EEG route if the aforementioned risk factors for a true seizure disorder are historically absent and if the routine EEG is normal. Indeed, you might question whether an EEG is needed at all if a staring spell looks fairly typical. It probably is not. All of us daydream once in a while. Some of us even sleep with our eyes open a few minutes at a time during the day. Life should be full of such little pleasures.

See if you can tell whether the following case involves a child with a seizure disorder or a seizure look-alike. A 4-year-old girl is seen at the Children's Hospital of Pittsburgh following seizure activity. The seizures are approximately 2 minutes in duration with a frequency of 10 to 15 episodes per day. During these episodes, the child stiffens and crosses her legs, holds onto furniture, and insists on maintaining an upright or supine position, but not a sitting position. There is no definite history of loss of consciousness or postictal sequelae, although the child did fall on 1 occasion, resulting in a broken tooth. Neurologic consultation by several neurologists reveal no neurologic defects. Findings from 5 EEGs, including 1 video EEG, a head CT scan, and a head MRI scan are all normal. Treatment with carbamazepine and valproic acid at therapeutic doses fails to control the seizures. With further questioning, it is found that these seizure episodes began shortly after the initiation of toilet training. Because she sometimes leaks stool during her "seizures," a pediatric gastroenterology consultation is sought. Your diagnosis?

The physical examination on this child ultimately disclosed a tubular mass in the left abdomen and a rectum impacted with firm stool. After evacuation by a series of enemas and chronic therapy with mineral oil (3 tablespoons/day) and Senokot (Purdue Frederick; 1 teaspoon at bedtime), this child had no further "seizure" activity. Not every pediatrician has seen this problem before, but virtually all pediatric gastroenterologists have. The phenomenon of seizure-like activity has a well-known descriptive name. It is the "doody dance."[1]

J.A. Stockman III, M.D.

Reference

1. Del Rosario JF, Orenstin SR, Crumrine P: Stool withholding masquerading as a seizure disorder. *Clin Pediatr* 37:201-204, 1998.

Complications of the Ketogenic Diet

Ballaban-Gil K, Callahan C, O'Dell C, et al (Montefiore Med Ctr, Bronx, NY; Albert Einstein College of Medicine, Bronx, NY)
Epilepsia 39:744-748, 1998   6–6

Background.—For more than 70 years, the ketogenic diet has been used successfully to treat epilepsy in children. Few serious complications have been reported. Complications that have been caused by the diet were documented.

Methods and Findings.—Fifty-two children treated in a 22-month period were monitored prospectively. Ten percent experienced serious adverse events after the diet was started. Four of these 5 children received valproate along with the diet, compared with only 25 of the 47 children without serious adverse events. Severe hypoproteinemia developed in 2 children within 4 weeks of diet initiation. One of these children also had lipemia and hemolytic anemia. Fanconi's renal tubular acidosis developed in a third child within 1 month of diet initiation. Two children had marked increases in liver function tests, one in the diet initiation phase and one 13 months later.

Conclusions.—Clinicians prescribing the ketogenic diet for the treatment of epilepsy in children must be aware of the potentially serious adverse effects that can occur. The ketogenic diet may interact with valproate.

▶ Ketogenic diets have been around for a long time and are now used as a last resort when conventional therapies fail in the treatment of refractory childhood epilepsy. Before this report appeared, ketogenic diets were thought to be relatively safe, although short-term complications had been reported on a few occasions. Previously reported complications have included dehydration, low blood sugar, vomiting, diarrhea, refusal to eat, kidney stones, recurrent infections, high uric acid levels, decreased calcium levels, acidosis, high cholesterol levels, and decreased amino acid levels. Now we see that about 10% of children also have other complications, some of which are potentially life threatening. Included in the list are severe hypoproteinemia, lipemia and hemolytic anemia, Fanconi's renal tubular acidosis, and serious disturbances in liver function.

It is not known why ketogenic diets cause potentially serious side effects. Then again, it is not normal for anyone to eat a diet that is extraordinarily low in carbohydrates and protein and high in fat. It's entirely possible that some of the complications recently reported are due to an interaction with recent vintage antiepileptics such as valproic acid.

Ketogenic diets have been around since before the Crash on Wall Street (the one in the '20s). Whether they represent voodoo medicine or whether they will remain a legitimate part of the therapeutic armamentarium for children with epilepsy remains to be seen. Clearly, the ketogenic diet candle is flickering. The passing of this treatment will not be mourned by many. I volunteer to drive the hearse.

J.A. Stockman III, M.D.

The Duration of Febrile Seizures and Peripheral Leukocytosis
van Stuijvenberg M, Moll HA, Steyerberg EW, et al (Sophia Children's Hosp, Rotterdam, The Netherlands; Erasmus Univ, Rotterdam, The Netherlands; Univ Utrecht, The Netherlands; et al)
J Pediatr 133:557-558, 1998   6–7

Introduction.—Peripheral leukocyte counts are often determined in children with seizures associated with fever to evaluate the source of the fever. It is suggested, however, that an increased leukocyte count might be explained by the seizure duration itself rather than by an infection. The leukocyte count may be increased by stress mechanisms, which may result from the seizure. Little is known about the diagnostic utility of peripheral leukocytosis in children with long-lasting febrile seizures. The association of the leukocyte count and the seizure characteristics in children with febrile seizures, irrespective of the underlying cause of the fever, was assessed.

Methods.—Two hundred three patients, aged 3 months to 5 years, who had a seizure associated with a fever in a 2-year period were studied. Their peripheral blood leukocyte counts were taken routinely to evaluate the fever. Leukocytosis was defined as a leukocyte count of 15.0×10^9 or more cells/L.

Results.—The most common type of seizure was the multiple type, followed by the focal type. In 61% of children, normal leukocyte counts were found. In patients with febrile status epilepticus, leukocyte counts after seizures lasting longer than 45 minutes were not significantly different. No clear association was found between blood leukocytosis or seizure duration in children with febrile seizures. Seizure duration may be the cause of misinterpretation of increased leukocyte counts.

Conclusion.—The underlying cause of fever should be evaluated by counting leukocytes in children with febrile seizures. A long-lasting febrile seizure should not be interpreted as the cause of leukocytosis.

▶ This is a terrific report. A terrific report can be defined as any report that reinforces ones own personal convictions. Such is the case here. White blood cell counts are of no use in helping to sort out infectious from noninfectious causes of febrile seizures. Seizures in and of themselves can raise the white blood cell count for a time. The duration of this period remains ill-defined in the literature. There is no difference in the level of the white blood cell count based on whether the seizure is relatively brief or substantially prolonged.

We thank our colleagues in The Netherlands for reminding us about how valueless it is to order a complete blood count (CBC) after a febrile seizure. Sure some will argue that a normal CBC will be reassuring, but we all know the lack of predictive value of a normal CBC ruling out serious infectious problems. The next time you get an urge to order a white count and differential in a child who has had a CBC, go get a cup of coffee. By the time you're done, perhaps the urge will have passed.

J.A. Stockman III, M.D.

The Rise and Fall of the Plantar Response in Infancy

Gingold MK, Jaynes ME, Bodensteiner JB, et al (West Virginia Univ, Morgantown)

J Pediatr 133:568-570, 1998   6–8

Introduction.—The normal newborn plantar response is extensor and is otherwise known as the Babinski sign. It is still not known when a persisting extensor response signifies a pathologic condition. It was not known when the normal flexor plantar response was reliably found in infants. Previous studies were conflicting in their results and physicians have disregarded the infant plantar response because of uncertainty regarding its significance. When the plantar response becomes reliably flexor was established in a group of normal infants who were monitored longitudinally with a standardized technique.

Methods.—One hundred sixty-nine infants had serial evaluation from 2 weeks to 12 months of age during their routine well-child visits. Pediatricians were instructed in how to use the technique for eliciting the plantar response. The infants were evaluated while awake, in supine position, with the head in midline, knee extended, and ankle and foot relaxed. To provide a noxious stimulus along the lateral aspect of the sole extending from the

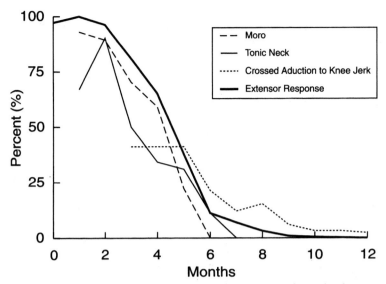

FIGURE 1.—Extensor plantar response plotted with other "primitive reflexes" that disappear with advancing age. (From Gingold MK, Jaynes ME, Bodensteiner JB, et al: The rise and fall of the plantar response in infancy. *J Pediatr* 133:568-570, 1998. Courtesy of Gingold M, Iannaccone S: Cerebral palsy and developmental disabilities, in Lazar R [ed]: *Principles of Neurologic Rehabilitation*. New York, McGraw Hill, 1998, pp 153-172. Reproduced with permission of The McGraw-Hill Companies.)

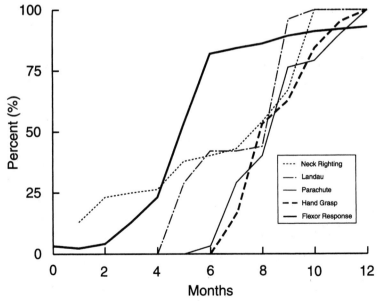

FIGURE 2.—Flexor plantar response plotted with other reflexes that develop with increasing maturity. (From Gingold MK, Jaynes ME, Bodensteiner JB, et al: The rise and fall of the plantar response in infancy. *J Pediatr* 133:568-570, 1998. Courtesy of Gingold M, Iannaccone S: Cerebral palsy and developmental disabilities, in Lazar R [ed]: *Principles of Neurologic Rehabilitation*. New York, McGraw Hill, 1998, pp 153-172. Reproduced with permission of The McGraw-Hill Companies.)

heel to the head of the 5th metatarsal, a wooden or plastic end of a cotton-tipped applicator was used. Extension of the great toe was scored as extensor. Flexion of the great toe was scored as a flexor response.

Results.—The plantar response was elicited in a standardized fashion, and at 2 months, it was extensor in 95.6% of the infants (Fig 1). At 4 months, it was extensor 64.8% of the infants; at 6 months, it was extensor in 10.9% of the infants; at 9 months it was extensor in 0.7% of the infants. At 12 months, it was not extensor in any of the infants.

Conclusion.—By 6 months of age, the plantar response becomes predominately flexor in normal infants (Fig 2). Other infantile reflexes are closely correlated with this maturation of response.

▶ I thought the title of this report was pretty nifty, almost a pun, or at least a play on words: "The Rise and Fall of the Plantar Response." Play on words or puns aside, it's nice to see a simply designed report that gives useful information to practitioners. So when is the flexor plantar response reliably found in normal infants? The answer is, by about 6 months of age. The plantar response of the extensor type in babies disappears at about the same time that other primitive reflexes disappear. The upgoing toe in normal infants merely reflects the immaturity of the brain and spinal column, an immaturity that should be gone in just about all babies at about 6 months from birth.

All this goes back to Dr. Babinski, of course. It was he who found that when there was lack of modulation of the reflex arch in the spine, occurring either because of pathology or immaturity, the extensor hallucis longus muscle points in the wrong direction. The Moro/tonic neck/crossed adduction to knee jerk/extensor response reflexes and the neck righting/landau/parachute/hand grasp/flexor response reflexes are like ships passing in the night. The former go away and are replaced by the latter, primitive being replaced by mature pretty much in all babies by no later than the end of the first half-year of life.

J.A. Stockman III, M.D.

Diagnostic Problems in Three Pediatric Neurology Practice Plans
Curless RG (Univ of Miami, Fla)
Pediatr Neurol 19:272-274, 1998   6–9

Background.—This author described differences in the diagnostic problems encountered among 3 different pediatric neurology practice plans over an 8-month period.

Methods.—Between October 1996 and June 1997, 1635 patients were seen at a government-supported clinic (n = 883), a clinic supported by a capitated contract (n = 598), or a private fee-for-service clinic (n = 154). Twenty-two diagnostic categories were created to describe the patient visits, and the frequencies of these diagnoses at each of the 3 practice plans were calculated and described.

TABLE 2.—Selected Diagnostic Categories

	1* (%)	2† (%)	3‡ (%)
Developmental syndromes (total)	14	41	23
ADD/ADHD	4	29	7
Paroxysmal disorders (total)	30	16	27
Epilepsy	26	10	22
Headaches (total)	12	21	9
Migraine	6	7	6
Categories >5% for at least one practice pain			
Neuromuscular disorders	7	1	8
Psychiatric disorders	2	6	3
Cerebral palsy	8	2	5
Miscellaneous	3	3	5

Note: Percentages are calculated from each category total.
*Government: n = 883.
†Capitated contract: n = 598.
‡Private fee-for-service; n = 154.
Abbreviation: ADD/ADHD, Attention deficit disorder/attention deficit hyperactivity disorder.
(Reprinted by permission of the publisher, from Curless RG: Diagnostic problems in three pediatric neurology practice plans. *Pediatr Neurol* 19:272-274. Copyright 1998 by Elsevier Science Inc.)

Findings.—In all 3 practice settings, the most common diagnoses were headache, epilepsy, and developmental delay (Table 2). Overall, the incidences of cerebral palsy and neonatal problems in the first 4 weeks of life were relatively low. The practice plans did differ in some ways, however. Patients attending the government-supported clinic tended to have more serious illness, and they typically required more evaluation, counseling, and therapy. This was particularly true for patients with primary brain neoplasms or neuromuscular disorders, who constituted 10% of the patients in the government clinic versus 8.4% in the fee-for-service clinic and 1.5% in the contract clinic. Generalized tonic-clonic seizures were also more commonly seen in the government clinic (50% of patients) than in the fee-for-service clinic (19%) or the contract clinic (15.5%). Patients attending the contract clinic were more likely to have developmental brain syndromes (41% vs 14% in the government clinic and 23% in the fee-for-service clinic), and these children were much more likely to have attention deficit disorder or attention deficit hyperactivity disorder (71% vs 30% in the other 2 clinics).

Conclusion.—Different pediatric neurology practice settings have differences in the proportions of various patient complaints.

Oral Fluid Therapy: A Promising Treatment for Vasodepressor Syncope
Younoszai AK, Franklin WH, Chan DP, et al (Ohio State Univ, Columbus)
Arch Pediatr Adolesc Med 152:165-168, 1998   6–10

Introduction.—A common complaint among teenagers is syncope, and the most common cause is vasodepressor syncope, also known as vasovagal syncope, accounting for 50% of all syncopal episodes in children.

Increased oral fluid intake is an alternative therapy to pharmacologic agents. The effectiveness of oral maintenance fluid therapy in patients with vasodepressor syncope was determined. The predictive value of the response to IV fluid with repeated tilt table testing in determining clinical outcome was also investigated.

Methods.—There were 58 patients with a positive baseline tilt table testing result who were treated with oral fluid therapy during a 5-year period in this retrospective review. An IV bolus of isotonic saline solution was given to patients with a positive tilt table test result. Those with a negative tilt table test result after the bolus were considered to be responders. Patients were prescribed a protocol of oral fluid therapy.

Results.—While receiving oral fluid therapy, 90% of patients had no recurrent syncope. After administration of the IV fluid, the mean arterial pressure seen with symptomatic events was lower during tilt table testing. After administration of the IV bolus, the heart rate increased during the tests in comparison with a dropped heat rate during the initial tests. The nonresponders had symptomatic episodes significantly later in the tilt table test when given fluids. A positive predictive value of 92% was seen in the response to IV fluid. The negative predictive value of clinical outcome was 11%.

Conclusion.—An effective treatment for vasodepressor syncope is oral fluid therapy. A high positive but a low negative predictive value of response to oral fluid therapy was found with fluid bolus response during tilt table testing. Oral fluid therapy is recommended as a primary intervention. Tilt table testing should be reserved for oral fluid therapy failures.

▶ Who would have ever believed that the Bezold-Jarisch reflex could be adequately modulated by drinking lots of fluid? If you have forgotten what the Bezold-Jarisch reflex is, it is the old-fashioned "vagal reflex" first noted by Bezold in 1867 and further elaborated on by Jarisch in 1948. Long before we ever heard of neurocardiogenic syncope, patients had symptoms of lightheadedness under certain circumstances, symptoms that were caused by the body's hypotensive response to stimulation of cardiac afferents, the so-called "vagal reflex." With the advent of the tilt test, we soon began to specifically diagnose neurocardiogenic syncope, also known as vasodepressor syncope.

Treatment of neurocardiogenic syncope has involved the use of mineralocorticoids, salt and some extra fluids, β-blockers, and disopyramide. Benefit from these has been pretty much hit or miss. Now comes the report abstracted here, which tells us that if you drink 64 oz of fluid a day, your chance of improving your neurocardiogenic syncope is about 90%. There is no simple, cheap therapy like nature's aqua.

So why does large-volume oral fluid therapy work? The authors of this report suggest that it expands your plasma volume. We can perhaps assume that that is correct, but please realize that the body is very efficient at regulating its own plasma volume, except at great extremes of overload or deprivation. The kidneys are quite efficient in peeing off what they do not need and of conserving when it is necessary to do so. This editor's theory is that drinking a lot of fluid to increase plasma volume has nothing to do with a reduction in neurocardiogenic syncope episodes. My bet is that patients who drink a lot just don't have time to get dizzy. They are either drinking or peeing. With all the movement involved with those 2 bodily functions, one is, indeed, in constant motion and never has a chance to pool fluids, lower blood pressure, or do anything like that. If this theory is correct, not only does the body not have time to have neurocardiogenic syncope, it also probably does not have time to sit through a 50-minute class, a 2-hour movie, or a car ride that takes any longer than a quick hop to the local mall.

J.A. Stockman III, M.D.

Pitfalls in the Diagnosis of Ventricular Shunt Dysfunction: Radiology Reports and Ventricular Size
Iskandar BJ, McLaughlin C, Mapstone TB, et al (Children's Hosp, Birmingham, Ala)
Pediatrics 101:1031-1036, 1998   6–11

Introduction.—One of the most common clinical problems in pediatric neurosurgery is shunt malfunction. Even for the experienced clinician, the diagnosis can be difficult and perplexing. With the advent of managed care, primary care physicians are being asked more frequently to evaluate patients with possible shunt malfunction. Because of their relative inexperience in reading cranial imaging and managing shunt patients, generalists tend to rely heavily on radiology reports in their assessments. The reliability of these reports in the diagnosis of shunt dysfunction was evaluated.

Methods.—Sixty-eight patients had 100 operations for shunt malfunction during an 8-month period, and all patients had evidence of catheter malposition, shunt blockage, disconnection, or valve pressure incompatibility. For each patient, the prospective radiographic interpretation of preoperative computed tomography and magnetic resonance imaging scans was reviewed.

Results.—No mention of shunt malfunction was made in 24% of the reports. The ventricular system was described in this report as "stable," "unchanged," "normal," "small," "smaller," "unremarkable," "slit," "negative," and "no hydrocephalus" (Figs 4 and 5). There was no additional comment to support a diagnosis of shunt malfunction. The same terms were used in an additional 9% of the reports, while also hinting at some other radiographic or clinical data that suggest the possibility of shunt failure, such as shunt disconnections seen on plain radiographs. Symptoms improved after surgery in all patients in this group.

Conclusion.—The diagnosis of shunt malfunction was not supported by a prospective radiologic interpretation of brain imaging in as many as one third of the patients who had shunt malfunction. Nonneurosurgeons would be reassured by a radiographic report that mentions or diagnoses shunt malfunction, although the neurosurgical community can assess the clinical situation to determine the need for surgery. Complex clinical

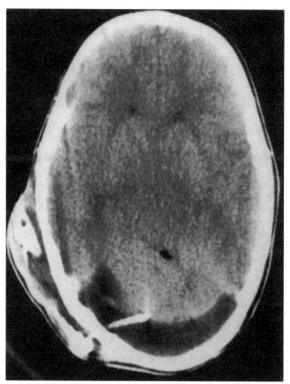

FIGURE 4.—Head CT scan showing small ventricles. Note the subgaleal fluid collection (*arrow*), which indicates in this case that the shunt was not working properly. (Reproduced with permission of *Pediatrics*, from Iskandar BJ, McLaughlin C, Mapstone TB, et al: Pitfalls in the diagnosis of ventricular shunt dysfunction: Radiology reports and ventricular size. *Pediatrics* 101:1031-1036, 1998.)

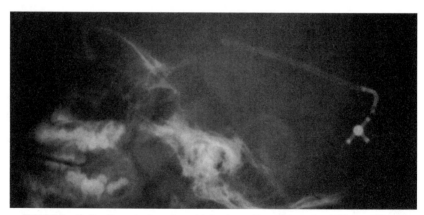

FIGURE 5.—Skull radiograph of a patient with "unchanged" ventricles on head CT scan. This patient has lateral as well as fourth ventricular catheters. Note the shunt disconnection distal to the three-way connector. (Reproduced with permission of *Pediatrics*, from Iskandar BJ, McLaughlin C, Mapstone TB, et al: Pitfalls in the diagnosis of ventricular shunt dysfunction: Radiology reports and ventricular size. *Pediatrics* 101:1031-1036, 1998.)

situations are being evaluated by nonneurosurgeons, who may rely on radiographic reports.

▶ Dr. Herbert E. Fuchs, associate professor of Surgery and head of Pediatric Neurosurgical Services, Duke University Medical Center, comments:

As the authors of this report point out, the diagnosis of ventricular shunt dysfunction is one of the most common problems in pediatric neurosurgery. Unfortunately, this diagnosis is not always straightforward, even for experienced pediatric neurosurgeons. In the managed care environment, primary care physicians are increasingly being asked to evaluate shunt patients, avoiding referrals to the higher-cost pediatric neurosurgeon. This approach has the potential for disaster, as pediatricians are generally not well versed in reading CT or MRI scans of the brain and may well rely on the radiologist's interpretation of the films. The authors demonstrate the pitfalls of this approach by retrospectively reviewing a series of 100 consecutive surgically treated cases of shunt malfunction and correlating the prospective radiology reports. Patients with small ventricles, which often did not dilate even with shunt malfunctions, were particularly problematic, even when other findings that might indicate shunt malfunction, such as subgaleal fluid collection or shunt disconnection, were noted on the reports.

The systematic approach of pediatric neurosurgeons to patients with potential shunt dysfunction includes personal review of current films and comparison with previous studies obtained at times of normal and impaired shunt function. It is critical to understand that although enlargement of the ventricular system indicates shunt malfunction, a lack of ventricular dilatation does not necessarily imply a functioning shunt. Such studies may include shunt tap, radionuclide shunt flow studies, intracranial pressure monitoring, and potentially even surgical exploration—all procedures that require a pediatric neurosurgeon.

I congratulate the authors for reviewing the seemingly mundane topic of shunt dysfunction and demonstrating the potential pitfalls in what many mistakenly view as a trivial diagnostic exercise but one that may become even more vital as our health care environment continues to change.

H.E. Fuchs, M.D., Ph.D.

The Guillain-Barré Syndrome and the 1992-1993 and 1993-1994 Influenza Vaccines
Lasky T, Terracciano GJ, Magder L, et al (Univ of Maryland, Baltimore; Ctrs for Disease Control and Prevention, Atlanta, Ga)
N Engl J Med 339:1797-1802, 1998   6–12

Background.—Between the 1991-1992 and 1993-1994 influenza seasons, the number of reports to the Vaccine Adverse Event Reporting System (VAERS) relating to vaccine-associated Guillain-Barré syndrome doubled (Fig 1). Although the VAERS indicates the number of cases that

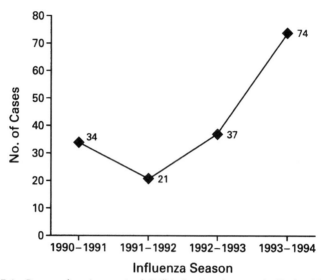

FIGURE 1.—Reports of vaccine-associated Guillain-Barré syndrome to the Vaccine Adverse Event Reporting System during the 1990-1991, 1991-1992, 1992-1993, and 1993-1994 influenza seasons. (Reprinted from *The New England Journal of Medicine*, from Lasky T, Terracciano GJ, Magder L, et al: The Guillain-Barré syndrome and the 1992-1993 and 1993-1994 influenza vaccines. N *Engl J Med* 339:1797-1802. Courtesy 1998, Massachusetts Medical Society. All rights reserved.)

were reported, it does not reveal the number of people at risk of vaccine-associated Guillain-Barré syndrome. These authors investigated the relative risk of having Guillain-Barré syndrome after an influenza vaccination during this period.

Methods.—A search of hospital discharge summaries from 4 states (Illinois, Maryland, North Carolina, and Washington) identified 273 adult patients in whom Guillain-Barré syndrome was diagnosed during the 1992-1993 or 1993-1994 influenza season (September 1 through February 28). Most of the patients were men (62%) and white (84%), and the mean age at hospital admission was 54 years. Of these 273 patients, 180 (66%) were interviewed by telephone to determine their vaccination histories, and the specific dates of vaccination were confirmed by contacting the person who provided the vaccine. Patients in whom Guillain-Barré syndrome developed within 6 weeks after they received an influenza vaccination were considered to have vaccine-associated disease. As a basis for comparing vaccine exposure, 1015 individuals in these 4 states were interviewed by means of a random-digit-dialing telephone survey to determine whether they had been vaccinated during these influenza periods.

Findings.—Vaccine-associated Guillain-Barré syndrome developed in 19 of the 273 patients (6.9%). In most of these patients (47%), the syndrome developed during the second week after vaccination, between days 9 and 12. Patients with vaccine-associated Guillain-Barré syndrome were significantly older than those without vaccine-associated disease (66 vs 55 years). When data were adjusted for age, sex, and influenza season, the overall adjusted relative risk of Guillain-Barré syndrome associated with vaccination was 1.7. Adjusted relative risks during the 1992-1993 and 1993-1994 seasons were 2.0 and 1.5, respectively.

Conclusions.—Although the number of cases of vaccine-associated Guillain-Barré syndrome increased markedly between the 1992-1993 and 1993-1994 influenza seasons, the associated risks did not increase significantly. The overall adjusted relative risk of 1.7 translates into about 1 additional case of Guillain-Barré syndrome for every 1,000,000 individuals who receive the influenza vaccine.

▶ It should come as no surprise that influenza vaccines still worry us when it comes to a potential for causing the Guillain-Barré syndrome. In the fall of 1976, when the swine flu virus vaccine was being used, a remarkable increase (somewhere between a four- and eightfold increase) in the number of cases of the Guillain-Barré syndrome was reported. Remember, at the time, the United States was on a roll with the recent introduction of many successful live virus vaccines, including polio, measles, German measles, and mumps vaccines. The report abstracted shows that even recently developed influenza vaccines continue to carry an increased risk of Guillain-Barré syndrome, albeit with a very low risk at this time. Within the last decade, only 1 to 2 additional cases of Guillain-Barré syndrome per 1 million vaccinated individuals were found. Since each year in the United States there are 20,000 to 30,000 deaths from influenza, the small chance of contracting a neurologic disorder appears to be outweighed by the benefits of the flu vaccine. As you might suspect, most of us remain cautious about flu immunization programs, a caution that is reinforced by the occasional new patient with Guillain-Barré syndrome who reports having received the flu vaccine in the previous few weeks.

Please remember that the influenza vaccine plays a relatively minor role in the causation of the Guillain-Barré syndrome. There are many more infectious things that ultimately produce this disorder. *Campylobacter jejuni* infection is one such entity. In as many as 30% of cases of Guillain-Barré syndrome, a preceding infection with *C. jejuni* can be detected serologically, even in the absence of prior gastrointestinal symptoms. Other antecedents of the Guillain-Barré syndrome include the Epstein-Barr virus, cytomegalovirus, human immunodeficiency virus, mycoplasma, *Shigella*, and *Clostridium*. Indeed, Georges Guillain himself reported cases that he thought were caused by the typhoid vaccine.

Why there is such an interesting relationship between organisms and vaccines and the Guillain-Barré syndrome remains something of a mystery. Some have suggested that infectious agents, including the live viruses used in vaccinations, share antigens with peripheral nerves. In all likelihood, the story is much more complex than that, particularly given the complexity of a patient's immune system. As one example of this, antibodies against ganglioside GM1 are consistently present in patients in whom the neurologic disorder develops after a bout of *Campylobacter* enteritis but are rarely present otherwise.[1]

As the controversy about flu vaccine continues, please remember that one contraindication to its use is a prior episode of Guillain-Barré, particularly if that episode occurred after a vaccination (especially with tetanus toxoid). Patients with Guillain-Barré syndrome should probably wait a long, very long, time to ever receive a flu vaccine after their neurologic difficulty unless contracting influenza would pose an extremely grave risk.

This commentary closes with a question. Have you had your flu vaccine this year?

J.A. Stockman III, M.D.

Reference

1. Sheikh KA, Nachamkin I, Ho TW, et al: *Campylobacter jejuni* lipopolysaccharides in Guillain-Barré syndrome: Molecular mimicry and host susceptibility. *Neurology* 51:371-378, 1998.

Investigation of Variant Creutzfeldt-Jakob Disease and Other Human Prion Diseases With Tonsil Biopsy Samples
Hill AF, Butterworth RJ, Joiner S, et al (St Mary's Hosp, London; Natl CJD Surveillance Unit, Edinburgh, Scotland; Inst of Psychiatry, London)
Lancet 353:183-189, 1999   6–13

Background.—The accumulation of an abnormal isoform of cellular prion protein (PrP^{Sc}) results in prion diseases. Prions replicate in lymphoreticular tissue before neuroinvasion, which suggests that lymphoreticular biopsy samples may enable early diagnosis by PrP^{Sc} detection. In its early stages, variant Creutzfeldt-Jakob disease (CJD) is difficult to distinguish from common psychiatric disorders, because the diagnosis relies on neuropathologic characteristics. Lymphoreticular tissues from a necropsy series were studied and tonsillar biopsy samples were assessed in a diagnostic investigation for human prion disease.

Methods.—Lymphoreticular tissue was acquired at necropsy from patients with prion disease as well as from neurologic and normal controls. The material included 68 tonsils, 64 spleens, and 40 lymph nodes. Tonsil biopsy specimens were also obtained from 20 patients suspected of having prion disease. Western blot analysis, PrP immunohistochemistry, or both were used to detect and type PrP^{Sc}.

Findings.—All lymphoreticular tissues obtained at necropsy from patients with neuropathologically confirmed variant CJD were positive for PrP^{Sc}. All such tissues from patients with other prion diseases and from controls were not positive. Also, PrP^{Sc} typing showed a consistent pattern ("type 4t") different from that in variant CJD brain (type 4) or in brain tissue from other CJD subtypes (types 1-3). Tonsil biopsy tissue was positive in all 8 patients with sufficient biopsy sample and a subsequent course consistent with variant CJD. Tonsil biopsy tissue from all patients in whom other diagnoses were later confirmed was negative.

Conclusions.—In the appropriate clinical context, a tonsil biopsy sample that is positive for PrP^Sc is diagnostic of variant CJD. This procedure obviates the need for brain biopsy. The pathogenesis of variant CJD may differ from that of sporadic CJD.

▶ Recall that acquired prion diseases, CJD, and kuru occur because of specific human exposure to prions through medical or surgical procedures or participation in cannibalism. A unique and "novel form of human prion disease, variant CJD, was recognised in the UK in 1996. Epidemiological studies argued for a link with bovine spongiform encephalopathy (BSE) and this was strongly supported by molecular strain typing and subsequently by transmission studies into both transgenic and conventional mice, confirming that variant CJD and cattle BSE are caused by the same prion strain." Even we here in the United States heard a lot about variant CJD, and many of us have lingering memories of the huge cattle slaughters that occurred at that time in Great Britain. In the last 4 years, most have come to accept that there is such a thing as variant CJD associated with the same prion that causes bovine spongiform encephalopathy, but the condition must be quite uncommon. Until this article appeared, definitive diagnosis of variant CJD remained neuropathologic, at postmortem or brain biopsy. Now we see that you can actually detect prions in affected patients by examining their tonsils. What remains to be learned is when prions first become detectable in human tonsils in affected patients. Once that is known, the need for brain biopsy in living patients will be obviated.

While we are on the topic of things related to infections and cattle, please be aware that there is new information about why it has only been in the last 50 years that we have recognized that cattle now harbor *Escherichia coli* 0157:H7. Since the second World War, cattle diets have shifted from hay to starchy grain feed. Investigators at Cornell recently studied 2 groups of cattle, 1 that was hay fed and 1 that was fed a processed corn grain diet. After 3 weeks of feeding the groups on the separate diets, 3 Cornell students tackled the not so pleasant task of removing fecal samples from the cows' rectums and determined their *E. coli* counts. In corn fed cows, *E. coli* flooded the digestive tract with more than six million *E. coli* organisms per gram of cow flop. Among hay fed animals, however, a mere 20,000 *E. coli* organisms per gram of stool were found. Furthermore, when *E. coli* was added to hay, cow's stomach acid easily inactivated the *E. coli*. This was not possible when *E. coli* was added to corn. The saga linking *E. coli* to cornmeal gives new meaning to the term "free range fed" that we frequently now see on restaurant menus. It doesn't take a hayseed to realize that natural foods must be better, even if we're only talking about cows.

J.A. Stockman III, M.D.

Leukotriene C₄-Synthesis Deficiency: A New Inborn Error of Metabolism Linked to a Fatal Developmental Syndrome

Mayatepek E, Flock B (Univ of Heidelberg, Germany)

Lancet 352:1514-1517, 1998   6-14

Background.—Leukotriene C_4 (LTC_4) is a potent lipid mediator with profound biologic effects on leukocyte chemotaxis, vascular permeability, smooth muscle tone, and mucus secretion. LTC_4 is synthesized (Figure) in eosinophils, mast cells, platelets, monocytes, and brain tissues, and it is normally found in the cerebrospinal fluid. These authors investigated LTC_4 synthesis and metabolism in an infant who died of a developmental syndrome of unknown cause.

> *Case Report.*—Infant, whose parents were first cousins, was evaluated at age 2 months because of muscular hypertonia and psychomotor retardation. Microcephaly was present, but organomegaly was absent. Results of standard blood biochemistry, glucose, lactate, karyotype, microbiological, fundoscopic, hearing, electrocardiographic, radiographic, and ultrasonographic tests were normal, and lysosomal-storage disorders and defects in the mitochondrial-respiratory chain, fatty acid oxidation, and pyruvate dehydrogenase metabolism were also ruled out. During the next 4 months the patient's condition worsened, and she died at 6 months.
>
> The patient's cerebrospinal fluid, plasma, urine, and peripheral blood monocytes were analyzed for the presence of leukotrienes. No levels of LTC_4 or its metabolites were detected in cerebrospinal fluid, plasma, and urine. Stimulation of monocytes failed to produce LTC_4, but stimulation did increase the synthesis of LTB_4. In addition, radio-high-pressure liquid chromatography was used to measure the formation of [³H]-LTC_4 from [³H]-LTA_4 in monocytes and platelets. In both monocytes and platelets, [³H]-LTC_4 could not be made from [³H]-LTA_4.

Conclusions.—This infant clearly was unable to synthesize LTC_4, which strongly suggests a deficiency in LTC_4 synthase. Confirmation that the defective LTC_4 synthesis was the cause of the fatal developmental syndrome in this infant, however, is at this point tentative and requires further investigation. These results do suggest that leukotriene analysis should be performed in patients with neurologic symptoms who might also have metabolic diseases.

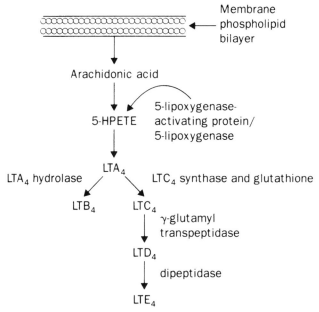

Metabolic pathway of leukotriene biosynthesis

FIGURE.—Metabolic pathway of leukotriene biosynthesis. (Courtesy of Mayatepek E, Flock B: Leukotriene C_4-synthesis deficiency: A new inborn error of metabolism linked to a fatal developmental syndrome. *Lancet* 352[9139]:1514-1517. Copyright 1998 by The Lancet Ltd.)

▶ Chances are that you will not be queried about LTC_4-synthesis deficiency. This report was selected for inclusion in the 2000 YEAR BOOK OF PEDIATRICS because this infant with a rapidly progressive neurologic disorder is the first child (or adult) in whom the unusual, and potentially important, disease has been recognized.

We've been hearing a lot about leukotrienes this past decade. We have become accustomed to think of them as inflammatory mediators. They play an important role in a variety of disease states, including asthma in childhood. What we have not known about leukotrienes is that they are found in cells other than eosinophils, mast cells, platelets, and monocytes. Human brain tissue also has the capacity to synthesize large amounts of leukotrienes. They are particularly made in the median eminence and other parts of the hypothalamus. Their role in the central nervous system is not known, but it is possible that they are messengers or modulators of central nervous system activity. All children and adults normally have evidence of leukotriene synthesis in their cerebrospinal fluid. The total absence of leukotrienes in the central nervous system of the baby who died of a developmental syndrome strongly suggests a link between the developmental problem and the leukotriene deficiency.

The more we learn about leukotrienes, the more we know how important they are. Stay tuned while we learn even more.

This is the end of the Neurology and Psychiatry chapter, so we will end with a question or two. First, it is said that with modern automobile technology, it is almost impossible to commit suicide by enclosing yourself in a garage with the motor running. Is that true? It is true that with catalytic converters, there is little likelihood that one will die of carbon monoxide poisoning under such circumstances. Please note, however, that this does not mean that people will not die as a result of inhaling exhaust fumes. A toxicologist at Guys Hospital has found that the number of people who are found dead in vehicles with catalytic converters has actually gone up over the last 28 years.[1] With the introduction of catalytic converters, the number of suicides caused by high concentrations of carboxyhemoglobin has fallen dramatically, but death may in fact result from oxygen deprivation and asphyxia.

In one British study of several scores of patients who committed suicide using exhaust fumes, the carboxyhemoglobin measurements ranged only from 2% to 24%, which is well below the potentially fatal level of about 40%. It is believed that these folks died from hypoxia because, although the automobile exhaust gases did not contain enough carbon monoxide to kill, they did not contain enough oxygen to keep anyone alive. The pathologist who has made these observations has also commented as follows: "As for the suggestion that the introduction of catalytic converters has lead to a reduction in the overall suicide rate, we should remember that when town gas was converted to carbon monoxide–free gas, the number of people who jumped in the canal went up."[1]

If it isn't one thing, it's another.

Second, did you ever wonder why there is such a wide variation across countries in the prevalence of major depression? Could it have anything to do with diet? If so, what diet? The World Health Organization estimates that major depression is the single greatest cause of disability worldwide. The annual prevalence of major depression shows a nearly 60-fold variation across countries, in a pattern similar to cross national differences in mortality from coronary artery disease, which suggests that similar dietary risk factors could be important. Recognizing that the essential fatty acids found in fish predict levels of CNS serotonin turnover, investigators studied the relationship between depression prevalence and fish consumption worldwide.[2] They found an indirect relationship between the prevalence of major depression and the annual fish consumption (pounds per person) throughout the world ($r = -0.84$). West Germany, for example, has one of the highest prevalences of depression. It is a country where the population, on average, eats less than 30 pounds of fish per person per year. Korea has half the prevalence of depression, a country that eats on average 110 pounds of fish per person per year. Japan has the lowest problem with depression throughout developed nations (1/50th the rate of West Germany), and it has the population that eats the most fish (148 pounds/yr).

When I was growing up, my mother always reminded me that fish was brain food. She might not have known exactly why, but she had it correct. The relationship between depression and fish ingestion is no fish story. If you don't want to swim with the fishes on a volitional basis, eat a few instead.

J.A. Stockman III, M.D.

References

1. Toseland PA: Catalytic converters and prevention of suicides. *Lancet* 353:244, 1999.
2. Hibblen JR: Fish consumption and major depression. *Lancet* 351:1213, 1998.

7 Child Development

More Awakenings and Heart Rate Variability During Supine Sleep in Preterm Infants
Goto K, Mirmiran M, Adams MM, et al (Stanford Univ, Calif; Oita Med Univ, Japan; Netherlands Inst of Brain Research, Amsterdam)
Pediatrics 103:603-609, 1999   7–1

Introduction.—An increased risk of sudden infant death syndrome (SIDS) is associated with prone sleeping. It is unknown how supine sleeping position reduced the rate of SIDS. In preterm infants with respiratory illness, however, it was generally believed that the prone position had greater advantages than the supine position. To reduce risk for SIDS, the American Academy of Pediatrics recommended that term infants and asymptomatic preterm infants sleep nonprone. Because of the lack of acute and long-term quantitative data on the effect of sleeping position on sleep and cardiorespiratory physiology in preterm infants, neonatologists and pediatricians are at a dilemma. Most preterm infants are discharged from a hospital at 36 weeks postconception, and a study was conducted comparing prone and supine sleep on infants at this age.

Methods.—Videosomnography was used to study 16 asymptomatic, preterm infants in both supine and prone sleeping positions at 36.5 ± 0.6 weeks postconceptional age. Using each infant as his or her own control, the sleep, respiratory, and heart-rate characteristics of the infants were compared between the 2 positions.

Results.—In the supine sleeping position, more awakenings were seen during all sleep states, such as arousals of 60 seconds or more; however, the sleeping position did not affect the overall total sleep and percent sleep state. The first quiet sleep was significantly shorter after each feeding in the supine position, with more heart-rate variability and awakenings than in the prone position. In the occurrence of arousals of less than 60 seconds or the incidence or severity of apnea and periodic breathing, there were no significant differences. There were no clinically significant apneas of 15 seconds or longer, bradycardia, or oxygen desaturations.

Conclusion.—The supine sleeping position had less quiet sleep and was associated with greater heart-rate variability during the first sleep cycle after feeding in 36-week postconceptional-age preterm infants. During all sleep states in the supine position, more awakenings were seen. More awakenings and a lower threshold for arousal may provide some benefit for the infant responding to a life-threatening event, and these data support the American Academy of Pediatrics recommendation for "Back to Sleep" for asymptomatic preterm infants. To address positional effect on the physiologic measures in preterm infants at an older age, further studies are necessary. The most healthy or advantageous sleep for newborns is still to be determined.

▶ After the better part of a decade putting babies to sleep on their backs, we still don't know what the precise mechanism is by which prone sleeping increases the risk for SIDS. Some have said that prone sleeping impairs cardiorespiratory control, causes hyperthermia, makes a baby rebreathe carbon dioxide, diminishes arousal, and increases orthosympathetic activity. One thing for sure, however, is that babies put to sleep on their backs, don't sleep as well as babies who sleep on their tummies. Their sleep is much lighter.

The issue with all this is pretty straightforward. We must continue to recommend that babies be put to sleep on their backs. At the same time, we should recognize that the long-term consequences of sleeping more lightly (and perhaps not sleeping as soundly) need to be looked at on a developmental and behavioral level. If we are raising a whole generation of fitful sleepers, we need to know what the outcome is sooner than later.

Please recognize that if we are raising a generation of "crybabies" because we put them to sleep on their backs, there is something that we can do about it. Expose them to the au de cologne of amniotic fluid. It has been shown that exposing a newborn crying baby to the odor of their own amniotic fluid significantly relieves the distress of being separated from their mothers. For example, in one investigation,[1] the distress of newborn babies was measured by determining the amount of time they cried while being exposed to various odors (amniotic fluid odors, breast milk odor, or no odor). Newborns who smelled their own amniotic fluid cried for just 29 seconds in a 1-hour period, significantly less than infants exposed to nothing or their mothers' breast milk. Crying overall was reduced by 90%. Infants exposed to their mothers' breast milk cried 15 times longer than those exposed to amniotic fluid, suggesting that babies who smell "food," but can't get it, are frustrated indeed.

One can imagine a whole variety of newborn perfumes based on the aroma of amniotic fluid. Perhaps a dab of amniotic liquor behind the ear before heel prick? A little on the wrist prior to a circumcision? Stranger things have happened in nature.[1]

J.A. Stockman III, M.D.

Reference

1. Larkin M: Smell recognition in the newborn. *Lancet* 351:1037, 1998.

Nervous Habits and Stereotyped Behaviors in Preschool Children

Gutermuth Foster L (Univ of Maryland, Baltimore)
J Am Acad Child Adolesc Psychiatry 37:711-717, 1998   7–2

Introduction.—Nervous habits and motor stereotypies are behaviors usually performed the same way every time; they are difficult to change and have an almost compulsive-like quality to them. Typical motor stereotypies are head and body rocking or hand flapping. Nervous habits are thumb sucking, nail biting, hair twirling, chewing an object, and picking at lips or sores. In schoolchildren developing typically, the frequency, age trends, and situational correlates of nervous habits (e.g., nail biting, thumb sucking, and motor stereotyped behaviors) were examined.

Methods.—There were 32 parent interviews and 100 teacher interviews in which the adults were asked about the behavior of children (ages 3 to 6 years) in their care. The interviews were semistructured and individually administered. The respondents reported on each child's behavior during the previous 2 weeks. They were asked when the nervous habits occurred.

Results.—More behaviors were reported by parents than teachers, with thumb sucking being the most prevalent (25%), followed by nail biting (23%). Among teachers' answers, a frequency of 4% was found in motor stereotypies, such as body rocking or hand flapping, and a frequency of 3% was noted in parent interviews. A decrease in picking at sores and lips occurred with age, according to reports by teachers. A decrease in all nervous habits occurred with age, according to parents. Structured times during the day and negative mood states were associated with nervous habits. Nervous habits were more likely to be displayed by girls than boys according to teacher interviews (Table 5).

Conclusion.—In typically developing preschool children, nervous habits and stereotypies are prevalent. Their presence appears to be a reflection of mood state. The habits are so common that they may serve an important

TABLE 5.—Sex Differences

Behavior	Teacher		Parent	
	Male	Female	Male	Female
Nervous Habits	13	42*	70	55
Sucking	2	23*	10	27
Bites Fingernails	2	10	30	23
Chews	0	4	0	0
Hair Twirl	2	4	10	5
Picks	4	10	0	9
Other Nervous Habit	6	8	20	5
Motor Stereotypy	2	6	0	5

*$P < .01$.

(Courtesy of Gutermuth Foster L: Nervous habits and stereotyped behaviors in preschool children. *J Am Acad Child Adolesc Psychiatry* 37[7]:711-717, 1998.)

function for developing children, perhaps helping the child cope with negative mood states, such as being nervous, upset, or angry.

▶ Nervous habits are fairly common. Take body rocking, for example. About 5% to 20% of children either currently body-rock or give a history of it. Thumb sucking, of course, is even more common; 1 in 5 to 1 in 3 children have seriously thumb-sucked. One in 10 preschool children bite their nails. Of school-aged children, 1 in 7 twist their hair on a regular basis. None of this is very surprising. What is surprising is the fact that so many of us persist with 1 or more nervous habits throughout life, well beyond the peak age at which most experience the habit.

This report doesn't provide serious new information about the frequency of nervous habits as they occur in children. It does tell us, however, that as children grow older, their habits become a bit more sophisticated. Hair twirling, sucking motions, etc., occur more frequently during periods of concentration. Visualize yourself. When you are pondering over a difficult problem at work, or at home, you may very well be apt to find yourself doodling or stroking your hair.

What cannot be found in the literature is the linkage between nervous habits in childhood and nervous habits in one's grown-up years. Presumably there is such a linkage. What happens when you are too old to suck on a binky, or don't have enough hair left to twirl? Do you become a doodler? Do you start finger tapping or foot tapping? Does chewing gum become an acceptable surrogate for nail biting? Chances are that the answer to these questions is yes. Chances are also that most people's habits will be carried with them to their grave.

Lastly, please recognize that fidgeting can be good for you. Fidgeting and staying on your feet may be linked to keeping slim.[1] Sixteen volunteers agreed to overeat by 1000 calories a day for 8 weeks. Although they all put on weight, the amount put on varied by a factor of almost 10. The differences in weight gain were almost exclusively explained by differences in non-exercise activity thermogenesis (NEAT). Fidgeting, moving around while maintaining one's posture when not lying down, and other involuntary movements all contributed to NEAT. Untested is whether biting your nails and swallowing the evidence contributes to weight loss or weight gain.

If there is a message in all this, it is that nail picking, hair twirling, foot tapping, and maybe even picking your nose all add up to calories burned. This is real NEAT.

J.A. Stockman III, M.D.

Reference

1. Reynolds PM, Saywer SJ: Non-exercise activity thermogenesis. *Science* 283:212-214, 1999.

Bullying in Schools: Self Reported Anxiety, Depression, and Self Esteem in Secondary School Children

Salmon G, James A, Smith DM (Warneford Hosp, Oxford, England)
BMJ 317:924-925, 1998   7–3

Purpose.—Bullying is apparently a major problem in secondary schools, particularly among boys. There are few data on the mental health problems associated with being bullied. This study assessed anxiety, depression, and self-esteem among secondary school children in relation to bullying.

Methods.—The investigators administered questionnaires regarding bullying, mood, anxiety, and self-esteem to 904 pupils at 2 U.K. secondary schools. The mental health outcomes were compared between children who were and were not bullied and those who were and were not bullies.

Results.—About 4% of children reported being bullied sometimes or more frequently, while about 3% reported bullying others sometimes or more frequently. Children who were bullied tended to be younger. Anxiety was higher for children who were bullied compared with their peers; for bullies, anxiety was similar or lower than for their peers. Being bullied was associated with a high lying score, while being a bully was associated with a high depression score. Both schools had bullying interventions in place, which may have had more impact on the direct bullying typically performed by boys than the indirect bullying more common among girls.

Conclusions.—This study demonstrates the mental health characteristics of secondary school children who are perpetrators and victims of bullying. Children who are bullied have high anxiety scores, while bullies have high depression scores. The prevalence of bullying in this study is lower than in previous reports, possibly reflecting the effectiveness of bullying interventions.

▶ Remember grade school and high school, particularly freshman year? There was always a class bully, and there was always one or more who were being bullied. For whatever reason, the personality disorders involved have never really been examined, at least until this report. We see that bullies are generally 12, 13, or 14 years old, as are those they pick on. Those picked on tend to be the more obviously anxious and insecure...no surprise. Unfortunately, this report gives us no insight into the short-term and long-term consequences of either bullying or being bullied. Are those who bully more likely to become adult sociopaths occupying a prison cell, or do they become the CEOs of Fortune 500 companies? Do those who are bullied develop more empathy for others? Do they become the more humane and sensitive among us? Do they become our poets...or are they the more frail in society?

Most types of adverse social interactions in grade school and high school occur in a manner readily visible to teachers. Now that we have our "100,000 new teachers," could we not assign to them the task of boxing the ears (as it were) of those who bully? Could they not be the sympathetic shoulder to those who have been harassed? There may be one other solution to the problem. Remember the film *My Bodyguard*? Having a buddy, a big buddy, even if you must pay for the service, is well worth the cost.

By the way, as far as those 100,000 new teachers is concerned, please note that there is little correlation between how much is spent each year on a public school student's education and his or her academic performance. For example, while the Washington, D.C. area spends more per student than anywhere in the country, the academic performance is among the nation's lowest. The following are the states/areas that spend the most money on their students according to 1998 national education statistics. Do you see any correlation with performance?

State	Expenditures * (per pupil)
1. District of Columbia	$10,180
2. New Jersey	$ 9677
3. New York	$ 9175
4. Alaska	$ 8882
5. Connecticut	$ 8473
6. Rhode Island	$ 7333
7. Pennsylvania	$ 6983
8. Massachusetts	$ 6959
9. Maryland	$ 6958
10. Wisconsin	$ 6717

*Expenditures for 1993-1994 academic year
(Data from *Digest of Education Statistics*, 1996.)

J.A. Stockman III, M.D.

Growth Deficits in Children With Attention Deficit Hyperactivity Disorder

Spencer T, Biederman J, Wilens T (Harvard Med School, Boston)
Pediatrics 102:501-506, 1998   7–4

Introduction.—A heterogeneous disorder of unknown cause, attention deficit–hyperactivity disorder (ADHD) may have an underlying pathophysiologic substrate caused by catecholamine dysregulation. Abnormalities in frontal networks may be implicated because these networks control attention and motor intentional behavior. Growth deficits have been associated with stimulants given to children with attention deficit–hyperactivity disorder. In preadolescence, height deficits have been reported. For adults, however, the heights were reported uncompromised. Stimulant-associated height deficits have not been explained by any consistent neurohormonal pathophysiology. There have been no replications of the initial associations of height and weight deficits.

Neuroendocrine Aspects.—Dysregulation of several neurotransmitter systems, particularly the catecholamines, is associated with attention deficit–hyperactivity disorder, and this may alter the neuroendocrine function and lead to growth delays. A review of the literature on neuroendocrine aspects of growth and treatment in ADHD and on growth in boys with this problem who underwent treatment with psychotronics was conducted. There were 124 boys with attention deficit–hyperactivity disorder in a controlled study.

Results.—When the boys with and without ADHD were compared, small but significant differences were found in height. The height deficits were seen in early but not in late adolescence, and the height deficits were not related to the use of psychotropic medications. In the children with attention deficit–hyperactivity disorder, there was no evidence of weight deficits compared with the controls. No relationship was found between short stature and malnutrition.

Conclusion.—Temporary deficits in height gain through midadolescence may be associated with attention deficit–hyperactivity disorder, but by late adolescence, the height may normalize. The disorder itself appears to mediate the effect, not the treatment.

Metabolic Abnormalities in Developmental Dyslexia Detected by ^{1}H Magnetic Resonance Spectroscopy
Rae C, Lee MA, Dixon RM, et al (Radcliffe Hosp, Oxford, England; Univ of Sydney, Australia; Radcliffe Infirmary, Oxford, England; et al)
Lancet 351:1849-1852, 1998   7–5

Introduction.—Enough evidence is available to indicate that developmental dyslexia has a neurobiological origin. Persons with dyslexia have altered lateral cerebral symmetry, impaired visual and auditory processing, disordered magnocells, and altered patterns of cerebral activation on verbal, visual, and auditory tasks. The most frequently suspected areas of the brain are the temporoparietal cortex and the cerebellum. Possible biochemical changes in the brains of persons with dyslexia were investigated.

Methods.—Localized proton magnetic resonance spectra were obtained bilaterally from the temporoparietal cortex and cerebellum in 14 men with well-defined dyslexia and 15 normal control subjects of similar age.

Results.—The ratio of choline-containing compounds (Cho) to N-acetylaspartate (NA) was significantly diminished in the left temporoparietal lobe in men with dyslexia, compared with normal control subjects. No difference was noted in the ratio of creatine (Cre)/NA in men with dyslexia. A nonsignificantly lower Cho/Cre ratio was observed, which suggests that the reduction in the Cho/NA ratio resulted from a decrease in Cho. The temporoparietal lobe ratio of Cho/NA was lower in men with developmental dyslexia on the left side, compared with the right side. Control subjects showed no contralateral differences in any ratio. Interruption of the metabolite ratios were not as clearly defined in the cerebellum of men with dyslexia. Significant reductions in the ratios of Cho/NA and Cre/NA in the right cerebellum and a trend toward a higher ratio of Cre/NA in the left cerebellum were noted. Significant contralateral differences in the Cre/NA ratio were observed in the dyslexic cerebellum. No correlation was noted between contralateral metabolic ratios and handedness in either group of research subjects.

Conclusion.—The observed differences in men with dyslexia and normal control subjects may reflect changes in cell density in the temporoparietal lobe in individuals with developmental dyslexia. The altered cerebral structural symmetry in dyslexia may be caused by abnormal development of cells or intracellular connections, or both. The cerebellum is biochemically asymmetric in men who are dyslexic, suggesting altered development of this organ. These differences offer direct evidence of involvement of the cerebellum in persons with dyslexia.

▶ As time passes, we are learning much more about the origins of dyslexia. Young adults with dyslexia may have both metabolic and structural brain alterations. In a way, these findings are consistent with prior evidence from positron emission tomography (PET) scanning, which has shown that the left temporoparietal lobe is potentially dysfunctional in dyslexia. A few postmortem studies of the brains of dyslexic men have revealed neuronal ectopias and dysplasias in these same areas.

In the abstracted article, MR spectroscopy studies of the brains of young adults revealed findings consistent with the PET studies. Patients with dyslexia apparently have a demonstrable difference in their overall brain cell density in affected areas of their cortex. Not only that, but abnormalities are also found in the cerebellum of these folks. The latter finding explains a great deal. Many individuals with dyslexia are often uncoordinated, have poor balance, and delayed motor milestones affecting crawling, walking, and learning to ride a bike. A recent fascinating observation is that antimotion sickness medications, which have been considered "cerebellar-vestibular stabilizers" and improve balance, have been shown to benefit reading performance in dyslexia. When all these findings are put together, some of the pieces of the puzzle of dyslexia begin to gradually fall into place.

A diagnosis of dyslexia is based upon educational and psychological tests that demonstrate large discrepancies between reading and spelling achievement and anticipated achievement based on age-defined and intelligence-defined norms. It seems clear now that dyslexia is much more complicated than a simple inability to read and write. Fingers are now pointing toward a developmental brain abnormality that may be structural, as well as functional, in origin.

While we're on the topic of educational achievement, can you name the top 10 cities or areas with the highest percentage of the population that has a college degree or better? Clue: The top area is where I reside, where there are more Ph.D.s per square mile than anywhere else on the planet. See the following table.

	Most Educated	
City/Area		% with 16+ Yrs. School
1. Raleigh/Durham/Chapel Hill, NC		40.6%
2. Seattle		37.9%
3. San Francisco		35.0%
4. Austin, Tex		34.4%
5. Washington, DC		33.3%
6. Lexington-Fayette, Ky		30.6%
7. Minneapolis		30.3%
8. Boston		30.0%
9. Arlington, Tex		30.0%
10. San Diego, Calif		29.8%

(Data from U.S. Census Bureau: *City and County Data Book*, 1994.)

By the way, there is a bottom 10 as well. The list is as follows:

	Least Educated	
City/Area		% with 16+ Yrs. School
1. Cleveland, Ohio		8.1%
2. Newark, NJ		8.5%
3. Detroit, Mich		9.6%
4. Santa Ana, Calif		10.6%
5. Las Vegas, Nev		13.4%
6. Miami, Fla		14.1%
7. Toledo, Ohio		14.1%
8. Milwaukee, Wis		14.8%
9. Akron, Ohio		14.9%
10. Stockton, Calif		15.0%

(Data from U.S. Census Bureau: *City and County Data Book*, 1994.)

J.A. Stockman III, M.D.

Persistence of Developmental Dyscalculia: What Counts? Results From a 3-Year Prospective Follow-up Study

Shalev RS, Manor O, Auerbach J, et al (Shaare Zedek Med Ctr, Jerusalem; Hebrew Univ-Hadassah, Jerusalem; Ben-Gurion Univ, Beer Sheva, Israel)
J Pediatr 133:358-362, 1998   7–6

Introduction.—Up to 6.5% of the normal school age population is affected by dyscalculia, a learning disability that is manifested by difficulty in acquiring arithmetic skills. Data on the prognosis of and usefulness of interventions in dyscalculia are lacking, yet there are indications that adequacy in arithmetic skills during childhood has an impact on future educational and professional achievement. The arithmetic ability and behavioral status of eighth-grade children given a diagnosis of dyscalculia in fifth grade were investigated. The short-term persistence of dyscalculia was determined, as well as the factors that may contribute to persistence.

Methods.—There were 3029 fourth-grade students, of whom 185 were classified as having dyscalculia. Intelligence quotient testing and arithmetic, reading, and writing evaluations were conducted on 140 of the children with dyscalculia. They were also assessed for attention-deficit/hyperactivity disorder throughout a 3-year period. When the children were in eighth grade, they were retested, and of these, 88% or 123 finished retesting.

Results.—Of the 123 children with dyscalculia, 95% had arithmetic scores that fell within the lowest quartile for their class. Three years later, 47% of the children were found to have persistent dyscalculia, scoring in the lowest 5% for their age group of 13- to 14-year-olds. The severity of the arithmetic disorder and arithmetic problems in siblings of the probands were factors that were significantly associated with persistence of dyscalculia. Socioeconomic status, gender, the presence of another learning disability, and educational interventions were factors that were not associated with persistence.

Conclusion.—Almost half of the affected children have a persisting course of dyscalculia, an outcome that is similar to that of other learning disabilities. These children performed poorly in arithmetic. Future studies should be conducted to determine the ultimate outcome of children with dyscalculia and the effect on education, employment, and psychological well being.

▶ I have to confess that I had not thought too much about the topic of dyscalculia before. In fact, when picking up this report, I thought that I was going to read something related to stones in the urinary tract. Developmental dyscalculia is a very specific form of learning disability isolated to the inability to acquire arithmetic skills. Like other forms of learning disabilities, the problem is a durable one. It tends not to go away if it is still present by the time a child is 9 or 10 years of age. Affected children may have the problem on an inherited basis. The problem is no less frequent than reading disabilities in the general childhood population. One in 20 will have it.

One last comment about developmental dyscalculia: Chances are that those with the learning disability will never become bookies. Bookies with developmental dyscalculia don't have what it takes to play the numbers. Avoid such individuals. Chances are if you don't, you'll get a "dyscount."

J.A. Stockman III, M.D.

8 Adolescent Medicine

Beach Week: A High School Graduation Rite of Passage for Sun, Sand, Suds, and Sex
Schwartz RH, Milteer R, Sheridan MJ, et al (Inova Hosp for Children, Falls Church, Va; Inova Health Systems, Falls Church, Va; Inova Fairfax Hosp, Falls Church, Va)
Arch Pediatr Adolesc Med 153:180-183, 1999   8–1

Background.—"Beach week" is a rite of passage for many adolescents in the 3 weeks after graduation from high school. These authors evaluated the role of alcohol, other drugs, and sex in the beach week experience among a group of female participants.

Methods.—The subjects were 59 female graduates of a suburban high school who completed a 33-item questionnaire regarding their risk-taking activities during beach week in 1996. Twenty-five of the subjects (42%) completed the survey during beach week, and the other 34 (58%) completed the survey 2 to 3 months later. The research assistant who administered the survey was also a 1996 high school graduate and was known and trusted by the subjects; she had also worked with the authors on a previous study. The research assistant also randomly measured breath alcohol levels as the 25 subjects who completed the survey during beach week entered and left several parties during the period.

Findings.—Before attending beach week, 16 subjects (27%) packed oral contraceptives, 10 (17%) packed male condoms, and 11 (19%) packed tear gas spray (to protect against assault). Twenty-nine subjects (49%) stayed in a hotel room that was coeducational. Before beach week, 13 of the subjects (23%) smoked 5 or more cigarettes/d; this number more than doubled during beach week, when 31 of the subjects (59%) smoked. All of the subjects had been drunk at least once before beach week; during beach week, most (44, or 75%) were drunk every day. Breathalyzer results for the 25 subjects who completed the survey during beach week showed that, at entry to a party, breath alcohol levels were typically 0.002 mmol/L or less. However, upon leaving the party, breath alcohol levels were 0.017 mmol/L or more in 15 subjects (60%), and between 0.01 and 0.015 mmol/L in an additional 8 subjects (32%). Only a few subjects reported first-time drug use (n = 2) or sex (n = 4) during beach week. Almost daily marijuana smoking was reported by 8 of 59 subjects (14%), and 9 subjects (15%) reported that they or a close friend required medical attention due to alcohol- or drug-related injuries or medical problems. Before beach week, 37 subjects (63%) had had sexual intercourse; 27 subjects (46%) reported having sex during beach week, typically with their steady boyfriend (18, or 67%). Most of the subjects having sex during beach week (86%) reported that they were drunk while having intercourse. Most of the subjects always (52%) or usually (22%) required their partner to wear a condom.

Conclusion.—Although the majority of respondents reported having sex, being drunk, and smoking cigarettes during beach week, there were abstainers. Parents of adolescents attending beach week must realize that these risk-taking behaviors are prevalent and should make sure their child has a medical insurance identification card. Other suggestions are including 1 adult chaperon for every 10 teenagers, setting a reasonable curfew, and requiring regular phone calls home during beach week.

▶ Meredith Stockman, one of the four Stockman children, who is now a college student, was asked to reflect on her personal experiences with "beach week." She comments:

The preceding article highlights the activities that do take place during beach week. Most of the findings mirrored what the beach week experience was like for my high school. There was coed rooming, there were parties, and most everyone received funding from parents. I was able to attend my beach week just after my high school graduation. Although I do believe that kids who attend beach week involve themselves in "risk-taking behavior," I do not believe that the behavior started there, nor do I think that it is the start of a major problem. It has become a week-long celebration of high school graduation and 1 last time to get together with friends before they go different ways.

If parents are concerned about what their kids may be getting themselves into at the beach, they should talk about it with them. They should let the kids know what worries they have and make sure the kids know what to do in case of an emergency. I believe that the "chaperoning" idea is an extremely poor solution, and the notion of a curfew would not be respected by any teen. I was lucky to have parents who trusted my judgement, respected my independence, and didn't give a second thought to my wishes for this graduation present.

As noted in the article, almost all of the participants in the survey saw beach week as a positive experience in retrospect. My experience at beach week was one that I will always remember. Looking back, I can see how if parents were given an inside look at beach week, they would cringe. But everyone who was there will look back and smile, and I will even go so far as to say that when I have kids, they will be the first ones to sign up.

M. Stockman

▶ Editorial note: It is easy now for Meredith to suggest that when she becomes a parent she will freely allow her children to participate in beach week without the same fears and concerns her own parents had. My bet is that then she will be just like her Mom (and Dad) and wish that she and her family were living somewhere in Kansas with no beaches within a thousand miles.

J.A. Stockman III, M.D.

Emergency Department Utilization by Adolescents in the United States
Ziv A, Boulet JR, Slap GB (Univ of Pennsylvania, Philadelphia; Children's Hosp of Philadelphia; Educational Commission for Foreign Med Graduates, Philadelphia)
Pediatrics 101:987-994, 1998   8–2

Introduction.—A previous study of adolescent health found unacceptably high rates of adolescent morbidity and mortality from injury, homicide, suicide, violence, sexually transmitted disease, and pregnancy. Overdependence on emergency services for crisis intervention and routine care may be seen among adolescents because of inadequate health insurance and underutilization of primary care services. The characteristics of adolescent visits to emergency departments have not been adequately described. A large nationally representative data set on emergency department visits by adolescents in 3 age groups (11-14 years, 15-17 and 18-21) was examined, with particular attention paid to number of visits, health insurance, presenting complaint, and diagnosis.

Methods.—There were 14.8 million adolescent visits in a nationally representative sample of 418 emergency departments in the United States in 1994. Records were examined to determine number of visits, health insurance, reasons for visits, urgency of visits, resulting diagnoses, and hospitalization rates.

Results.—In 1994, adolescents accounted for 15.4% of the population and 15.8% of emergency department visits. In emergency department visits, older adolescents (18-21 years) were overrepresented relative to their population proportion (6.85% of visits and 5.3% of population). There was underrepresentation of younger adolescents (11-14 years) (4.6% of visits and 5.9% of population). Among 11- to 21-year-olds, lack of health insurance was more common (26.2%) than among either children (13.6%) or adults (22.7%). Uninsured visits were found in 40.5% of the 18- to 21-year-old male patients and in 27.6% of the female patients. Adolescents had more injury-related visits than children (28.6% vs 23.1%) or adults (18.2%). Among all adolescent age-sex subgroups, injury was the leading reason for visits, accounting for up to 42% of male visits and up to 27.2% of female visits. Among female patients aged 18 to 21 years, digestive reasons ranked first (18.8%). Up 5.3% of visits resulted in hospitalization across all adolescent age-sex subgroups, and up to 52.5% of the visits were urgent.

Conclusion.—During adolescence, utilization of emergency departments increases and health insurance decreases, suggesting that adolescents with inadequate health insurance may be relying heavily on emergency departments for their health care. Nonemergency primary care sites would be more useful for treating most adolescent problems, inasmuch as most adolescent visits to emergency departments are not urgent.

▶ Dr. Christoph Lehmann, instructor, Department of Pediatrics, Johns Hopkins University, Baltimore, Md, comments:

Although adolescence is supposedly the healthiest time in our lives, providing health care to adolescents is a complicated and time-consuming art. Adolescents' morbidity and mortality stem in large part from their tendency to engage in high-risk behaviors. Consequently, detection and counseling of high-risk attitudes and addressing the specific needs of adolescents must be important goals in the delivery of health care. Emergency departments that are intended to provide acute care might not be able to meet this objective. Nevertheless, as Ziv et al. demonstrated, adolescents visit emergency rooms an estimated 14.8 million times annually.

Based on a national survey, this study provides some fascinating insights into which adolescents use the emergency room and what may motivate them. Applying new recommendations for age definition, the authors found an overuse of emergency department services among older adolescents and blacks. Suspecting that inadequate insurance coverage may lead to a lack of identified primary care providers and emergency department overuse, the authors examined the adolescents' insurance status. Adolescents using the emergency department were uninsured at a higher rate than adolescents in the general population. Furthermore, the authors demonstrated an alarming increase in the number of uninsured, especially among older males, who lost public or private coverage at a staggering pace and had the highest uninsured rate among all age groups. Although injury was the most common reason for visiting the emergency department, a large proportion of visits was related to common medical illnesses.

Adolescents seem to be using the emergency departments for some primary care functions. The adolescent users of emergency departments experience a decline in identified primary care sources with age.[1] If lack of insurance is truly the barrier to seeking health care in a primary care setting, it might be a costly obstacle for individuals and for society. Illness that otherwise could have been prevented or treated earlier may result in higher costs and loss of function or life.

C.U. Lehmann, M.D.

Reference

1. Lehmann CU, Barr J, Kelly PJ: Emergency department utilization by adolescents. *J Adolesc Health* 15:485-490, 1994.

Premenstrual Symptoms: Prevalence and Severity in an Adolescent Sample
Cleckner-Smith CS, Doughty AS, Grossman JA (Visiting Nurses Assoc of Rockford, Ill; Univ of Illinois, Rockford; Univ of Illinois at Chicago)
J Adolesc Health 22:403-408, 1998   8–3

Background.—This study examined the prevalence and severity of premenstrual symptoms in a teenaged population.

Study Design.—The study group consisted of 75 adolescent girls, aged 13 to 18 years, with regular menses, recruited from a private day school in a small midwestern town. The average gynecologic age was 40.3 months. More than 90% of the participants identified themselves as white. Patients were given demographic sheets and the validated Premenstrual Assessment Form (PAF) to evaluate changes in mood, behavior, and physical condition in the 7 days before onset of bleeding for 3 menstrual cycles.

Findings.—All participants reported at least 1 premenstrual symptom. Moderate symptoms were reported by 88%, severe by 73%, and extreme by 56%. The most commonly reported symptoms were food cravings, breast swelling, abdominal discomfort, mood swings, feelings of stress, and dissatisfaction with appearance (Table 1). A minority of teenagers reported violence, absence from school, or suicidal thoughts. Girls younger than 15 had significantly less intense symptoms than older teenagers.

Conclusions.—Premenstrual symptoms of at least moderate intensity were reported by 88% of adolescents in this sample. Adolescents who were at least 41 months postmenarche reported more intense premenstrual symptoms. A minority of teenaged girls reported aberrant behavior and suicidal thoughts as premenstrual symptoms.

▶ Frank Oski, former chair of pediatrics at SUNY Syracuse and Johns Hopkins and editor/coeditor of the YEAR BOOK OF PEDIATRICS until shortly before his death in 1996, once noted that "...when the training bra goes on, the trouble begins." I don't think Frank was talking about premenstrual symptoms, but as the father of Jane and Jessica (now a pediatrician and a lawyer, respectively), he probably knew what he was talking about when it came to the travails of parenting teenaged girls. Before the report abstracted appeared, even this editor was not aware (despite experiences with three teenaged daughters of his own) that premenstrual symptoms were so pervasive and potentially so severe. Only about 1 in 10 youngsters seem to get by with mild or no premenstrual symptoms. The rest have moderate or severe complaints in terms of signs and symptoms.

The table shows why being 15 to 18 years of age and having an XX chromosome composition is problematic on a periodic basis. Dickens' words apply equally to the middle of the second decade of life: "It was the best of times, it was the worst of times."

J.A. Stockman III, M.D.

TABLE 1.—Premenstrual Symptoms Reported by Severity Level (n = 75)

| | Participants | | | |
	Moderate	Severe	Extreme	Total (%)
Mood changes				
Low mood/loss of pleasure				
Feel tearful	9	9	14	41.3
Feel depressed	8	11	11	40.0
Want to be alone	8	11	11	40.0
Feel sad or blue	8	13	9	38.7
Feel lonely	12	11	6	38.7
Decrease in self-esteem	9	9	9	36.0
Feel empty	12	3	7	29.3
Endogenous depressive features				
Feel worse in A.M.	9	5	10	32.0
Less desire to talk/move	11	6	6	30.7
Lability				
Mood swings	8	10	16	45.3
Rapid mood swings	13	7	3	30.7
Atypical depressive features				
Crave specific foods	16	12	13	54.7
Mood swings	8	10	16	45.3
Increased appetite	12	10	5	36.0
Feels sleepy	4	13	8	33.3
Rapid mood changes	13	7	3	30.7
Physical changes				
Signs of water retention				
Abdominal discomfort/pain	17	8	10	46.7
Feel bloated	7	10	8	33.3
Breast pain or swelling	11	5	3	25.3
General physical discomfort				
Abdominal discomfort/pain	17	8	19	46.7
Backaches, joint, or muscle pain	7	13	11	41.3
Headaches or migraines	8	10	8	34.7
Autonomic physical changes				
Feel cold	18	6	5	38.7
Urinate frequently	10	6	3	25.3
Fatigue				
Decreased energy	14	8	3	33.3
Feeling of weakness	8	9	5	29.3
Tired legs	9	8	4	28.0
Behavior changes				
"Hysteroid" features				
Dissatisfied with appearance	11	13	11	46.7
Sensitive to rejection	13	9	3	33.3
Hostility/anger				
Outbursts or irritability	12	10	7	38.7
Intolerant/impatient	9	10	2	28.0
Social withdrawal				
Wants to be alone	8	11	11	40.0
Less desire to talk/move	11	6	6	30.7
Stay at home	9	5	6	26.7
Avoid social activities	9	5	4	24.0
Impaired social functioning				
Family notes mood changes	10	11	8	38.7
Tend to nag	16	12	12	30.7
Stay at home	9	5	6	26.7
Avoid social activities	9	5	4	24.0
Miss school	6	6	5	22.7
Anxiety				
Feel under stress	12	13	9	45.3
Miscellaneous mood/behavior changes				
Feeling overwhelmed	16	7	5	37.3
Drink more coffee/tea	8	7	11	34.7
Feel insecure	8	14	1	30.7

Sleep Schedules and Daytime Functioning in Adolescents
Wolfson AR, Carskadon MA (College of the Holy Cross, Worcester, Mass)
Child Dev 69:875-887, 1998   8–4

Background.—During adolescence, sleep and waking behaviors change significantly. This study investigated the relationship among adolescents' sleeping habits, demographic characteristics, and daytime functioning.

Methods and Findings.—A Sleep Habits Survey was distributed to 3120 high school students at 4 public high schools in 3 school districts in Rhode Island. For adolescents between the ages of 13 and 19 years, self-reported total sleep times declined by 40 to 50 minutes. Sleep loss resulted from increasingly later bedtimes. Rising times were more consistent across ages. Students who described themselves as struggling with or failing in school slept about 25 minutes less on school nights and went to bed an average of 40 minutes later than students who were doing well in school. Students with worse grades also had greater weekend delays in sleep schedule than those with better grades. The daytime functioning of groups with adequate sleep habits was compared with that of groups with less adequate sleep habits. The group with short school-night total sleep, defined as less than

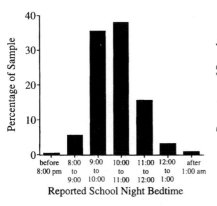

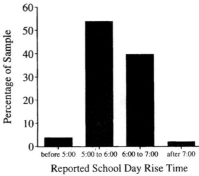

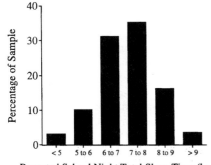

FIGURE 1.—Sample distributions of sleep patterns. (Courtesy of Wolfson AR, Carskadon MA: Sleep schedules and daytime functioning in adolescents. *Child Dev* 69:875-887, 1998.)

6 hours 45 minutes, and weekend bedtime delays, defined as more than 120 minutes, had increased daytime sleepiness, depressive mood, and sleep/wake behavior problems compared with students sleeping more than 8 hours 15 minutes with less than a 60-minute weekend delay (Fig 1).

Conclusions.—Most of the adolescents in this survey did not get enough sleep. Such sleep loss appears to interfere with daytime functioning.

▶ This report is clear evidence that when teenagers ambulate into school, they really are *somnobulating*. They are sleepwalking. The reason is obvious. Most are in a chronic sleep-deprived state. Evidence suggests that teenagers need as much sleep each night as those in middle childhood. Data suggest that the average teenager needs about 9.2 hours of sleep each night.[1] Nonetheless, the average teenager in this study of more than 3000 high school students sleeps just 7 hours, 4 minutes each night during the week and 8 hours and 38 minutes each night on weekends. Apparently, just 15% of teenagers sleep 8.5 hours or more on school nights. Even with sleeping in an extra few minutes on a weekend, it is impossible for them to make up for the sleep deprivation that has occurred during the week.

Chances are pretty good that there is little or nothing that will change the problem of sleep deprivation during one's teens, despite the fact that sleep deprivation can seriously affect academic performance. One thing that schools can do is to not put the teenager at a disadvantage over younger students. All too frequently in crowded schools, there is a staggered start time. Teenagers are usually asked to be the first ones there when the doors open in the morning. If you've ever seen a school that operates this way, the senior students look like zombies at 7:30 AM.

While we're on the topic of things related to sleep, here are a few more facts. First, teenagers aren't the only ones who are sleep-deprived these days. The Federal Highway Safety Administration of the U.S. Department of Transportation tells us that long-haul truck drivers get little sleep as well. On the surface, the federal regulations regarding long-haul truck drivers seem fairly appropriate (in the United States, drivers can drive a total of just 10 hours without having 8 hours off; in Canada, it's 13 hours without 8 hours off), but in reality that is not enough time to sleep. It would appear that with their 8 hours off, they don't sleep all that much. When carefully studied, long-haul truck drivers averaged just 5.18 hours in bed per day (with 4.78 hours of actual sleep) when following federal guidelines for maximal driving hours. The same drivers, when they are not hauling on the road, get about 7.1 hours of shut-eye a day.[2] To say this differently, many truck drivers are rolling hazards.

Using a cellular phone while driving produces a similar hazard.[3] Retelmeier and Weinstein tell us that cellular calls in the United States each day account for about 984 reported automobile collisions, 1729 total collisions, 2 deaths, 317 persons with injuries, 99 years of lost life expectancy, 161 lost quality years, $1 million dollars in health care costs, and $4 million dollars in property damage and other costs.

Finally, it has been documented that sustained wakefulness for just 17 hours decreases driving performance about as much as having a blood-alcohol concentration of 0.05%, the legal limit for driving in many countries such as France, The Netherlands, Norway, and Finland.[4] The 0.05% level is generally considered to be produced by the rapid ingestion of two 45-mL (1.5-oz) drinks of spirits. To put all this differently, the average resident on call for a 36-hour stretch shouldn't be getting behind the wheel. Program directors should be providing a chauffeur, or at least a taxi cab, to take them home at the end of a tour of duty.

This commentary ends with a quiz. What is the origin of the word *somnolence*? Somnolence, of course, refers to sleepiness or drowsiness. The origin of this word comes from the Latin *Somnus*. Somnus is the god of sleep. Somnus is also the brother of Death and a son of Night. All of these gods are distant relatives of Nike; no, not the shoe, but the goddess of victory, also known as Athena. Just think, we could all be wearing Athenas instead of Nikes.

J.A. Stockman III, M.D.

References

1. Carskadon MA, Harvey K, Duke P, et al: Pubertal changes in daytime sleepiness. *Sleep* 2:453-460, 1980.
2. Mitler MM, Miller JC, Lipsitz JJ, et al: The sleep of long-haul truck drivers. *N Engl J Med* 337:755-761, 1997.
3. Retelmeier DA, Weinstein MC: Cost effectiveness of regulations against cellular phone use while driving. *Med Decis Making* 19:1-8, 1999.
4. Dawson D, Reid K: Fatigue, alcohol and performance impairment. *Nature* 388:235, 1997.

Alcohol Use Beliefs and Behaviors Among High School Students
Feldman L, Harvey B, Holowaty P, et al (East York Health Unit, Toronto)
J Adolesc Health 24:48-58, 1999   8–5

Background.—The beliefs and behaviors regarding alcohol use of Canadian students in grades 9 through 13 were examined in a cross-sectional study.

Methods.—Three urban Canadian schools were selected for this survey. Ultimately 1236 students (628 males and 608 females) in grades 9 through 13 (ages, from 14 years and younger to 18 years and older) provided evaluative data for a response rate of 87%. The survey addressed sociodemographics and lifestyle issues, including alcohol use beliefs and behaviors of the students, their parents, and their peers.

Findings.—Five percent of respondents did not describe their level of alcohol use. Of those who did, 24% had never tasted alcohol. Another 22% had tasted alcohol but were not current drinkers. Of the remaining half, 39% reported current moderate drinking (<5 drinks on 1 occasion at least once a month) and 11% reported current heavy drinking. Males were much more likely to be heavy drinkers than females (15% vs 6%), and the incidence of moderate or heavy drinking in males increased dramatically between grades 9 and 12 (from 29% to 70%). Certain risk behaviors were significantly associated with current heavy drinking, including sexual activity (71% of heavy drinkers were sexually active), current smoking (47%), and driving while intoxicated (45%). The most common reasons students gave for drinking were "to get in a party mood" (18%), "because I enjoy it" (16%), and "to get drunk" (10%). Current heavy drinkers were more likely than moderate drinkers to drink "to get drunk" (22% vs 7%). The most common reasons for not drinking were "bad for my health" (25%), religious reasons (13%), and upbringing (13%).

Upbringing also influenced the drinkers' behaviors: in homes in which the father drank daily, 22% and 46% of students were heavy and moderate drinkers, respectively, and in homes in which the mother drank daily, 31% and 44% of students were heavy and moderate drinkers, respectively. The alcohol use of friends was also an influence on an individual's drinking behavior: 60% and 14% of heavy and moderate drinkers, respectively, reported that all their friends drank, whereas 56% of students who never drank and 27% of students who were not current drinkers reported that none of their friends drank. Ethnicity also played a role in alcohol use in that more students who reported their ethnicity as Canadian were heavy drinkers than were European or Asian students.

Conclusion.—Alcohol use is a significant problem in urban Canadian adolescents in grades 9 through 13. Heavy drinkers were at increased risk for driving while drunk, smoking, and being sexually active, and, typically, they had friends and parents who drank. Thus, the roles of peers and parents in adolescent alcohol use must be considered in safe alcohol use programs targeted to this population.

▶ It's incredible to think that teenagers in this study have such beliefs about alcohol and its use. Although this report is from Canada, similar findings would probably be seen south of the border as well. You are probably not aware of this, but the highest U.S. spending on alcohol (for both adults and adolescents) is found in Long Island, New York, and in San Jose, California (based on consumer spending surveys), where the yearly amount spent for booze per capita is $427. Washington, DC, Anchorage, Alaska, and Honolulu, Hawaii, are also cities in which one finds much higher than average yearly spending per capita on liquor.[1]

By the way, there is no correlation between level of education and levels of alcohol consumption. For example, Alaska has the highest percentage of the U.S. population with a high school diploma (86.6%), but also has one of the highest alcohol consumption rates in the country. Contrarily, Mississippi has the lowest percentage of the U.S. population with a high school diploma (64.3%), but is only about average in its alcohol consumption. I don't know what such statistics mean, except that there is no accounting for statistics these days.

J.A. Stockman III, M.D.

Reference

1. Krantz L: Cities: Most spending on alcohol. *The Definitive Guide to the Best and Worst of Everything.* Paramus, NJ, Prentice-Hall, 1997, pp 84-85.

Self-Assessment of Sexual Maturation in Adolescent Females With Anorexia Nervosa

Hick KM, Katzman DK (Univ of Toronto)
J Adolesc Health 24:206-211, 1999   8–6

Background.—The feasibility and accuracy of anorexic teenaged girls' self-assessment of sexual maturation have not been investigated. The accuracy of such self-evaluation and the desired stage of pubertal maturity in adolescent girls with anorexia nervosa were reported.

Methods.—Forty consecutive adolescent girls with anorexia nervosa were provided standardized figure drawings of Tanner's sexual maturation stages and asked to determine their own current and desired pubertal development. Two investigators then independently assessed pubertal development.

Findings.—Agreement between physicians and patients was 30% for the developmental stage of breasts and 50% for pubic hair. Patients underestimated their breast development 3.4 times as often as they overestimated it. They overestimated pubic hair development 1.5 times as often as they underestimated it. In a multivariate probit analysis, inaccuracy in self-assessment of breast development was correlated inversely with a desire for sexual maturity. Ninety percent of the patients said that their desired stage of breast development was equal to or more mature than their present stage. Eighty percent of the patients said their desired stage of pubic development was equal to or more mature than their current stage.

Conclusion.—Anorexic teenaged girls' self-assessment of sexual maturity using standardized figure drawings of Tanner's stages is inaccurate. Girls desiring a sexually immature body were most likely to be inaccurate in their self-assessment.

▶ It has been known for some time that if you ask adolescents about their secondary sexual characteristics, they will be quite accurate in their description, so accurate that the self-assessment is virtually identical with a physician's Tanner stage examination. This is true when a child is of normal height and weight. It is true even when the child is unusually obese. It is true whether the child is advanced or somewhat behind in terms of sexual maturation, assuming all other things are normal. The self-assessment, however, is not accurate if one is dealing with a young lady with anorexia nervosa. Adolescent females with this disorder are notoriously inaccurate in their assessment of their Tanner breast stage and their pubic hair stage. They tend to underestimate their breast stage of development and overestimate their pubic-hair stage.

These findings are not too terribly surprising, but they do indicate that such an inaccurate self-assessment profile probably correlates with a strong desire for sexual immaturity and a moderate degree of emaciation. Indeed, the thinner these girls were, the worse their ability, or desire, to accurately assess their degree of sexual maturation.

So what do we learn from all this? One thing is fairly obvious. Before this report appeared, researchers had routinely allowed self-assessment to substitute for a physical examination in studies that required some knowledge of a study subject's sexual maturation. Although this is still possible, the buyer must beware when the study subject has anorexia nervosa. Another lesson learned, perhaps, is that you can learn a fair amount about your patient with anorexia nervosa by such a self-assessment instrument. The more inaccurate such an assessment is, the more likely it is that the child is in greater difficulty. Whether this is a strict correlation or not remains to be proven, but the phenomenon probably is true.

While we're on the topic of sexual maturation, please recognize that the age at which puberty begins has been falling steadily for several centuries, and that trend continues as this millennium ends. Herman-Giddens and colleagues report that at age 7 years, 27.2% of African American girls and 6.7% of white girls now have evidence of breast development, pubic hair, or both.[1] African American girls have onset of menses at 12.1 years and white girls at 12.9 years, not significantly younger than previously reported.

So what does all this mean? It means that we have to lower the age for the indications of investigation of suspected precocious puberty. The recommendation now is that an evaluation should be performed in girls with pubic hair or breast development before 6 years of age and in boys with any sign of puberty before 7 years of age.[2]

J.A. Stockman III, M.D.

References

1. Herman-Giddens ME, Slora EJ, Wasserman RC, et al: Secondary sexual characteristics and menses in young girls seen in office practice: A study from the pediatric research in office settings network. *Pediatrics* 99:505-512, 1997.
2. Elders MJ, Scott CR, Frindik JP, et al: Clinical workup for precocious puberty. *Lancet* 350:457-458, 1997.

Fine-needle Aspiration of Breast Masses: A Review of Its Role in Diagnosis and Management in Adolescent Patients
Pacinda SJ, Ramzy I (Baylor College of Medicine, Houston; Methodist Hosp, Houston)
J Adolesc Health 23:3-6, 1998
8–7

Objective.—Fine-needle aspiration (FNA) is an accepted technique for evaluation of breast masses in women. However, there is little information on the use of this technique in adolescent girls, a group in which open biopsy may interfere with breast maturation and development. This study

TABLE 1.—Summary of Results of 59 Aspirates
(in 47 Female and 4 Male Patients)

Aspiration Biopsy Diagnosis	Cases (*n*)	Cases With Open Biopsy (*n*)
Fibroadenoma	28	11
Juvenile fibroadenoma	2	2
Benign ductal epithelium	12	1
Benign cyst fluid	2	
Inflammation	3	
Lactational changes	6	
Gynecomastia	3	
Unsatisfactory aspirate	3	

Note: No false-positive or false-negative diagnoses were encountered in any of the 56 satisfactory aspirates.

(Reprinted by permission of Elsevier Science Inc., from Pacinda SJ, Ramzy I: Fine-needle aspiration of breast masses: A review of its role in diagnosis and management in adolescent patients. *J Adolesc Health* 23:3-6. Copyright 1998 by the Society for Adolescent Medicine.)

reports an experience with FNA for evaluation and management of breast masses in adolescent girls.

Methods and Findings.—The 15-year review included 325 FNAs performed in 302 patients aged 21 years or younger at 4 university clinics. Fifty-nine FNAs of the breast were performed in the 51 patients, 47 of whom were females. The breast was the most commonly aspirated organ in female patients. Fibroadenomas accounted for 49% of breast aspirates in females; there were no cases of breast cancer or phyllodes tumor. The FNA procedure was followed by surgical biopsy in 14 cases, revealing 11 fibroadenomas, 2 juvenile fibroadenomas, and 1 case of ductal hyperplasia with adenosis (Table 1). All other masses had the clinical and cytologic appearance of fibrocystic changes or benign cysts, and were followed up clinically.

Conclusions.—Breast masses are the most common indication for FNA in adolescent girls, and fibroadenoma is the most commonly diagnosed lesion. By far, most masses in the adolescent breast are benign. FNA provides a useful and reliable tool in the conservative management of these masses.

▶ FNA of breast tissue would not even be a consideration in the adolescent age group if it weren't for the rare possibility of a breast mass because of a cancer. Although no malignancies were found in this series of 59 breast aspirations, about 1 in 1000 breast cancers do present in the teenage years. It would take a very large series to document the effectiveness of FNA in uncovering such malignancies. Since the technique itself is so benign, it does seem wise to use it to exclude malignancy and to make more common diagnoses, such as fibroadenoma.

Lumps and bumps in the breast are scary issues for teenagers and equally frightening to their parents. It's nice to know that a simple FNA can alleviate fears while avoiding the problems of a surgical biopsy. Surgical biopsies carry no serious morbidity, but when performed on an immature breast, they may cause deformity or asymmetry of the breast, and other cosmetic sequelae. At a minimum, a surgical biopsy leaves a scar, which unlike a tattoo, is generally unacceptable to a teen.

In the report abstracted, all aspirates were performed by cytopathologists. They are the experts, and the procedure is best left to them because the processed material must be immediately smeared onto glass slides and stained. Surgeons and gynecologists commonly do such aspirations as well.

J.A. Stockman III, M.D.

Identifying Women With Cervical Neoplasia: Using Human Papillomavirus DNA Testing for Equivocal Papanicolaou Results

Manos MM, Kinney WK, Hurley LB, et al (Northern California Kaiser Permanente Med Group, Oakland; Johns Hopkins Med Inststitutions, Baltimore, Md)

JAMA 281:1605-1610, 1999   8–8

Background.—A Papanicolaou (Pap) test finding of atypical squamous cells of undetermined significance (ASCUS) is difficult to interpret. Although only 5% to 10% of women with ASCUS have serious cervical disease, more than one third of high-grade squamous intraepithelial lesions (HSILs) in screening populations are found by ASCUS Pap test results. This study determined whether human papillomavirus (HPV) DNA testing of residual material from liquid-based Pap tests and referral of HPV-positive patients directly to colposcopy is sensitive in detecting underlying HSILs in women with ASCUS Pap results compared with repeat Pap testing.

Methods and Findings.—Nine hundred ninety-five women with Pap results of ASCUS consented to participate in the study. Nine hundred seventy-three had a definitive histologic diagnosis as well as an HPV result. Sixty-five women (6.7%) had HSIL or cancer diagnosed histologically. The HPV test was positive in 89.2% of women with histologic findings positive for HSILs. The specificity of the HPV test was 64.1% in this group. Repeat Pap testing was abnormal in 76.2%. Based on HPV testing alone or repeat Pap testing alone, about 39% would have been referred to colposcopy. The sensitivity of HPV DNA testing for HSILs was comparable to or greater than that of the repeat Pap test. An HPV-based algorithm including the immediate colposcopy of HPV-positive women, then repeat Pap testing of all others, was estimated to have a sensitivity of 96.9%.

Conclusion.—Among women with Pap results of ASCUS, HPV DNA testing of residual specimens obtained for routine cervical cytology may help identify those with underlying HSILs. By testing the specimen acquired at initial screening, most high-risk patients can be identified and referred for colposcopy after a single screening.

▶ If you care for adolescents, this report is on your "must read" list, even if you yourself are not doing routine Pap smears as part of your practice.

Things are changing fairly quickly in our understanding of the evaluation of the role of Pap smears and HPV testing these days.

As many as 2 to 3 million women (including teenagers) are given a diagnosis (post–Pap smear) of ASCUS. Although 90% to 95% of such Pap smears do not represent anything significant, 5% to 10% of women with ASCUS harbor underlying HSILs. The latter are the precursors to cervical cancer and must be managed vigorously. Some 39% of the total number of cases of HSILs are found on ASCUS follow up, so finding ASCUS remarkably elevates the probability that something serious is going on. The rub, however, is how to find the 1 in 20 to 1 in 10 with ASCUS who has a significant lesion without going whole hog (immediate colposcopy) on these 2 to 3 million women each year.

What the investigators in the above report tell us is that if you have ASCUS and are also found to be HPV negative, the risk of finding anything serious on colposcopy is small. Thus, combining Pap smears with HPV screening for those with abnormal Pap smears affords a higher degree of specificity to our procedures for cervical cancer screening techniques. To say this differently, women with ASCUS who have not become infected with the HPV virus are much less likely to have a high-grade lesion. It seems likely that at some time in the future, screening will consist of the historical Pap smear that goes back some 40-plus years *and* saving a part of the specimen for HPV testing if necessary. Those who have abnormal Pap smears and who are HPV-positive will go immediately to colposcopy. Those who are HPV-negative with abnormal Pap smears showing ASCUS can be followed with repeated Pap smears.

If colposcopy is performed and a cervical premalignant lesion is found (the usual one is known as cervical intraepithelial neoplasia)—an occurrence that is increasingly being noted in teenagers these days—3 outpatient treatment options are now used in this country: cryotherapy, laser vaporization, and the loop electrosurgical excision procedure. Each of these approaches has its own staunch supporters and critics. Proponents of cryotherapy have emphasized its reliability; ease of use; low complication rate; low cost; and the potential that leaving a large, dead viral load of HPV within disrupted cells may improve the immune response to the causative agent of the premalignant lesion. Laser therapy, on the other hand, is truly ablative and easily tailored to the specific size of the patient's lesions. It is, however, costly. It also requires more training and skill than the other 2 procedures. Proponents of the loop electrosurgical excision procedure emphasize the fact that with this procedure you have tissue specimens that you can analyze to be certain that patients do not have more aggressive lesions than you had initially thought. High cost and the potential for unintentional removal of an excessive amount of cervical tissue are the main disadvantages of the loop electrosurgical excision procedure.

If you want to read more about the status of Pap smears and HPV testing as well as the various ways of managing cervical lesions, read the excellent reviews of these topics by Cox.[1,2] Also, see the article and commentary that follow (Abstract 8–9).

J.A. Stockman III, M.D.

References

1. Cox JT: Evaluating the role of HPV testing for women with equivocal Papanicolaou testing findings. *JAMA* 281:1645-1647, 1999.
2. Cox JT: Management of cervical intraepithelial neoplasia. *Lancet* 353:857-859, 1999.

A Study of 10 296 Pediatric and Adolescent Papanicolaou Smear Diagnoses in Northern New England

Mount SL, Papillo JL (Univ of Vermont, Burlington; Fletcher Allen Health Care, Burlington, Vt)
Pediatrics 103:539-545, 1999   8–9

Background.—Differences in the biological maturity of the immune system and cervix may increase adolescents' risk for the development of squamous intraepithelial lesions (SILs). Pediatric and adolescent Papanicolaou (Pap) smear diagnoses were analyzed to determine the prevalence rates of SILs and infectious and reactive processes in this age group.

Methods.—A total of 10,296 Pap smear diagnoses from patients aged 10 to 19 years obtained during 1 year were reviewed. Diagnoses were classified by the Bethesda system. Almost all the girls were white and lived in rural or suburban regions of 3 New England states. The percentage of abnormal smear findings was compared with that from older age groups.

Findings.—Seventy percent of the girls had normal Pap smear findings. Benign cellular change was noted in 16.4%, atypical squamous cells of undetermined significance in 9.8%, SILs in 3.8%, and atypical glandular cells of undetermined significance in 0.06%. Infectious processes were evident in 14.6% of the smears. Among women aged 20 to 29 years, 11.8% had infectious processes, and 3.5% had SILs. Among women older than 30 years, 8.4% had infectious processes, and 1.3% had SILs. Thus, patients aged 10 to 19 years had the highest rate of infectious processes and SILs (Figs 1 and 2).

Conclusion.—The high rate of abnormal Pap smear results of an infectious and precancerous nature in this young age group may reflect a high level of sexual activity among adolescent girls. Early cervical Pap smear screening in sexually active girls is important.

▶ Samantha Stockman, a recent college graduate, middle daughter of the editor, and congressional aid in Washington, DC, comments:

This article clearly demonstrates the importance of implementing early cervical Pap smear screening in adolescents and young adults. Awareness might shed some light for those who do not truly understand the need for early detection and why the prevention of cancer is so important. Frequent Pap smears at an early age can help detect forms of SILs that can lead to cancer in later life. Early detection is critical for adolescents and young

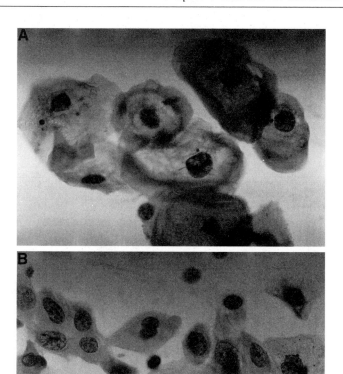

FIGURE 1.—**A**, squamous intraepithelial lesion (SIL), low grade, Papanicolaou-stained cervical smear of a 14-year-old; original magnification, ×1000. **B**, SIL, high grade, Papanicolaou-stained cervical smear of a 16-year-old; original magnification, ×1000. (Reproduced by permission of *Pediatrics*, from Mount SL, Papillo JL: A study of 10 296 pediatric and adolescent Papanicolaou smear diagnoses in northern New England. *Pediatrics* 103:539-545, 1999.)

adults, who may not realize that they are vulnerable to certain viruses that affect the cervix and can lead to the development of cancer.

My own experience with the issue has made me more aware of the need for young adults to have routine pelvic examinations and Pap smears. Most sexually active young women never see themselves as being at risk for contracting a virus that could lead to a life-threatening disease. Adolescents are often consumed with worry about protecting themselves from the high profile sexually transmitted diseases that they hear most about in the media, but not many know of the high risks of contracting human papilloma virus (HPV) and what that can mean to their health in later life.

Adolescents receiving suspicious Pap results after a routine examination are often very confused. Thoughts can range from worries about everything

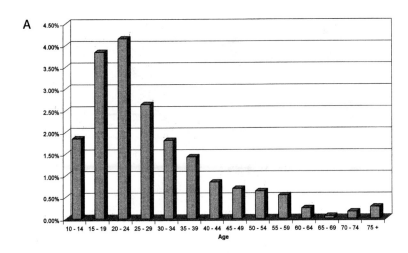

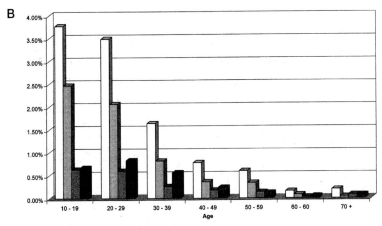

☐ Total SIL ☐ Low Grade SIL ☒ SIL - Grade Uncertain ■ High Grade SIL

FIGURE 2.—Percentage of squamous intraepithelial (SIL) diagnoses graphed by 5-year (**A**) and 10-year (**B**) groupings, with percentage of SIL low grade, SIL high grade, and SIL grade undetermined. (Reproduced by permission of *Pediatrics*, from Mount SL, Papillo JL: A study of 10 296 pediatric and adolescent Papanicolaou smear diagnoses in northern New England. *Pediatrics* 103:539-545, 1999.)

from AIDS to cancer because many young people are unaware of exactly what Pap smears test for. When I received a suspicious result, I was extremely confused. I was told that the dysplasia shown might be caused by HPV. I was told that HPV is very hard to diagnose and, because dysplasia of the cervix is usually a signal of its presence, I most likely had the virus. Because the dysplasia that HPV causes can lead to cervical cancer, I was worried about my health and went through with the suggested procedures to remove the dysplasia. The emotions accompanying this experience made me realize how prevalent these risks are in our society and that if it could happen to me, it has happened and will continue to happen to millions of women.

S. Stockman, B.S.

Evaluation of Vaginal Infections in Adolescent Women: Can It Be Done Without a Speculum?
Blake DR, Duggan A, Quinn T, et al (Johns Hopkins Univ, Baltimore, Md)
Pediatrics 102:939-944, 1998   8–10

Introduction.—Sexually transmitted diseases are common in adolescents. The seeking of care may be delayed by teenagers because of their fear of the pelvic examination and the use of the speculum. The Food and Drug Administration has recently approved the use of urine-based nucleic acid amplification tests for the diagnosis of *Neisseria gonorrhea* and *Chlamydia trachomatis*. Microscopic evaluation of fluid taken from the vagina can also be used for diagnosis of vaginal infection, and in theory, this method does not require a speculum. Whether the etiology of vaginal infections can be diagnosed without the use of a speculum was determined.

Methods.—For the diagnosis of trichomoniasis, bacterial vaginosis, and vulvovaginal candidiasis, vaginal specimens were collected from 686 women, aged 12 to 22 years, before and during speculum exam in a 1-year period. Blinded microscopic evaluation was used to evaluate paired vaginal specimens. The collection method sensitivities were compared. The proportions of infections detected by 1 method that were also detected by the other method were assessed.

Results.—Speculum methods had a sensitivity of 75% and nonspeculum methods had a sensitivity of 77% for trichomoniasis. For bacterial vaginosis, the speculum method had a sensitivity of 64% and the nonspeculum method had a sensitivity of 68%. For vulvovaginal candidiasis, the speculum method had a sensitivity of 85% and the nonspeculum method had a sensitivity of 80%. Of the infections identified by the nonspeculum method, the speculum method identified 88% of trichomoniasis, 90% of bacterial vaginosis, and 81% of vulvovaginal candidiasis. Of the infections detected by the speculum method, the nonspeculum method identified 91% of the trichomoniasis, 95% of the bacterial vaginosis, and 76% of the vulvovaginal candidiasis.

Conclusion.—Adequate diagnosis of vaginal infections can be conducted without a speculum. It may be possible to perform evaluations for uncomplicated genitourinary complaints without using a speculum, once urine-based diagnosis of gonorrhea and chlamydia becomes well established.

▶ This will be the last entry in the YEAR BOOK OF PEDIATRICS for a while on the topic of how you can do an evaluation for vaginal infections without using a speculum. The advantages of a "noninvasive" examination or evaluation for such infections is obvious. Many teenagers delay seeking care for sexually transmitted diseases because of real or perceived discomfort at the time of a standard vaginal exam, which includes the use of a speculum. If all one is doing such an examination for is to screen for vaginal infections, such an examination also takes more time than urine-based nucleic acid amplification tests. Such tests have been approved by the Food and Drug Administration for the diagnosis of both *N. gonorrhoea* and *C. trachomatis*. Such tests are equally as or even more sensitive in detecting infection than endocervical culture. Sensitivity and specificities range are in excess of 90% for the detection and diagnosis of these infections. Some patients may be culture negative, but may show evidence of recent infection by having a positive urine-based test—another plus.

The data seem perfectly clear. You can skip the vaginal examination if you are only screening for infection. Obviously a vaginal exam is necessary if you are also screening for cervical dysplasia or cancer. No one has yet figured out how to do a "Pap smear" on urine. For more on the topic of chlamydia infections in young females, see the abstract that follows, which tells us that somewhere between 12% and 15% of female military recruits are expected to be chlamydia positive on urine screening.

J.A. Stockman III, M.D.

Chlamydia trachomatis Infections in Female Military Recruits
Gaydos CA, Howell MR, Pare B, et al (Johns Hopkins Univ, Baltimore, Md; Walter Reed Army Inst of Research, Washington, DC; US Army Med Dept Activity, Fort Jackson, SC; et al)
N Engl J Med 339:739-744, 1998   8–11

Introduction.—More than 4 million urogenital *Chlamydia trachomatis* infections occur each year. Women bear the burden of disease, with consequences ranging from pelvic inflammatory disease to ectopic pregnancy and infertility. It is recommended to screen young, sexually active women because many infected women are asymptomatic. DNA-amplification assays performed on urine specimens can be used to detect *C. trachomatis* with high sensitivity. Female military recruits were screened to determine the extent of infection, to assess the feasibility of a screening program, and to find which epidemiological correlates would be useful to implement an effective chlamydia-control program.

Methods.—There were 13,204 new female U.S. Army recruits from 50 states who had urine samples taken for screening by ligase chain reaction for *C. trachomatis* infection. The recruits filled out a questionnaire to help determine potential risk factors. Criteria for a screening program were identified by multivariate analysis.

Results.—Among the recruits, the overall prevalence of chlamydia infection was 9.2%, with a peak of 12.2% among the 17-year-olds (Fig 1). Among recruits from 5 southern states, the prevalence was 15% or more. The following independent risk factors were associated with infection: having had vaginal sex (odds ratio for infection, 5.9), being 25 years old

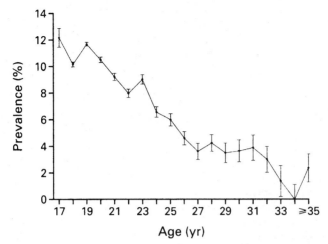

FIGURE 1.—Mean (± SE) age-specific prevalence of chlamydial infection among 13,204 female army recruits, according to ligase-chain-reaction assays of urine specimens. (Reprinted by permission of *The New England Journal of Medicine*, from Gaydos CA, Howell MR, Pare B, et al: *Chlamydia trachomatis* infections in female military recruits. *N Engl J Med* 339:739-744. Copyright 1998, Massachusetts Medical Society. All rights reserved.)

or younger (3.0), being black (3.4), having had more than 1 sex partner in the previous 90 days (1.4), having had a new partner in the previous 90 days (1.3), having had a partner in the previous 90 days who did not always use condoms (1.4), and having had a sexually transmitted disease (1.2) (Table 3). Up to 95.3% of the infected women would have been identified by a program screening those who are 25 years old or younger.

TABLE 3.—Multivariate Analysis of Factors Independently Associated With Chlamydial Infection in Female Army Recruits

Risk Factor	Odds Ratio (95% CI)*
Age ≤25 yr	3.0 (2.3-4.0)
Black race†	3.4 (2.9-3.8)
Other (nonwhite, nonblack) race†	1.7 (1.4-2.1)
Having ever had vaginal sex	5.9 (3.2-10.6)
Having had >1 sex partner in previous 90 days‡	1.4 (1.2-1.7)
Having had a new sex partner in previous 90 days§	1.3 (1.1-1.6)
Having had a partner who did not always use condoms in previous 90 days¶	1.4 (1.1-1.6)
Having ever had a sexually transmitted disease	1.2 (1.0-1.4)

*CI, confidence interval.
†Reference group, white participants.
‡Reference group, participants who did not have more than 1 sex partner, who answered that they did not know, or for whom data were missing.
§Reference group, participants who did not have a new sex partner, who answered that they did not know, or for whom data were missing.
¶Reference group, participants who had a partner who always used condoms.
(Reprinted by permission of *The New England Journal of Medicine*, from Gaydos CA, Howell MR, Pare B, et al: *Chlamydia trachomatis* infections in female military recruits. *N Engl J Med* 339:739-744. Copyright 1998, Massachusetts Medical Society. All rights reserved.)

Conclusion.—The prevalence of chlamydial infection is high among female military recruits. Infection, transmission, and the sequelae could be reduced by a control program screening female recruits, who are 25 years old or younger, with urine DNA-amplification assays.

Efficacy of Home Sampling for Screening of *Chlamydia trachomatis*: Randomised Study

Østergaard L, Andersen B, Olesen F, et al (Aarhus Univ Hosp, Denmark)
BMJ 317:26-27, 1998   8–12

Background.—*Chlamydia trachomatis* commonly causes urogenital infections and may result in female infertility and ectopic pregnancy. This randomized study investigated the efficacy of home sampling for screening of *C. trachomatis* among adolescents.

Methods.—Seventeen high schools in 1 county were randomly assigned to 2 screening groups. In the home sampling group, girls were asked to collect 2 urine samples and 1 vaginal flush sample, and boys were asked to collect 1 first void urine sample. These samples were mailed from the home to a microbiology department at a university. In the control group, physicians or the local clinic for sexually transmitted diseases offered students the testing. A questionnaire and information on *C. trachomatis* infection were distributed to students in both groups. Students returning the questionnaire who were also sexually active were designated eligible responders.

Findings.—Forty-eight percent of the girls in the home sampling group responded, compared with 38% of the girls in the control group. Thirty-four percent of the boys in the home sampling group and 19% in the control group responded. In the home sampling group, 93.4% of the eligible female responders were tested, compared with 7.6% in the control group. Rates of detected infection were 4.6% and 0.6%, respectively. In the home sampling group, 97.3% of the eligible male responders, compared with 1.6% in the control group, were tested. Detected infection rates were 2.5% and 0.4%, respectively.

Conclusions.—The efficacy of *C. trachomatis* screening is more effective when high school students can collect their own samples at home and mail them directly to a laboratory than when students must see a physician. Home sampling may decrease the prevalence of and the number of complications from *C. trachomatis*.

▶ Switching sexes for a second regarding urogenital infections, what would you do in the following scenario? You are having lunch with a colleague of yours, a urologist, who relates an interesting story to you. He has seen 4 adult males in consultation for an internist who was unable to make a diagnosis based on these patients' symptoms. All 4 individuals had recently returned from travels overseas. All 4 had identical symptoms. The complaint was that of an alteration in their ejaculates. There was a change in color to yellow, a reduction in volume, and a reduction in viscosity to the consistency of water. The internist had treated all 4 individuals on the suspicion that they had either prostatitis or non-gonococcal urethritis, but the symptoms and signs did not abate. What would be your diagnosis?

Well, as it turns out, all 4 men in question were real and were members of a church group that had recently returned from travels to Africa. There, they swam in a freshwater lake, Lake Malawi, and soon developed their symptoms upon return. A careful examination of seminal fluid from all 4 showed the same findings: a polymorph infiltrate along with *Schistosoma haematobium* ova. The number and motility of spermatozoa were unaffected. All this was reported in a recent issue of the *British Medical Journal*.[1] The most common change in the ejaculate is not a change in color to yellow, but rather that of hematospermia in such infected patients. Obviously, a reported alteration in semen is an unusual presenting symptom. Such changes following exposure to *S. haematobium* have been reported previously. There is no reason to think that teenagers might not develop similar symptoms under the same circumstances.

With *C. trachomatis* one of, in fact, the most common cause of female infertility and ectopic pregnancy, all the world has waited for a simple diagnostic test for this organism. That test came along just a few years ago with the ability to detect *C. trachomatis* by amplification of DNA either from urine or vaginal secretions. With this technology, culture becomes unnecessary. The rub, however, is getting the teenager or adult woman into the office or clinic for obtaining and processing the sample.

If a patient won't come to you, at least their urine can, thanks to Uncle Sam and the U.S. Postal Service. It's as easy as pie. A sample of urine (male or female) dropped in the local outgoing mailbox will survive well and suffers no loss of diagnostic abilities (unless the mail carrier loses the specimen).

Now there is no excuse for missing *C. trachomatis* infections. Neither sleet, nor rain, nor snow, nor dark of night shall be a deterrent.

J.A. Stockman III, M.D.

Reference

1. McKenna G, Schousboe M, Paltridge G: Subjective change in the ejaculate symptoms of infection with *Schistosoma haematobium* in travelers. *BMJ* 315:1000, 1997.

A Controlled Trial of Nonoxynol 9 Film to Reduce Male-to-Female Transmission of Sexually Transmitted Diseases
Roddy RE, Zekeng L, Ryan KA, et al (Family Health Internatl, Durham, NC; Ministry of Public Health, Yaoundé, Cameroon)
N Engl J Med 339:504-510, 1998   8–13

Background.—Whether nonoxynol 9 is both a microbicide and a spermicide is unknown. The efficacy of nonoxynol 9 film in reducing male-to-female transmission of sexually transmitted disease (STD) was investigated.

Methods.—A total of 1292 HIV-negative female prostitutes in Cameroon were enrolled in the double-blind, placebo-controlled study. The women were assigned randomly to the use of a film containing 70 mg of nonoxynol 9 or placebo, to be inserted into the vagina before intercourse. The women were also given condoms for their partners' use. Colposcopy was performed every month. In addition, endocervical specimens for gonorrhea and chlamydia infection were tested with DNA probes, and HIV testing was done each month. The women were treated for curable STDs.

Findings.—The nonoxynol 9 and placebo groups had HIV infection rates of 6.7 and 6.6 per 100 woman-years, respectively. Genital lesion rates were 42.2 and 33.5 per 100 woman-years, respectively. The rate of gonorrhea was 33.3 per 100 woman-years in the nonoxynol 9 group and 31.1 per 100 woman-years in the placebo group. The chlamydia infection rates were 20.6 cases and 22.2 cases per 100 woman-years, respectively. Condoms were reportedly used during 90% of sexual acts.

Conclusions.—The use of nonoxynol 9 vaginal film did not decrease the rates of new HIV, gonorrhea, or chlamydia infection in this group of prostitutes. As expected, the occurrence of genital ulcers was increased among nonoxynol 9 users.

▶ The results of this report are disappointing, but probably predictable. A number of studies over the years have shown that a variety of STDs could be reduced with the use of the spermicide, nonoxynol 9. This nonionic detergent not only disrupts the cell membrane of sperm cells, but also that of epithelial cells to which bacteria and viruses attach. It may also disrupt the cell membranes of bacteria and viruses. Nonoxynol 9 is not a uniformly perfect agent in preventing STDs, however. We see that it does little to reduce the rate of HIV infection, gonorrhea, or chlamydia infection, at least in prostitutes in Cameroon. What to do with this information in our pediatric practices is unclear. Certainly condoms should be used on every conceivable occasion (pardon the pun). Even though the average teenager in the United States is not likely to be as sexually active as a prostitute in Cameroon, whatever benefit nonoxynol 9 affords would seem to be worth going for. It will help reduce the risk of STD, although not in a perfect fashion. It will help reduce the risk of conception, albeit not in a perfect fashion either. There is little reason not to try to obtain whatever benefit it can produce.

Nonoxynol 9 may not work well to reduce STDs, but it is okay as a contraceptive. In case you are interested in the birth rates (high and low) of countries throughout the world and in the cities in our country, see the interesting tables that follow:

Countries		U.S. Cities	
Highest Birth Rates (per 1000)		Highest Birth Rates (per 1000)	
Niger	52.5	La Puente, Calif	64.8
Uganda	51.8	Miami, Fla	49.5
Angola	51.3	Gaithersburg, Md	49.2
Mali	50.8	Watsonville, Calif	49.2
Guinea	50.6	Whittier, Calif	44.1
Malawi	50.5	Palmdale, Calif	44.1
Somalia	50.2	Lake Worth, Fla	43.0
Afghanistan	50.2	Bakersfield, Calif	42.4
Cote d'Ivoire	49.9	Madera, Calif	41.3
Yemen	49.4	Jacksonville, NC	40.3
Lowest Birth Rates (per 1000)		Lowest Birth Rates (per 1000)	
Spain	9.7	Danville, Ill	18.0
Italy	9.8	Longview, Wash	18.0
Germany	9.9	Baltimore, Md	18.0
Greece	9.9	Greenville, SC	18.0
Japan	10.1	Rochester, NH	18.0
Bulgaria	10.3	Charlotte, NC	18.0
Slovenia	10.5	Manchester, NH	18.0
Russian Federation	10.9	Worcester, Mass	18.0
Estonia	11.0	Jacksonville, Fla	18.0
Croatia	11.3	Hampton, Va	18.0
Romania	11.3		

(Data from U.S. Census Bureau *County and City Data Book*, 1994, and *Statistical Abstract of the United States*, 1996.)

J.A. Stockman III, M.D.

Saliva Test as Ovulation Predictor

Braat DDM, Smeenk JMJ, Manger AP, et al (Univ Hosp Nijmegen, The Netherlands; St Antonius Hosspital, Nieuwegein, The Netherlands)
Lancet 352:1283-1284, 1998   8–14

Objective.—The use of mini-microscopes to assess microscopic ferning in saliva samples has become a proposed method of predicting a woman's fertile period. Proponents believe ferning is correlated with 17β-estradiol concentrations. This test has become widely available and is recommended by infertility specialists and patient groups. A prospective study examined its reliability.

Methods.—The study included 30 women with regular menstrual cycles in whom the day of ovulation was confirmed by ultrasound and serum luteinizing–hormone measurements or by basal body temperature. Each morning, a dried drop of saliva from each subject was examined for ferning using either a mini-microscope or a normal light microscope.

Results.—Examination using the mini-microscope was 53% sensitive and 72% specific for predicting the fertile period. For light microscopic examination, sensitivity was 86% and specificity 14%. Positive results were achieved using the same test in postmenopausal women and in men. Ferning was unrelated to saliva 17β-estradiol concentration.

Conclusions.—Microscopic examination of saliva to detect ferning is not a reliable test to predict a woman's fertile period. Its use should therefore be discouraged.

▶ The YEAR BOOK OF PEDIATRICS rarely reports on negative data. In this case, however, the data do seem worthy of comment because it is a common belief that one can examine the saliva to tell when a woman is "fertile."

For some time now, demand for self-tests to predict the time of fertility has been increasing. Although the urine luteinizing hormone test seems to be the most effective predictor of ovulation, inexpensive small microscopes have been used to predict fertile days by detecting microscopic ferning in saliva drops. The theory is that ferning of saliva correlates with 17 β-estradiol in serum or saliva and, therefore, with the fertile period. The mini-microscope has been proposed as a reliable tool for natural family planning, as well as for the prediction of the fertile period. This type of microscope can be found in any average toy store. In many parts of the world, infertility specialists and patient groups have widely recommended such self-diagnostic home tests on saliva.

So just how good is saliva in telling when the best time is for conception? It is not worth a spit! It is not very good, especially since most men will test positive. Does this mean that men are always ready to procreate? Yes, but true, true unrelated. In any event, saliva ferning just isn't sufficiently sensitive or specific to do the job if a couple really wants to be assured of the highest chance of success in their timing of intercourse. A plain old body temperature chart works just as well, if not slightly better.

J.A. Stockman III, M.D.

Depot Medroxyprogesterone Acetate (Depo-Provera) and Levonorgestrel (Norplant) Use in Adolescents Among Clinicians in Northern Europe and the United States
Cromer BA, Berg-Kelly KS, van Groningen JP, et al (Ohio State Univ, Columbus; Univ of Goteberg, Sweden; Univ of Leiden, The Netherlands; et al)
J Adolesc Health 22:74–80, 1998   8–15

Background.—Even though depot medroxyprogesterone acetate (Depo-Provera, or DMPA) and levonorgestrel (Norplant) implants were generally approved earlier in The Netherlands, Sweden, and Great Britain than in the United States, practitioners in these Northern European countries seem to underprescribe these contraceptives for adolescents. The authors undertook this study to examine differences between these 4 countries in attitudes and practices related to the use of DMPA and levonorgestrel in adolescents.

Methods.—The authors developed a questionnaire to explore attitudes and practices relating to the prescription of DMPA and levonorgestrel for

TABLE 2.—Clinicians' Uses of and Preferences for DMPA and
Levonorgestrel in Adolescents

	Sweden (n = 282)	U.S. (n = 548)	Holland (n = 197)	Great Britain (n = 126)
DMPA use [% yes (n)]	39 (110)	81 (440)*	33 (66)	86 (108)*
Levonorgestrel use, [% yes (n)]	34 (96)	70 (382)*	0	35 (44)
DMPA in top three, choices [% (n)]	10 (28)	68 (374)*	24 (46)	59 (74)*
Levonorgestrel in top three choices [% n)]	5 (14)	41 (222)*	0	3 (4)

*Chi-square > 100, P < .0001.
Abbreviation: DMPA, depot medroxyprogesterone acetate.
(Reprinted by permission of Elsevier Science Inc., from Cromer BA, Berg-Kelly KS, van Groningen JP, et al: Depot medroxyprogesterone acetate [Depo-Provera] and levonorgestrel [Norplant] use in adolescents among clinicians in Northern Europe and the United States. *J Adolesc Health* 22:74-80. Copyright 1998 by the Society for Adolescent Medicine.)

adolescents, taking into account each country's health care delivery system. They sent the questionnaires to appropriate clinics or practitioners (physician, nurse practitioner, nurse midwife, physician assistant). Questionnaires were sent to 500 physicians in The Netherlands (197 of whom responded), 181 clinics in Sweden (282 practitioners responded), 500 physicians in Great Britain (108 of whom responded), and 1000 practitioners in the United States (548 of whom responded).

Findings.—Significantly more practitioners in Great Britain and the United States prescribed DMPA and included DMPA in their top 3 choices for contraception in adolescents than did practitioners in Sweden and The Netherlands (Table 2). In addition, adolescents in Great Britain and the United States were significantly more likely to ask about DMPA than were their peers in Sweden and The Netherlands. Significantly more U.S. practitioners prescribed levonorgestrel and included levonorgestrel in their top 3 choices for contraception in adolescents than did practitioners in the other 3 countries (note that this implant is not licensed in The Netherlands). In addition, U.S. adolescents were significantly more likely to ask about DMPA than were their peers in other countries. The most common circumstance in which either of these 2 methods was prescribed was noncompliance with other methods. Practitioners were also asked about their "worst fears" with these 2 contraceptive methods. The most common responses for DMPA were infertility and failure to use condoms. (Significantly more practitioners in Sweden voiced these concerns.) The most common responses for levonorgestrel were failure to use condoms and breakthrough bleeding. (Again, significantly more Swedish practitioners voiced these concerns.)

Conclusions.—Significant differences in attitudes and practices surrounding the use of DMPA and levonorgestrel in adolescents exist among these 4 countries. The highest levels of enthusiasm are found among U.S. and British practitioners. These results may be explained in part by the low compliance rates with oral contraceptives in the United States and the

United Kingdom and the high compliance rates in Swedish and Dutch adolescents.

▶ It is easy to see why DMPA and Norplant are becoming increasingly more popular these days. Both methods of contraception have been found suitable by care providers who advise adolescents and young adults about contraceptive methods. In comparison with oral contraceptive pills, they are more effective in preventing pregnancy, largely because they are "forget-me-not" methods of prophylaxis against pregnancy. As this report tells us, acceptance of DMPA and Norplant is greater here than in many parts of the world. This may, in part, be due to the fact that we are a somewhat wealthier nation and are perhaps willing to pay the higher tab that comes with these two forms of hormonal contraception.

Please note that none of these forms of contraception are bullet proof. There are disadvantages to each one. Regarding oral contraceptive pills, they must be taken every day. They may also cause unwanted menstrual cycle changes. Other unwanted side effects include headaches, decreased libido, depression, etc., in some users. A downside to Norplant is its significant expense. While the putting in of Norplant may be covered by insurance, its removal rarely is, even when medically indicated. Another problem with Norplant is that many teenagers and adults blame every little sign and symptom they develop that is unrelated to the contraceptive on the Norplant. DMPA, while having many advantages, does have some disadvantages. Its effects are delayed. Patients also must return every 3 months for repeat injections. Once stopped, fertility doesn't always promptly return. Thus, those who wish to become pregnant ASAP may be plumb out of luck.

On a slightly different topic, the controversy about routine Papanicolaou (Pap) smear screening in adolescents continues. Given the high percentage of sexually active adolescents and of those with a history of sexual abuse, the high prevalence of sexually transmitted diseases (HPV specifically) and smoking, and the recent study suggesting a much higher degree of cervical dysplasia than previously appreciated in teenagers, one can strongly argue for continuing Pap smear screening for adolescents as an essential part of preventive health care. This is the position taken by Emans et al.[1] The concern of those who advise against such Pap smear screening is that youngsters who want to avoid the required examinations might be the ones who would accept screening for sexually transmitted diseases by noninvasive techniques if there were no need for a speculum examination related to a Pap smear.

In a world of unintended consequences, what we don't want are teenagers shying away from a good thing, Pap smears, because we ask for more than they are willing to deliver.

Before we close this commentary having to do with sexual activity in adolescents, were you aware that those who are not sexually active have a significantly higher risk of dying young? 'Tis true. In this case, more is more. In a study of 918 men aged 45 to 59, death from coronary artery disease was 50% lower in a group of men who had orgasms 100 times or more per year in comparison with those who did not.[2] Specifically, the odds ratio for total mortality in men who experienced 100 orgasms per year was 0.64. For men who had infrequent orgasms, the adjusted odds ratio for coronary artery disease and death was 2 times greater than average. It is entirely possible that some of our teenagers, based on these findings, would likely become Methuselahs.

Information such as this is interesting, but the conclusions probably have little to do with true linkages between coronary artery disease and the frequency of orgasm. Then again, this finding that those who are more sexually active live longer is a basic violation of the principle that less is more—more or less.

J.A. Stockman III, M.D.

References

1. Perlman SE, Kahn JA, Emans SJ: Should pelvic examinations and Papanicolaou cervical screening be part of preventive health care for sexually active adolescent girls? *J Adolesc Health* 23:62-67, 1998.
2. Smith GD: Sex and death: Are they related? Findings from the caerphilly cohort study. *BMJ* 315:1641-1645, 1997.

Early Sexual Initiation: The Role of Peer Norms
Kinsman SB, Romer D, Furstenberg FF, et al (Children's Hosp of Philadelphia; Univ of Pennsylvania, Philadelphia)
Pediatrics 102:1185-1192, 1998   8–16

Background.—Adolescents who initiate unprotected sexual intercourse at an early age are at increased risk of negative health outcomes. Numerous factors influence an adolescent's decision to initiate sexual intercourse; the affect of peer norms on sexual initiation in sixth graders was assessed.

Methods.—The study included 1389 sixth-grade students attending 14 public schools in Philadelphia who completed surveys at the beginning (time 1) and the end (time 2) of the school year. Half were boys and half were girls, with a mean age at time 1 of 11.7 years. About half (55%) were African American, 22% were white, 12% were Latino, and 3% were Asian. The 40-item questionnaire assessed whether the child intended to initiate sexual intercourse in the upcoming year, what the child's risk behaviors were, the child's perceptions of his or her peers' risk behaviors, and the child's perceptions of peer norms about sexual initiation.

Findings.—Almost one third—416 children, or 30%—had already initiated sexual intercourse at time 1. Another 74 (5%) initiated sexual intercourse during the sixth-grade year, while 873 (63%) did not. These latter 2 groups (initiated vs never) were investigated further. At time 1, half of the children in the initiated group reported that they intended to initiate sexual intercourse during the sixth grade. Compared with children who had never had sex, children who initiated sex during the study were significantly more likely to be older (mean age at time 1, 11.9 vs 11.6 years), to be boys (58 vs 37), to be African American (70 vs 51), to attend poorer schools (87 vs 85), and to live in an area with a higher proportion of single-parent homes (45 vs 41). Children in the initiated group were also more likely to have used alcohol and participated in a fight, and they reported that more of their peers drank alcohol and smoked at 13 to 14 years. They also reported that more of their peers had already initiated sexual intercourse, and more children in this group believed that a sexually experienced boy, aged 12 years, would gain respect among his peers. Three models were developed to test the links between intention and behavior, peers and behavior, and peers and intention. The strongest predictor of sexual initiation was the intent to do so at time 1 (odds ratio, 2.33), and the strongest predictor of intention was the belief that most of one's peers had already initiated intercourse (odds ratio, 2.5).

Conclusions.—For many adolescents, the decision to initiate early sexual intercourse is planned. The perceptions of peers' behaviors play a significant role in the perception of the norm, and in the intent to initiate sexual relations. Pediatricians who hope to delay their patients' sexual initiation must focus on both the norms and behaviors of the patient's cohorts, and the patient's own perceptions and behaviors.

▶ Fascinating report. We see that the image that many of us have, so erroneously stereotypic, that first sexual encounters are often precipitous and unplanned is indeed a myth. The first encounter, it would appear, is a calculated, planned, premeditated event—fornication in the first degree. It is hardly an experiment. It is a deliberate step to gain social acceptance as well as a little pleasure. While this may not be the first scenario for all teens, it is for most. By the way, the sampling that was done was of those youngsters who were in the sixth grade.

So what's the good news? The good news is that for the first time in decades, sexual activity is leveling off and may be decreasing among certain groups of teenagers, particularly among white teenage males. At the same time, condom use has increased and the level of unprotected intercourse (without condoms) has fallen. Despite this semblance of good news, data from the Population Studies Center, The Urban Institute in Washington show that a significant fraction of teenagers continue to have unprotected sexual intercourse, putting them at risk of HIV infection, sexually transmitted diseases, and unintended pregnancies.[1] In the aggregate, recent findings are encouraging and suggest that public health and educational initiatives to improve sexual and contraceptive behaviors of American teenagers have been moving in the right direction. However, they also warn us that more improvements are needed, particularly to protect the health of African American and Hispanic youths.

J.A. Stockman III, M.D.

Reference

1. Sonenstein FL, Ku L, Lindberg LD, et al: Changes in sexual behavior and condom use among teenage males: 1988 to 1995. *Am J Public Health* 88:956, 1998.

Homicide Rates Among US Teenagers and Young Adults: Differences by Mechanism, Level of Urbanization, Race, and Sex, 1987 Through 1995

Fingerhut LA, Ingram DD, Feldman JJ (Natl Ctr for Health Statistics, Hyattsville, Md)
JAMA 280:423-427, 1998   8–17

Introduction.—Between the mid-1980s and the early 1990s, homicide rates for individuals aged 15 through 24 years increased. These rates declined between 1993 and 1994. The homicide rate for this age group remains high despite the declines; the rate in 1995 was 71% higher than a decade earlier. Most homicides are committed with firearms. Homicide trends from 1987 through 1995 were examined for individuals aged 15 through 24 years by urbanization level.

Methods.—Firearm and nonfirearm homicide rates and average annual percentage changes by 5 urbanization levels, race, and sex were measured in those 15 through 24 years old whose cause of death was homicide. The 5 urbanization strata were core, or counties with the primary central city of a metropolitan statistical area of 1 million or more; fringe, or remaining counties within a metropolitan statistical area of 1 million or more; medium, counties with a metropolitan statistical area of 250,000 to 999,9999; small, counties in a metropolitan statistical area of less than 250,000; and nonmetropolitan, counties not in a metropolitan statistical area.

Results.—Among all 5 urbanization strata, the average annual firearm homicide rates in this age group increased between 10.7% in small counties and 19.8% in fringe counties from 1987 to 1991. From 1991 and 1993, in core counties, the rate increased 3.3%, and in small counties the increase was 11.7%. From 1993 to 1995, the rates in fringe counties declined by 4.4%, and in medium counties the decline was 15.3%. In the nonmetropolitan counties, firearm homicide rates among this age group was 6.5 per 100,000 by 1995, and in small counties, the rate was 7.3 per 100,000. In the fringe strata, the rate was 9.6 per 100,000. In the medium strata, the rate was 13.3 per 100,000. In the core stratum, it was 33.5 per 100,000. Nonfirearm homicide rates were stable or increased during 1987 through 1990. In all 5 strata, the nonfirearm homicide rates declined from 1990 through 1995. The decline was an average of 3.7% to 8% per year. In 1995 the nonfirearm homicide rates ranged from 2.1 to 4.7 per 100,000 across the strata.

Conclusion.—Among individuals 15 through 24 years of age, firearm and nonfirearm homicide rates began to decline between 1993 and 1995. All urbanization strata and white and black males and females are all showing these declines. Between 1987 and 1993, there had been a steady increase in those rates.

▶ The data from this report speak for themselves. Let's hope that the decline in homicide among U.S. teenagers and young adults continues well into the current millennium. In 1995, homicides accounted for 21% of all deaths among individuals 15 to 24 years old, compared with 12% of all deaths in 1985. Firearms continue to be the instruments with which most homicides are committed, with the proportion of homicides resulting from the use of firearms actually increasing from 66% in 1985 to 84% of all homicides in 1995. Thus, further reductions in the homicide rate will be made most effectively by getting rid of guns. Once the firearm problem is solved in this country, we can then worry about the switchblades, baseball bats, and steel-tipped shoes.

This is the last entry in the Adolescent Medicine chapter, so we will close with a question having to do with adolescent and young adult women. How would you answer the following? It has been suggested that women who are in close proximity to other women in a working environment or in other close environments (dorms, etc.) tend to have menstrual cycles with about the same length. How is this possible?

This may have something to do with human pheromones. Human pheromones exist and, at the very least, seem to influence the length of women's menstrual cycles.[1] Pheromones are chemicals secreted by one member of a species that influence the physiology or behavior of others in the same species. About 25 years ago, it was shown that women living together in a college dormitory developed synchronized menstrual cycles. This may well be caused by pheromone production. Investigators collected samples of odorless compounds from the armpits of 9 healthy women with normal menstruation during distinct phases of the menstrual cycle. They then exposed 20 similar women to the aroma of these samples and found that compounds secreted during the late follicular phase accelerated the preovulatory surge of luteinizing hormone of recipient women, shortening their menstrual cycles. Compounds collected later in the cycle, at ovulation, had the opposite effect.

To say all this differently, the menstrual cycle may not be regulated only by internal mechanisms, but also it is affected by a woman's environment. One wonders what studies of pheromones from the axilla of males during bonding experiences such as backwoods fishing trips might show. Probably a simultaneous urge to have another beer.

J.A. Stockman III, M.D.

Reference

1. McClintock M, Stern K: Human pheromones. *Nature* 392:177-179, 1998.

9 Therapeutics and Toxicology

Accidental and Suicidal Adolescent Poisoning Deaths in the United States, 1979-1994
Shepherd G, Klein-Schwartz W (Univ of Maryland, Baltimore; Univ of Texas, Dallas)
Arch Pediatr Adolesc Med 152:1181-1185, 1998   9–1

Background.—Death due to poisoning (both accidental and intentional) is a tragic problem in adolescents. This study describes the incidence and specific causes of deaths due to poisoning in adolescents in the United States between 1979 and 1994.

Methods.—National mortality data were extracted from the Center for Disease Control and Prevention (CDC)'s website, Wonder, on the Internet. This website provides access to national databases that include demographic characteristics of individuals who died and the cause of their deaths (based on ICD-9 codes). All deaths of children aged 10 to 19 years between January 1, 1979, and December 31, 1994, were identified and analyzed.

Findings.—During this 16-year period, a total of 7936 adolescents died of poisoning; 4129 of the deaths were suicides and 3807 were accidental. Although mortality rates for accidental poisonings remained relatively stable, suicide rates decreased in the 1990s. The adolescents most likely to die of poisoning were male (male:female ratio 1.8:8), white (whites vs blacks, 1.47/100,000 vs 0.78/100,000 individuals), and 15 to 19 years old (compared with 10- to 14-year olds, 2.36/100,000 vs 0.28/100,000). Slightly more poisoning deaths in males (2661 of 5032 deaths, or 52.9%) were accidental, whereas more deaths in girls (1748 of 2094, or 60.5%) were due to suicide. The type of substance involved differed between adolescents aged 10 to 14 years committing suicide (drugs [excluding alcohol], 85.3%; gases or vapors, 12.1%) and those aged 15 to 19 years (gases or vapors, 51.4%; drugs [excluding alcohol], 45.4%). The type of substance involved also differed between adolescents 10 to 14 years old dying of accidental poisoning (gases or vapors, 51.0%; drugs [excluding alcohol], 22.4%) and those who were 15 to 19 years old (gases or vapors, 43.9%; drugs [excluding alcohol], 38.5%). Overall, 3725 deaths (46.9%)

were attributable to gases or vapors; of these, 3034 deaths (81.4%) were due to carbon monoxide (i.e., 38.2% of all deaths). Of the 4211 deaths (53.1%) attributable to drugs or alcohol, 3468 (82.3%) deaths were due to drugs and 743 (17.7%) deaths were due to alcohol.

Conclusions.—Poisoning deaths are more common in white males 15 to 19 years old. Interventions to manage depression, to educate adolescents about drug abuse, to encourage the use of carbon monoxide detectors in the home, and to encourage carbon monoxide shut-off switches in motor vehicles could reduce the number of poisoning deaths in this population.

▶ This report summarizes the entire nation's experience with death from poisoning in adolescents. The database used to provide this information was extracted from the CDC's *Wonder* Web site. In case you weren't aware, the National Center for Health Statistics collects and publishes data on deaths. In addition, specific demographic characteristics of those who died and what caused the death are provided. Exploring this database can be a fascinating experience and well worth your time. The database may be found at: *http://wonder.cdc.gov.*

Before the report appeared, this editor was not aware that inhalation of toxic gases constituted such a huge proportion of both accidental deaths and deaths by suicide. Deaths caused by poisonous gases are roughly equivalent in number to deaths from all other poisonous materials. Most accidental deaths from inhalant poisons are related to inhalation of the fluorinated hydrocarbon refrigerant, Freon. Presumably, such deaths result from inhalant abuse. Carbon monoxide gas inhalation is the most common poisoning with respect to intentional suicide. Accidental carbon monoxide poisoning also occurs and may be related to faulty oil and gas heating units, fires, and poor ventilation of buildings. Intentional suicide from carbon monoxide more often than not results from sitting in an automobile, with the engine running, within a closed space.

In case you are not aware, it's getting harder and harder to intentionally kill one's self with carbon monoxide. The reason is that we are producing relatively "clean" automobiles. Catalytic converters decrease the carbon monoxide content of automobile exhaust gases from about 3.5% to 0.5%, also removing oxides of nitrogen and sulfur. Data from Scotland show a remarkable decline in the number of suicides attributable to carbon monoxide poisoning, presumably as a consequence of the required installation of catalytic converters into new cars. (All cars sold in the United Kingdom since December 31, 1992, have had to have catalytic converters.) Catalytic converters have been installed on cars sold in the United States for many more years. To kill yourself with any degree of assurance, you might try a '53 DeSoto.

No one thought that one of the spin effects, a positive effect of the "Clean Air Act" would have been a reduction in suicide-related deaths from carbon monoxide poisoning. We should be grateful for such an unintended consequence.[1]

Lastly, be aware that the classical physical examination finding of a cherry-red appearance is actually not all that common with carbon monoxide poisoning. Cherry-red discoloration of the skin and mucous membranes is an often-quoted sign of such poisoning. A veterinarian was recently reported who suspected carbon monoxide poisoning in a dog because of its "cherry-red conjunctiva."[2] As it turns out, only about 1 case in 100 in a prospective study showed such discoloration.[3] The fact that many care providers don't know much about skin color and carbon monoxide was recently illustrated in a report from Italy, where physicians were asked how often *rossa caligo* (cherry red) is seen with such poisoning. Only 6% of physicians gave the correct prevalence (1%), and 10% thought this sign was present in all patients. When shown pictures of cherries ranging from dark blue to bright red (bing to maraschino), 1 in 4 associated the cherry-red color with purple and dark blue shades and 1 in 4 with bright red.[4]

J.A. Stockman III, M.D.

References

1. Kendell RE: Catalytic converters and prevention of suicides. *Lancet* 352:1525, 1998.
2. Bignall J: Looking the dog in the eye. *Lancet* 345:852, 1995.
3. Gorman DF, Clayton D, Gilligan JE, et al: A longitudinal study of 100 consecutive admissions for carbon monoxide poisoning to the Royal Adelaide hospital. *Anaesth Intens Care* 20:311-316, 1992.
4. Simini B: Cherry-red discoloration and carbon monoxide poisoning. *Lancet* 354:1154, 1998.

Caffeine Withdrawal in Normal School-age Children

Bernstein GA, Carroll ME, Dean NW, et al (Univ of Minnesota, Minneapolis; Neuropsychiatric Research Inst, Fargo, ND; Univ of Florida, Gainesville; et al)
J Am Acad Child Adolesc Psychiatry 37:858-865, 1998   9–2

Background.—American children 8 to 12 years old who drink caffeine have a mean daily caffeine intake of 54.6 mg/day, which is more than the amount of caffeine contained in a 12-oz soft drink. Caffeine increases sympathetic stimulation and circulating catecholamine levels, and the effects of its withdrawal in adults include depression, anxiety, fatigue, and headache. This study evaluated the effects of caffeine withdrawal in children.

Methods.—Thirty children between 8 and 12 years old (17 boys and 13 girls; mean age, 10.1 years) who consumed at least 10 mg caffeine daily were enrolled. Mean daily caffeine consumption was 38.5 ± 31.4 mg. At baseline, they completed self-reports of symptoms of caffeine side effects and performed attention, motor performance, processing speed, and memory tests. Then they drank three 12-oz beverages each day for 13 days, either Coca-Cola (caffeine content 120 mg/day; n = 5) or Mountain Dew (146 mg/day; n = 25) brand soft drinks, while abstaining from other caffeine-containing products. Self-reports and tests were repeated after 7 days of soft drink consumption, and on day 14 they switched to a non-caffeinated soft drink for 1 day. Self-reports and tests were repeated on day 14 during caffeine withdrawal, and again after they had resumed their normal diet for 7 days (i.e., return to baseline). Compliance was confirmed by measuring mean salivary caffeine levels.

Findings.—Between the 4 measurements, there were significant differences in responses on the Test of Variables of Attention (TOVA). During the 11-minute TOVA, they are exposed to two stimuli and should press a button when the target stimulus appears. Response times were significantly better during the baseline and caffeine conditions than during the caffeine withdrawal and return to baseline conditions (452.6 and 459.4 vs 523.0 and 521.3 msec, respectively). Practice effects were apparent for commission errors on the TOVA and for motor performance, processing speed, and memory tests, because scores were significantly lower at baseline than during any of the other 3 conditions. Symptoms of caffeine withdrawal did not differ significantly between the caffeine consumption and caffeine withdrawal conditions.

Conclusions.—At caffeine withdrawal and up to 1 week after, attention decreased significantly as measured by a visual continuous performance attention task. Thus caffeine withdrawal seems to have detrimental effects on attention for these children. However, no differences in withdrawal symptoms were found, and a practice effect obscured any differences that may have existed in performance times during the various test conditions.

▶ Caffeine is a mixed blessing for teenagers. It's been suggested that caffeine may be efficacious for treating symptoms of attention-deficit hyperactivity disorder, both in children and adolescents. Studies on this are somewhat conflicting, but it is clear that children will show a significant improvement in attention with fewer omissions on various performance tests when they have recently consumed caffeine. Most teenagers have long recognized that a can of Coke in the morning before an exam seems to help them. At the time of finals, the product Jolt (double the caffeine, double the sugar), if you can still find it, is even more desired.

The rub is coming off caffeine. Symptoms of caffeine withdrawal include fatigue, drowsiness, depression, and occasionally headaches. Virtually all the children in this report were found to have testing abnormalities following withdrawal of caffeine that they were taking as part of the investigation. The daily dose of caffeine ingested during this study was approximately 3 to 4 times greater than the children's baseline intake of 38.5 mg/day and 2.7 times greater than the average daily intake for caffeine-consuming children in the United States. It seems that the average child consumes about the amount of caffeine in one regular Coke or Mountain Dew. In this study, everyone had to drink about 3 cans of these nectars a day for 2 weeks.

Between Coca-Cola, Mountain Dew, Dr. Pepper, and Jolt, we are creating a population of teenagers who are "all juiced up" with very little in the way of where to go. A little more sleep at night and a little less caffeine would probably produce the same academic outcome.

J.A. Stockman III, M.D.

Positron Emission Tomographic Evidence of Toxic Effect of MDMA ("Ecstasy") on Brain Serotonin Neurons in Human Beings

McCann UD, Szabo Z, Scheffel U, et al (Natl Inst of Mental Health, Bethesda, Md; Johns Hopkins Med Insts, Baltimore, Md)

Lancet 352:1433-1437, 1998   9–3

Background.—Experimental evidence suggests that (±)3,4-methylenedioxymethamphetamine (MDMA, or "Ecstasy") could damage brain serotonin (5-HT) neurons in humans. These authors used positron emission tomography (PET) to compare the status of brain 5-HT neurons in users of MDMA with that in control subjects.

Methods.—The subjects were 14 patients (9 men and 5 women; mean age, 26.6 years) who had previously used MDMA and 15 age- and sex-matched control subjects who had never used this drug. Patients had used MDMA at a mean dose of 386 mg for a mean of 4.60 years but had been abstinent at enrollment (as confirmed by blood and urine samples) for a mean of 19 weeks. The radioligand [^{11}C]McN-5652 selectively labels the 5-HT transporter, which is a structural component of 5-HT neurons in the human brain. This radioligand was used in PET imaging for all subjects, then 5-HT transporter binding was compared between the 2 groups.

Findings.—Compared with the control subjects, the patients had significantly lower global and regional distribution volumes for [^{11}C]McN-5652 binding (Fig 3), suggesting that fewer 5-HT transporter sites were present.

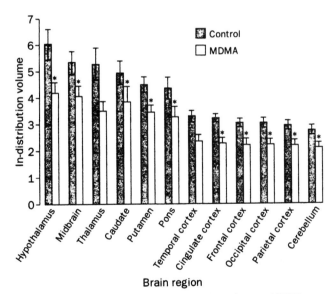

FIGURE 3.—Differences in regional brain distribution volumes between MDMA users and control subjects. Data are mean (SE). *Asterisk* indicates $P < .05$. (Courtesy of McCann UD, Szabo Z, Scheffel U, et al: Positron emission tomographic evidence of toxic effect of MDMA ["Ecstasy"] on brain serotonin neurons in human beings. *Lancet* 352[9138]:1433-1437. Copyright 1998 by The Lancet Ltd.)

Furthermore, there was a significant correlation between greater previous MDMA use and greater loss of 5-HT transporter sites.

Conclusion.—Patients who used MDMA had global and regional dose-related reductions in 5-HT transporter sites in the brain. These changes in brain 5-HT were present in some patients even after they had stopped using MDMA for several years. Thus, the recreational use of MDMA puts the user at risk of development of 5-HT neural injury in the brain.

▶ Finally, we have hard evidence that a recreational drug, in this case "Ecstacy," produces readily documentable structural and functional brain abnormalities, abnormalities that are likely to be permanent. These findings confirm earlier animal studies in which MDMA had been given to primates. The studies showed that the doses of MDMA that produce neurotoxic brain injury in nonhuman primates overlap with the doses currently used recreationally by some of us humans.

Recall the ad of the early 90s showing an egg frying in a pan with an actor suggesting an analogy to ones brain on drugs. Now, with PET scanning, we know that that is exactly what happens, at least when it comes to MDMA. Is a moment of MDMA worth a lifetime of disability? It would have to be an awfully good "high" for one to want to take such a risk. The "down" after such a high is a long, long spiral of brain rot.

Lastly, on the subject of illicit drugs, see if you can figure out what is going on here: A teenager on a flight from South America becomes ill. During the flight he did not take any food or drink. On arrival at the airport in Miami, he is unable to stand. He is perspiring and complains of abdominal pain. He is agitated and hallucinating. He has no psychiatric history. When seen in the emergency room, he has dilated pupils, and a plain film of the abdomen shows numerous spherical packages. It seems obvious that he was a "body packer." In fact, he fesses up to having ingested 102 latex condom packages, each containing 5 g of cocaine. This patient's urine is strongly positive for cocaine with a concentration more than 3 mg/L. However, because he is clinically stable, a decision is made to treat him with diazepam and to follow him clinically. He is also given lactulose and liquid paraffin as a laxative. After a period of initial stability, his condition quickly deteriorates. Death results from cardiac arrhythmias. An autopsy shows his gastrointestinal tract to be filled with cocaine packages, more than half of which have ruptured. The question is, what was done wrong as part of this patient's care?

"Body packing" refers to the swallowing of narcotics, usually wrapped within latex condoms. The purpose is obvious: to transport them illegally. Once transported, the condoms are recovered from the stool and the narcotics retrieved. The management of patients with ruptured packages is tricky. Narcan (Du Pont Merck) can hardly keep up with the load of narcotic. If a patient is asymptomatic or otherwise clinically stable, it is usually best to allow the packages to be passed naturally, although some encourage passage with the use of various agents to "move things along." Sorbitol or lactulose with activated charcoal are the preferred agents. Surgery should be considered if there are symptoms of intoxication of a serious nature. In the patient described above, the mistake was treating the patient with liquid paraffin in mineral oil. Older handbooks on clinical toxicology suggest the use of paraffin as a purgative. The rub is that, with the associated mineral oil, latex dissolves. Exposure of latex to mineral oil causes a decrease in the strength and flexibility of latex within a period of just 15 minutes.[1] It is suspected in the case described above that so many latex packages ruptured because of the administration of the paraffin/mineral oil mixture.[2] Body packers are well aware of the risks of their illegal activities. Since a single package generally contains more than 3 g of cocaine, rupture of just 1 package is potentially fatal.

J.A. Stockman III, M.D.

References

1. White N, Taylor K, Lyszkowski A, et al: Dangers of lubricants used with condoms. *Nature* 335:19, 1988.
2. Visser L, Stricker B, Hoogendoorn M, et al: Do not give paraffin to packers. *Lancet* 352:1352, 1998.

Cost-effectiveness Analysis of Lead Poisoning Screening Strategies Following the 1997 Guidelines of the Centers for Disease Control and Prevention

Kemper AR, Bordley WC, Downs SM (Univ of North Carolina, Chapel Hill)
Arch Pediatr Adolesc Med 152:1202-1208, 1998   9–4

Background.—Mean blood lead (BPb) levels in US preschoolers have decreased dramatically since the mid-1970s, from 0.72 μmol/L between 1976 and 1980 to 0.13 μmol/L between 1990 and 1994. Given these declining levels, the Centers for Disease Control and Prevention (CDC) has recommended that each state develop its own plan for screening children less than 2 years old on the basis of local lead exposure conditions. This study estimated and compared the cost-effectiveness of 4 different screening strategies for identifying 1-year-old children with lead poisoning.

Methods.—The CDC recommends that venous lead levels should be checked in children with a BPb level of 0.48 μmol/L or more. Thus, a decision tree model was constructed to evaluate the accuracies and costs of 4 screening strategies to detect a BPb level of 0.48 μmol/L or more: universal screening of (1) venous or (2) capillary BPb levels and targeted screening of (3) venous or (4) capillary BPb levels in children at risk. Three hypothetical cohorts of 100,000 1-year-old U.S. children were created to analyze communities with a high, moderate, or low prevalence of lead poisoning. The models included the costs of screening, evaluation, treatment, and follow-up testing and treatment but not indirect costs (e.g., lost parental wages, transportation costs, etc.).

Findings.—The only strategy that detected all BPb levels of 0.48 μmol/L or more in all 3 cohorts was universal venous screening. Universal capillary screening was the next most effective strategy, detecting between 93.2% and 95.5% of the cases. Targeted venous testing identified between

77.3% and 77.9% of the cases, and targeted capillary testing identified between 72.7% and 72.8% of the cases. In the cohort with a high prevalence of lead poisoning, universal venous testing minimized the cost per case ($490). In the cohorts with a low or moderate prevalence of lead poisoning, targeted venous testing minimized the costs per case ($729 and $556). In all 3 cohorts, regardless of whether universal or targeted screening was used, costs per case were lower with venous testing than with capillary testing.

Conclusions.—In communities with a high prevalence of lead poisoning, universal venous screening is clearly the most accurate and least expensive means of identifying children with elevated BPb levels. In communities in which the prevalence of lead poisoning is low or moderate, however, the added accuracy of universal venous screening (100%) must be considered in light of its increased costs ($800 in low-prevalence areas, $579 in moderate-prevalence areas). Whichever testing strategy is chosen—universal or targeted—venous testing is more accurate and less expensive than capillary testing.

▶ In the early part of the last decade, both the CDC and the American Academy of Pediatrics had in place recommendations for universal screening of all children for lead poisoning. At the time, data suggested that the average BPb level of the American child was hovering at about 15 µg/dL. It had also been shown that neurocognitive deficits began to be measurable at BPb leads that were in excess of 10 µg/dL. For this reason, it seemed wise to make sure that every American child had a "safe" BPb level. Within a very short period of time, however, BPb levels began to fall, in part as a consequence of the elimination of leaded automobile fuels here in the United States. Now, the average BPb level in the United States is under 3 µg/dL. Because of this decline, screening recommendations were changed in the mid-1990s. The current recommendation is to screen only those children who are identified as being at increased risk of lead poisoning. Such children include those who live in aging housing, those who have a sibling with lead poisoning, and those who have a friend with lead poisoning. Also, the CDC recommends universal screening in areas where the prevalence of elevated BPb levels greater than 10 µg/dL is at least 12%.

What we learn from this report is that when lead screening is indicated, it will detect all cases of lead poisoning and is a cost-effective strategy in high-prevalence populations. Also, it is cheaper to do this by obtaining a venous blood sample than by obtaining blood by a capillary technique. With the capillary technique, even minor contamination of the skin will cause erroneously high values. Such falsely high values are expensive in terms of both dollars and time.

Lastly, as good a job as we are doing here in the United States at reducing blood-lead levels, terrible problems still exist elsewhere. India is a good example of a country where much work remains to be done. A study done in 6 Indian cities indicates that more than 50% of children younger than 12 years old have blood-lead concentrations higher than the recommended maximum, 10 µg/dL. More than 12% of the children tested had concentrations of 20 μg/dL or more. Urban children were found to have higher blood-lead levels than rural children, possibly as a result of automobile pollution. In India, lead-free gasoline is mandatory only in Delhi, where ambient air lead concentrations have fallen by 70% since the use of lead-free gasoline was enforced.[1]

For more on the topic of lead poisoning, see the article that follows, which deals with the declining blood levels found during childhood these days and the impact of BPb on cognitive function.

J.A. Stockman III, M.D.

Reference

1. Sharma AM: Alarming amounts of lead found in Indian children. *Lancet* 353:647, 1999.

Declining Blood Lead Levels and Changes in Cognitive Function During Childhood: The Port Pirie Cohort Study
Tong S, Baghurst PA, Sawyer MG, et al (Queensland Univ, Brisbane Australia; Adelaide Women's and Children's Hosp, Australia; Royal Children's Hosp, Melbourne, Australia; et al)
JAMA 280:1915-1919, 1998   9–5

Background.—Most studies have found a significant relationship between increased exposure to environmental lead at an early age and decreased cognitive performance. The purpose of this study was to determine whether cognitive performance improves when the lead exposure is reduced.

Methods.—The subjects were 375 children living near a large lead smelter, who were followed up from birth to age 11 to 13 years. Blood lead concentrations were measured at 2 years and at 11 to 13 years. Cognitive performance was assessed at 2 years (by means of the Bayley Mental Development Index), 4 years (by means of the McCarthy General Cognitive Index), and at 7 and 11 to 13 years (by means of the Wechsler Intelligence Scale).

Findings.—Mean blood lead concentrations decreased from 1.02 μmol/L at age 2 years to 0.38 μmol/L at age 11 to 13 years. At all ages, children with the highest blood lead (BPb) concentrations had lower cognitive scores. To determine whether the effect of an elevated BPb concentration is transient, the cognitive performances of the children with the greatest versus the least decreases in BPb concentrations were compared. Cognitive performance in both groups was statistically the same.

Conclusions.—A decline in BPb concentrations between ages 2 and 11 to 13 years was not associated with an improvement in cognitive performance at ages 11 to 13 years. Thus, the neurocognitive effects of increased lead exposure at an early age appear to be persistent.

▶ These data tell us two things. They tell us that BPb levels have declined, and they tell us that the natural decline in BPb levels within a given child does not necessarily correlate with a change for the better in IQ. In this Port Pirie series, without anything being done, a BPb level at age 2 averaging 21 μg/dL will be expected to decline to less than 8 μg/dL within 10 years. Unfortunately, IQ does not go up as blood lead levels go down.

If you have some curiosity about where Port Pirie is and why it is important when it comes to lead, Port Pirie is in South Australia. It is the site of one of the largest lead smelting facilities in the Southern Hemisphere. Starting in the late 1970s, children in the Port Pirie area came under very close observation to be certain that they did not have lead poisoning. At the time, many children had BPb levels that were considered "safe," levels that we now know can cause cognitive deficits. Thus, these children were followed up without intervention. Fortunately, their IQ was measured along with other developmental assessments. The Port Pirie area has provided us with data showing that even minor elevations of lead can cause cognitive impairments, impairments that do not disappear when BPb levels fall on their own.

If you think severe lead poisoning from extraordinarily high BPb concentrations is no longer seen in children, you are wrong. Just recently, the case of a 3-year-old child with a BPb concentration of 550 μg/dL was reported. The youngster lived in Chicago, in older housing that had peeling paint. The child also had pica. At the time of this high BPb level, the child had a Glasgow coma score of 8. With intensive chelation, the BPb level was reduced over a period of 5 days to between 50 and 60 μg/dL. She responded extremely well, although there was no assessment of neurocognitive functioning.[1]

Sometimes when dealing with lead poisoning cases, you might have to be a detective. Try out the following scenario to test your snooping skills. You practice in an impoverished, older section of a city. For that reason, you do routine blood-lead screening on most of your patients at appropriate ages. An 8-year-old boy is found to have a blood-lead of 53 μg/dL. As part of this youngster's management, you do a careful history. It turns out that he lives in subsidized housing, but his home is almost brand new. Neither he nor anyone else in his family has any unusual hobbies. The father is a carpenter. He spends a lot of time with his son fishing. What should you "fish around" for as additional possible sources of lead in this boy?

If you have one question to ask, ask whether the boy uses his teeth, rather than plyers, to clamp down on his fishing sinkers when baiting his lines. The case described is a real one. When the patient was evaluated, a plain film of the abdomen showed multiple small lead sinkers which the child had swallowed accidentally while preparing his fishing lines. The plain films estimated that there were 20 to 25 sinkers scattered throughout his gastrointestinal tract. The treatment of this child was quite complicated. A nasogastric tube was placed and many volumes of polyethylene glycol solution were given to irrigate the gastrointestinal tract. This worked for most of the sinkers, but 7 remained. Colonoscopy took care of 4, but 3 small sinkers were beyond the reach of the endoscope. Oral chelation was begun, and after several additional days, the final sinkers were passed.

The lesson to all this is pretty straightforward. If you're "hooked" on fishing and like to bring young children with you, it would be wise to do the equivalent of a sponge count (i.e., a sinker count) with each cast. By the way, this was the first reported case of lead poisoning resulting from ingested fishing sinkers.[2]

J.A. Stockman III, M.D.

References

1. Gordon RA, Roberts G, Amin Z, et al: Aggressive approach in the treatment of acute lead encephalopathy with an extraordinarily high concentration of lead. *Arch Pediatr Adolesc Med* 152:1100, 1998.
2. Mowad E, Haddad I, Gemmal DJ: Management of lead poisoning from ingested fishing sinkers. *Arch Pediatr Adolesc Med* 152:485-488, 1998.

Treating the Snakebitten Child in North America: A Study of Pit Viper Bites
Lopoo JB, Bealer JF, Mantor PC, et al (Univ of Oklahoma, Oklahoma City)
J Pediatr Surg 33:1593-1595, 1998   9–6

Introduction.—About 90% of the 8000 venomous snakebites that occur each year are from the Crotalidae (or pit viper) family of snakes, which consists of copperheads, rattlesnakes, and cottonmouths. There is still debate over the proper medical management of venomous snakebites, particularly in children, with some recommending that all snakebitten children be admitted for care. The history of children seen after venomous snakebites was analyzed to evaluate the efficacy, morbidity, and cost-effectiveness of standard treatment.

Methods.—The records of 37 snakebitten children seen in a 10-year period were analyzed for demographic data, signs of envenomation, use of specific therapies (antivenin, blood products, or surgery), complications, length of hospitalization, and cost of care.

Results.—A major envenomation was found in 54% of the children, which was demonstrated by systemic symptomatology, laboratory analysis, or need for surgery. Full recoveries occurred in all children, with 92% receiving only supportive care. Eight hours was the average time before they were seen at an emergency department, where all children with major envenomation and those requiring specific therapies, such as clotting factors or surgery, were identified. The identified treatment algorithm includes observing the child for escalating signs of toxicity, with supportive care such as wound care, tetanus prophylaxis, and intravenous hydration. If severe local envenomation, such as coagulopathy, intractable nausea or vomiting, or parasthesia, decreased capillary refill, pain to passive motion, or decreased pulses, is identified, the patient should be admitted to the

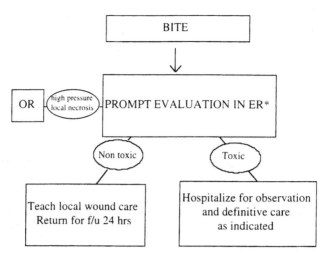

FIGURE 3.—Pit viper bite treatment algorithm. *Emergency room evaluation includes chemistry, coagulation panel, and compartment pressures if indicated. (Courtesy of Lopoo JB, Bealer JF, Mantor PC, et al: Treating the snakebitten child in North America: A study of pit viper bites. *J Pediatr Surg* 33:1593-1595, 1998.)

hospital (Fig 3). An average of $2450 was spent for care of each child, with most of the cost being attributed to the length of hospitalization.

Conclusion.—If no signs of major envenomation are noted within 8 hours of the bite, most snakebitten children can be cared for safely and cost-effectively as outpatients. Most children completely recover with minimal supportive care.

▶ Hospital administrators are going to like this article, particularly in this era of managed care. What is described is the minimalist approach to the care and management of snakebites in children. We see in this series that the majority of snake bites are caused by copperheads, with rattlesnake bites contributing a minor role. We learn that signs and symptoms of envenomation, if they are going to present, present within the first 6 to 8 hours. This means that the emergency room is the appropriate setting to observe children with snakebites. Hospitalization is necessary only if signs of systemic or severe local envenomation are identified. These signs and symptoms include coagulopathy, intractable nausea/vomiting, or a compartment syndrome. Patients with these findings, although requiring admission, may not need antivenin. In fact, the authors strongly argue against antivenin therapy, except in the most severe cases. The reason for this nihilist approach is because of the extraordinarily high frequency of allergic reactions to antivenin, which sometimes further complicate the clinical status of a patient. If you can avoid hospitalization, the cost of managing a patient with a snakebite should run no more than a few hundred dollars. If the patient is put into the hospital, even if it's for overnight, multiple 4-digit costs will be incurred.

Snakes and spiders are God's revenge on man. Few things are more disgusting or are more capable of inducing tachycardia.

J.A. Stockman III, M.D.

Use of Misoprostol During Pregnancy and Möbius' Syndrome in Infants
Pastuszak AL, Schüler L, Speck-Martins CE, et al (Univ of Toronto; Universidade Federal do Rio Grande do Sul, Porto Alegre, Brazil; Unidade de Genetica, Brazil; et al)
N Engl J Med 338:1881-1885, 1998   9–7

Introduction.—Used to prevent and treat gastrointestinal lesions induced by nonsteroidal anti-inflammatory drugs and upper gastrointestinal ulceration, misoprostol is a synthetic prostaglandin E_1 analogue. When used during pregnancy, it may cause vaginal bleeding, stimulate uterine contractions, and endanger fetal survival. In the elective induction of abortion, misoprostol has been combined with mifepristone. Up to 75% of women who attempt abortion in Brazil use misoprostol because elective abortions are prohibited and the drug can be obtained over the counter. Unfortunately, up to 80% of women who use this drug as an abortifacient continue their pregnancies to term. Möbius' syndrome (congenital facial paralysis with or without limb defects) has been reported in infants whose mothers took misoprostol. The frequency of misoprostol use during the first trimester of pregnancy was compared in mothers of infants with Möbius' syndrome and those of infants with neural-tube defects.

Methods.—There were 96 infants with Möbius' syndrome and 96 infants with neural-tube defects. Möbius' syndrome was first diagnosed in the infants at a mean age of 16 months, and neural-tube defects were

TABLE 2.—Clinical Manifestations in Infants With Möbius' Syndrome Who Were Exposed to Misoprostol and Those Who Were Not Exposed

Manifestation	Exposed (N=47)	Not Exposed (N=49)	P Value
	No. (%)		
Bilateral facial-nerve (cranial nerve VII) paralysis	34 (72)	36 (73)	0.92
Abducens-nerve (cranial nerve VI) paralysis	39 (83)	37 (76)	0.52
Other cranial-nerve palsy	10 (21)	8 (16)	0.72
Limb defects			
All types combined	31 (66)	28 (57)	0.50
Club feet only	25 (53)	18 (37)	0.21
Limb reduction*	6 (13)	10 (20)	0.64
Orofacial anomalies	18 (38)	11 (22)	0.16
Mental retardation	26 (55)	26 (53)	0.99
Other defects	15 (32)	14 (29)	0.89

*Limb reduction was present with or without other manifestations.
(Reprinted by permission, from Pastuszak AL, Schüler L, Speck-Martins CE, et al: Use of misoprostol during pregnancy and Möbius syndrome in infants. *N Engl J Med* 338:1881-1885. Copyright 1998, Massachusetts Medical Society. All rights reserved.)

diagnosed within 1 week of birth. The frequency of misoprostol use by mothers of these infants during the first trimester was noted.

Results.—It was found that 49% of the mothers of infants with Möbius' syndrome used misoprostol in the first trimester of pregnancy, whereas 3% of the mothers of infants with neural-tube defects used misoprostol in the first trimester of pregnancy. Clinical manifestations of Möbius' syndrome were bilateral facial nerve paralysis, abducens nerve paralysis, other cranial nerve palsy, limb defects, orofacial anomalies, mental retardation, and other defects (Table 2). Of the mothers with infants who had Möbius' syndrome and who took misoprostol, 20 took the drug orally, 20 took it both orally and vaginally, 3 took it vaginally, and 4 did not report how they took it.

Conclusion.—An increased risk of Möbius' syndrome in infants is associated with attempted abortion with misoprostol.

▶ The possibility of a relationship between misoprostol use during pregnancy and Möbius' syndrome in babies may seem so far off the wall to you that you wonder how such a putative relationship ever made it into *The New England Journal of Medicine.* If you think for a few minutes, however, about what might be going on, all of this makes some sense, but a little background is in order.

Misoprostol has been around for some time. It is generally used to prevent and treat the type of gastrointestinal ulcerations and gastritis caused by nonsteroidal inflammatory drugs. It is contraindicated in pregnancy because it is well known to stimulate uterine contractions and bleeding, endangering fetal survival. The combination of misoprostol and mifepristone or methotrexate has been used for some time for the elective induction of abortion. In some areas of the world, including Brazil (the country of origin of this report), where elective abortions are prohibited, as many as 75% of women who attempt an abortion use misoprostol. This drug can be obtained over the counter without a prescription. The rub, however, is that in 4 out of 5 women who attempt such an abortion the pregnancies will continue. Thus, if there is any teratogenic consequence of misoprostol use, that consequence will soon become obvious.

So what is the possible relationship with Möbius' syndrome? Recall that Möbius' syndrome is a bilateral or unilateral facial-nerve paralysis. Babies with Möbius' syndrome have the typical "expressionless face." This is a potentially lifelong problem. It is, indeed, biologically plausible that exposure to misoprostol might cause Möbius' syndrome. The syndrome may be due to vascular disruption of the subclavian artery during the fourth to sixth weeks of embryonic development. Environmental insults, including failed abortion, prolonged rupture of membranes, and chorionic villus sampling, have been implicated in its pathogenesis. Misoprostol exposure during the first 2 months of pregnancy could cause an ischemic event in the embryonic brain stem that might result in Möbius' syndrome. As an example of this possible pathophysiology, two cases of maternal antenatal splenic rupture resulting in hypotension have been reported after the birth of an infant with Möbius' syndrome. In these cases, the mothers were 18 and 14 weeks pregnant at the time of the accident. Both infants had hypoxic-ischemic brain stem damage. Thus, the relationship between early intrauterine events, including those that decrease blood flow to a baby's brain, and Möbius' syndrome, makes sense.

There is no way of telling what proportion of babies with Möbius' syndrome in this country may have the disorder as a consequence of maternal use of the teratogenic agent, misoprostol. In Brazil, in one half of affected babies the syndrome seems to be the result of misoprostol administration during pregnancy. In any event, should you see a baby with Möbius' syndrome, at least think of the possibility of such a relationship. A star for your forehead if the connection is found.

J.A. Stockman III, M.D.

Effects of Prenatal and Postnatal Methylmercury Exposure From Fish Consumption on Neurodevelopment: Outcomes at 66 Months of Age in the Seychelles Child Development Study
Davidson PW, Myers GJ, Cox C, et al (Univ of Rochester, NY; Republic of Seychelles Ministry of Health, Victoria, Mahé; Ctrs for Disease Control and Prevention, Atlanta, Ga; et al)
JAMA 280:701-707, 1998   9–8

Background.—All fish contain various levels of methylmercury. Studies suggest that methylmercury levels as low as 10 ppm can cause neurologic toxicity in humans. However, studies have also found that methylmercury poisoning is rare in populations that depend on fish as a major part of the diet. This study assessed the methylmercury levels and neurological development of children from Seychelles, where 85% of the population eats fish every day.

Methods.—Seven hundred eleven mother-child pairs from the Republic of Seychelles, an archipelago in the middle of the Indian Ocean, were studied. At enrollment, the mothers ate an average of 12 fish meals per week. To determine prenatal methylmercury exposure, the total mercury concentration was measured in a segment of maternal hair representing growth during pregnancy; this measure correlates well with fetal methylmercury blood levels. To determine postnatal methylmercury exposure, the total mercury concentration was measured from a hair close to the scalp of the child at 66 months of age. Total mercury concentrations were also analyzed in the fish typically consumed. At age 66 months, the children underwent a test battery to measure 6 primary skills: cognitive ability, expressive and receptive language ability, reading ability, arithmetic ability, visual-spatial ability, and social and adaptive behavior.

Findings.—Median total mercury levels in the fish ranged from 0.004 to 0.75 ppm, with most medians ≤ 0.025 ppm. Mean prenatal total mercury levels in the mother's hair during pregnancy were 6.8 ± 4.5 ppm, and mean postnatal total mercury levels in the child's hair at 66 months were 6.5 ± 3.3 ppm. There was no significant association between maternal total mercury levels and those in the children. The children's performance on the neurodevelopmental test battery showed no damaging effect of either prenatal or postnatal methylmercury exposure. In fact, their test results were comparable to those expected of healthy U.S. children. Furthermore, test scores did not differ significantly between children with high (>12 ppm) and low (≤3 ppm) levels of methylmercury exposure.

Conclusions.—For these Seychellois children, eating a diet dependent largely on ocean fish had no deleterious effect on neurodevelopment through 66 months of age. The methylmercury levels in the fish that these children eat were similar to levels found in fish eaten in the United States. The authors conclude that the risk of methylmercury poisoning at the levels of fish consumption found in the United States is small, and does not offset the health benefits of eating fish.

▶ There are lots of ways to be exposed to mercury these days. For example, take the situation of those who work around crematoria. Hair samples from groundskeepers of crematoria show a 50% higher mercury level than one might expect, based on occupations that have no known exposures to mercury. Those who actually work inside crematoria (administrators and cremation operatives), have approximately twice the hair mercury content of control subjects. What is happening is fairly obvious. Dental amalgam consists of 50% metallic mercury. Those dealing with amalgam, such as dentists, have a small but real potential for exposure to mercury. The risk is somewhat higher, however, in occupations in which amalgam is incinerated. The mercury either remains in the ashes of a deceased person after cremation, or more likely, it enters the environment via the smoke output of a crematorium. In countries such as Great Britain, where about 70% of all corpses are cremated, the average crematorium emits between 5 and 6 kg of mercury per year. The health implications of such mercury exposure have not been carefully documented. Some countries, such as Sweden, have recognized this as a potential problem for crematorium workers and require the installation of selenium filters in crematoria. Such filters remove 80% to 85% of mercury from the emissions of crematoria.[1]

Did you also know that *all* fish contain methylmercury? Did you know that frequent consumption of ocean fish can lead to methylmercury hair levels in excess of 10 ppm and as high as 50 ppm? We're not talking about fish from Lake Michigan here. We're talking about Charley the Tuna from the North Atlantic. The results of this report, however, suggest that eating a lot of fish does not impair the intellectual development of children, at least if you live on the archipelago of the Republic of Seychelles in the Indian Ocean where virtually everyone consumes a fish or more a day that contains an average 0.5 to 0.25 ppm of methylmercury.

So, can you have your fish and eat it too? The answer is yes and no. Eating a lot of fish is probably okay if you are Seychellois. There is a very real possibility that the Seychellois population is in some way buffered against the adverse consequences of in utero exposure to low levels of mercury, perhaps because of some other protective effect of a high level of fish consumption. Eat enough fish and you may be taking the antidote, as it were, for the retardation problem associated with methylmercury. The U.S. situation is very different. Most people don't eat an enormous amount of fish, but they might eat fish that contains significantly more mercury. On average, the species of fish consumed in the United States have mercury concentrations of about 0.13 ppm. Some local freshwater sources of fish in the United States have much higher mercury concentrations. Forty-one states issue fishing advisories based on mercury contamination, and 11 states advise specific limitations on fish consumption from all water bodies within those state limits. Data gathered from the mid-1990s from the northeast states show that average mercury concentrations were more than 0.5 ppm in 20% to 100% of samples and more than 1 ppm in 2% to 25% of samples.[2] In Wisconsin, the mercury concentration of walleye (the most commonly sought after game fish) averages 0.5 ppm with some individual fish values greater than 3 ppm.

It would appear that the gills of Wally the walleye are a wonderful device for sucking in and concentrating methylmercury from lakes, ponds, and streams. Given the child development health consequences of methylmercury and polychlorinated biphenyls (PCBs), also found in fish, you wonder whether fish can any longer be considered "brain food." Finally, on the other hand, if you're fishing off Navy Pier in Chicago for your daily sustenance, think twice, if your mind is still functioning. The rub from methylmercury and PCBs is not significant if you are talking about ocean fish.

This is the final entry in the Therapeutics and Toxicology chapter, so we will close with an interesting poisoning case: A 48-year-old chemistry professor is admitted to Dartmouth-Hitchcock Medical Center with a 5-day history of progressive deterioration in balance, gait, and speech. She has lost 15 lbs over 2 months and has experienced brief episodes of nausea, diarrhea, and abdominal discomfort. On physical examination, the patient is thin but otherwise appears healthy. The examination shows moderate, upper-extremity dysmetria, dystaxic handwriting, a widely based gait, and mild "scanning speech." Routine laboratory test results are normal. A CT and MRI of the head have normal results. CSF findings are also unremarkable. Over the ensuing days, a tingling in the fingers is noted, along with brief flashes of light in both eyes. Neuropsychiatric testing reveals marked deficits in all areas. There is papilledema. The patient's neurologic status continues to deteriorate, and the patient dies. The only significant history is that approximately 10 months before her death, the patient was known to have spilled several drops of liquid from the tip of a pipette onto the dorsum of her gloved hand while transferring a substance from a container to a capillary tube. Name the substance.

This saga of a chemistry professor is a true one. The patient was sufficiently lucid enough at the time of admission to recall that she had spilled several drops of dimethylmercury onto a gloved hand while transferring a small amount of the liquid in a laboratory. She cleaned up the spill first and then removed her protective gloves. It was not evident that the methylmercury had eroded the gloves or had in any way penetrated them. What this chemist failed to recognize was that dimethylmercury is so dangerous that even a misuscule amount can quickly permeate common latex gloves and form a toxic vapor after a spill. This was first noted a long time ago. When dimethylmercury was initially synthesized, the two laboratory assistants who helped in its preparation died. That was in 1865. Nearly 100 years later, another laboratory worker died after synthesizing the compound for an experiment. He had a rapid downhill course very similar to that of the patient at Dartmouth.

Just to show you how toxic dimethylmercury is, the Dartmouth professor had a blood concentration of mercury equal to 4000 µg/L, which represents about 16.8 m of mercury in the blood. Only 5% of methylmercury remains in blood, thus her total body mercury content was 336 m. Since dimethylmercury has a density of 3.2 g/mL, this amount of mercury was contained in only 0.11 mL of liquid dimethylmercury. Routine laboratory gloves are easily penetrated by dimethylmercury within 15 seconds.

To read more about this case, see the report of Nierenberg.[3] The patient in question was well for almost half a year following her exposure to what ultimately turned out to be a lethal dose of dimethylmercury. Despite aggressive chelation therapy and other supportive therapies she died, as has happened with patients similarly exposed to this extraordinarily toxic substance.

J.A. Stockman III, M.D.

References

1. Maloney SR, Phillips EA, Mills A: Mercury in the hair of crematoria workers. *Lancet* 352:1602, 1998.
2. Northeast States for Coordinated Air Use Management: Mercury and northeastern freshwater fish: Current levels and ecological impact, in *Mercury: A Framework for Action.* New York, Natural Resources Defense Council, 1998.
3. Nierenberg GW, Nordgren RE, Chang MB, et al: Delayed cerebellar disease and death after accidental exposure to dimethylmercury. *N Engl J Med* 338:1672-1676, 1998.

10 The Genitourinary Tract

Current Findings in Diagnostic Laparoscopic Evaluation of the Nonpalpable Testis
Cisek LJ, Peters CA, Atala A, et al (Harvard Med School, Boston)
J Urol 160:1145-1149, 1998   10–1

Background.—Although laparoscopy is widely used to localize the nonpalpable testis, critics note that as many as 60% of these patients have inguinal testes or remnants, and thus inguinal exploration alone is all the patient would have required. These authors review the literature and report their experience with the use of diagnostic laparoscopy.

Methods.—During a 4-year period, the authors found 263 nonpalpable testes in 225 patients who were scheduled for diagnostic laparoscopy. Patients ranged from 1-month- to 21-years-old (median age, 14.5 months), and 15 were older than 10-years-old. Operative reports were examined to determine the findings with the patient under anesthesia and at laparoscopy, the surgical approach used, the position and size of the testes, and the character of the vas deferens and spermatic vessels. Furthermore, a search of the OVID citation database during the same period identified 24 articles reporting sufficient positional classification data about 1311 testes.

Findings.—Of the 263 nonpalpable testes found by the authors, 46 testes (18%) in 40 patients were palpable when the patient received anesthesia before laparoscopy. These patients' testes were considered missed during the office exam, which did not undergo laparoscopy and were not included in analysis. Another 2 patients were excluded because of incomplete examination information. Thus statistical analyses are based on 215 testes in 183 patients, of which 61% were viable. A nonpalpable testis on the right side was significantly more likely to be viable than a testis on the left (69% vs 54% viable). No testis distal to the internal ring with an atretic vas and atretic vessels was viable, whereas 45% of those with a normal appearing vas and vessels were viable. The testes were precanalicular in 48.8% of cases, distal in 40%, and transinguinal in 11.2%. Inguinal exploration alone could have identified 45.7% of the testes, and in 34% of these cases, laparoscopy provided little additional information over that obtainable by inguinal exploration alone. Nonethe-

TABLE 3.—Localization of Testes During Laparoscopy in
Current Literature and in Our Series

	No. Literature (%)[1-3, 6-26]		No. Present Series (%)	
Precanalicular:				
Intra-abdominal	486	(37)	84	(39)
Intra-abdominal vanishing	213	(16)	21	(10)
Transinguinal	14	(1)	24	(11)
Distal:				
Inguinal	188	(14)	26	(12)
Inguinal remnant	381	(29)	53	(25)
Other	8	(1)	7	(1)
Nondiagnostic	21	(2)		
Totals	1,311	(100)	215	(100)

(Courtesy of Cisek LJ, Peters CA, Atala A, et al: Current findings in diagnostic laparoscopic evaluation of the nonpalpable testis. *J Urol* 160[3]:1145-1149, 1998.)

less, laparoscopy found a viable testis distal to the inguinal ring in 12.6% of the testes, which were considered missed on examination. Laparoscopy also found precanicular vanishing testes in 9.8% of cases. Overall, laparoscopic findings were able to avoid unnecessary abdominal surgery in 13.2% of the cases. Furthermore, without information provided by laparoscopy, the conventional surgical incision to explore the inguinal region would have been less than optimal in two thirds of cases. The authors' findings were similar to those in the literature (Table 3).

Conclusions.—Palpating the testis with the patient under anesthesia avoided unnecessary laparoscopy for 40 patients (46 testes). Thus taking this extra step before laparoscopy is well worth the time. In addition, laparoscopy avoided unnecessary surgery in 13.2% of the cases. However, about one third of patients did not benefit from laparoscopy over inguinal exploration alone.

▶ Another report showing how boys can be so troublesome. In this case, it's the boy with the non-detectable testis. Is it there, or isn't it there? Is it a vanishing testis? Is it a yo-yo testis? Is it simply residing in the inguinal canal? A number of techniques have been suggested to avoid the necessity of a laparoscopic evaluation when there is a possibility of a viable testis sitting distal to the inguinal ring not detected on physical examination. The use of human chorionic gonadotropin stimulation, inguinal ultrasound and computerized tomography have been advocated for this purpose. Such approaches have decreased the number of viable testes found in the inguinal area at the time of inguinal surgical exploration or laparoscopy to approximately 10% to 15% of nonpalpable testes cases. When a careful examination using anesthesia is performed before committing to laparoscopy, you can further reduce the number of nonpalpable testes that are actually in the inguinal canal by about 20%. Unfortunately, these studies do not diagnose vanishing testes, frequently do not localize intra-abdominal testes, and seldom provide localization of atrophic testes.

Laparoscopy allows the definitive diagnosis of the intra-abdominal vanishing testis, and it is informative regarding testis location in virtually all cases. It contributes to the management of nonpalpable testis in 2 ways. It identifies intra-abdominal vanishing testis, replacing extensive open intra-abdominal exploration with a brief, minimally morbid diagnostic procedure. Furthermore, abdominal exploration would have been required to confirm an absent testis in about 3% of the cases in the series reported. Thus, laparoscopy seems to remain a valuable diagnostic tool for evaluating the nonpalpable testis. The problem with laparoscopy in children seems to be the learning curve required on the part of the urologist. It is a complex skill that must be mastered to be comfortable with the "ins and outs" of the gonads of little boys.

J.A. Stockman III, M.D.

Epididymitis in Children: The Circumcision Factor?
Bennett RT, Gill B, Kogan SJ (Duke Univ, Durham, NC; Montefiore Med Ctr, Bronx, NY; Cornell Univ, White Plains, NY)
J Urol 160:1842-1844, 1998   10–2

Objective.—Whereas some studies have found an increased risk of urinary tract infection in uncircumcised boys, no one has evaluated the relationship between epididymitis and circumcision. The circumcision status of 36 consecutive patients younger than 18 years with acute epididymitis was retrospectively reviewed.

Methods.—Between 1987 and 1992, epididymitis was diagnosed in 36 boys, aged 10 weeks to 20 years, out of 128 patients (group 1) with acute scrotal inflammation. In all patients with epididymitis, the involved testis was in the scrotum. The circumcision status was also determined in a group of 43 patients (group 2) treated for epididymitis and discharged. The New York State hospital discharge figures for circumcision in newborns provided group 3, and the circumcision rate in 200 consecutive pediatric emergency room patients was included as group 4.

Results.—The numbers and percentages of circumcised patients in each group were 9 (25%) in group 1, 11 (26%) in group 2, 70% in group 3 (number was not applicable), and 131 (65%) in group 4. Compared with groups 3 and 4, significantly fewer group 1 and 2 patients were circumcised.

Conclusion.—Whereas acute epididymitis is rare in prepubertal boys, a significant number of uncircumcised boys in this study were found to have the infection, suggesting that the presence of a foreskin is a risk factor for epididymitis.

▶ This is an interesting little report. It extends our understanding of what it means to be circumcised or not. It seems fairly clear that there is an increased risk of urinary tract infection in young uncircumcised boys; that much we now know to be true.[1] These authors have extended circumcision status to an increased risk of epididymitis.

Epididymitis in childhood is not a frequent problem; nor is it readily diagnosed unless one thinks of it first. The most common clinical presentations of acute epididymitis are pain, swelling, and redness of the skin of the scrotum. The majority of times, an enlarged tender epididymis can be felt, separate from a normal-appearing testis. In young boys, however, the testis and the epididymis are usually indistinguishable and form a large, tender swollen mass, making the diagnosis of epididymitis vs. torsion of the testis somewhat difficult. Fever is not always present. A cremasteric reflex is. If confusion exists between the diagnosis of epididymitis and torsion of the testis, a radionuclide technetium pertechnetate scrotal scan or a Doppler study is obviously in order and usually readily differentiates the two problems.

Acute epididymitis has a biphasic age distribution. It occurs either in infancy or in boys older than 7 years. When it occurs in infants, it is more likely to be associated with underlying anomalies of the genitourinary tract. It can also be a sign at this young age of infection elsewhere associated with a septicemia. It is frequently associated with infection in the urine itself.

This is the first series ever to link circumcision status to the prevalence of epididymitis in children. Given the fact that almost three quarters of the cases of epididymitis are associated with the uncircumcised state (in the population in which 70% are circumcised), there seems to be no doubt that having an intact foreskin is a risk factor for epididymitis.

So what is the punch line here? Is this one more piece of evidence to suggest that all boys should be circumcised? That would be a stretch, since the occurrence of epididymitis during childhood is so low. One would have to do a whole lot of circumcisions just to prevent one case of epididymitis. Nonetheless, it is important to remember this association.

For more on the topic of epididymitis, testicular torsion, and torsion of the testicular appendages, see the article that follows.

J.A. Stockman III, M.D.

Reference

1. Wiswell TE, Hachey WE: Urinary tract infections (UTIs) and the uncircumcised state: A meta-analysis. *Pediatr Res* 31:103A, 1992.

A Retrospective Review of Pediatric Patients With Epididymitis, Testicular Torsion, and Torsion of Testicular Appendages
Kadish HA, Bolte RG (Univ of Utah, Salt Lake City)
Pediatrics 102:73-76, 1998   10–3

Introduction.—Scrotal pain, swelling, or a mass presenting to the emergency department is a potential surgical emergency, although not usually life-threatening. The most common causes of scrotal swelling are epididymitis, testicular torsion, and torsion of appendix testis. Differentiating

TABLE 1.—Historical Features in Pediatric Patients with Epididymitis, Testicular Torsion, and Torsion Appendix Tests

Historical Features	(N) = Number of Patients in Each Group		
	EPD (64)	TT (13)	TAT (13)
Duration of symptoms			
<12 hours*	20 (31%)	9 (69%)	8 (62%)
12-24 hours	14 (22%)	1 (8%)	1 (8%)
24-72 hours	21 (33%)	2 (15%)	4 (31%)
>72 hours	9 (14%)	1 (8%)	0 (0%)
Similar pain in past	13 (20%)	1 (8%)	0 (0%)
Fever	12 (19%)	1 (8%)	1 (8%)
Nausea/vomiting	10 (16%)	4 (31%)	0 (0%)
Dysuria	9 (14%)	0 (0%)	0 (0%)
Sexual activity	2 (3%)	0 (0%)	0 (0%)
History of trauma	14 (22%)	1 (8%)	3 (23%)

*Statistically significant when epididymitis is compared to testicular torsion or torsion appendix testis.
Abbreviations: EPD, epididymitis; *TT,* testicular torsion; *TAT,* torsion appendix testis.
(Reproduced by permission of *Pediatrics,* from Kadish HA, Bolte RG: A retrospective review of pediatric patients with epididymitis, testicular torsion, and torsion of testicular appendages. *Pediatrics* 102:73-76, 1998.)

among these can be difficult. Depending on the disease process, treatment options differ dramatically, ranging from observation to surgery. Historical features, physical examination findings, and testicular color Doppler ultrasound were compared for diagnostic efficacy in pediatric patients with epididymitis, testicular torsion, and torsion of appendix testis.

Methods.—The study included records of 90 boys younger than 18 years diagnosed with epididymitis, testicular torsion, or torsion of appendix testis, which were retrospectively reviewed. Data were analyzed concerning the patient's age, duration of pain, history of similar pain in the

TABLE 2.—Physical Examination Findings in Pediatric Patients with Epididymitis, Testicular Torsion, and Torsion Appendix Testis

Physical Examination	(N) = Number of Patients in Each Group		
	EPD (64)	TT (13)	TAT (13)
Temperature >38.1°C	7 (11%)	1 (8%)	0 (0%)
Normal testicular lie*	64 (100%)	7 (54%)	13 (100%)
Tender epididymis*	62 (97%)	3 (23%)	0 (0%)
Absent cremasteric reflex*†	9 (14%)	13 (100%)	0 (0%)
Tender testicle*†	44 (69%)	13 (100%)	4 (31%)
Scrotal erythema/edema	43 (67%)	5 (38%)	1 (8%)
"Blue dot sign"	0 (0%)	0 (0%)	3 (23%)
Isolated tenderness† (superior pole of testis)	0 (0%)	0 (0%)	13 (100%)

*Statistically significant when epididymitis is compared to testicular torsion.
†Statistically significant when torsion appendix testis is compared to testicular torsion.
Abbreviations: EPD, epididymitis; *TT,* testicular torsion; *TAT,* torsion appendix testis.
(Reproduced by permission of *Pediatrics,* from Kadish HA, Bolte RG: A retrospective review of pediatric patients with epididymitis, testicular torsion, and torsion of testicular appendages. *Pediatrics* 102:73-76, 1998.)

past, history of fever, nausea, vomiting, dysuria, sexual activity, and trauma (Table 1).

Results.—Except for duration of symptoms, historical features did not differ among the 3 groups: 64 with epididymitis, 13 with testicular torsion, and 13 with torsion of appendix testis. Tender testicle and an absent cremasteric reflex were evident in the boys with testicular torsion. Fewer boys with epididymitis had a tender testicle (69%) or an absent cremasteric reflex (14%) when compared with the testicular torsion group (Table 2). A tender epididymitis was seen in 97% of boys with epididymitis, and scrotal erythema/edema was seen in 67% of boys with epididymitis. Tender epididymitis was seen in only 23% of boys with testicular torsion and scrotal erythema/edema was seen in 38% of those with testicular torsion. Decrease or absent blood flow was seen in 8 boys with Doppler utlrasound, 7 of whom were diagnosed with testicular torsion. A salvageable testicle at the time of surgery was found in 10 of 13 boys with testicular torsion.

Conclusion.—To distinguish between epididymitis, testicular torsion, and torsion of appendix testis, the physical examination is helpful. A testicular torsion was more likely among boys with a tender testicle and an absent cremasteric reflex than epididymitis or torsion of appendix testis. The most sensitive physical finding for diagnosing testicular torsion was an absent cremasteric reflex. In the evaluation of the acute scrotum when physical findings are equivocal, color Doppler ultrasound is a useful adjunct.

▶ This article confirms the physical findings from the previous abstract, which attempts to distinguish between epididymitis and testicular torsion. Statistically, a child presenting with an acutely painful scrotum is more likely to have a testicular torsion or a torsion of the appendix testis than he is to have epididymitis. Some things help and some things do not help in sorting out these diagnoses. Historical factors, signs and symptoms, such as fever, nausea, vomiting, dysuria, sexual history, and a history of trauma, are not particularly helpful in differentiating epididymitis, testicular torsion, and torsion appendix testis. On the other hand, some physical examination findings are of significant assistance in the differential diagnosis. Those with testicular torsion are likely to have a tender testis. The testis may not be in its normal position (may be riding high in a torsion). An absent cremasteric reflex strongly favors a torsion. In the article abstracted, all 13 patients with testicular torsion had an absent cremasteric reflex.

This is not the only report to document the value of looking for a cremasteric reflex in the differential diagnosis of acute scrotal swelling. Of 245 boys with a painful swollen scrotum, Rabinowitz found that no patient with a normal cremasteric reflex had a testicular torsion.[1] He concluded that the presence of a cremasteric reflex is the single most valuable clinical finding in ruling out testicular torsion. The findings of the study abstracted strongly support this conclusion. An additionally important finding was that a urinalysis is not helpful since only 15% of patients with epididymitis were found to have an abnormal urinalysis.

So what should you do the next time you see a child who presents with an acutely swollen and tender scrotum? If the physical findings seem clear (for example, an absent cremasteric reflex and an unequivocally tender testis), the gurney should be pushed toward the operating room immediately. If things are less clear, a quick as possible testicular scan or Doppler ultrasound are the diagnostic tools of choice. The Doppler ultrasound, in particular, has an extremely high sensitivity and specificity in separating out the causes of an acute scrotum. It would seem wise to recommend a Doppler ultrasound on all children with an acute scrotum if there is some question about what is going on unless this would result in an inordinate delay.

By the way, do you know the origin of the word "cremaster?" It is from the Greek, *kremasté*, a suspender, from *kremannynai*, to hang. So, fellas, the next time you put your pants on, but can't find your belt, reach for the *kremastés*.

J.A. Stockman III, M.D.

Reference

1. Rabinowitz R: The importance of the cremasteric reflex in acute scrotal swelling in children. *J Urol* 132:89-90, 1984.

Acute Scrotum: An Exceptional Presentation of Acute Nonperforated Appendicitis in Childhood
Méndez R, Tellado M, Montero M, et al (Complejo Hospitalario "Juan Canalejo," La Coruña, Spain)
J Pediatr Surg 33:1435-1436, 1998   10–4

Background.—The vast majority of children who have acute appendicitis have abdominal pain as their main symptom, and genitourinary complaints are unusual. This case report describes a boy with appendicitis whose presenting signs were right hemiscrotal swelling and pain.

Case Report.—Boy, 8 years, brought to the emergency department complaining of right scrotal pain and swelling, diffuse abdominal pain, nausea and vomiting, and low-grade fever of 12 hours' duration. The right hemiscrotum was painful, hyperemic, and edematous (Fig 1), and the cremasteric reflex was absent. The right lower quadrant of the abdomen was soft, with no rebound or guarding, and no inguinal hernia or hydrocele was noted. The suspected diagnosis was right testicular torsion, and the child was taken to the operating room, where the scrotum was incised. The processus vaginalis was patent, but the presence of seropurulent fluid prompted surgeons to perform a right transverse laparotomy. This procedure revealed an unperforated, gangrenous retrocecal vermiform appendix, which was removed. Afterward, warm saline

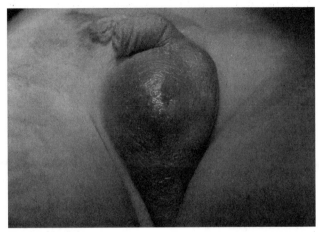

FIGURE 1.—Hyperemic, edematous, and painful right hemiscrotum. (Courtesy of Méndez R, Tellado M, Montero M, et al: Acute scrotum: An exceptional presentation of acute nonperforated appendicitis in childhood. *J Pediatr Surg* 33:1435-1436, 1998.)

was used to irrigate the peritoneum, and antibiotics were given for 1 week. Two months after the appendectomy, a herniotomy was performed.

Conclusions.—This boy's appendix was retrocecal, and the gangrenous tip near the ureter may have caused the inguinal pain. This report joins 14 others in the literature describing a child with acute appendicitis who presents with acute scrotal signs or symptoms. This entity must also join the list of differential diagnoses in children with inflammation of the lower abdomen and scrotum.

▶ Wow. Who would have thought that an 8-year-old presenting with a hyperemic, edematous, and painful right hemiscrotum and absence of the cremasteric reflex would have appendicitis as the cause? That is, however, exactly how this 8-year-old youngster presented. There are several other reports of acute appendicitis presenting in exactly the same way. Presumably in this case, the processus vaginalis was patent. Please remember that in such cases, when everything is cleared up, someone is going to have to go back in and correct the potential hernia that these patients also happen to have.

The moral in all this is straightforward. The next time you see an "acute scrotum," think beyond the possibility of testicular torsion, torsion of the testicular appendix, epididymitis, and orchiditis. In rare circumstances, other etiologies, such as thrombosed scrotal veins, bleeding into a testis in Henoch-Schönlein purpura, and an inflamed appendix can be the culprit.

On a slightly different note, a controversy rages about the value of pathologic evaluation of excised surgical tissue. Some have argued that there is no reason to send an obviously inflamed appendix to the pathology lab. Those who believe in such a minimalist approach should read the report of a 10-year-old girl who presented with an elevated temperature, anorexia, and right lower quadrant abdominal pain. A diagnosis of appendicitis was made and an inflamed appendix was removed. The diagnosis was changed to adenocarcinoma of the appendix after a pathologist examined the appendix.[1] This unusual pathology confirms the importance of subjecting all resected specimens of an appendix to histologic examination and ensuring that the subsequent report is actually seen. These rare cases of malignancies within an appendix presenting as an appendicitis require more aggressive surgical treatment than simply an appendectomy.

One last note having to do with pathologic evaluation of surgical specimens. In a study of 7924 hernia sacs submitted to the Pathology Department at the Children's Hospital of Philadelphia, not a single pathologic abnormality was found other than a hernia sac.[2] Unlike the resected appendix, submission of a hernial sac appears to be a waste of time, at least from the pathologist point of view.

J.A. Stockman III, M.D.

References

1. Driver CP, Bowen J, Bruce J: Adenocarcinoma of the appendix in a child. *J Pediatr Surg* 33:1437-1438, 1998.
2. Wenner WJ, Gutenberg M, Crombleholme T, et al: Pathological evaluation of the pediatric inguinal hernia sac. *J Pediatr Surg* 33:717-718, 1998.

Risk of Testicular Cancer With Cryptorchidism and With Testicular Biopsy: Corhort Study

Møller H, Cortes D, Engholm G, et al (Danish Natl Research Found, Copenhagen; Natl Univ Hosp, Copenhagen)
BMJ 317:729, 1998   10–5

Background.—A previous study suggested that men undergoing surgery for cryptorchidism have a greatly increased relative risk for subsequent testicular cancer. A cohort of men who had undergone surgery for undescended testes at 1 center was investigated to further define this possible risk.

Methods and Findings.—Eight hundred thirty patients were treated for a total of 1026 undescended testes between 1971 and 1992. An open surgical biopsy sample was obtained from all testes at that time. Seven cases of testicular neoplasia occurred overall. One occurred before a biopsy sample was obtained from the contralateral testis, 3 were diagnosed by histologic assessment at the time of surgery for cryptorchidism, and 2 occurred in previously biopsied testes. The last case was a contralateral cancer found in a man previously operated on for unilateral cryptorchidism. The relative risk among men who had a testicular biospy in 1 or both testes was 2.0. The 2 cases occurring in biopsied testes corresponded to a relative risk of 2.2.

Conclusions.—These findings in men undergoing surgery for cryptorchidism do not support previous findings of a significant increased risk of testicular cancer in biopsied testes. In the current series, the risk increased moderately.

▶ For some time a popular belief has been that biopsying a testis brought down at the time of orchiopexy causes the testis to have a somewhat increased risk of malignancy over the already expected higher rate of malignancy common to undescended testes. What little data exists in the literature suggest the simple act of biopsy multiplies 10-fold the subsequent risk of cancer development.

Well, it would appear that some old spouse's (using "wive's" is no longer politically correct) tales just aren't so. Based on a large series of men operated on for cryptorchidism, investigators from Denmark found little, in fact nothing, to support earlier findings of a greatly increased risk of testicular cancer in biopsied testes. On the contrary, the data now suggest only a moderately increased (twofold to fourfold) risk of testicular cancer in biopsied testes, along the same order of risk found in the unbiopsied testes of those treated for cryptorchidism.

On a different note, this chapter has little on the common topic of childhood enuresis. How would you deal with the following query? A woman has recently delivered twins. At the first postpartum visit, she and her husband ask what the chance is that these babies will have a problem with enuresis; both parents were enuretic as children. How would you respond?

This turns out to be a quite complex question. Several studies suggest an important role of genetic factors in enuresis. The familial occurrence of bed-wetting is well recognized, and 77% of children suffer from enuresis if both parents were enuretic as children. This is reduced to 44% when only 1 parent has a positive history of enuresis. Inheritance through a single recessive gene has been suspected in children with primary enuresis. As far as this couple and their twins are concerned, there is probably a very high chance that these babies will be enuretic. In addition to the above statistics, a long term twin study has revealed some interesting information about the occurrence of nocturnal enuresis.[1] When looking at thousands of identical and nonidentical twin pairs, if 1 identical twin has enuresis, there is a 40% to 50% chance that the other will have the same problem, independent of parent status. For nonidentical twins, this likelihood decreases to 20%. Interestingly, if a twin, when becoming an adult, still has enuresis, there is a 25% chance that the corresponding twin will also have adult persisting enuresis.

To say all this differently, if 2 parents have enuresis and have identical twins, the family will need a sturdy Maytag and lots of bed sheets.

J.A. Stockman III, M.D.

Reference

1. Hublin C, Kaprio J, Partin EN: Nocturnal enuresis in a nationwide twin cohort. *Sleep* 21:579-585, 1998.

Prenatal and Postnatal Management of Hyperprostaglandin E Syndrome After Genetic Diagnosis From Amniocytes

Konrad M, Leonhardt A, Hensen P, et al (Philipps Univ, Marburg, Germany)
Pediatrics 103:678-683, 1999   10–6

Introduction.—A hereditary tubulopathy mimicking long-term furosemide treatment, hyperprostaglandin E syndrome is an antenatal variant of Bartter syndrome. Autosomal recession is the mode of inheritance, and the syndrome causes excessive saluresis and polyurea leading to polyhydramnios and preterm delivery. Because polyhydramnios occurs in a number of maternal and fetal disorders, prenatal diagnosis of hyperprostaglandin E syndrome is often missed, leading to serious dehydration and electrolyte imbalances for the infant in the first weeks of life. A rational approach to perinatal management of infants with hyperprostaglandin E syndrome would be helpful. The prenatal molecular genetic diagnosis of hyperprostaglandin E syndrome with identification of mutations in the ROMK gene in a female fetus were reported.

Methods.—Two siblings were affected by hyperprostaglandin E syndrome, and the clinical and laboratory findings during pregnancy and the neonatal period were reviewed. Single-strand conformational analysis and direct sequencing were performed with mutational analysis of the ROMK channel gene (*KCNJ1*) from amniocytes.

Results.—The clinical diagnosis of hyperprostaglandin E syndrome was confirmed at 26 weeks of gestation with compound heterozygosis of the fetus in *KCNJ1* (D74Y/P110L). Further progression of polyhydramnios was prevented with indomethacin therapy from 26 to 31 weeks, without major adverse effects. The neonatal course was uncomplicated, in contrast to the elder brother, who was diagnosed at the age of 2 months. There could be prevention of hypovolemic renal failure after excessive renal loss of salt and water. There was no severe nephrocalcinosis.

Conclusion.—The natural course of hyperprostaglandin E syndrome is beneficially affected by genetic diagnosis and subsequent prenatal indomethacin therapy. This course especially helps with polyhydramnios and could prevent extreme prematurity. With early diagnosis postnatally, there is a chance to provide effective water and electrolyte substitution before severe volume depletion.

▶ Craig B. Langman, M.D., Division of Nephrology, Children's Memorial Hospital, Chicago, comments:

This innovative paper on what seems at first glance a rather esoteric subject presents several interesting areas for direct comment to the practicing pediatrician. In the end, it may serve as a model for many future encounters in our community.

The past few years have seen the emergence of the understanding of many disorders of salt and water metabolism at the molecular level, where specific gene mutations have been linked intimately to the expression of a well-known clinical disorder.[1,2] As has often been the case for other diseases, the genes that have been responsible for disturbed electrolyte and mineral metabolism have not been those that would be predicted *a priori* to be involved. For example, the gene encoding the renal chloride channel, CLCN5, has been linked to a wide variety of clinical renal disorders, including low molecular weight proteinuria alone in Japanese schoolchildren, X-linked nephrolithiasis with renal failure in some kindreds, and Dent's disease in others still.[3] Thus, the knowledge of a single gene mutation in a given situation may not necessarily provide the clinician with certainty of the clinical disturbance that may ensue as its consequence.[4] On the other hand, other gene mutations appear to produce more homogeneous clinical disease in the kidney. Obviously, we are in the infancy of our knowledge of predicting disease from gene mutations, and of the still largely unknown effects of disease-enhancing or disease-retarding genes.

For the clinician faced with a situation in which an inherited disorder of salt and water metabolism is a possible outcome in the fetus, the difficult problem remains whether to obtain amniocytes by early amniocentesis or chorionic villous sampling for direct genetic analysis of relevant gene(s), given the known level of bad outcome to an existing pregnancy from such a procedure.[5] Even more problematic is knowing the gene mutation may or may not yield sufficient information to predict the clinical outcome. Yet more vexing is many inherited diseases of salt and water metabolism, once known, have variable responses to conventional treatment.

In the study abstracted, the authors explored the possibility of a genetic mutation only after it appeared that a clinical syndrome (HPS) was duplicated, heralded by polyhydramnios. They took a leap of some faith in administering oral nonsteroidal anti-inflammatory drugs (popularly called NSAIDs) to the mother with an affected fetus, but watched for significant adverse effects as well as the desired effects to reduce or hold constant amniotic fluid levels until fetal lung maturity was assured.

Would such knowledge of other gene defects for specific disorders of electrolytes, water, or mineral metabolism lead any of us to similar choices? I think the approach offered by these investigators is rational when a uniform clinical disease is *almost always* associated with a unique gene disturbance that can be detected *almost always* and when treatment exists that has *routinely* modified the course of the disease under study. Many readers will likely face the issue in their practice lifetime, as both the Human Genome Project nears completion in the early part of the next millennium and innovative therapies for monogenic disorders increase dramatically year by year. Pay close attention to studies like this for further guidance in this emerging area of pediatrics: fetal therapeutics.

C.B. Langman, M.D.

References

1. Scheinman SJ, Guay-Woodford LM, Thakker RV, et al: Mechanisms of disease: Genetic disorder of renal electrolyte transport. *N Engl J Med* 340:1177-1187, 1999.

2. Bichet DG: Nephrogenic diabetes insipidus. *Am J Med* 105:431-442, 1998.
3. Thakker RV: The role of renal chloride channel mutations in kidney stone disease and nephrocalcinosis. *Curr Opin Nephrol Hypertens* 7:385-388, 1998.
4. Lloyd SE, Pearce SH, Fisher SE, et al: A common molecular basis for three inherited kidney stone diseases. *Nature* 379:445-449, 1996.
5. Collins VR, Webley C, Sheffield LJ, et al: Fetal outcome and maternal morbidity after early amniocentesis. *Prenat Diagn* 18:767-772, 1998.

Increasing Incidence of Childhood Class V Lupus Nephritis
Sorof JM, Perez MD, Brewer ED, et al (Baylor College of Medicine, Houston; Texas Children's Hosp, Houston)
J Rheumatol 25:1413-1418, 1998   10–7

Background.—Up to three fourths of children with systemic lupus erythematosus (SLE) develop nephritis within 5 years of SLE onset. Results of immunosuppressive or surgical therapy in patients with World Health Organization (WHO) class V lupus nephritis (LN) have varied. These authors characterized the incidence, frequency of transformation to another class, and outcomes of class V LN in pediatric patients.

Methods.—From January 1985 to July 1997, 97 renal biopsies from 60 children with suspected LN were reviewed. There were 8 boys and 52 girls, with a mean age at first biopsy of 13.2 ± 3.7 years. Of particular note were the histologic WHO class at presentation, any transformations to a different WHO class over time, and treatments (including oral prednisone, IV pulse methylprednisolone, and IV cyclophosphamide). The data were grouped into 3-year intervals to determine any changes in trends over time.

Findings.—On the first biopsy, 17 of 60 patients (28%) had class V LN; at the most recent biopsy, 22 (37%) had class V disease. Of 27 patients who had serial biopsies, histologic transformation occurred in 18 (67%); 19% of transformation were to a less proliferative lesion, 22% to a more proliferative lesion, and 19% to a membranous lesion. No patient with class V disease converted to a class II, III, or IV lesion. When data from 1995 to the present were compared with data from the preceding 9 years, class V LN was significantly more common since 1995. From 1987 through 1994, 8 of 46 initial biopsies (17%) had class V LN, whereas between 1995 and 1997, 9 of 14 initial biopsies (64%) had class V disease. The difference was also significant for all biopsies combined (including repeat biopsies): 15 of 74 biopsies (20%) before 1995 had class V disease compared with 12 of 23 biopsies (52%) since 1995. These changes in prevalence were not accounted for by differences in age at presentation, age at biopsy, time to biopsy, or type of treatment across the 12-year period. Information on renal outcome was available for 48 of the patients; 20 had class V disease and 28 had non-class V LN. The 2 groups did not differ in the incidence of death or renal dysfunction (1 of 20 vs 6 of 28). Patients whose first biopsy showed class V disease had normal renal function at the last follow-up visit (mean, 4.7 ± 3.2 years).

Conclusions.—This study found a significantly higher prevalence of class V LN than has been reported, and a significant (almost fourfold) increase in the incidence of class V disease since 1995. Whereas serial biopsies often showed a transformation of histologic classification, no patient with class V LN experienced any lesion regression. These high levels of class V disease have practical clinical implications for the care of children with LN, because physicians must balance the need to prevent the progression of renal disease with the risks of aggressive immunosuppression.

▶ Dr. Noosha Baqi, acting director of the Division of Pediatric Nephrology at the State University of New York Health Science Center at Brooklyn, comments:

The WHO histopathologic classification of LN is an indispensable tool for predicting the prognosis of LN and determines the physician's treatment choices. Class IV disease is an active diffuse proliferative nephritis requiring aggressive therapy, while class V disease or membranous LN has had a better reported prognosis in terms of renal and patient survival and was not treated aggressively until recently.[1] This report is important because it is one of the largest studies in children with 60 patients followed throughout approximately 5 years and 97 renal biopsies for analysis. It also presents a curious and apparently inexplicable finding, which is the increased frequency of class V LN in the last 3 years. Given the paucity of recent data on children with LN, there may be a shift to more class V disease. Only multi-center studies can assess the validity of this finding. For the general pediatrician involved in the care of a child with LN, this may translate into less aggressive immunosuppressive regimens. For the child with lupus, it may mean less morbidity from the disease and its treatment. Transformation between lupus classes is a well-known phenomenon. Again, earlier identification of disease and more aggressive therapies may be responsible for almost equal numbers of transformation to less severe lesions. Prospective, controlled randomized trials of the National Institutes of Health (NIH) in the adult population have concluded that systemic use of IV cyclophosphamide in conjunction with oral steroids provides the best outcome in SLE patients at risk for the development of renal failure.[2,3] There are no comparable studies in pediatric patients nor any data on long-term outcome. In general, pediatric nephrologists tend to follow the NIH guidelines for proliferative nephritis with the use of IV cyclophosphamide. The efficacy of this therapy needs to be studied in pediatric patients. Perhaps even more importantly, we should look at the part socioeconomic factors play. SLE is more prevalent in the African American and Hispanic populations, which are communities that rely largely on publicly funded medical care. The payment source of medical care has been shown to significantly influence prognosis.[4] Thus, improved medical services and early identification of disease combined with less toxic therapies may lead to better patient and renal survival in this disease.

N. Baqi, M.D.

References

1. Yang LY, Chen WP, Lin CY: Lupus nephritis in children: A review of 167 patients. *Pediatrics* 94:335-340, 1994.
2. Austin HA, Klippel JH, Balow JE, et al: Therapy of lupus nephritis: Controlled trial of prednisone and cytotoxic drugs. *N Engl J Med* 314:614-619, 1986.
3. Balow JE, Austin HA, Muenz LR, et al: Effect of treatment on the evolution of renal abnormalities in lupus nephritis. *N Engl J Med* 311:491-495, 1984.
4. Ginzler EM, Diamond HS, Weiner M, et al: A multicenter study in the outcome in systemic renal erythematosus. *Arthritis Rheum* 25:601-610, 1982.

The Natural History of Microalbuminuria in Adolescents With Type 1 Diabetes
Gorman D, Sochett E, Daneman D (Univ of Toronto)
J Pediatr 134:333-337, 1999   10–8

Background.—Previous researchers have reported that the presence of microalbuminuria (MA) predicts progression to overt diabetic nephropathy in 50% to more than 80% of adults with type I diabetes. Five percent to 20% of adolescents with type I diabetes reportedly have MA. The natural history of urinary albumin excretion in adolescents and the predictors of the onset and progression of MA in this population were investigated.

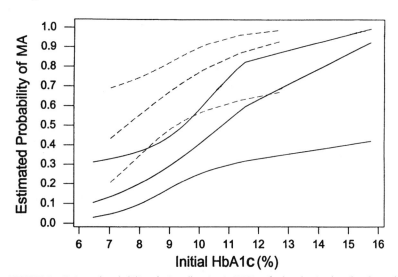

FIGURE 1.—Estimated probability of microalbuminuria (*MA*) at final evaluation based on hemoglobin (Hb) A1c level at initial assessment with upper and lower 95% confidence intervals. *Broken line* represents those initially microalbuminuric (n = 28); *solid line* represents normoalbuminuric group (n = 47). Two lines are parallel and linear, with significantly higher probability of MA at final evaluation in those initially microalbuminuric ($P < .001$). (Courtesy of Gorman D, Sochett E, Daneman D: The natural history of microalbuminuria in adolescents with type 1 diabetes. *J Pediatr* 134:333-337, 1999.)

Methods.—The records of 76 adolescents were reviewed. All patients had had their albumin excretion rate (AER) determined in the first decade of their diabetes. Patients were monitored for a mean of 6 years after initial AER testing. Patients with MA were compared with initially normoalbuminuric patients matched for age, sex, and diabetes duration.

Findings.—Twenty-eight patients initially had MA. Thirty-two percent regressed, 36% had persistent MA, and 32% progressed. In 5 of the 9 patients with progression, overt proteinuria developed. Of the 47 patients initially normoalbuminuric, MA developed in 30% and overt proteinuria in 6%. In a multiple regression analysis, initial AER and hemoglobin A1c measured at the same time independently predicted MA status at follow-up (Fig 1).

Conclusion.—In about two thirds of adolescents with type I diabetes, MA detected in the first decade of disease will persist or progress in the second decade. In one third of those initially normoalbuminuric, new MA will develop. Metabolic control influences the appearance, persistence, or progression of MA. Thus, MA screening early in the course of type I diabetes is necessary in this population.

▶ Data from the adult literature suggest that should a diabetic adolescent leave the second decade of life with MA, there is greater than an 80% chance of progression to overt renal disease. It is also not just the presence or absence of albumin, it is the amount of albumin as well that makes a difference. It is also clear that the likelihood of having MA is directly correlated with the degree of diabetes control as documented by hemoglobin A1c levels.

The question that remains is whether all diabetic teenagers should be screened for MA. The answer is "yes" if you intend to use that information in some useful way and "no" if not. If a patient is already being managed as tightly as possible and is as well controlled as one would hope for, screening for MA will do nothing that will change the management of your patient. If, on the other hand, you need more convincing evidence to convince a patient that better control is needed, there is nothing more powerful than being able to say to patients that they are already showing evidence of MA and that they need to take better care of themselves and their kidneys.

By the way, data from Canada clearly suggest that home-based management of type I diabetes is as effective for newly diagnosed insulin-dependent diabetes in children as is initial hospitalization for education and insulin management, followed subsequently by outpatient clinics or office-visit-setting contacts with patients.[1]

J.A. Stockman III, M.D.

Reference

1. Doughtery G, Schiffrin A, White D, et al: Home-based management can achieve intensification cost effectively in type 1 diabetes. *Pediatrics* 103:122-128, 1999.

Procalcitonin is a Marker of Severity of Renal Lesions in Pyelonephritis

Benador N, Siegrist C-A, Gendrel D, et al (Children's Hosp, Geneva; Hôpital Saint-Vincent-de-Paul, Paris; Institut Gustave-Roussy, Villejuif, France)
Pediatrics 102:1422-1425, 1998   10–9

Background.—Febrile urinary tract infection (UTI) is a common problem in children. The clinical findings of fever or flank pain and laboratory markers such as serum leukocyte counts and C-reactive protein (CRP) do not reliably distinguish acute pyelonephritis, which requires more aggressive therapy, from lower UTI, especially in young children. The authors attempted to distinguish acute pyelonephritis from lower UTI by measuring serum procalcitonin (PCT) levels, a recently reported marker of infection.

Methods.—Eighty children, aged 1 month to 16 years, admitted for suspected pyelonephritis were included in the study. Serum CRP, leukocyte counts, and PCT concentrations were measured. Using ^{99m}Te–dimercaptosuccinic acid scintigraphy, renal involvement was evaluated in the first 5 days after admission. If the first result was abnormal, the examination was repeated.

Findings.—Mean PCT levels were .38 µg/L in lower UTI and 5.37 µg/L in pyelonephritis. Mean leukocyte counts were 10,939 and 17,429/mm³, respectively, and CRP levels were 30.3 and 120.8 mg/L. When inflammatory markers were correlated with renal lesion severity ranked by scintigraphy, a highly significant association with plasma PCT levels was noted. However, CRP showed a borderline significant association, and leukocyte counts showed no association. Patients without vesicoureteral reflux had an average PCT of 5.16 µg/L, which was comparable to that in patients with reflux, with a mean PCT of 5.76 µg/L. For predicting renal lesions at admission, the sensitivity and specificity of CRP were 100% and 26.1%, respectively. The sensitivity and specificity of PCT were 70.3% and 82.6%, respectively.

Conclusion.—Serum PCT concentrations appear to be increased significantly in children with UTI and renal parenchymal involvement. This marker may help identify patients at risk for severe renal lesions.

▶ Wouldn't it be nice to say that we have come a long way in terms of knowing precisely how to manage a child with a UTI? If you really think we have come a long way, why do we see articles such as this still appearing in the literature? The reason why is obvious. There remains no easy way to tell pyelonephritis from lower UTI in a febrile child with infected urine. Given the absence of good study data, there is currently no agreement on the optimum route of administration of antibiotics, the duration of treatment, or the requirement that somebody be hospitalized with a febrile UTI. The only "gold standard" for distinguishing pyelonephritis from a lower UTI is an abnormal dimercaptosuccinic acid scan, which is expensive and also not available in every institution.

Surrogates for the gold standard have proven to be less than adequate. Some time ago, a variety of inflammatory markers or mediators were studied to see whether they could substitute for the dimercaptosuccinic acid scan. CRP, in particular, has been the most extensively investigated. Although CRP elevations are highly sensitive, they are not sufficiently specific to routinely recommend them as the technique for differentiating upper UTI from lower UTI. PCT, a propeptide of calcitonin is also an inflammatory mediator. Although having less sensitivity than CRP, it has a much greater specificity (>80%). This mediator alone, however, cannot be used to identify all renal lesions as some 30% of patients with upper UTIs will have normal PCT levels.

Thus, the search continues for the perfect differentiator between sites of UTI. In some ways, CRP and PCT are quite complementary in terms of sensitivity and specificity. One wonders whether studies will be performed that allow the strengths and weaknesses of each to balance one another as part of a screening panel. One test has a high sensitivity but only modest specificity. The other test has moderate sensitivity and high specificity. One would think that the 2 in combination might prove to be the pot of gold at the end of the rainbow when it comes to a noninvasive, relatively inexpensive assessment of the site of an infection in the urinary tract.

Before this commentary is ended, an update on the role of juices in the management of UTI is in order. Clearly cranberry juice will lower bacterial adhesion in the urinary tract and can be useful for preventing recurrence of infection. Grapefruit juice will not do this, although it is good for other purposes because it alters the metabolism of cyclosporine, permitting lower amounts of this expensive medication to be administered as an immunomodulatory agent in those who have had a kidney transplanted. If you like to drink a lot of grapefruit juice, however, be aware of some potential problems related to excessive ingestion of the latter. The Nurses' Health Study has recently reported in the *Annals of Internal Medicine* that those who take too much of the sour stuff may have an increased tendency to develop kidney stones.[1] The risk of stone formation is increased 28% above baseline in those who drink just one 8-oz serving of grapefruit per day. The risk is increased 20% in those who drink non-diet soda. Water is essentially a neutral risk factor for kidney stones. If you really want to decrease your risk, take 8 oz of wine a day. The chance of stone recurrence in wine drinkers is one third that of those who drink water instead.

Intuition would tell you that anything tasting as sour as grapefruit juice can't be good for you. If you want to decrease your risk of UTI without casting your kidneys in stone, stick to cranberry juice. The bogs will like you for it.

J.A. Stockman III, M.D.

Reference

1. Grapefruit juice and renal stones (editorial). *Ann Intern Med* 128:534-540, 1998.

Mycoplasma hominis Parasitism of *Trichomonas vaginalis*
Rappelli P, Addis MF, Carta F, et al (Univ of Sassari, Italy)
Lancet 352:1286, 1998   10–10

Background.—Vaginal infection during pregnancy carries an elevated risk of intrauterine growth retardation, preterm birth, and perinatal morbidity and mortality. Vaginal infection with *Trichomonas vaginalis* may be associated with concomitant *Mycoplasma hominis*. This study examined the co-occurrence of vaginal infection with *T. vaginalis* and *M. hominis*.

Methods and Results.—*T. vaginalis* isolates from Italian and African women were incubated for 7 days or 3 months and then tested with a specific polymerase chain reaction for *Mycoplasma* spp. Just 2 of the 37 isolates were negative for *Mycoplasma* in both short-term and long-term cultures. There was no evidence of in vitro contamination. All of the mycoplasmas identified were of the species *M. hominis*. Further in vitro studies found that *M. hominis* was the only organism capable of infecting a *Mycoplasma*-free *T. vaginalis* isolate. *M. hominis* not only infected *T. vaginalis* cells but replicated along with them. *T. vaginalis* cells infected with *M. hominis* transmitted the infection to human epithelial cells, which in turn transmitted *M. hominis* to *T. vaginalis*.

Conclusions.—This study shows an association between vaginal infection with *M. hominis* and *T. vaginalis*. The 2 pathogens share a single route of transmission, and *M. hominis* appears capable of parasitizing and replicating in association with *T. vaginalis*.

▶ At a recent resident morning report in the department of pediatrics at the University of North Carolina, Chapel Hill, a 3-day-old infant with a scalp abscess was presented. The infant was born by cesarean section after a long trial of labor. It appeared that the scalp may have become infected as a result of a digital examination as the infant was crowning. This resulted in a small abrasion. Everyone seemed surprised when the organism turned out not to be *Staphylococcus aureus*, but, rather, a *Mycoplasma* species. The latter has been described before, on rare occasions, as a cause of skin abscess in the neonatal period. From this report, we see that *Mycoplasma* organisms in the vagina rarely exist independently and are often a parasite of another organism, such as the sexually transmitted *T. vaginalis*.

Prior studies of pregnant and nonpregnant women have shown an association between *T. vaginalis* and *M. hominis* infections. In an area of Africa with a high prevalence of trichomoniasis, it has been noticed that antimycoplasma antibodies are found in an unexpectedly high number of women with antitrichomonas antibodies.[1] Electromicroscopy has also shown that *Mycoplasma* organisms exist within food vacuoles of protozoa such as *Trichomonas*, thus cinching the probability that *T. vaginalis* can take on hitchhikers.

To say all this differently, *T. vaginalis* is the Trojan horse of the genitalia, depositing *Mycoplasma* species at will in the vagina. The latter can infect not only women but also their babies and their sexual partners.

Beware of such horses bearing gifts with strings attached!

J.A. Stockman III, M.D.

Reference

1. Germain M, Crohn MA, Hilliar SL, et al: Genital flora in pregnancy and its association with intrauterine growth retardation. *J Clin Microbiol* 32:2162-2168, 1994.

Refined Microscopic Urinalysis for Red Blood Cell Morphology in the Evaluation of Asymptomatic Microscopic Hematuria in a Pediatric Population

Ward JF, Kaplan GW, Mevorach R, et al (Children's Hosp, San Diego, Calif)
J Urol 160:1492-1495, 1998   10–11

Background.—Refined microscopic urinalysis for the detection of dysmorphic red blood cells (RBCs) has been used in children and adults with a known source of hematuria. The clinical value of this approach in children with an unknown source of hematuria was investigated.

Methods.—Forty-four children aged 12 years or younger were studied. All had been referred for assessment of asymptomatic microscopic hematuria showing 4 or more RBCs per high-power field. A first morning urine sample was obtained and analyzed by refined urinalysis for RBC morphology. Standard assessments were also done until the source of hematuria was determined.

Findings.—Refined urinalysis demonstrated pure dysmorphic RBCs in 22 children, pure isomorphic RBCs in 8, and mixed isomorphic/dysmorphic RBCs in 14. The presence of dysmorphic RBCs had a sensitivity and specificity of 83% and 81%, respectively, in correctly predicting a glomerular source of hematuria. The presence of isomorphic RBCs predicted a uroepithelial source of hematuria with a sensitivity and specificity of 25% and 22%, respectively. Hematuria and 2+ proteinuria were 100% sensitive and 83% specific in predicting glomerulotubular hematuria.

Conclusions.—Refined microscopic urinalysis is a costly test that offers little additional information in the evaluation of microscopic hematuria in children. A careful history and physical examination with microscopic urinalysis and dipstick for proteinuria provide the same amount of diagnostic information.

▶ The subject of this report is now an old one. For more than 20 years, various reports have suggested the potential clinical use of an examination of urine RBC morphology to differentiate patients with glomerular disease from those with lower urinary tract disease. There are two ways to do this. One way consists of determining the proportion of abnormally shaped RBCs in the urine by phase-contrast microscopy or in stained smears of the urinary sediment. The other way consists of determining the mean corpuscular volume of RBCs in the urine using electronic blood cell counters, the same ones used to do a complete blood count (CBC). Patients with glomerular bleeding tend to have low red cell mean corpuscular volumes in their urine. In this report, the method used was a cytologic examination of first-morning voided urine, an examination performed by a seasoned pathologist who was looking for evidence of deformed RBCs. We see that the sensitivity and specificity with this approach are not good enough to add significant additional information to a patient's evaluation. The thought was that if one could determine that glomerular disease accounted for a particular patient's hematuria, that patient could be referred to a nephrologist. Contrarily, if the evaluation suggested lower urinary tract problems, that patient could be referred to a urologist. Would that life be so simple.

By the way, it was Addis who first described the presence of dysmorphic RBCs in urine samples from patients with glomerular disease. That was in 1948. More than 50 years later, while we've learned a lot about RBC morphology in the urine, we must recognize that RBC morphology cannot be proposed as a uniformly sensitive or specific test in pinpointing the source of hematuria. It is just one of several tools, including a history and physical examination, that must be used to try to determine a cause of hematuria in children. Also an issue is whether a primary care physician should undertake an extensive evaluation for an ill-defined hematuria or whether a referral to a seasoned pediatric nephrologist or pediatric urologist might be more cost-effective. Obviously this depends a great deal on the experience of the primary care physician.

This is the last entry in the Genitourinary Tract chapter, so we'll close with a quick quiz. You are treating a patient with an overactive bladder. Specifically, this patient has a phenomenon called *detrusor hyperreflexia*, which causes the bladder to spontaneously empty before reaching full capacity. How might peppers be used to treat your patient? "Peppers?" you say? It turns out that pepper extracts are being used these days to treat such overactive bladders. The pepper extract in question is capsaicin. Capsaicin is an active ingredient in hot peppers of the genus Capsicum. People who enjoy "hot" foods will recognize some of the pharmacologic effects of capsaicin, including burning of the skin and mucous membranes (irritation) upon contact, followed by a gradual diminishing of the intensity of irritation after several contacts to the point of insensitivity. It has now been shown that if chili pepper extracts are instilled into the bladder of humans who have bladder hyperreflexia, capsaicin will modulate the afferent branch of the micturition reflex, allowing for a larger bladder capacity before the urge to void. Desensitization of the bladder sensory nerves also occurs and may be useful as part of the management for painful bladder conditions such as interstitial cystitis. A single installation in the bladder for these conditions results in improvement or correction of the problem for as long as 6 months, during which time the original condition may resolve to the point that reinstallation is not necessary.

There is an obvious problem with instilling chili pepper extract into the bladder. Just like with chilies in the mouth, there is an initial burning sensation that can be quite significant before desensitization ocurs. To get around this problem, a more potent form of capsaicin has been found that acts very quickly. It is known as *resinifera toxin*, a naturally occurring analog of capsaicin. What makes resinifera particularly appealing is that it is 1000-fold more potent but has significantly less acute toxicity and pain. For more on the topic of hot tamales in the bladder, see the editorial by Chancellor.[1]

J.A. Stockman III, M.D.

Reference

1. Chancellor MB: Should we be using chili pepper extracts to treat the overactive bladder (editorial)? *J Urol* 158:2097, 1997.

11 The Respiratory Tract

Sleep-Disordered Breathing and School Performance in Children
Gozal D (Tulane Univ, New Orleans, La)
Pediatrics 102:616-620, 1998   11–1

Objective.—It has been suggested that up to 2% of children have obstructive sleep apnea syndrome (OSAS). Failure to recognize and treat OSAS in this age group causes significant morbidity, but the possible cognitive consequences are not known. This study examined the incidence and academic consequences of sleep-associated gas-exchange abnormalities (SAGEA) in children.

Methods.—The prospective study included 297 urban public school first-graders with school performance in the lowest 10th percentile of their class. All these children underwent home screening for OSAS; this consisted of a parental questionnaire and a single night recording of pulse oximetry and transcutaneous partial pressure of carbon dioxide. Parents were advised to seek medical attention for children with a diagnosis of SAGEA. The children's school grades for the year before and the year after screening for OSAS were analyzed.

Results.—Fifty-four children were found to have SAGEA, an incidence of 18%. Twenty-four of these children were treated with tonsillectomy and adenoidectomy, and parents did not seek treatment for the remaining 30 children. Treated children showed an overall improvement in their grades during the second grade, from 2.43 to 2.87. The untreated children showed no improvement, nor did children who did not have SAGEA.

Conclusions.—This study finds a high frequency of SAGEA among first-graders with poor academic performance. These children show academic improvement after treatment for their OSAS. The results suggest that children with developmental or learning difficulties should be evaluated for sleep-related symptoms, and early evaluation for sleep-disordered breathing is in order.

▶ This is an intriguing report. If the conclusions are correct, the findings could have profound implications for our educational processes. What the authors did here was to screen for OSAS at home, using a combination of a parent questionnaire and a recording of a child's pulse oximetry/partial pressure of carbon dioxide during sleep. It would appear that as many as 1 in 5 children show evidence of OSAS, presumably related to enlarged tonsils. When the tonsils are removed, academic achievement scores go up.

It should be stressed that school grades provide only a relatively rudimentary assessment of cognitive, behavioral, and learning capabilities. Before the results of this report are translated into wholesale tonsillectomies, we should wait for more elaborate investigations that substantiate these very interesting findings. Nonetheless, these researchers are probably correct. Families that snore together probably do stay awake together. Families that snore together probably also have difficulty graduating from grade school together.

By the way, the word *snore* is from the Danish word: *snorke*, meaning making funny noises with one's nose. We have 4 dogs at home, 2 of whom are pugs who *snorke* a lot during their sleep. As lovable as they are, they are not the brightest. Perhaps a little canine CPAP would be in order.

J.A. Stockman III, M.D.

Factors Associated With the Transition to Nonprone Sleep Positions of Infants in the United States: The National Infant Sleep Position Study
Willinger M, Hoffman HJ, Wu K-T, et al (NIH, Bethesda, Md; Harvard Med School, Boston; Univ of Southern California, Los Angeles; et al)
JAMA 280:329-335, 1998   11–2

Introduction.—The leading cause of postneonatal infant mortality in the United States is sudden infant death syndrome (SIDS). During the decade before 1992, the rate of sudden infant death syndrome changed little, despite significant declines in overall infant mortality. Factors associated with increased risk of SIDS have been low birth weight, preterm birth, young maternal age, high parity, late or no prenatal care, smoking, and substance abuse. Previous studies found a strong association between placement of infants in the prone position (on their stomachs) for sleep and SIDS. Within 2 years after a public information campaign to have mothers place their infants in the supine position (on their backs), sudden infant death rates dropped 50% or more. This study sought to determine the typical sleep positions of infants younger than 8 months, as well as the factors associated with the placement of infants in a supine or prone position and the changes that occurred after recommendations were made to lay the infants in a supine position.

Methods.—A telephone survey of the 48 contiguous states of the United States was conducted between 1992 and 1996. During these years, about 1000 interviews were conducted with nighttime caregivers of infants born within the last 7 months.

Results.—In each wave of the survey, 97% of respondents placed their infants to sleep in a specific position. In 1992, before the campaign, 70% of caregivers placed the infants in the supine position, whereas in 1996 24% of caregivers placed them on their backs. In 1992 13% of caregivers placed the infants on their backs, and this rose to 35% in 1996, whereas 15% placed them on their sides in 1992, and this rose to 39% in 1996. Maternal race reported as black, mother's age 20 to 29 years, region reported as the mid-Atlantic, mothers with a previous child, and infant age younger than 8 weeks were significant predictors of prone placement. Compared with the other age groups, infants aged 8 to 15 weeks were significantly more likely to be placed nonprone over time.

Conclusion.—Between 1992 and 1996, the prevalence of infants placed in the prone sleep position declined by 66%. During this period, SIDS declined approximately 38%; however, causality cannot be proved. Efforts to promote the supine sleep position should be aimed at groups at high risk of prone placement to achieve further reduction in prone sleeping.

▶ This report is one of many dealing with factors associated with sleep position in infants here in the United States. It has been just 8 years since the American Academy of Pediatrics (AAP) Task Force on Infant Positioning and SIDS published its recommendation that healthy, full-term infants be placed in the lateral or supine position to sleep. That immediately started a controversy based on medical concerns about the change to prone sleeping. Between 1992 (the initial task force report) and 1996, additional information on the health outcomes in infants who slept in a nonprone position led to a consensus that risk-reduction efforts should be strengthened and actually accelerated. A coalition was formed among the U.S. Public Health Service, the AAP, the Association of SIDS Program Professionals, and the SIDS Alliance for the Planning, Development, and Implementation of a "Back to Sleep" National Public Education Campaign, which was launched in June 1994. While all this was going on, the National Institute of Child Health and Human Development began to carefully track population-based studies on sleep practices and the impact on SIDS. The article abstracted here reports on data from one of these studies, the National Infant Sleep Position Study, which observed infants vis-á-vis their sleep position between 1992 and 1996.

Since the National Institutes of Health started tracking SIDS and its relationship to sleep position, a variety of interesting data have emerged. First, and most obvious, is the description of the decline in SIDS deaths, which does seem to be attributable to the change in sleep position. Second, the observation has been made that lateral sleep position is not as good as the supine position. Babies tend not to stay on their sides and have a 50-50 chance of winding up on their stomachs. Infants placed to sleep in the lateral position are 1.84 times more likely to die of SIDS than infants placed to sleep in the supine position. Because of this, in November 1996, the AAP revised its sleep position statement to emphasize that supine is the preferred position, although lateral may be an acceptable alternative.

Continuing with the topic of infant sleep position, have you ever wondered what happens to the skin temperature of babies who are placed to sleep in the prone as opposed to the supine position? It was only recently that data appeared documenting that the prone position may increase temperature around the head of a baby. Investigators in France studied a 4-month-old baby to examine what the effect of sleep position is on skin temperature. Temperature probes were placed in the supracephalic, peritemporal, and the submandibular areas. There was an increase in temperature in the immediate vicinity of the head in the prone position. This was reflected in a +1°C increase in the supracephalic area. Other increases seen were: +2.1°C in the peritemporal area and +3.5°C in the submandibular area. These findings, by the way, were repeated on a baby-like mannequin that was ventilated with air heated to 37°C (98.6°F) internally by inflating the chest. The mannequin showed virtually identical rises in temperature in the surface about its head when it was placed prone.

So what does all this mean? It probably means nothing more than when you sleep on your belly, the skin in and about your head becomes hot, most likely because of poor ventilation. In itself this would mean little, except for the fact that some authors consider temperature to be a major factor in SIDS. This finding could provide a theoretical link supporting epidemiologic evidence that the prone position and hyperthermia are risk factors for SIDS.[1]

J.A. Stockman III, M.D.

Reference

1. Oriot D, Berthier M, Saulnier J-P, et al: Prone position may increase temperature around the head of the infant. *Acta Paediatr* 87:1005-1007, 1998.

Chest Radiograph in the Evaluation of First Time Wheezing Episodes: Review of Current Clinical Practice and Efficacy

Roback MG, Dreitlein DA (Univ of Colorado, Denver)
Pediatr Emerg Care 14:181-184, 1998   11–3

Background.—Asthma or reactive airways disease and bronchiolitis are the most common diagnoses in children with wheezing. However, other possibilities need to be considered, particularly in first-time wheezing (FTW) episodes. The clinical use and value of chest radiographs in the workup of children with FTW episodes as evaluated in an emergency department were studied.

Methods.—The clinical findings in 121 patients with FTW undergoing chest radiography were compared retrospectively with those in 177 patients not undergoing chest radiography. Twenty-four percent of the patients had significant radiographic findings (findings expected to change management), and 76% did not.

Findings.—Patients undergoing radiography were older than those who did not (39 and 20 months, respectively), had lower pulse oximetry (89.7% and 92.7%, respectively), and were less likely to have a family history of asthma or a history of atopy. Children with localized wheezes, localized rales, and localized reduced breath sounds were also more likely to undergo chest radiography. Factors associated with positive findings on radiography were increased temperature, absence of family history of asthma, and the presence of localized wheezes or rales.

Conclusions.—Emergency department physicians do not routinely obtain chest radiographs in children with FTW episodes. The use of such radiography was associated with increased temperature, no family history of asthma, and localized wheezes or rales on ausculatory examination.

▶ Chances are that you are not one of those who do a chest x-ray in a child who wheezes for the first time, or are you? If you are, stop. This is not the first study to show how ineffective and unreliable the chest x-ray is in assisting you in the management of such children. Believe the studies. It is true that "all that wheezes is not asthma," and that some popular textbooks, including *Rudolph's Pediatrics*, state that chest x-rays should be performed at the initial evaluation of all patients with asthma. Nonetheless, you can be selective in your use of the radiology department. Absence of a family history of allergy/asthma, unexplained fever, or focal chest findings on physical examination might lead you toward a chest x-ray and that would be fine. The same would be true for a history of choking (potential aspiration of a foreign body).

While we're on the topic of foreign bodies, in the old days, one never got too excited about any child who swallowed a penny because, presumably, everything would come out in the end, so to speak. We should be more wary now. What has changed is that the traditional copper penny was replaced in 1982 with a zinc core which has a very thin copper coating. The zinc is highly digestible by acid and can cause problems such as ulcers, anemia, and damage to the kidneys, liver, and bone marrow. A 2½-year-old boy was recently brought to the Duke University Medical Center when he complained of an upset stomach 4 days after he had swallowed an unknown foreign object. An x-ray film of his abdomen revealed a small metallic disc with holes in it in his stomach. The radiologist thought the object was probably a small battery, but when the child underwent fiberoptic gastroscopy, a severely corroded 1989 penny was retrieved. Stomach acid had eaten away some 72% of the coin in just a few short days. The patient had an acute ulcer in the gastric mucosa where the penny had been. The ulcer itself healed within a few days without treatment. It should be noted that the amount of zinc this child ingested was probably only equivalent to 3 or 4 over-the-counter zinc lozenges, far in excess of a therapeutic dose of zinc for a child this size, but hardly toxic.[1]

Whoever said that a penny doesn't buy what it used to is wrong. A penny will buy you a whole lot of trouble, if it sits in your stomach too long.

J.A. Stockman III, M.D.

Reference

1. Jefferson T: A penny for your thoughts. *JAMA* 281:122, 1999.

Cystic Fibrosis, Young's Syndrome, and Normal Sweat Chloride

Wellesey D, Schwarz M (Princess Anne Hosp, Southampton, England; Royal Manchester Children's Hosp, England)
Lancet 352:38, 1998   11–4

Introduction.—Clinicians need to be aware that children with chronic lung disease and normal sweat chlorine tests may have Young's syndrome, a chronic sinopulmonary disease with azoospermia. The cases of 2 brothers with Young's syndrome who were treated inappropriately for asthma for several years are reported.

Patient Histories.—Both brothers were treated for asthma into their adult years. They both had diminished lung function and substantial lung impairment as adults as well as azoospermia. Chest radiographs revealed that both brothers had bronchiectatic changes consistent with cystic fibrosis. Brother A moved away and was re-evaluated at the age of 27 years. His sweat test remained negative, and he continued to experience azoospermia. His treatment was changed, and he subsequently showed a marked improvement in lung function and well-being. The other brother continued to be treated for asthma. Genetic testing revealed that both brothers were heterozygous for the ΔF508 mutation on the *CFTR* gene. When cystic fibrosis was suspected, further genetic analysis revealed that both brothers had the Q1291H mutation. This confirmed a diagnosis of cystic fibrosis in both patients.

Discussion/Conclusion.—The substitution of a guanine base by a cytosine at the last nucleotide of exon 20 in the Q1291H mutation leads to abberant splicing of the mRNA. The *CFTR* mutations have been considered as a cause for Young's syndrome in earlier reports. Results have been inconsistent; yet few mutations, if any, included the Q1291H mutation. Suspicion of Young's syndrome in chronic lung disease, even with negative sweat chloride, will help prevent inappropriate asthma treatment in patients with these sometimes mild forms of cystic fibrosis.

▶ This article is one of those little gems in the literature that, despite being only half of a journal page in length, provides us significant insight into a clinical dilemma that previously had no explanation. In this case, the dilemma is how some individuals otherwise look and act like they might have cystic fibrosis, but have a normal sweat chloride test. The term "Young's syndrome" was described a couple of decades earlier. It is a syndrome characterized by sinopulmonary disease accompanied by azoospermia. Some have suggested that this syndrome is actually more common than cystic fibrosis. Patients with Young's syndrome have negative sweat chloride tests. As this article shows, some patients with sinopulmonary disease and azoospermia actually have atypical cystic fibrosis. By this is meant that they are carriers of the ΔF508 mutation, but also have an additional mutation, uncommon to the clinical picture of cystic fibrosis, but which, in conjunction with the ΔF508 mutation, produces some of the signs and symptoms of cystic fibrosis, although with a negative sweat chloride test.

If you should ever see a child or teenager with a sinopulmonary disorder consistent with cystic fibrosis, but the sweat chloride test is negative, do not rule out the possibility of cystic fibrosis totally. A comprehensive mutation analysis of the *CFTR* gene may give you the correct diagnosis when the sweat chloride test will not.

J.A. Stockman III, M.D.

Cystic Fibrosis Newborn Screening: Impact on Reproductive Behavior and Implications for Genetic Counseling
Mischler EH, Wilfond BS, Fost N, et al (Med College of Wisconsin, Milwaukee; Univ of Arizona, Tucson; Univ of Wisconsin, Madison; et al)
Pediatrics 102:44-52, 1998   11–5

Background.—Screening of newborn infants for cystic fibrosis (CF) remains controversial. To examine the medical and psychosocial impact of newborn CF screening, a randomized controlled trial was conducted in Wisconsin between 1985 and 1994.

Study Design.—The Wisconsin CF Neonatal Screening Project was a randomized trial of early diagnosis through CF neonatal screening. In the first 6 years of this study, analysis of immunoreactive trypsinogen (IRT) with sweat test confirmation was used to screen infants. Of the 220,862 infants in the early treatment group, 369 had an elevated IRT and 46 were found to have CF. There were 10 patients with false negative IRTs. During the last 3 years of the study, DNA analysis was added (IRT/DNA) to improve accuracy. There were 104,308 children randomized to the early treatment group, with 132 positive screening tests and 21 diagnoses of CF. There was 1 false negative finding. Infants in the early diagnosis group were contacted within the first 8 weeks, and the rest were not contacted for 4 years. All 135 families who had a child with CF were offered genetic counseling. A questionnaire on knowledge and attitudes toward CF and reproductive decisions was sent to all families 3 months after the sweat test, 1 year after, and in June of 1994.

Findings.—In families who had a child with CF, 95% initially understood that there was a 1:4 chance of CF in subsequent children. There was good retention of this information at follow-up. After the 1994 assessment, 52% of the families had not conceived more children. In those couples in whom CF was diagnosed in their first child, 70% did conceive more children. There were 43 more pregnancies in 31 families. Prenatal diagnosis was used by 26% of these families for 21% of these pregnancies. CF was detected in 3 pregnancies; all were carried to term. Among those with false positives findings, more than 95% of the families did not understand initially that their children did not have CF. Follow-up assessment demonstrated that many of these families were still thinking frequently about the test results after 1 year. One year later, more than half of the families with false positive findings did not understand that they were at increased risk of bearing a child who had CF.

Conclusions.—In a large series of families who had a child with CF, neonatal CF screening did not have a significant impact on their reproductive behavior. Some parents were confused about the results of testing, even after genetic counseling, but most parents understood and retained information provided during genetic counseling. However, most of these families did not use prenatal screening for subsequent pregnancies. More research is needed on genetic counseling methods and their impact on knowledge and behavior.

▶ The concept of screening newborn infants for CF has long had its advocates and its opponents. This report will be interesting reading for both, since those who are supportive of neonatal screening will see enough in this report to support their views. The same thing will be true of those who oppose CF screening in the newborn period. On the plus side, with modern-day molecular screening techniques, coupled or not with serum testing for immunoreactive trypsinogen, one can adequately screen for this disorder.

One can counsel families of affected infants about the subsequent risks of future pregnancies. At the same time, neonatal screening does carry with it false positive reactions, which need to be sorted out by sweat testing. This results in a fair amount of parental anxiety, and even a year or more later such babies frequently carry, at least in their parents' minds, a defect. Although the principal reason for doing newborn screening is to provide genetic counseling for future pregnancies, it would appear that most parents of a child with CF will go ahead and have more children, and the large majority of the latter pregnancies will be allowed to come to term, even if CF is diagnosed in utero in a subsequent pregnancy. What all this means is straightforward. Although we certainly can, and probably should, do neonatal screening for CF, in an imperfect world the outcome is not always as some intend.

In a world of good intentions, CF is screening gets a solid "B." More homework is needed for an "A+."

J.A. Stockman III, M.D.

Intermittent Administration of Inhaled Tobramycin in Patients With Cystic Fibrosis
Ramsey BW, for the Cystic Fibrosis Inhaled Tobramycin Study Group (Univ of Washington, Seattle; et al)
N Engl J Med 340:23-30, 1999   11–6

Background.—Traditional treatment for periodic exacerbations of *Pseudomonas aeruginoa* endobronchial infection in persons with cystic fibrosis (CF) consists of parenteral antipseudomonal antibiotics for 7 to 21 days. However, pulmonary function still declines, by about 2% per year, and 90% of such patients eventually die of lung disease. Long-term antibacterial therapy may help maintain pulmonary function. Two multicenter, double-blind, placebo-controlled studies of intermittent inhaled tobramycin in patients with CF and *P. aeruginosa* infection were reported.

Methods.—Five hundred twenty patients, aged a mean of 21 years, were assigned to 300 mg of inhaled tobramycin or placebo twice a day for 4 weeks, followed by 4 weeks of no study drug. Patients were given treatment or placebo in 3 on-off cycles for a total of 24 weeks. End points included pulmonary function, *P. aeruginosa* density in sputum, and hospitalization.

Findings.—Patients given inhaled tobramycin had a mean increase in forced expiratory volume in 1 second of 10% at week 20 compared with baseline, whereas patients given placebo had a 2% decline in forced expiratory volume in 1 second. In tobramycin recipients, *P. aeruginosa* density declined by a mean of 0.8 $\log_{10}$ CFU/g of expectorated sputum between weeks 0 and 20, compared with an increase of .3 $\log_{10}$ CFU/g in the placebo recipients. Tobramycin recipients were 26% less likely to be hospitalized than placebo recipients. Inhaled tobramycin was unassociated with detectable ototoxic or nephrotoxic effects or with drug accumulation in serum. In the tobramycin group, the proportion of patients with *P. aeruginosa* isolates for which the minimal inhibitory concentration of tobramycin was 8 μg/mL or greater was 25% at baseline and 32% at week 24. In the placebo group, this proportion decreased from 20% at week 0 to 17% at week 24.

Conclusion.—In this study, intermittent administration of inhaled tobramycin improved pulmonary function, reduced *P. aeruginosa* density in sputum, and decreased the risk of hospitalization in patients with CF. Active treatment was also tolerated well.

▶ It has been over 50 years since antibiotics have been used in a widespread manner to manage some of the complications of CF. Although concerns still linger about the risks of antibiotic resistance as a result of frequent exposure to antimicrobials, there is no choice but to use them as often as is necessary to preserve lung function. Given the fact that, even now, the average patient with CF will lose about 2% of lung function per year, anything that improves on the status quo will be welcomed. Thus, if intermittent administration of inhaled tobramycin helps in this regard, its use should be embraced.

The data from this report, although promising, are still somewhat preliminary. We will need to see more substantiation of effectiveness, particularly to be certain that individual patients do not become refractory to the benefits of tobramycin. Also, recognize that tobramycin must be administered by means of a jet nebulizer to produce particle sizes of about 4 μm. This device was chosen to deliver the drug to the site of infection which is within the airways rather than within the alveoli. The approach used minimizes antibiotic delivery to the alveolar surface, and, thus, there may be some appropriate and desired limitation of systemic absorption.

The trick these days with CF is to keep patients well enough, long enough to be afforded the ultimate benefits of gene therapy. Since the discovery of the gene encoding CF, there has been much excitement about the possibility of gene therapy, which has now reached the stage of phase I clinical trials in older patients. These trials are getting down to younger and younger ages. Recognize, for example, that although the baby born with CF has normal lungs at birth, evidence of inflammation and lung changes are present as early as 4 weeks of age. Thus, if gene therapy is going to be used, it should be used sooner rather than later.

Until recently, the only gene therapies that have been employed very early in children have been part of the treatment of adenosine deaminase deficiency, but as of the past year, over 100 patients with CF have received the gene in gene therapy trials. We will not know for some time exactly how effective such therapy will be. In the meantime, good nutrition, aggressive use of antibiotics, and meticulous physical therapy are the keys to keeping patients alive. If you want to read more about the status of gene therapy for CF, see the excellent review of this topic by Jaffe et al.[1]

J.A. Stockman III, M.D.

Reference

1. Jaffe A, Bush A, Geddes DM, et al: Prospects for gene therapy in cystic fibrosis. *Arch Dis Child* 80:286-289, 1999.

Effect of Prolonged Methylprednisolone Therapy in Unresolving Acute Respiratory Distress Syndrome: A Randomized Controlled Trial
Meduri GU, Headley AS, Golden E, et al (Univ of Tennessee, Memphis)
JAMA 280:159-165, 1998   11–7

Background.—To date, no pharmacologic therapy has effectively modified the clinical course of acute respiratory distress syndrome (ARDS). Mortality remains higher than 50%. The value of prolonged methylprednisolone treatment in patients with unresolving ARDS was studied.

Methods.—Twenty-four patients with severe ARDS were enrolled in the randomized, double-blind, placebo-controlled trial. In all patients, the lung injury score had failed to improve by the seventh day of respiratory failure. Sixteen patients were given methylprednisolone at an initial dose of 2 mg/kg per day. The remaining 8 patients were given placebo. Treatment duration was 32 days. Four patients with lung injury score who did not improve by at least 1 point after 10 days of treatment were crossed over (blindly) to the alternative group.

Findings.—By treatment day 10, methylprednisolone recipients had reduced lung injury score, improved ratio of PaO_2 to FIO_2, reduced multiple organ dysfunction syndrome score, and successful intubation compared with placebo recipients. Intensive care unit mortality was 0 in the methylprednisolone group and 62% in the placebo group. Hospital-associated mortality was 12% and 62%, respectively. The 2 groups had similar rates of infection per day of treatment. Pneumonia was commonly detected in the absence of fever.

Conclusions.—Prolonged methylprednisolone therapy in patients with unresolving ARDS improves lung injury score and multiple organ dysfunction syndrome score. Mortality is also significantly reduced. Timing of methylprednisolone administration affected treatment response. Few clinically important complications were associated with methylprednisolone.

▶ The ARDS has also been commonly called the *adult* respiratory distress syndrome, presumably to differentiate it from the type of problem we see in our premature intensive care nursery. ARDS, however, is not just a problem of adults; it can affect children, and commonly does as a complication of a variety of illnesses associated with the rapid development of diffuse injury to the terminal portions of the respiratory tract resulting in a exudative pulmonary edema. ARDS is associated with a very high mortality, ranging from 35% to 65% in mixed aged studies. Severe hypoxemia (i.e., an oxygenation ratio of PaO_2 to fraction of inspired oxygen [FIO_2] of < 200) is the hallmark of the syndrome, but most fatalities result from associated conditions, especially multiple organ failure and sepsis, and less commonly from intractable respiratory failure.

The usual circumstance under which ARDS occurs is as a consequence of direct lung injury, such as pulmonary infection, or indirect lung injury, such as observed in sepsis or a host of other non-pulmonary conditions. Early ARDS is associated with a local and systemic inflammatory response, with high levels of inflammatory mediators in the bronchoalveolar lavage fluid. Soon after this initial acute lung injury, lung repair and remodeling occurs and is associated with high levels of growth factors and a marked increase in collagen synthesis, so much so that if the patient survives, he or she might develop fibrosing alveolitis. The injury is also aggravated by high pressure mechanical ventilation.

Attempts to pharmacologically blunt the early inflammatory response thought to contribute to the lung injury have targeted various steps of the inflammatory process. Agents such as steroids, anticytokine therapy, antioxidants, cyclooxygenase inhibitors, and prostaglandins have all been tried. Unfortunately, none of these approaches has been established as both safe and effective. The results of randomized trials of the early introduction of high-dosed steroids in ARDS have also been disappointing.

This study examining the prolonged use of methylprednisolone therapy in unresolving ARDS suggests it may never be too late to try steroids. While early therapy doesn't work, late introduction of steroids just might. The problem with the trial involving the late introduction of steroids relates to the small numbers of patients in this study. Given this limitation, the beneficial effects of steroids must be interpreted with caution, and these results must be confirmed in a larger trial before steroid therapy gains widespread acceptance in unresolving ARDS. Nevertheless, this trial provides a strong impetus for further testing of a new approach in an area that needs desperately innovative therapeutic strategies.

Whoever said that no one should ever die without being afforded the benefit of steroids? For more on the topic of steroid therapy and ARDS, see the excellent commentary by Brun-Buisson and Brochard.[1]

J.A. Stockman III, M.D.

Reference

1. Brun-Buisson C, Brochard L: Corticosteroid therapy in acute respiratory distress syndrome: Better late than never? *JAMA* 280:182-183,1998.

Tobacco and Alcohol Use Among 1996 Medical School Graduates
Mangus RS, Hawkins CE, Miller MJ (Oregon Health Sciences Univ)
JAMA 280:1192-1193, 1195, 1998   11–8

Introduction.—The health-related behavior of medical professionals has drawn considerable attention in this era of prevention and health promotion. Addiction of physicians to chemical substances has long been a concern, although it is a problem that can afflict any person. Although tobacco use has declined among physicians in the last 50 years, alcohol intake has remained steady. The prevalence of tobacco use and the patterns of alcohol consumption among medical students graduating in 1996 was assessed.

Methods.—Questionnaires were placed in the campus mailboxes of 1,001 graduating medical students. Of these, 549 (55%) were returned. Questions about overall general health status, practices, social and professional relationships, and demographics, were asked in the questionnaire, which took about 10 minutes to complete.

Results.—Respondents were aged from 23 to 47 years. Smokers were found among 2% of the graduating students, with 13% who reported ever having been smokers. A history of previous smoking was more common with increased age. Eighteen percent of students reported frequent alcohol use (3 or more days a week), and 21% of students reported at least 1 episode of binge drinking (5 or more drinks in one sitting) in the past 30 days. Both of these behaviors were significantly more likely to have been exhibited by men students than women students. More than 2 drinks at each drinking session was consumed by 18% of respondents. Binge drinking was more likely to be reported by white students than by any of the other racial groups. Alcohol intake was believed to have increased among 18% of women and 11% of men while in college.

Conclusion.—An important decline in the prevalence of tobacco use was found among medical students in this survey. The patterns of physician alcohol intake have remained steady or have shown a slight increase. Alcohol is consumed by younger physicians with the same frequency and in the same amounts as their age-related peers. In contrast to the intake of the general population, alcohol intake among physicians tends to increase with age.

▶ It's astounding how far we've come educating medical students about the hazards of smoking. It would appear that just 2% of those exiting our ivy clad halls of medicine partake of the dirty weed. We are good role models indeed.

Alcohol is another story. Would you believe that almost 20% of medical students report frequent alcohol use? Even more alarming is that 1 in 5 also report at least 1 episode of binge drinking in the last month. It is easy to see why 50% of all medical students graduate in the bottom half of their class.

J.A. Stockman III, M.D.

Increased Levels of Cigarette Use Among College Students: A Cause for National Concern
Wechsler H, Rigotti NA, Gledhill-Hoyt J, et al (Harvard School of Public Health, Boston; Harvard Med School, Boston; Univ of California, Los Angeles)
JAMA 280:1673-1678, 1998   11–9

Background.—Each year the Monitoring the Future Study provides information about the number of adolescents in high school who smoke. Data indicate that the prevalence of smoking in this population has increased since 1991. However, data on changes in smoking incidence over time in the college population are lacking. These authors surveyed 116 representative United States 4-year colleges in 1993 and again in 1997 to characterize changes in cigarette use in college students.

Methods.—The questionnaire created for the 1993 College Alcohol Study also gathered information on the number of cigarettes smoked in the previous 30 days and in the previous year. This survey was completed by 15,103 students (70% response rate) in 1993 and by 14,251 students (60% response rate) at the same colleges in 1997. The 1997 survey also asked about the respondent's age at first tobacco use and the number of attempts to quit smoking.

Findings.—Between 1993 and 1997, there was a 27.8% increase in the prevalence of current cigarette smoking (within the past 30 days; from 22.3% to 38.5%). The prevalence of current smoking increased at 99 of the 116 colleges surveyed (85%), and the increase was statistically significant at 27 of these schools (23%). Significant increases in current cigarette smoking occurred for almost all demographic groups, including males (23.4%), females (31%), African Americans (42.7%), whites (31.2%), Asians/Pacific Islanders (22.5%), those less than 24 years of age (29.8%), those 24 years of age and older (18.5%), freshmen (28.4%), sophomores (20.7%), juniors (32.4%), and seniors (21.6%). Furthermore, significant increases in current cigarette smoking occurred across the colleges regardless of their characteristics (commuter vs noncommuter, public vs private, etc.). Most prominently, the incidence of current smoking rose faster at public colleges (33.1%, vs 16.8% at private schools) and in the North Central (35.2%) and West (32.3%) regions.

According to the 1997 survey, 11% of smokers had their first cigarette at age 19 years or younger and 28% began to smoke at age older than 19 years, that is, when they were in college. Half the current smokers had tried to quit smoking in the previous year, and almost 1 in 5 (18%) had made 5 or more attempts to quit.

Conclusion.—In almost all demographic groups and in all types of schools, cigarette smoking is on the rise in United States colleges. More than a quarter of the current smokers began smoking after they entered college. Nonetheless, many of these young smokers are trying to kick their nicotine habit. Thus, smoking cessation programs and other interventions targeted specifically to college students are needed at a national level.

▶ Some of us had thought that we were beginning to win the war on cigarettes—apparently not so when it comes to college students. The fact that college students are smoking more and more relates to Murphy's Rule No. 97: IQ and practical intelligence are inversely related. In a short, recent 4-year period, cigarette smoking has grown by almost 30% among our collegiate progeny.

That's the bad news. The good news is that a fair percentage of college smokers only begin to start smoking when they enter college and many (almost half) recognize the problem they have gotten into and will try to quit smoking. Thus, we have an opportunity to put into place targeted programs on college campuses to either prevent smoking, or to help students quit smoking, once begun. The college years are not the only time when young people recognize that smoking is a bad habit. Among 485 smoking high schoolers in San Jose, California, more than half reported 1 or more attempts to quit smoking.[1]

Other bad news related to tobacco smoke includes the recognition that children in a family in which there are 2 or more household smokers are more than twice as likely to have middle ear disease in the first few years of life.[2] So that's the bad news. What is the good news when it comes to smoking? There isn't much. One minor benefit (or debit, depending on the circumstances) of smoking is a decreased pregnancy rate. Women who smoke during adolescence have a 50% lower chance of becoming pregnant as an adolescent, and when they do become pregnant, the delay in onset of pregnancy is some 22.6 months.[3] Who would have ever thought that putting something in your mouth would be a partially effective contraceptive?

The last bit of news is that, if you are a bartender in a state that has banned smoking, your health has been significantly improved.[4] Such bartenders now no longer wheeze, cough, or hock up sputum, all presumably because of the enlightenment of their state legislatures in banning smoking in public places. Manufacturers of spittoons, take heed.

On a slightly different note, it has been said that Europeans are more willing to tolerate second-hand smoke and are less supportive of clean indoor air regulations than are Americans. It has also been said that because of this, we here in the United States, where such regulations are becoming increasingly common in hotels and restaurants, should be expecting to see fewer and fewer Europeans wanting to be tourists on our shores. Actually, the data do not support this. For many years, the tobacco industry has warned states that contemplate enacting laws mandating smoke-free restaurants that they were only shooting themselves in the foot in terms of foreign tourism. Secret research conducted for the Phillip Morris Company in 1989, however, shows that this belief is incorrect. Phillip Morris polled 1000 people in each of 10 European countries and found that smokers were more accepting of the smoke-free restaurant ordinances than were Americans.[5] Also, a comparison of hotel revenues and tourism rates before and after passage of 100% smoke-free restaurant ordinances shows that passage of the ordinances is associated with either a statistically significant increase in hotel revenues or no change in revenues in the overwhelming majority of localities where such ordinances are instituted.[6] International tourism in the latter report was either unaffected or actually increased following implementation of smoke-free ordinances.

If Jerome Kern were to write *Smoke Gets In Your Eyes* again, and if MTV were to do a musical video of it, you can bet that it wouldn't be shot in an American bistro.

Lastly, why is it that some can easily give up cigarette smoking and others cannot? The answer lies in one's genes. People who carry allele 9 of the dopamine transporter gene (*SLC6A3*) are less likely to be smokers. While the correlation between starting to smoke and the *SLC6A3-9* genotype is a weak one, not so weak is the ability to stop smoking if you have this genotype. People with the allele 9 are 1.5 times more likely to have given up smoking than those without it. Apparently it is hard to stay hooked on smoking if you have this genotype.[7]

J.A. Stockman III, M.D.

References

1. Rojas ML, Killen JD, Haydel KF, et al: Nicotine dependence among adolescent smokers. *Arch Pediatr Adolesc Med* 152:151, 1998.
2. Adair-Bischoff CE, Sauve RS: Environmental tobacco smoke and middle ear disease in preschool aged children. *Arch Pediatr Adolesc Med* 152:127-133, 1998.
3. Fiscella K, Kitzman HJ, Cole RE, et al: Delayed first pregnancy among African-American adolescent smokers. *J Adolesc Health* 23:232-237, 1998.
4. Eisner MD, Smith AK, Blanc PD: Bartenders' respiratory health after establishment of smoke-free bars and taverns. *JAMA* 280:1909-1914, 1998.
5. Phillip Morris, International Web Site: Tobacco issues 1989: How today's smokers and non-smokers in Europe feel about smoking issues. October, 1989. Available at: *http://www.pmdocs.com*.
6. Glantz SA, Charlesworth A: Tourism and hotel revenues before and after passage of smoke-free restaurant ordinances. *JAMA* 281:1911-1918, 1999.
7. Senior JA: The need for a cigarette: Does it reside in the genome? *Lancet* 353:384, 1999.

12 The Heart and Blood Vessels

Prevalence of Sudden Cardiac Death During Competitive Sports Activities in Minnesota High School Athletes
Maron BJ, Gohman TE, Aeppli D (Minneapolis Heart Inst Found; Univ of Minnesota, Minneapolis)
J Am Coll Cardiol 32:1881-1884, 1998   12–1

Introduction.—A variety of underlying and usually unsuspected structural cardiovascular diseases are the cause of sudden deaths on the athletic field. The frequency of such deaths is still unknown but would be useful in designing the most effective preparticipation screening strategies. A high school student population was studied to determine deaths caused by cardiovascular disease and to establish reliable estimates of the frequency of these catastrophic events.

Methods.—In Minnesota, the precise number of participants and deaths caused by cardiovascular diseases was ascertained over a 12-year period based on an insurance program for catastrophic injury or death. This insurance program was mandatory for all student athletes competing in interscholastic sports. Covered were 27 high school sports, 651,695 student athlete participants, and 1,453,280 overall sports participants.

Results.—There were 3 sudden deaths caused by cardiovascular disease in grades 10 to 12 over the 12-year period (Table 1). One death was the result of anomalous origin of the left main coronary artery from the right sinus of Valsalva. Another was caused by congenital aortic valve stenosis (with bicuspid valve), and the third was caused by myocarditis. The athletes were male, white, and 16 or 17 years of age. One competed in basketball and the other 2 in cross country/track. Per academic year, the calculated risk for sudden death was 1:500,000 participations and 1:217,400 participants. The estimated risk over a 3-year high school career for a student athlete was 1:72,500.

Conclusion.—In a population of high school student athletes, the risk of sudden cardiac death was small, in the range of 1 in 200,000 per year. In male athletes, this risk was higher. The limitations implicit in structuring productive and cost-effective, broad-based preparticipation screening strategies for high school athletes are underlined by the rare occurrence of sudden cardiac death in competitive sports.

TABLE 1.—Profiles of Sudden Cardiac Deaths in Minnesota High School Athletes

No.	Age at Death (Years)	Year of Death	Race/ Gender	Sport	Circumstances of Collapse	Heart Weight (g)	Time of Day	Diagnosis
1	16	1990	W/M	Cross-country	During warm-up, stretching exercises	460	3 PM	Anomalous left main coronary artery
2	16	1993	W/M	Cross-country	Early during 5-K race	385	10 AM	Myocarditis
3	17	1996	W/M	Basketball	Minutes after entering game became fatigued; removed self from game; collapsed on bench	—	6 PM	Aortic valvular stenosis (bicuspid valve)

(Reprinted with permission from the American College of Cardiology, from Maron BJ, Gohman TE, Aeppli D: Prevalence of sudden cardiac death during competitive sports activities in Minnesota high school athletes. *J Am Coll Cardiol* 32:1881-1884, 1998.)

▶ If you want to know the prevalence of cardiac disease among those engaging in competitive high school sports, Minnesota is the state to examine. The reason is that the Minnesota State High School League has an extensive database on medical illness in high schoolers who compete in sporting activities. The league is a voluntary, nonprofit association of schools (independent of the Board of Education) that is responsible for a variety of administrative functions related to student athletes within the 440 public and private high schools of Minnesota. The league provides a mandatory insurance program covering catastrophic injury or death for all student athletes engaged in interscholastic sporting programs at both the junior varsity and varsity levels. The database that has been accumulated over the last decade and a half provides a rich source of information about all kinds of problems in high schoolers, including data on deaths caused by cardiovascular diseases.

So what is the chance that an otherwise healthy teenage athlete will suddenly die as a result of cardiovascular problems while competing in an interscholastic sporting event? It turns out that the prevalence of sudden death in such circumstances is about 1 in 200,000 individual participants per academic year and about 1 in 130,000 male athletes. If you look at this in the context of an average 3 years of high school interscholastic athletic activity, the overall risk for sudden death is just about 1 in 70,000, a relatively reassuring figure suggesting that despite all of the hype by the news media—which has given substantial visibility to isolated catastrophic events—these events are still quite rare.

Despite the rarity of cardiac events on the playing field, full preparticipation screening is still necessary. Unfortunately there are no well-established procedures for determining whether amateur athletes with cardiovascular disease are eligible to participate in competitive sports, particularly at the college level. Organizations such as the National Collegiate Athletic Association do not have standards for excluding athletes with heart disease, but do permit member institutions to establish physical qualifications and assign responsibility to team physicians for making all such medical determinations. In 1994, a consensus panel known as the 26th Bethesda Conference (sponsored by the American College of Cardiology) addressed the medical eligibility criteria for participation in competitive sports in a systematic, prospective fashion and provides specific, unbiased recommendations with respect to more than 70 specific cardiovascular abnormalities.

By the way, in the Minnesota experience, there were just 3 deaths in high schoolers from cardiovascular events. One death was from an anomalous origin of the left main coronary artery from the right sinus of Valsalva; 1 death was from myocarditis, and 1 death was from congenital aortic valve stenosis. Only the last would have been detectable by a preparticipation screening.

As pediatricians, we should be generally familiar with what to do should there be an untoward event, cardiac-wise, occurring on the playing field. The chance of something happening, as noted above, is quite small and actually much less than would be the call for assistance, say, on an airliner these days. American Airlines was the first airline to carry full cardiac arrest equipment including defibrillators on any of its aircrafts. By mid-1998, all of their planes had such equipment. On that carrier alone, in a 1-year period, defibrillators were used 65 times, although primarily as monitors. One patient did have his life saved as a result of having a readily available defibrillator. Flight attendants are trained to use the equipment without the involvement of a physician. Such involvement is purely voluntary.[1] Thus, if you're the type of physician who hasn't been near a defibrillator in years, you may render assistance, but at the same time, you may want to let the flight attendant deliver the shock. Also, please note that physicians who do assist in medical emergencies on airliners are the ones who make the decision about the need for the plane to land at the nearest airport because of a medical emergency. Such decisions are those, and those alone, of the involved physician. Pilots are obligated to accept such decisions unless the safety of other passengers would be put at risk.

J.A. Stockman III, M.D.

Reference

1. McKenas DK: Letter to the editor. *N Engl J Med* 339:928, 1998.

Profile of Preparticipation Cardiovascular Screening for High School Athletes
Glover DW, Maron BJ (St Luke's Hosp, Kansas City, Mo; Minneapolis Heart Inst Found)
JAMA 279:1817-1819, 1998   12–2

Objective.—Interest in preparticipation screening for competitive high school athletes is increasing because of reports of sudden death in young athletes as a result of unsuspected cardiovascular disease. Preparticipation screening procedures available to high school athletes were assessed for adequacy.

Methods.—Guidelines, requirements, and screening measures of high school athletic associations from 50 states and the District of Columbia were reviewed and compared with the 1996 American Heart Association (AHA) consensus panel guidelines on screening.

Results.—Whereas all jurisdictions except Rhode Island require an examination before athletic participation, 8 states do not have recommended history and physical questionnaire guidelines. Important cardiovascular items were included in 0 to 56% of the state forms, and only 26 states required parental verification and approval of histories. Specific heart problems were addressed on only 5% to 37% of physical examination forms. Of 39 states with history and physical examination questionnaires, 16 had not revised their forms in more than 5 years and 6 had not revised their forms in more than 10 years. Seventeen of 43 states' forms contained at least 9 of 13-AHA recommended items. Five of 50 states requiring preparticipation screening had no specific recommendations or requirements regarding examiners. Eleven states allow for practitioners with little or no cardiovascular training, and 25 allow examination by nonphysicians. Only 33 states recommend annual preparticipation screening.

Conclusion.—Preparticipation as it is currently being practiced in U.S. high schools is unlikely to screen out potentially lethal cardiovascular problems effectively. Critically important guidelines are often missing. It is recommended that national standards be developed for preparticipation screening of high school athletes.

▶ Dr. Richard Liberthson, associate professor of Pediatrics, Harvard Medical School, and pediatrician and physician in Medicine, Massachusetts General Hospital, Boston, comments:

Drs. Glover and Maron are to be commended for bringing to our attention the surprising inadequacy of current state-approved guidelines for preparticipation screening of U.S. high school athletes. Their survey reveals significant inadequacy in most states compared with the 1996 American Heart Association recommendations, and 8 states have no guidelines.[1]

Sudden cardiac death in the young athlete is rare and has numerous causes.[2] Many at high risk can be identified by a discerning history and clinical examination; thus, many who have cardiomyopathy, myocarditis, Marfan's syndrome, precocious coronary artery disease and high-risk preoperative and postoperative congenital heart lesions can be appropriately counseled. Other sudden-death-prone entities are more covert, and even sophisticated cardiologic assessment may fail to detect and prevent sudden death in these cases. Certainly, highlighting the risks associated with substance abuse (including steroids) and the dangers of eating disorders will spare some.

It is unlikely that any screening effort can prevent all sudden deaths in young athletes. Clearly, however, optimal screening would prevent some deaths and would allow identified individuals to be referred for appropriate medical supervision.

Large-scale implementation of screening protocols are costly, to be sure. However as cited by Drs. Glover and Maron, in most states guidelines and personnel are already in place and need only modification. It would thus seem appropriate to upgrade both training of examiners and questionnaire content to at least the level recommended by the 1996 American Heart Association Consensus Panel.[1] Conversely, to not do so would seem hard to defend. Prevention of even a few premature deaths would justify the quality upgrade, and an added benefit of these improvements would be the reassurance they provide to students and families and to the school and athletic personnel and physicians.

R. Liberthson, M.D.

References

1. Maron BJ, Thompson PD, Puffer JC, et al: Cardiovascular preparticipation screening of competitive athletes. *Circulation* 94:850-856, 1996.

2. Liberthson RR: Sudden death from cardiac causes in children and young adults. *N Engl J Med* 334:1039-1044, 1996.

Physiologic Left Ventricular Cavity Dilatation in Elite Athletes

Pelliccia A, Culasso F, Di Paolo FM, et al (Univ La Sapienza, Rome; Minneapolis Heart Inst Found)
Ann Intern Med 130:23-31, 1999   12–3

Introduction.—Cardiac morphologic changes such as increased left ventricular cavity dimension, wall thickness, and calculated mass have been associated with long-term athletic training and have been referred to as "athlete's heart." It may be difficult to know the difference between athlete's heart and structural heart disease, and the identification of certain cardiovascular disease may constitute the basis for disqualifying an athlete from competing. Echocardiography was used to systematically evaluate the morphologic characteristics and physiologic limits of left ventricular cavity enlargement associated with intensive and long-term athletic condition in highly trained athletes.

Methods.—There were 1309 elite athletes (957 men and 352 women) ranging in age from 13 to 59 years who participated in 38 different sports. Measurements were taken of the left ventricular cavity dimension with echocardiography, and the determinants were measured through multivariate statistical analysis.

Results.—There was a wide variance of left ventricular end-diastolic cavity dimension. Women had a mean of 48 mm and a range of 38 to 66 mm. Men had a mean of 55 mm and a range of 43 to 70 mm. The dimensions were generally within accepted normal limits ($\leq$54 mm) for 55% of the participants. In 14% of participants, the left ventricular cavity was substantially enlarged, based on an arbitrary clinical cut-point of 60 mm. These athletes had global left ventricular systolic function within normal limits and no regional wall-motion abnormalities. For up to 12 years, the athletes were free of cardiac symptoms and impaired performance. Greater body surface area and participation in certain endurance sports, such as cycling, canoeing, and cross-country skiing, were the major determinants of cavity dimension (Fig 2).

Conclusion.—In almost 15% of participants, the left ventricular cavity dimension was strikingly increased to a degree compatible with primary dilated cardiomyopathy. This cavity dilatation is most likely an extreme physiologic adaptation to intensive athletic conditioning, in the absence of systolic dysfunction. Little is known about the long-term consequences and significance of this marked left ventricular remodeling of the athlete's heart.

▶ Some years back in the YEAR BOOK OF PEDIATRICS, we commented on a report on cardiac septal measurement in highly trained athletes. As the muscle in the heart gets bigger in these athletes, the septal measurements

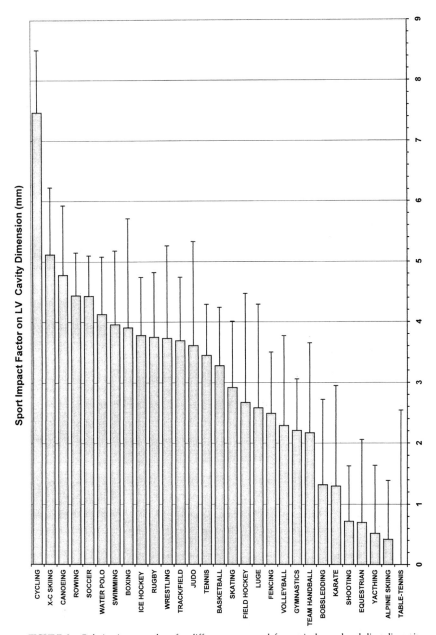

FIGURE 2.—Relative impact values for different sports on left ventricular and end-diastolic cavity dimension. The *bars* show the individual sport regression coefficients and the 95% upper confidence indexes. These impact values were calculated relative to the reference sport (table tennis; regression coefficient, −2.96), which was then set at zero. This figure included the 29 sporting disciplines represented in the study sample with more than 10 participants. (Courtesy of Pelliccia A, Culasso F, DiPaolo FM, et al: Physiologic left ventricular cavity dilatation in elite athletes. *Ann Intern Med* 130:23-31, 1999.)

that are normally used to determine whether someone has hypertrophic cardiomyopathy, do indeed reach high enough numbers that the differentiation of the athlete's heart from the abnormal heart becomes somewhat difficult. At the same time the muscle hypertrophies, the size of the left ventricle during diastole also increases as the heart gets ready to deliver a larger amount of blood with each systole. As this report shows, the size of the left ventricular cavity can be so large that the technical definition of dilated cardiomyopathy is met. Indeed, many (14%) do. Imagine having a left ventricle whose size measures in excess of 70 mm!

It is clear that certain types of sporting activities carry a greater likelihood of developing the athlete's heart. Cycling, cross-country skiing, canoeing, and rowing head the list. As you might suspect, these types of exercises are somewhat more "isometric" than are some others. That is the suspected link. What happens when someone stops being an expert cyclist, cross-country skier, canoer, or rower, is another interesting question. What becomes of that big heart? Does it return to normal size, or will it look like the skeletal muscles of flabby aging wrestlers? Jesse Ventura, can we echo your heart to find the answer?

If you're into exercise, but want to do just enough to lower your risk of heart disease and not so much as to ever develop the kind of enlarged hearts seen in elite athletes, all you really have to do is take a walk in a park for an hour each week. Or, you could spend an hour mowing, raking, or weeding in the garden. Such minimal activity provides substantial protection against sudden cardiac death from myocardial ischemia.[1] Even I would find such minor activity acceptable to keep in shape. Round is a shape, isn't it?

J.A. Stockman III, M.D.

Reference

1. Howards M, Berman S, Samuels J, et al: Exercise and the risk of cardiac events. *Ann Intern Med* 159:686-690, 1999.

Distribution of and Factors Associated With Serum Homocysteine Levels in Children: Child and Adolescent Trial for Cardiovascular Health

Osganian SK, Stampfer MJ, Spiegelman D, et al (New England Research Insts, Watertown, Mass; Harvard Med School, Boston; Natl Heart, Lung, and Blood Inst, Bethesda, Md; et al)
JAMA 281:1189-1196, 1999
12–4

Background.—Evidence suggests that homocysteine is a risk factor for cardiovascular disease in adults. However, little is known about homocysteine levels in children. The distribution of serum homocysteine levels in children was determined, as well as the association between these levels and several other characteristics such as serum concentrations of folic acid and vitamins B_{12} and B_6.

Methods and Findings.—Data on 3524 United States children, aged 13 and 14 years, were analyzed in this cross-sectional analysis. The range of homocysteine values was 0.1 to 25.7 μmol/L. Geometric mean homocysteine levels were significantly greater in boys than in girls, in blacks than in whites or Hispanics, in multivitamin nonusers than in users, and in smokers than in nonsmokers. Homocysteine levels were not significantly correlated with serum lipid levels or family history of cardiovascular disease. In addition, they were only weakly associated with body mass index and systolic blood pressure. After adjustment in a multivariate analysis, homocysteine levels continued to be independently correlated with sex, race, serum folic acid and vitamin B_{12} levels, and systolic blood pressure.

Conclusion.—Although the distribution of homocysteine levels in children is markedly lower than in adults, a small percentage of children may still be at increased risk for future cardiovascular disease. Serum folic acid may be important in determining homocysteine concentrations in children.

▶ The plot thickens when it comes to the relationship between homocysteine levels and cardiovascular health. The thickening agent involved is the child. Now we learn that even children are not immune to the potential that an elevated homocysteine level could eventually affect their well being.

It has been known for some time that an elevation in homocysteine in blood is one of several adverse cardiovascular risk factors. Homocysteine is formed during the conversion of methionine to cysteine. Its main metabolic pathways require folic acid, vitamin B_{12}, and vitamin B_6. The lower the levels of vitamin B_6 and B_{12} and folic acid, the higher the levels of homocysteine. Even a normal person's homocysteine levels can be significantly reduced by taking folic acid. It would appear that a small but significant percentage of children are at potentially elevated risk for future cardiovascular disease as a result of elevated homocysteine levels. Although, overall, children's levels of homocysteine are less than those of adults, some kids are as bad off as their geriatric counterparts. The reason why is related to poor folate intake.

While on the topic of cardiovascular risk factors, the dairy industry is on a high these days. The reason is that a large prospective study of egg consumption has concluded that eating up to 1 egg a day is unlikely to have any substantial overall impact on the risk of heart disease or stroke among healthy men and women. Eggs have really gotten a bad rap in the last 20 years. As a result, in men, the average egg consumption declined from 2.3 eggs per week in 1986 to 1.6 eggs per week in 1990. In women, the average egg consumption declined from 2.8 eggs per week in 1980 to 1.4 eggs per week in 1990. Notable, however, is the fact that those who eat eggs, while consuming more dietary cholesterol and protein, eat significantly less in the way of carbohydrates. It is speculated that the consumption of eggs instead of carbohydrate-rich foods might raise high-density lipoprotein cholesterol levels and decrease blood glycemic and insulinemic responses. Please also recognize that eggs contain unsaturated fats, essential amino acids, folate, and a whole variety of B vitamins.

So can you have your egg and eat it too? Chances are that yes, you can have up to an egg a day without incurring any substantial overall increased risk of heart disease if you lead a healthy lifestyle otherwise. Take, however, the average person at your corner Waffle House. There you find the proto-typical overweight male not eating just eggs, but eggs with bacon and hash browns fried with lard (with a side of waffles and pancakes), and if right-handed, the left hand is alternately holding a cup of caffeinated coffee and a cigarette. In such circumstances, it is hard to say that eating an egg a day, either way, makes much difference. A daily diet of Egg McMuffins is prob-ably not much better.[1]

J.A. Stockman III, M.D.

Reference

1. Hu FB, Stampfer MJ, Rimm EB: A prospective study of egg consumption and risk of cardiovascular disease in men and women. *JAMA* 281:1387-1394, 1999.

Prevalence and Extent of Atherosclerosis in Adolescents and Young Adults: Implications for Prevention From the Pathobiological Determi-nants of Atherosclerosis in Youth Study
Strong JP, for the Pathobiological Determinants of Atherosclerosis in Youth Research Group (Louisiana State Univ, New Orleans; et al)
JAMA 281:727-735, 1999   12–5

Background.—Atherosclerosis, the underlying cause of coronary heart disease, has been reported even in young adults. The extent and severity of atherosclerosis in adolescents and young adults in the United States were investigated.

Methods and Findings.—Data on 2876 persons, aged 15 to 34 years, who died of external causes and underwent autopsy between June, 1987 and August, 1994 were analyzed. In the 15- to 19-year-old group, intimal lesions appeared in all aortas and in more than half of the right coronary arteries. The prevalence and extent increased with age. Fatty streaks were more extensive in black persons than in white persons; however, raised lesions did not differ between these 2 racial groups. Raised lesions in the aorta were similar in men and women, but women had fewer raised lesions in the right coronary arteries. The proportion of raised lesions among total lesions was greater in the right coronary artery than in the aorta.

Conclusions.—This study shows that atherosclerosis begins in youth. Between 15 and 34 years of age, the prevalence and extent of fatty streaks and clinically significant raised lesions increased rapidly. Primary preven-tion of atherosclerosis must begin in childhood or adolescence.

▶ This past year has been an interesting one. Not only did we learn that statins, the cholesterol lowering agents, could be safely and effectively used to lower a teenager's cardiac risk factors, but we also learned that virtually all teenagers, even those without high cholesterols, etc., already have inti-mal lesions in their aortas and half have abnormal coronary arteries. The most common early lesions are fatty streaks. There is no longer a question of when the primary prevention of heart disease should occur. It is in childhood. This conclusion is really not a surprise. It was back in 1986 that *JAMA* republished the landmark article, a 1953 study by Enos et al.,[1,2] reporting atherosclerosis in young American soldiers killed in the Korean War.

So what does all this mean? It means that each and everyone exiting adolescence has some risk factors for the development of atherosclerosis even if he doesn't smoke, even if he doesn't drink, and even if his total cholesterol is 150. The trick would be to find out during early to mid-adulthood if our coronaries are "normal." Treadmill stress tests are not particularly sensitive for this purpose. There are no good blood tests that are sensitive markers of endothelial damage. Noninvasive US is great at picking up arterial wall lesions in some places in the body such as the neck, but it fails miserably when it comes to the heart. The same is true of MRI. The hottest new thing is electron-beam (or "ultrafast") CT. This differs from conventional CT in that the x-ray source does not need to be rotated around the patient, allowing much faster acquisition of information. It allows the early detection of calcification in atherosclerotic plaques. A large majority of such plaques do have calcium within them.

In the last few years, electron-beam CTs for detecting coronary artery disease have taken off like a rocket. They have become the mammogram of the heart, as it were. News reports in the lay press as well as mass media advertising have promoted the test to the general public, and many CT centers now perform electron-beam CTs permitting patients to self-refer themselves (i.e., the patient schedules the test for him- or herself and receives the results directly without consulting a physician). Many of these centers (most hospital-affiliated and free-standing) rely on self-referred patients for the majority of the volume of their procedures. The average cost of scanning with electron-beam CT is approximately $475. There are currently about 50 electron-beam CT scanners here in the United States. Most are operated in association with hospitals, but the industry projects that the number of scanners in clinical use will double within 1 or 2 years. It's easy to see why the test is appealing; it is noninvasive, has very low radiation exposure, is fast (under 15 minutes), and is quite simple.

Chances are that few of us will be ordering electron-beam CTs for children. It is good to know, however, that the disease that starts more on our watch as pediatricians may be detected during adult life early enough to prevent major coronary events. Also, it may not be too early to think about electron-beam CT scanning for kids with abnormal coronary arteries, such as those who have recovered from Kawasaki disease, to determine if they are developing calcified atherosclerotic plaques. You can bet that we are going hear a great deal more about all of this, including its implications to pediatric care, in the not-too-distant future. To learn more about electron-beam CTs, read the superb commentary of Taylor and O'Malley.[3]

J.A. Stockman III, M.D.

References

1. Enos WF, Holmes RH, Beyer J: Coronary artery disease among United States soldiers killed in action in Korea. *JAMA* 152:1090-1093, 1953.
2. Enos WF, Holmes RH, Beyer J: Coronary artery disease among United States soldiers killed in action in Korea (Landmark article). *JAMA* 256:2059-2062, 1986.
3. Taylor HA, O'Malley PG: Self-referral of patients for electron-beam computed tomography to screen for coronary artery disease. *N Engl J Med* 339:2018-2019, 1998.

Efficacy and Safety of Lovastatin in Adolescent Males With Heterozygous Familial Hypercholesterolemia: A Randomized Controlled Trial
Stein EA, Illingworth DR, Kwiterovich PO Jr, et al (Med Research Labs, Highland Heights, Ky; Metabolic and Atherosclerosis Research Ctr, Cincinnati, Ohio; Oregon Health Sciences Univ, Portland; et al)
JAMA 281:137-144, 1999   12–6

Introduction.—The underlying cause of marked increase in early coronary artery disease is elevated circulating low-density lipoprotein cholesterol levels found in familial hypercholesterolemia, a dominant genetic disorder. The risk of clinically overt coronary artery disease is up to 50% by age 50 years in men with untreated heterozygous familial hypercholesterolemia. It is considered medically appropriate to begin lipid-lowering treatment in select children with heterozygous familial hypercholesterolemia; however, the proper age to begin such treatment is still unknown. Statins have been shown to reduce total cholesterol and low-density lipoprotein cholesterol. Adolescent boys with severe heterozygous familial hypercholesterolemia were evaluated to assess the lipid-lowering efficacy of lovastatin and its effect on growth, sexual maturation, and biochemical, nutritional, and endocrine parameters.

Methods.—There were 132 boys aged 10 to 17 years with heterozygous familial hypercholesterolemia who were randomized to receive lovastatin or placebo. In the first 24-week period, lovastatin was increased at 8 and 16 weeks; during the second 24-week period, the dosage remained stable. Lovastatin was administered at a dose that began at 10 mg/day, with a forced titration at 8 weeks to 20 mg/day and at 16 weeks to 40 mg/day.

Results.—There was a significant decrease in low-density lipoprotein cholesterol levels among the boys receiving lovastatin. With a dose of 10 mg/day, there was a 17% decrease; with a dose of 20 mg/day, there was a 24% decrease, and with a dose of 40 mg/day, there was a decrease of 27%. At 48 weeks, the level remained 25% lower than baseline. The lovastatin and placebo groups had no difference in growth and sexual maturation, testicular volume, serum hormone levels, or biochemical parameters of nutrition throughout the study. Significant differences in safety parameters could not be detected because the study was underpowered. Lovastatin treatment resulted in a reduction in serum vitamin E levels, which was consistent with reductions in the levels of low-density lipoprotein choles-terol, the major carrier of vitamin E in the circulation.

Conclusion.—The low-density lipoprotein cholesterol–reducing effec-tiveness of lovastatin was confirmed in this study of adolescent boys with heterozygous familial hypercholesterolemia. During 48 weeks, no signifi-cant differences between lovastatin and placebo were seen in the compre-hensive clinical and biochemical data on growth, hormonal, and nutri-tional status. Further study is necessary.

▶ Our knowledge of whether we can effectively and safely treat children with heterozygous familial hypercholesterolemia using statins has been hampered by reports that have been very modest in size. Because the prevalence of this disorder is only approximately 0.2% in the population, it is difficult to study large numbers of patients to detect adverse effects that are low in frequency. Fortunately, this study gives us good information, because it is the largest and longest placebo-controlled trial of any lipid-lowering drug used in an adolescent population. Furthermore, the authors chose an age group that was at a critical stage in growth and development, so if there was going to be any evidence of clinical and/or biochemical disturbance, it would likely have been picked up. None was detected.

Heterozygous familial hypercholesterolemia is no laughing matter. Among the boys enrolled in this study, 1 in 5 had already lost a father to a coronary event. The biochemical abnormality is known to cause a risk of clinically obvious coronary artery disease of 20% by age 40 years and 50% by 50 years. Earlier methods of reducing low-density lipoprotein cholesterol in the teen population have not proven to be very effective. Diet therapy low in saturated fat and cholesterol has a relatively small effect on reducing low-density lipoprotein cholesterol. Bile acid sequestrants have been around for well over 2 decades. These agents are safe, but their impact on low-density lipoprotein cholesterol is fairly modest. This plus the fact that most teens, and even adults, find their use so noxious means that long-term compliance is abysmal. Alternative therapy in the form of nicotinic acid is rarely used in childhood and adolescence because of tolerance problems. Fibric acid de-rivatives have met a similar fate. Thus, statins hold the greatest promise because they are simply a matter of taking a pill a day. In this report, at least, there were virtually no significant side effects.

Gene therapy may be the answer to some problems related to cholesterol abnormalities. Investigators are actively working on therapies that could effectively and permanently turn on low-density lipoprotein liver receptors. Also, while on the topic of gene therapy, investigators from Boston have reported on 16 patients (all adults) with severe refractory angina, all of whom had had coronary artery bypass graft or percutaneous transluminal coronary angioplasty. To stimulate new blood growth, the patients received a direct myocardial injection of the gene for vascular endothelial growth factor via a minithoracotomy. Symptoms improved in all 16 patients and nitroglycerin use dropped from an average of 60 tablets a week to just 2.5 tablets per week. Sixty percent of the patients are entirely free of angina.[1]

For better or worse, we are what we are because of our genes, especially when some of us, cardiac-wise, have a gene pool without much of a deep end. Whether gene therapy will ultimately prove to be the magic bullet for most diseases or whether we will find out that it's not nice to fool Mother Nature is the challenge of this millennium.

J.A. Stockman III, M.D.

Reference

1. Husten L: Gene therapy door opened wider (editorial). *Lancet* 352:1603, 1998.

Reduced Fetal Growth Rate and Increased Risk of Death From Is-chaemic Heart Disease: Cohort Study of 15 000 Swedish Men and Women Born 1915-29
Leon DA, Lithell HO, Vågerö D, et al (London School of Hygiene and Tropical Medicine; Univ of Uppsala, Sweden; Stockholm Univ)
BMJ 317:241-245, 1998   12–7

Background.—Previous research has suggested that cardiovascular disease, particularly ischemic heart disease, is inversely associated with birth weight. To date, no one has attempted to systematically study whether it is the rate of fetal growth that underlies the correlation of size at birth with cardiovascular mortality. The current cohort study examined whether fetal growth rate is associated with death from ischemic heart disease.

Methods.—All 14,611 babies born at the Uppsala Academic Hospital in Sweden between 1915 and 1929 were followed up to the end of 1995. Follow-up data on 97% of the cohort were obtained.

Findings.—Cardiovascular disease was associated inversely with birth weight among males and females, although the correlation was significant only for the males. A 1000-g increase in birth weight among males was correlated with a proportional decrease of 0.77 in the rate of ischemic heart disease. This effect was attenuated slightly after adjustment for socioeconomic circumstances at birth and in adulthood. Compared with the lowest quartile of birth weight for gestational age, males in the second, third, and fourth quartiles had an ischemic heart disease death rate of 0.81, 0.63, and 0.67, respectively.

Conclusions.—These data are persuasive evidence of an association between size at birth and death from ischemic heart disease in men. Methodologic artifact or socioeconomic confounders cannot explain this correlation. Variation in fetal growth rate, rather than size at birth, appears to be the causal factor.

▶ This editor read this report from London and Sweden at least 3 times to try and see any plausible explanation why being smaller than expected at birth causes premature death of coronary artery disease. No real explanation is offered, so we are left to our own devices in determining why an inverse relationship exists between birth weight and longevity. This is the one and only study that has examined this potential problem. Needless to say, those individuals followed in this report were born many decades ago, and it is entirely possible that low birth weight for gestational age babies born now may not experience the same premature demise.

This is the last entry in the Heart and Blood Vessels chapter dealing with risk factors for coronary artery disease, so we'll close with a few fast facts about such factors. First, data now suggest that garlic does not lower cholesterol levels. In a randomized controlled trial comparing tablets containing garlic powder with a placebo administered for some months, there was no effect of garlic on cholesterol, triglycerides, or lipoprotein profiles.[1] Please note that the patients involved in this study were single adults who remained single, perhaps a biological (and logical) consequence of the garlic.

Next, recent data have suggested that you can drink coffee and not be worried about the possibility of an increased risk of myocardial infarction, at least here in the United States. Recent studies have suggested that if there is any association between coffee drinking and myocardial infarction, it occurs in Europe, where 10 to 12 cups of coffee a day are quite commonly ingested. Contrarily, there are excellent data now that suggests tea drinkers have a significantly lower risk of heart attack, perhaps a 50% reduction in risk. It is suggested that tea may be beneficial because it contains flavonoids, which reduce platelet aggregation and inhibit LDL-cholesterol oxidation. Flavonoids are a hot area of nutrition research, partly because tea makers want to tout their product as a good choice.[2] Next, if you want to remain trim, don't move to New Orleans. New Orleans leads the United States with the most obese people. It is a city where just under 40% of all adults tip the scales at well above the mean. If you're wondering where the fewest obese people are found, it's in Denver, where just 22% of adults challenge the weight scales. If you want a full rundown on the ponderosity of most cities in the country, see *USA Today*.[3]

Lastly, if you think you are avoiding fat by going to Chinese restaurants, you may be thinking wrong, depending on what you order. For example, if you order sweet and sour pork or Kung Pao chicken, you would be ordering dishes with 71 and 76 grams of fat, respectively. That is a full 40 g of fat more than a McDonald's biscuit with sausage and egg. When dining Oriental style, stick with steamed rice. Your heart will love you for it.

J.A. Stockman III, M.D.

References

1. Garlic fails to lower cholesterol levels (editorial). *Arch Intern Med* 158:1189-1194, 1998.
2. Wehrwein P: More evidence that tea is good for the heart. *Lancet* 353:384, 1999.
3. Hellmich N: New Orleans tops scales for obesity. *USA Today*. March 4, 1997; Life section:1D.

Diagnostic Accuracy of Pediatric Echocardiograms Performed in Adult Laboratories

Stanger P, Silverman NH, Foster E (Univ of California, San Francisco)
Am J Cardiol 83:908-914, 1999   12–8

Background.—The diagnostic accuracy of echocardiography in children has never been evaluated. The accuracy of pediatric echocardiograms performed and evaluated in adult laboratories was compared prospectively with evaluations in pediatric laboratories.

Methods.—Data were obtained from 66 patients, aged 1 day to 18 years, undergoing adult-laboratory echocardiography in community hospitals or private offices before assessment by a pediatric cardiologist. Sixty-five of these patients later underwent echocardiography in a university hospital pediatric laboratory.

Findings.—Eighteen patients had no cardiac disease; 42 had simple lesions; 5 had intermediate lesions; and 1 had a complex lesion. In 25 patients with 46 procedure-proved diagnoses, the most important error in adult-laboratory echography was major in 44%, moderate in 28%, and minor in 12%. In pediatric-laboratory echocardiography, the most important error was major in none, moderate in 4%, and minor in 4%. Among 41 patients with 62 duplicate-observer–verified diagnoses, the most important error in adult-laboratory echography was major in 12%, moderate in 29%, and minor in 12%, compared with no errors in pediatric-laboratory echocardiography. In 53% of the adult-laboratory echocardiograms, the most important error was major or moderate; 71% of these were interpretive, 17% technical, and 11% both. The incidences of error were unassociated with patient age, year of study, the use of color Doppler, or complexity of diagnoses. In 29 of these 35 patients, pediatric-laboratory echograms altered clinical management, including 12 operations and 2 averted operations. In 3 of the 29, delayed diagnoses were correlated with fixed pulmonary vascular disease, hypoxemic spells, and vascular collapse with severe metabolic acidosis.

Conclusion.—The incidence of diagnostic errors in pediatric echocardiography done in community-based adult laboratories is high, despite a preponderance of simple diagnoses or no heart disease. In this series, at least 3 delayed diagnoses were associated with clinical problems.

▶ This report really comes as no surprise, although it is disturbing to see that adult cardiologists are willing to undertake the practice of pediatric cardiology, even in the limited sense of performing echocardiography, given the high error rates involved. The average adult cardiologist is more than 20 times more likely to make an error in performing or reading an echocardiogram of a child than is a pediatric cardiologist. An echo is not an echo, is not an echo. Its interpretation requires complete familiarity with a different anatomy, physiology, and echocardiographic appearance and different Doppler characteristics of the various congenital cardiac anomalies and of normal pediatric hearts. It is as easy for adult cardiologists to overread as to underread, given the extent of their training and the profound variations that are normally found in pediatric patients. A seasoned pediatric cardiologist is familiar with all of these issues.

So why do kids wind up in an adult cardiac laboratory? In some cases, the parents make the choice because of proximity to their home. In others, the pediatrician has had a relationship with a colleague treating adults and has no reason to think that the colleague has inadequate skills in interpreting pediatric studies. In other cases, the health care provider dictates the referral line. In each of these situations, with a little bit of work (and advocacy for children), correct referral lines should be able to be established.

If you are fortunate enough to drive a Maserati, chances are that you would not take it to your local Kia dealer to have it serviced. Children should be thought of as being analogous to a fine automobile. When their carburetor is on the fritz, the correct subspecialist should be in order. That is a pediatric cardiologist well seasoned in echocardiographic interpretations.

While we're on the topic of technology and cardiology, do you know when the stethoscope became a routine part of the diagnostic armamentarium of care providers in this country? Well, it was about 1910 when the stethoscope first became an essential tool of the practicing physician. Auscultation of the heart and lungs had become a trademark of physicians' highly skilled physical examination just about that time. In addition, the stethoscope was the one medical tool that had not passed on into the hands of nursing staff. That didn't happen until around the 1950s, when nurses acquired stethoscopes in conjunction with the gradual acceptance of the nurse's role in the measurement of blood pressure. Please note that when nurses were "permitted" to use stethoscopes, this was done somewhat begrudgingly. Physicians made sure that great care was exercised to avoid any confusion between the nurses' tool and the physicians' tool. The new nursing stethoscopes of the '50s and '60s came with names such as *assistascope* and *nurse-o-scope*. The latter were made of lightweight, pastel-colored materials to clearly distinguish such instruments from the heavy, black tools that were in the exclusive domain of physicians. Apparently, more serious tools implied more serious practices, helping to avoid the appearance of overlap between the nursing profession and the practice of medicine by physicians.[1]

J.A. Stockman III, M.D.

Reference

1. Krenner CJ: The rise of the stethoscope. *Ann Intern Med* 128:488-490, 1998.

Using Fetal Nuchal Translucency to Screen for Major Congenital Cardiac Defects at 10-14 Weeks of Gestation: Population Based Cohort Study

Hyett J, Perdu M, Sharland G, et al (King's College Hosp, London; Guy's Hosp, London)
BMJ 318:81-85, 1999   12-9

Purpose.—Prenatal diagnosis of most major congenital cardiac defects can be made at around 20 weeks' gestation, but it is difficult to identify high-risk pregnancies requiring referral to a specialist center. The current screening approach consists of a 4-chamber view of the heart at 16 to 22 weeks' gestation. US measurement of the fetal nuchal translucency at 10 to 14 weeks' gestation may be a more sensitive approach. This method of screening for major congenital cardiac defects was evaluated in a population-based cohort study.

Methods.—The retrospective analysis included 29,154 singleton pregnancies with a chromosomally normal fetus. All underwent US examination at 10 to 14 weeks' gestation, including measurement of the fetal nuchal transparency thickness. The diagnostic performance of this measurement in screening for major cardiac defects was evaluated.

Results.—Fifty fetuses with major defects of the heart and great arteries were identified, for a prevalence of 1.7/1000 pregnancies. On US examination, 1822 pregnancies had fetal nuchal translucency thicknesses above the 95th percentile of normal. Twenty-eight of these fetuses had major congenital cardiac defects. Using the 95th percentile as the cutoff, measurement of nuchal translucency thickness had a positive predictive value of 1.5% and a negative predictive value of 99.9%.

Conclusions.—US examination at 10 to 14 weeks' gestation identifies increased fetal nuchal translucency thickness in 55% of fetuses with major abnormalities of the heart and great vessels. The good diagnostic performance of this measurement suggests that it may be useful as an indication for specialist fetal echocardiography.

▶ If you hadn't heard about fetal nuchal translucency, now you have. If you missed, for some reason, reading about this relatively new observation linking the finding to congenital heart disease, you'll hear about it soon somewhere else. It is that significant an observation. When you think about it, you wonder why the observation has not been made earlier.

Fetuses in utero are like infants, children, and older folks in that edema, if it's going to develop, will develop in dependent areas. During the first trimester of pregnancy, fluid collects behind the neck of the fetus, much as it does in dependent areas, such as the ankles, in later life. This occurs partly because of the fetus' tendency to lie on its back and partly because of the laxity of the skin of the neck. As with ankle edema, this accumulation of fluid can represent several pathological processes, including heart failure. There is a brief opportunity between 10 and 14 weeks' gestation (when the fetal lymphatic system is developing and the peripheral resistance of the placenta is high) to detect abnormal fluid collections. Fluid collecting behind the neck can be detected as nuchal translucency by ultrasound scanning, and it can be measured. There are tight normative ranges for this measurement on ultrasound scanning. The more fluid has accumulated, the greater the risk of an abnormality being present. The opportunity to do such a screening rapidly evaporates after 14 weeks, when the lymphatic system is sufficiently developed to drain away any excess fluid, and changes to the placental circulation result in a drop in peripheral resistence. So after this time, any abnormalities causing fluid accumulation will usually correct themselves and thus go undetected if one is measuring nuchal translucency. The finding of nuchal translucency is not specific for heart disease. Several abnormalities cause the accumulation of fluid in the neck of fetuses. Chromosomal abnormalities—for example, Down syndrome—can do this. Chromosome 21 contains the gene that codes for type VI collagen. In trisomy 21, 1 subunit of this collagen can be overexpressed, resulting in connective tissue that has a more elastic composition. Also, if a fetus fails to move, there will be tissue fluid accumulation in subcutaneous areas such as of the neck. Neuromuscular abnormalities will do this. One example is arthrogryposis, which causes contractures and flexion deformities and can be fatal. Other causes of fluid accumulation are intrathoracic and extrathoracic compressive syndromes. If the thoracic cage is abnormally narrow or an intrathoracic lesion is present (such as a diaphragmatic hernia), the vessels in the fetus' head and neck become congested and neck edema occurs. Likewise, if heart failure occurs secondary to congenital cardiac anomalies or cardiac dysfunction, such as from arrhythmias, more extravascular fluid will form. The advantage of assessing nuchal translucency is that it is so easy to measure. If the amount of translucency is particularly high, the likelihood of some type of fetal abnormality, perhaps including a congenital heart defect, becomes more likely. Such patients should be referred to centers that are expert at fetal echos in order to allow the greatest likelihood of a defect's being determined. If no heart lesion can be found, the mother probably should be offered chorionic villus sampling and a repeat scan a couple of weeks later to exclude chromosomal or major physical anomalies. Fetuses with thick necks will not just require a large collar size. They may need expert consultation by a pediatric cardiologist well versed in prenatal echoes.

To read more on the topic of fetal nuchal translucency, see the excellent commentary by Burger.[1] You will see that a downside of the technique is that many normal fetuses will be referred, depending on what standard deviation above the range of normal is chosen for measuring nuchal translucency. The more sensitive the standard, the less specific the findings, causing too many normal pregnancies to be further evaluated.

J.A. Stockman III, M.D.

Reference

1. Burger A: Science commentary: What is fetal nuchal translucency? *BMJ* 318:85, 1999.

Pediatric Cardiac Surgery: The Effect of Hospital and Surgeon Volume on In-hospital Mortality

Hannan EL, Racz M, Kavey R-E, et al (State Univ of New York, Albany; State Univ of New York, Syracuse; Columbia-Presbyterian Hosp, New York; et al)
Pediatrics 101:963-969, 1998   12–10

Background.—An inverse relationship between adverse outcomes for certain types of patients and the amount of experience of health care providers in treating such patients has been documented. The relationship between in-hospital mortality and both surgeon and hospital volume for pediatric cardiac surgery in New York State between 1992 and 1995 was retrospectively analyzed.

Study Design.—Information came from the part of New York's Cardiac Surgery Reporting System database dedicated to pediatric cardiac surgery, which comprises all 7169 pediatric cardiac surgeries performed from 1992 to 1995 in New York State in the 16 hospitals with certificate of need approval. The risk-adjusted mortality rates for hospital and surgeon volumes ranges were calculated with adjustments for severity of illness.

Findings.—After controlling for severity of illness, hospitals with annual pediatric cardiac surgery volumes of fewer than 100 cases had significantly higher mortality rates than hospitals with volumes of 100 or more. Surgeons with annual volumes of less than 75 cases had significantly higher mortality rates than surgeons with annual volumes of 75 or more.

Conclusions.—Both the annual hospital and the surgeon volume were found to be significantly related to in-hospital mortality of cardiac surgery patients in this population-based retrospective cohort study, even after controlling for patient age, procedure complexity, and other clinical risk factors. These differences persisted even when only low-complexity pediatric cardiac procedures were considered.

▶ Dr. C. Mavroudis, chief of Cardiovascular-Thoracic Surgery, Children's Memorial Hospital, Chicago, comments:

Hannan and associates examined the relationship between annual pediatric cardiac surgery volume and in-hospital mortality for 7169 cases reported in New York State between 1992 and 1995. The authors controlled for severity of disease and clinical risk factors and concluded that centers performing greater than 100 cases per year had a lower overall mortality (5.95%) than did centers which performed less than 100 cases per year (8.26%). Similar and corresponding findings were noted for individual surgeons performing less than or greater than 75 cases per year. This well-designed and nicely performed study confirms many obvious biases that increased volume results in better and more efficient outcomes. Inherent, although not discussed, in this article is the likelihood that higher volume centers will have the "critical mass" and clinical expertise of pediatric anesthesiologists, intensivists, cardiologists, nurses, and medical personnel that support such an enterprise. While it is true that complications are made or avoided in the operating room, it is also true that competent postoperative care will impact favorably on the clinical outcomes. Large cities have many medical schools, each with its own vision of comprehensive clinical services, which usually include pediatric cardiac surgery, pediatric solid organ transplantation, and other low-volume and high-tech subspecialties. If the level of care is to be improved, combined services involving multiple medical schools have to evolve. The quid pro quos of such relationships will require careful negotiations and enlightened leadership. As always, the guiding principle should be demonstrable quality of care for our patients. This article demonstrates obvious conclusions. How these data will be used to improve quality of care remains to be seen.

C. Mavroudis, M.D.

Comparison of Cost and Clinical Outcome Between Transcatheter Coil Occlusion and Surgical Closure of Isolated Patent Ductus Arteriosus
Prieto LR, DeCamillo DM, Konrad DJ, et al (Cleveland Clinic Found, Ohio)
Pediatrics 101:1020-1024, 1998   12–11

Objective.—Transcatheter closure of the patent ductus arteriosus (PDA) with Gianturco coils was retrospectively compared with surgical repair at the Cleveland Clinic Foundation.

Methods.—Procedural and recovery costs for 36 patients, aged 13 months to 28 years, who underwent coil occlusion or surgical closure of uncomplicated PDA between August 1993 and June 1996 were determined. Patients were excluded if they had other serious coexisting medical conditions.

Results.—The average cost of coil occlusion was a significant 38% lower than the cost of surgery ($5273 vs $8509). Respective costs for inpatient hospital stays were $398 versus $2566, and the costs of professional services were $1506 versus $2782 (Table). Technical costs were similar, even though hourly costs for the catheterization laboratory averaged twice those of the operating room. Median duration of the transcatheter coil occlusion was 150 minutes, and median duration of surgery was

TABLE.—Comparison for Coil and Surgical Patients

	Coil Patients (N = 24)	Surgical Patients (N = 12)	P Value
Professional	$1506 ± 703	$2782 ± 516	<.001
Technical	$2156 ± 797	$2151 ± 736	NS
Postprocedure tests	$ 245 ± 177	$ 327 ± 160	.05
Hospital stay	$ 398 ± 217	$2566 ± 626	<.001
Miscellaneous	$ 969 ± 874	$ 684 ± 329	NS
Total	$5273 ± 1940	$8509 ± 1615	<.001

Note: Results expressed as mean and SD.
(Reproduced with permission from *Pediatrics*, from Prieto LR, DeCamillo DM, Konrad DJ, et al: Comparison of cost and clinical outcome between transcatheter coil occlusion and surgical closure of isolated patent ductus arteriosus. *Pediatrics* 101:1020-1024, 1998.)

165 minutes. Patient outcomes were similar in both groups, although 4 patients (17%) in the coil group versus no patients in the surgery group had residual leaks at an average of 6 months, as detected by echocardiography performed on all coil group patients and 5 (42%) of the surgery patients. There were no other short-term or long-term complications in either group and no deaths.

Conclusion.—Transcatheter coil occlusion for PDA is as safe and effective as surgery and is much less expensive.

▶ Nonsurgical treatments for congenital heart disease have been around for a while now. It was almost 50 years ago that the first attempts were made at transcatheter treatments of valvular heart disease. Such approaches were put on the map by William Rashkind, who in 1966 perfected the balloon atrial septostomy technique as part of the palliation of transposition of the great vessels. Since then, a variety of transcatheter therapies have become more or less established as part of the routine armamentarium of the pediatric interventional cardiologist. Among these therapies are pulmonary balloon valvotomy, balloon angioplasty of coarctation of the aorta, endovascular stent therapy (for various vascular obstructions), transcatheter atrial septal defect occlusion devices, and, as we see in this report, PDA embolization.

Many techniques have been developed to close PDAs. The longest-standing one, of course, is surgical ligation (first performed in 1939). In 1967, the first PDA occlusion device was used in the form of a conically shaped polyvinyl alcohol foam. This device was termed the Ivalon plug. The problem with the Ivalon plug was that it required a very large catheter sheath to insert the plug, and younger patients were not eligible for the procedure. This problem was corrected in 1979, when Rashkind developed his PDA occluder. Still the sheath size was still somewhat large for the tiniest of newborns. Also, some 7% of the patients had clinical evidence of residual ductal patency. Worst yet, in most series, 10% of the patients had embolization of the Rashkind plug to either the aorta or the pulmonary artery. Such patients required surgical recovery of the device.

Approximately 8 years ago, the Gianturco coil for occlusion of the PDA was introduced. This coil is made of stainless steel wire into which are incorporated Dacron strands to enhance ductal thrombosis and closure. The coil has several major advantages. It is readily available. It costs considerably less than other occluders. The sheath sizes used for delivery are extremely small and perfectly applicable to the wide range of pediatric population. A PDA Coil Registry, begun early in the last decade, accumulated data on well over 1000 coil embolization procedures from more than several dozen centers. The vast majority of patients have been adequately treated. The most common complication of coil closure is embolization of the coil through the ductus to the pulmonary arteries. In most cases, the coil can be retrieved by a transcatheter snare. The incidence of coil embolization is now quite low, given the fact that most individuals who are using this technique have had extensive experience.

Transcatheter closure of PDAs initially was not considered cost-effective. For example, the mean cost of the Rashkind PDA device closure strategy was $11,466 per patient, in comparison with $8838 per patient for surgical repair. This difference was due in part to the higher cost of the device, the cost of cardiac catheterization and angiography before implantation, reimbursement policies, and the cost of treating residual shunts or complications associated with the device. As we see in the report abstracted from Cleveland, however, coil occlusion does carry a significantly lower cost than surgical closure ($5273 vs $8509). None of the patients in this series had a serious complication that would add on extra costs.

Some still consider the surgical approach to PDA closure to be the gold standard. The reason is that surgical mortality and morbidity are virtually nonexistent, but morbidity with coil occlusion is also very, very low. Neither surgical closure nor transcatheter closure seems to be associated with an increased risk of bacterial endocarditis. The occurrence of endocarditis with a silent PDA is also low (just one case reported in the last 13 years).[1]

Unless a patient wishes to have a surgical scar, it would seem that the choice between transcatheter coil occlusion and surgical closure would favor the former, on a cost basis if nothing else. To read more about the topic of transcatheter therapy for a variety of congenital heart disease types, see the excellent review of this topic by Mendelsohn and Shim.[2]

Lastly, recognition that PDAs exist has been around for a long time. The ductus arteriosus was first mentioned by Galen in the second century. The continuous "machinery" murmur that we now know is due to a PDA was described in 1900 by Gibson in Edinburgh. In 1907, Munro in Boston wrote of the possibility of ligating a PDA, but never undertook the procedure because anesthetic techniques at the time were thought to be so risky as to negate any possible benefits from this potential surgical procedure. Surprisingly, the first attempt to close a PDA was not made until 30 years later, and even more surprisingly, it was done on a case made difficult by the added complication of subacute bacterial endocarditis. This first attempt was made by a surgeon in Boston by the name Streider. The year was 1937 and the procedure was not successful. The first successful closure of an uninfected PDA was carried out in 1938 on a 7½-year-old child by Robert Gross, who, as a young surgical resident in Boston, appeared to have been unaware of Streider's earlier, unsuccessful attempt in the same city. Now we consider closing PDAs with relatively noninvasive techniques. We certainly have come a long way.[3]

J.A. Stockman III, M.D.

References

1. Balzer DT, Spray TL, McMullin D, et al: Endocarditis associated with a clinically silent patent ductus arteriosus. *Am Heart J* 125:1192-1193, 1993.
2. Mendelsohn AM, Shim D: Inroads in transcatheter therapy for congenital heart disease. *J Pediatr* 133:324-333, 1998.
3. Hurt R: Historical vignette: Patent ductus arteriosus. *Pediatr Cardiol* 19:245, 1998.

Congenital Heart Disease Caused by Mutations in the Transcription Factor *NKX2-5*

Schott J-J, Benson DW, Basson CT, et al (Harvard Med School, Boston; Brigham and Women's Hosp, Boston; Harrisburg Hosp, Pa; et al)
Science 281:108-111, 1998   12–12

Background.—Cardiac development is a complex process, relying on the integration of cell commitment, morphogenesis, and excitation-contraction coupling. Several transcription factors have been implicated in this process. This study identified mutations in the transcription factor *NKX2-5* as a cause of congenital heart disease.

Methods and Findings.—Mutations in the gene encoding the homeobox transcription factor *NKX2-5* were implicated in nonsyndromic human congenital heart disease. A dominant disease locus associated with cardiac malformations and atrioventricular conduction abnormalities was mapped to chromosome 5q35, which is the location of *NKX2-5*, a *Drosophilia tinman* homolog. Three different *NKX2-5* mutations were evident: 2 that are likely to impair binding of *NKX2-5* to target DNA, resulting in haploinsufficiency, and 1 that may augment target-DNA binding.

Conclusions.—The identification of human mutations that cause congenital heart disease provides a complementary approach to gene ablation studies and helps define gene defects that perturb subsequent stages of cardiac development. The current data show that *NKX2-5* is important in regulating septation during cardiac morphogenesis. *NKX2-5* also appears to be important for maturation and maintenance of atrioventricular node function throughout life.

▶ Investigators are fast on the trail of genetic mutations that cause serious cardiac abnormalities such as the Holt-Oram syndrome, atrial-septal defects, cardiomyopathy, long QT syndrome and other arrhythmias. People were shocked when Boston Celtics star Reggie Lewis collapsed on the basketball court in the summer of 1993, but his death had a familiar ring. Every few years a well-known young athlete drops dead without warning during a sporting event, the victim of an undetected genetic heart condition.

Until about 9 or 10 years ago, none of the genes at fault had yet been identified. Then there was an explosion of information about mutations that directly impair the heart—an explosion that still hasn't settled down. Some of the gene mutations actually affect the formation of the heart structure such as described in the article abstracted. Mutations in these genes may cause abnormalities such as an atrial septal defect. Other genetic defects cause alterations in protein pores within the heart that control the electrical conductants of cardiac rhythm. Mutations in myosin and other proteins involved in muscle contraction are at the root of the problem of hereditary cardiomyopathies.

If you put together all of the hereditary disorders that affect the heart, including the long QT syndrome, at most perhaps 0.2% of the population is affected, but as we learn more about what causes structural heart disease, the percentage is increasing. Take the long QT syndrome. Hereditary long QT syndrome affects 1 in 10,000 people, but for those affected, the risk of death can be as high as 50% over a 10-year period. Unfortunately, one third of people who die of this syndrome have the first and last episode as one event. We now know that some commonly prescribed antibiotics, antihistamines, and antifungal agents increase the chance of heart arrhythmias, and the discovery of the channel defects causing the long QT syndrome has made it clear why. Most of these drugs affect a particular potassium channel that is abnormal in about 30% of patients with the long QT syndrome. Such drugs therefore pick out those who otherwise might be at risk for sudden death from this inherited arrhythmia.

If you have forgotten what the Holt-Oram syndrome is, it is a rare hereditary condition that causes defects between the atria and, sometimes, the ventricles, in addition to arm and hand defects. The genetic defect in this disorder is due to an abnormality in the gene known as *TBX5*. This gene defect is also found in fruit flies. The gene has been subtitled the "Tin Man" gene because, like the Tin Man in *The Wizard of Oz*, fruit fly embryos that lack both copies of the gene have no hearts at all.

There are no human homozygous Tin Man types among us, for obvious reasons. Theoretically, however, it is likely that more than 1 baby has been conceived and expired soon thereafter with a double genetic defect that would cause that conceptus to have no heart (an interesting bit of trivia).

Chances are we will be hearing a great deal more about some of the genes that cause heart defects. If you want to read an interesting review of this topic, see the superb summary by Barinaga.[1]

J.A. Stockman III, M.D.

Reference

1. Barinaga M: Tracking down mutations that stop the heart. *Science* 281:32-34, 1998.

Failure to Diagnose Congenital Heart Disease in Infancy
Kuehl KS, Loffredo CA, Ferencz C (Children's Natl Med Ctr, Washington, DC; Univ of Maryland, Baltimore)
Pediatrics 103:743-747, 1999   12–13

Background.—Physiologic changes in the circulation after birth can mask the signs of some congenital cardiovascular malformations (CCVMs) in early infancy. Factors predicting failure to diagnose congenital heart disease in newborns were investigated.

Methods.—Data were obtained on 4390 infants with CCVMs identified between 1981 and 1989 in a population-based study of the Baltimore-Washington metropolitan area. Eight hundred infants died before 1 year of age, including 76 before heart disease was diagnosed. The characteristics of these infants were compared with those of infants who died after cardiac disease was diagnosed.

Findings.—Factors associated with the death of infants with CCVMs and with death before diagnosis included infant birth weight, gestational age, intrauterine growth retardation, and chromosomal anomaly. Diagnoses of coarctation of the aorta, Ebstein's anomaly, atrial septal defect, and truncus arteriosus were overrepresented, especially in infants without associated malformations. Although paternal education level was associated with failure to diagnose congenital heart disease during life, other sociodemographic characteristics of the family were not.

Conclusion.—Diagnosing CCVMs in infants requires close observation during the neonatal period. Infants with undiagnosed CCVMs may be at increased risk if discharged from the hospital within the first 2 days of life.

▶ As the time that babies have been allowed to stay in the hospital post partum has shortened, similarly shortened is the time such babies have to clinically manifest evidence of congenital heart disease, should they have it. Thus, it becomes incumbent upon each of us to use our utmost clinical skills to rule out heart disease in the nursery. In this report, of all infants with cardiovascular malformations who died in the first week of life, 25% did not have the cardiac lesion identified before discharge. If one takes the entire first year of life, some 10% of those with CCVMs will die without a correct diagnosis ever having been made.

Please do not think that the problem of failing to diagnose CCVMs in infancy is unique to pediatricians here in the United States. A retrospective study of all cases of structural heart disease diagnosed within the first 12 months of life in Great Britain showed that routine neonatal examination failed to detect more than half of babies with heart disease. Examination at 6 weeks of age missed a full third of babies.[1]

If CCVMs are missed in the immediate neonatal period, please remember that you have other later opportunities to pick them up, assuming a child has not died or been seen with overt clinical evidence of a problem. A recent report from Great Britain shows us that at the 6- to 8-week routine baby examination, about one baby in 100 will have a murmur heard and about one quarter of these babies will have evidence of structural heart disease.[2] To say this differently, there are numerous opportunities to diagnose CCVMs, and if you miss them in the first month or so of life, keep looking for them at the 6-week to 2-month examination. Given the fact that missed heart disease is one of the major causes of malpractice litigation for pediatricians, it is important to remember all these statistics.

J.A. Stockman III, M.D.

References

1. Wren C, Richmond S, Donaldson L: Presentation of congenital heart disease in infancy: Implications for routine examination. *Arch Dis Child Fetal Neonatal Ed* 80:F49-F53, 1999.
2. Gregory J, Emslie A, Wyllie J: Examination for cardiac malformations at six weeks of age. *Arch Dis Child Fetal Neonatal Ed* 80:F46-F48, 1999.

Culture-negative Endocarditis Caused by *Bartonella henselae*
Baorto E, Payne M, Slater LN, et al (Washington Univ, St Louis; Univ of Oklahoma, Oklahoma City; Stanford Univ, Calif; et al)
J Pediatr 132:1051-1054, 1998   12–14

Background.—*Bartonella henselae* is the organism responsible for cat-scratch disease. This article describes a child with endocarditis caused by *B. henselae*.

> *Case Report.*—Girl, 4 years, previously healthy, with a ventricular septal defect, bicuspid aortic valve, and repaired coarctation of the aorta presented with fever, fatigue, bilateral lower extremity swelling, and epistaxis. The family had 2 cats and several kittens. On examination, the patient had a harsh grade 3/6 systolic murmur, and rheumatoid factor was positive at a dilution of 1:1280. A chest radiograph revealed cardiomegaly. Echocardiography demonstrated aortic insufficiency, aortic stenosis, and a bicuspid aortic valve. Blood cultures were negative. The patient underwent a Ross procedure and repair of the ventricular septal defect. The resected valve was cultured but was sterile. Pathologic examination revealed acute and chronic inflammation with calcifications. The patient was discharged. One week later, a sample of serum from day 3 of hospitalization was found to contain elevated levels of antibodies to *B. henselae*. This was confirmed by reculturing, immunohistochemical analysis, and polymerase chain reaction analysis of the excised valve. Outpatient antibiotic therapy was continued with ceftriaxone, erythromycin, and rifampin. Antibody titers remained elevated for at least 5 months. The patient remains stable after 18 months of follow-up.

Conclusions.—Clinicians should be alert to *B. henselae* as a potential cause of apparent culture-negative endocarditis in children.

▶ *Bartonella endocarditis*—the 24th reason why cats are injurious to your health. It wasn't so bad when *B. henselae* was first described. That was in 1990, when it was thought to be a cause of bacillary angiomatosis, relapsing bacteremia with fever, and peliosis hepatis. These were unusual problems generally seen only in immunocompromised individuals, folks usually infected with HIV. Unfortunately, *B. henselae* can affect the immune component as well. The most common manifestation in healthy children is cat-scratch disease, which in and of itself is usually self-limited. On occasion, cat-scratch disease is complicated by ocular involvement (Parinaud's oculoglandular syndrome, retinitis, or optic neuritis), meningoencephalitis, or disseminated infection with persistent fever and visceral involvement. To these more serious complications may be added endocarditis in childhood, the subject of this report. In parts of Canada and France, *Bartonella* is estimated to account for as much as 3% of all cases of infective endocarditis in adults. The diagnosis is usually pretty easy: there is a known history of underlying valvular disease or murmur and a history of recent contact with cats or kittens. The next time you see a child with fever of undetermined origin who has a heart murmur and who has a cat or kitten, think *Bartonella* endocarditis. Thus far, all adults who have been reported with this infection have required valve replacement. A fair percentage of these patients will have negative blood cultures. Needless to say, part of the treatment, or prophylaxis of the next episode, is getting rid of the cat.

With respect to infectious organisms and heart disease, recent research has shown that *Chlamydia* proteins have been found in almost 80% of coronary artery plaque formations in adults with coronary heart disease. In fact, clinical trials are now under way to determine whether prolonged antibiotic therapy of those with serious coronary artery disease might, in fact, reduce the incidence of heart attack or other untoward clinical events. Thus far, 6 months into these trials, no diminished risk has been found. However, compared with controls, there has been observed a decrease in the number of inflammatory mediators in the circulation of antibiotic-treated patients, suggesting that some benefit may be seen over the long haul. To read more about infections as a cause of artery clogging plaques, see the "News Focus" editorial that appeared recently in *Science*.[1]

Continuing the theme of things that can infect the heart, see if you can get the correct diagnosis for the following case. A previously healthy adult male, a professional hunter, is initially seen with high fever and altered mental status. This hunter frequently dressed meat from wild pigs, although he had not done so for the preceding 6 months. Four days before his admission, the patient felt weak and developed abdominal pain, nausea, vomiting, chills, fever, diarrhea, and left upper extremity weakness. Physical examination reveals that the patient is anxious and disoriented. He has an oral temperature of 40°C. An MRI of the brain shows areas of microinfarction. Lumbar puncture has unremarkable results. Over the course of several days, a murmur develops in the patient, and petechiae are noted on his feet. Splinter hemorrhages are present under his fingernails. An echocardiogram reveals two large vegetations on his mitral valve. Name the organism.

This patient has what is known as *boar hunter's endocarditis*. In this case, the organism was *Actinobacillus suis*. *A. suis* is rarely a cause of endocarditis in humans, but is a frequent pathogen of the heart in pigs, horses, and other animals. Veterinarians and animal handlers are known to be at increased risk for infection with this organism. By the way, the fellow in question required a mitral valve replacement and, 6 months following surgery, was doing perfectly fine and was out boar hunting again. Nothing boring about boar hunting, is there?

J.A. Stockman III, M.D.

Reference

1. Gura T: Infections: A cause of artery-clogging plaques? *Science* 281:35-37, 1998.

Supraventricular Tachycardia in Infancy: Evaluation, Management, and Follow-up
Etheridge SP, Judd VE (Univ of Utah, Salt Lake City)
Arch Pediatr Adolesc Med 153:267-271, 1999   12–15

Background.—Though supraventricular tachycardia (SVT) is common in infants, some have no recurrence after its initial presentation. Furthermore, about 30% lose SVT inducibility by 1 year of age. Initial SVT features, tachycardia characteristics, and esophageal electrophysiology (EP) data were studied to determine whether they would predict which infants need no antiarrhythmic medication and which will have no inducible SVT at 1 year of age.

Methods and Findings.—Thirty-three infants, aged 3 months or younger, with SVT from August 1995 to October 1997 at one medical center underwent esophageal EP study at diagnosis and at 1 year of age. In all infants, the SVT was controlled. At initial EP, the mechanism of SVT was found to be atrioventricular node re-entry in 15% and orthodromic reciprocating tachycardia by an accessory atrioventricular connection in 85%. Eleven infants had SVT control by propranolol hydrochloride, 10 had SVT control by amiodarone, and 6 needed more than 1 medication. Five infants never needed medication. One was lost to follow-up. Seventy-six percent of the children who reached 1 year of age were free of medication and SVT at follow-up. Eleven of the 16 patients without clinical SVT who underwent a follow-up esophageal EP were found to have inducible SVT. Thus, overall, 24% of the 1-year-olds studied no longer had clinical or inducible SVT.

Conclusions.—In all infants in the current series, SVT control was possible. Clinical episodes of SVT were uncommon after discharge, although most still had inducible SVT at the age of 1 year. None of the initial clinical or EP findings predicted clinical course or continued SVT.

▶ It's nice to see that the outcome of babies with SVT is so good. This does not mean that babies with this arrhythmia may not initially be at death's door. Indeed, some do die during the initial episode if not promptly diagnosed and managed. As often as not, an icebag on the head is all that is needed, however.

While on the topic of arrhythmias, how would you deal with the following? You are at a Little League baseball game. The pitcher throws a wild fastball, that strikes the batter squarely in the middle of the chest. The batter goes down, totally passed out, but recovers quickly.

You know that some youngsters and adults will die when struck in such a manner. Most survive such minimal trauma, but why do others die? Why, after being hit in the chest by a baseball, a hockey puck, or other similar object, do some athletes remain briefly conscious, even active, before they suffer cardiac arrest and die?

Sudden death due to low-energy chest-wall impact is also known as commotio cordis.[1] Death from such low-energy blows occurs only when they are delivered to the precordium during a narrow time window on the upstroke of the electrocardiographic T wave. The blow does this by causing ventricular fibrillation.

One of the first reported occurrences of this phenomenon happened on August 1, 1970, when a healthy, athletic, 42-year-old man collapsed immediately after being struck in the chest by a cricket ball during a match in Louisville, Kentucky.[2] A team member who was a physician immediately began cardiopulmonary resuscitation, and the patient was transported to a nearby hospital but was pronounced dead on arrival. An autopsy showed no evident cause of death though it was presumed to have resulted from cardiac arrhythmia. A cricket ball, similar to a baseball, is very firm and is made of rubber with layers of cork and leather covering. Measuring 3 inches in diameter and weighing 5.5 oz, it is hit with a wooden bat at high impact, as in baseball. Cricket players typically do not wear padding over the chest.

Obviously, brains and hearts are different. The former can sustain a concussion. The latter cannot, at least not without flipping a few arrhythmias.

J.A. Stockman III, M.D.

References

1. Bokenkamp R, Paul T: Sudden death due to low-energy chest-wall impact. *N Engl J Med* 339:1398, 1998.
2. Haq CL: Letter to the editor. *N Engl J Med* 339:1399, 1998.

Orthostatic Intolerance in Adolescent Chronic Fatigue Syndrome
Stewart JM, Gewitz MH, Weldon A, et al (New York Med College, Valhalla)
Pediatrics 103:116-121, 1999   12–16

Introduction.—Characteristics of chronic fatigue syndrome include debilitating fatigue lasting at least 6 months, cognitive difficulties, pharyngitis, tender lymphadenopathy, muscle pain, joint pain, headache, sleep disturbance, and postexercise malaise. This may be related to orthostatic intolerance, which encompasses many problems, including syncope, autonomic failure, and the orthostatic tachycardia syndrome. Adolescents may be particularly prone to orthostatic intolerance because of their high state of modulation of the autonomic nervous system. Patients with chronic fatigue syndrome were studied with head-up tilt and compared with patients who had a history that was compatible with neurally mediated syncope and with normal control subjects.

Methods.—There were 26 adolescents, ages 11 to 19 years, with chronic fatigue syndrome included in the study. Their heart-rate and blood-pressure responses to head-up tilt were compared with adolescents referred for the evaluation of simple faint as well as with 13 normal healthy control children of similar age.

Results.—Typical faints with an abrupt decrease in blood pressure and heart rate associated with loss of consciousness were seen in 4 of 13 control subjects and in 18 of 26 simple faint patients. A normal head-up tilt response was found in 1 chronic fatigue syndrome patient. Severe orthostatic symptoms were found in 25 of 26 chronic fatigue syndrome patients, with 7 of 25 having syncope, 15 having orthostatic tachycardia with hypotension, and 3 having orthostatic tachycardia without significant hypotension. In 18 of 25 patients, acrocyanosis, cool extremities, and edema indicated venous pooling. Comparable acral or tachycardiac findings were not found in any of the control or simple faint patients.

Conclusion.—In adolescents, orthostatic intolerance is highly related to chronic fatigue syndrome. A partial autonomic defect may contribute to symptomatology because it was found that the orthostatic intolerance of chronic fatigue syndrome often had heart-rate and blood-pressure responses that were similar to responses in the syndrome of orthostatic tachycardia.

▶ These investigators are on to something. Many of the symptoms of chronic fatigue syndrome are similar, if not identical, in part, to the type of orthostatic intolerance commonly referred to as neurally mediated hypotension or cardiogenic syncope. It will be interesting to see how effective the treatments are for neurocardiogenic syncope if such treatments are applied to the management of chronic fatigue syndrome. Low-dose propranolol, fludrocortisone, and large-volume water just might do the trick for those with chronic fatigue syndrome. If you're up to your ears with such patients, you might try some of these therapies. A recent report shows that drinking large volumes of water, in fact, is a very potent pressor for those with neurocardiogenic syncope.[1] Also, in some patients with chronic fatigue syndrome, low-dose hydrocortisone reduces fatigue levels in a very dramatic way.[2]

In case you were not aware of this, the measurement of blood pressure as part of the physical examination will soon be a century old in the United States. While traveling in Europe in 1901, U.S. surgeon Harvey Cushing saw a new blood pressure cuff instrument in clinical use in a hospital in Pavia, Italy. The instrument, a version of the modern blood pressure cuff, had been devised by the Italian physician, Scipione Riva-Rocci a few years earlier. Cushing cajoled Riva-Rocci into making a gift to him of one of these cuffs, and he brought it back with him to Johns Hopkins Hospital in Baltimore. There, Cushing began to espouse its use. He had a difficult time, however. In 1903, when he traveled to Boston to speak at Harvard Medical School about the virtues of the new cuff, he was somewhat shunned, although those at the Massachusetts General Hospital, Children's Hospital, and Boston City Hospital did agree to a clinical trial of the value of blood pressure measurement. When the trial was completed a year later, the verdict went against the new cuff. Not dismayed, Cushing continued to push for routine blood pressure measurement. Studies of hospital charts in the early part of this century show that measurement of blood pressure began to be part of the patient record as a routine beginning in 1910 and shortly thereafter.

Please note that what Harvey Cushing did was not the type of blood pressure recording that we do now. His method was a determination of blood pressure based on that pressure necessary to occlude the radial artery (sort of a systolic blood pressure). Measurement of both the systolic and diastolic blood pressure based on modern auscultation techniques was first described by Nikolai Korotkoff, the Russian physician, in the early part of this century. It took a little while, however, for physicians to switch over from palpation of the radial artery to auscultation methods of blood pressure determination.

By the way, before blood pressure could actually be physically measured, physicians did practice an art of physical examination that could give them some sense of how healthy the blood flow was. As part of medical school training in the 1800s, it was expected that all exiting students would become expert at radial pulse palpation. They learned that careful palpation of the radial pulse would reveal valuable information about the force of blood flow. A standard U.S. medical text on physical examination published in the late 19th century advised a physician to palpate the patient's radial pulse for "the fullness of the vessel...the tension of the artery....the size of the [pulse] wave...the force of the wave...[and] the duration of the wave."[3] When blood pressure cuffs were first introduced, many well-known physicians indicated that the information derived from palpation of the pulse was much better than that obtained with a blood pressure cuff and could never be obtained mechanically by use of the latter instrument.

New technologies have lots of barriers to overcome. When it comes to change, many of us are from Missouri, the "Show-Me State."

J.A. Stockman III, M.D.

References

1. Jordan J, Shannon JR, Grogan E, et al: A potent pressor response elicited by drinking water. *Lancet* 353:723-724, 1999.
2. Cleare AJ, Heap E, Malhi GS, et al: Low-dose hydrocortisone in chronic fatigue syndrome: A randomised crossover trial. *Lancet* 353:455-458, 1999.
3. Gibson CA, Russell W: Physical diagnosis: A guide to methods of clinical investigation. New York, Appleton, 1891, p 94.

Syncope Recurrence in Children: Relation to Tilt-test Results
Salim MA, Ware LE, Barnard M, et al (Univ of Tennessee, Memphis; LeBonheur Children's Med Ctr, Memphis, Tenn)
Pediatrics 102:924-926, 1998   12–17

Introduction.—Syncope is a common complaint of children, and its incidence peaks in midadolescence. Neurocardiogenic syncope is the most prevalent form in children with a normal heart. To establish the diagnosis of neurocardiogenic syncope, tilt testing is used widely. It reproduces the orthostatic stress that led to syncope and is used as an indicator for treatment. Patients with a negative tilt test are often discharged from further follow-up. For syncope in children, the recurrence rate is unknown. The intermediate-term outcomes of children with syncope were examined by comparing the recurrence of syncope in children with a positive versus a negative tilt test.

Methods.—There were 45 children, of whom 20 had a negative tilt test and 25 had a positive test. Chart review, a mailed questionnaire, or telephone interview were conducted to determine the recurrence of syncope through follow-up.

Results.—Fifteen children whose tilt test was negative and 25 whose tilt test was positive were available for follow-up. In the positive–tilt test children, recurrent syncope was significantly greater (13 of 25) than in the negative–tilt test children (2 of 15). The syncope-free group and the recurrent syncope group had no differences with respect to duration of symptoms, age at initial syncope, age at tilt test, or duration of follow-up, nor did the tilt-positive or tilt-negative groups. More syncopal episodes were seen among children with a positive tilt test and those with recurrent syncope before their evaluation than either the group with no recurrent syncope or those with a negative tilt test.

Conclusion.—After either a negative or a positive tilt test, syncope may recur. For the tilt-positive children, however, the recurrence rate is higher. Recurrent syncope occurred in those who received either volume expansion, β-blockers, or both. No single agent or combination of agents was found to be completely effective in the prevention of recurrent syncope.

▶ Dr. David Driscoll, professor of Pediatrics, and head, Section of Pediatrics, Mayo Clinic and Foundation, Mayo Medical School, Rochester, Minn, comments:

Syncope is a common event in children. In a population-based study, we recently reported an incidence of syncope in children of 72 to 126 per 100,000 population. In general, syncope has very benign implications, but in the very rare patient, it can herald the presence of an important, potentially life-threatening condition. An important issue, therefore, is to define the appropriate evaluation of these patients that identifies the rare patient at risk for a catastrophic event, but yet is cost effective and not inappropriate for the vast majority of patients with benign syncope.

Where does tilt table testing fit into the appropriate evaluation of these patients? It is clear that the physiologic and pathophysiologic responses to tilt table testing have allowed identification of several underlying mechanisms for syncope. These include cardioinhibitory, vasodepressor, and mixed cardioinhibitory-vasodepressor forms of syncope. Categorization of patients based upon the pathophysiologic mechanism of the syncope might allow better treatment selection and assessment of the results of treatment. As Salim et al. so nicely demonstrate, the results of tilt table testing may be helpful in better defining the natural history of patients with different types of syncope. It is clear that tilt table testing is a useful *research* tool for studying this problem. It is not yet clear that tilt table testing has a cost-effective useful role in the *clinical* management of individual patients.

D. Driscoll, M.D.

Age- and Sex-related Differences in Clinical Manifestations in Patients With Congenital Long-QT Syndrome: Findings From the International LQTS Registry

Locati EH, Zareba W, Moss AJ, et al (Univ of Rochester, NY; Univ of Milan, Italy; Univ of Pavia, Italy; et al)
Circulation 97:2237-2244, 1998   12–18

Background.—Patients with congenital long-QT syndrome (LQTS) have prolonged ventricular repolarization, leading to syncope and unexpected death caused by malignant ventricular arrhythmias. This autosomal disorder is more prevalent among females than males. The diagnosis is made on the basis of QT interval duration, which varies significantly by age and sex. This study examined the effects of patient age and sex on the clinical manifestations of LQTS.

Methods.—Patients were identified from the International LQTS Registry. The analysis included 479 probands and 5275 family members, with ECG data available on all probands and 53% of family members. Based on a $QT_c > 440$ ms, 37% of these family members were designated as effective. Clinical end-points for the analysis were syncope, nonfatal cardiac arrest, and unexplained sudden death before age 40. Age and sex differences in clinical manifestations were analyzed in the overall study population, and among 162 patients with various known LQTS gene mutations.

Results.—Seventy percent of the probands and 58% of the affected family members were female. Among subjects with LQTS gene mutations, 71% of probands and 62% of symptomatic family members were female. At the time of the initial clinical manifestation of LQTS, mean age was 8 years for male probands versus 14 years for female probands. Nearly three fourths of male probands had their first clinical event by the age of 15 years, compared with about half of female probands. Hazard ratio for clinical events among female probands, with adjustment for QT_c duration, was 0.48 by age 15 years versus 1.87 by age 15 to 40 years. For female family members, these hazard ratios were 0.58 and 3.25, respectively. Male carriers of the LQT1 mutation had a clinical event rate of 69%, compared with 32% for female carriers. For LQT2 and LQT3 carriers, the event rate did not vary by age or sex.

Conclusions.—This study finds significant sex-related differences in the onset of clinical manifestations in families with LQTS. Males with this congenital syndrome are at greater risk of cardiac arrest up to puberty, but females are at greater risk in adulthood. This age-sex pattern is also present in LQT1 gene carriers. The reduced incidence of clinical events in males may be related to their more prominent reduction in QT_c duration after puberty; the mechanism of these differences is unknown. The results suggest that women with LQTS should be considered for prophylactic therapy even if they have never experienced cardiac events.

▶ In the 1999 YEAR BOOK OF PEDIATRICS the purported relationship between the prolonged QT syndrome and sudden infant death syndrome was reviewed. In this study from the International Registry on the LQTS, we see that women at the other end of the age spectrum are at significantly higher risk than men as young adults in terms of dying from this disorder. Boys run into problems early and girls late. The diagnosis of LQTS is more common in girls and women later in life after a series of repetitive nonfatal events, whereas LQTS in boys presents an earlier onset of fatal cardiac events. Young effected males should be considered at extremely high risk of potentially serious consequences from their LQTS. The longer a boy survives, the risk of sudden death decreases because many will have a spontaneous shortening of the QT interval during and after puberty. Affected females, even free of cardiac events, should be considered for prophylactic therapy because of the persistent risk of first events and torsade de pointes in adult life.

If you are not aware of the potential effect of a commonly used drug, cisapride, on the QT interval in children, you probably should be. Cisapride is a compound that stimulates motor activity in all segments of the gastrointestinal tract by the release of acetylcholine from the enteric nervous system. It has been used in various gastrointestinal conditions, including gastroesophageal reflux, functional dyspepsia, gastroparesis, chronic pseudoobstruction syndrome, and chronic constipation. After the Food and Drug Administration (FDA) approved its use in the United States in 1993, possible cardiac side effects were suggested when some adults experienced palpations, tachycardia, and extrasystole during treatment with this drug. Symptoms resolved after discontinuation of cisapride. No other cause could be identified. Several recent cases report cardiac side effects (arrhythmias associated with a prolonged QT interval) in patients taking cisapride. The arrhythmias involved were torsade de pointes and second-degree heart block, both of which are known to occur in patients with congenital or acquired QT prolongation. Some of the cases described involved children.

Between September 1993 and April 1996, the FDA's MedWatch program reported 34 patients with torsade de pointes and 23 with prolonged QT interval who were using cisapride. Some of these patients were children and one was an adolescent. There were several deaths and more than a dozen cardiac arrests. Somewhat more than half of these patients were also taking medications of the imidazole class or macrolide antibiotics. A recent report of the effects on cisapride on the QT interval of children showed about 13% taking this drug had significant prolongation of the QT interval with repolarization abnormalities. While the incidence of such abnormalities is low, when the QT interval is prolonged to greater than 440 msec, it would be wise to reduce or stop the cisapride.[1]

This commentary closes with two clinical pearls related to cardiac rhythm issues. First, beware of cellular phones if you have a pacemaker. All cellular phones are dangerous for pacemaker patients. The only way to safely use them is to make sure that a turned-on phone is never juxtaposed to the pacemaker itself. During a study of 200 patients with pacemakers who were monitored to determine whether there was any interference created by digital and analog cellular phones, the Global System for Mobil Communications system cellular phone interfered with pacing 97 times in 43 patients (21.5% of times actually used). During tests on the Total Access of Communication System cellular telephones, there were 60 cases of pacing interference in 35 patients (17.5% of times used).[2] If there is a lesson in all this, it would be that Ma' Bell's rotary phones, if you can still find one, are the way to go if your heart is hardwired, even though your phone may not be.

Second pearl, tell your patients with LQTS to be careful around phones, doorbells, and alarm clocks. Researchers have recently identified a genetic mutation that causes some with LQTS to be unusually sensitive to auditory stimuli such as alarm clocks or doorbells. The defect is in the HERG gene.[3] When the phone rings, some will pass out!

J.A. Stockman III, M.D.

References

1. Khongphatthanayothin A, Lane J, Thomas D, et al: Effects of cisapride on QT interval in children. *J Pediatr* 133:51-56, 1998.
2. Santucci PA, Haw J, Trohman RG, et al: Interference with an implantable defibrillator by an electronic antitheft-surveillance device. *N Engl J Med* 339:1371-1374, 1998.
3. Husten L: When a ring at the doorbell can be fatal. *Lancet* 353:473, 1999.

Prevention of Cardiac Hypertrophy in Mice by Calcineurin Inhibition
Sussman MA, Lim HW, Gude N, et al (Children's Hosp Med Ctr, Cincinnati, Ohio, Univ of Texas, Dallas; Case Western Reserve Univ, Cleveland, Ohio; et al)
Science 281:1690-1693, 1998   12–19

Introduction.—An inherited form of heart disease that affects 1 in 500 individuals is hypertrophic cardiomyopathy. In young people, it has been cited as the most frequent cause of sudden death. It is defined by a generalized enlargement of the myocardium, and it can progress to heart dilation, functional insufficiency, and failure. Cardiac hypertrophy has been initiated by calcineurin, a calcium-regulated phosphatase, when it was expressed in a constitutively active form in the heart of transgenic mice. There may be a link between calcium concentration and a calcium-regulated signaling molecule in the heart. It was determined whether calcineurin plays a pivotal role in signaling maladaptive hypertrophy in response to alterations in calcium handling in the heart.

Methods.—Four transgenic mouse models of cardiomyopathy were treated, as well as a rat model of pressure-overload hypertrophy with the calcineurin inhibitors cyclosporin and FK506. A mouse model of dilated cardiomyopathy caused by cardiac-specific overexpression of the actin-capping molecule tropomodulin was tested.

Results.—In the pathogenesis of hypertrophic cardiomyopathy, calcineurin plays a critical role. In mice that were genetically predisposed to develop hypertrophic cardiomyopathy as a result of aberrant expression of tropomodulin, myosin light chain-2, or fetal β-tropomyosin in the heart, administration of the calcineurin inhibitors cyclosporin and FK506 prevented disease.

Conclusion.—For certain forms of human heart disease, calcineurin inhibitors merit investigation as potential therapeutics. However, adverse effects associated with long-term therapy have been reported, thus new calcineurin inhibitors may need to be developed. For example, cardiac transplant patients who received such therapy had nephrogenic toxicity and hypertension.

▶ The more we learn about hypertrophic cardiomyopathy, the great deal more we know. Several cardiomyopathies are caused by genetic mutations in contractile proteins. These proteins are organized into repetitive units known as sarcomeres. For example, such mutations have been identified encoding the following genes: beta-myosin heavy chain, cardiac troponin T, alpha tropomyosin, myosin-binding protein C, myosin light chains, and cardiac alpha actin. In order for the sarcomere to do its function in contracting, it requires a basal concentration of intracellular calcium. It has been suggested that mutations in sarcomeric proteins lead to increases in intracellular calcium in order to maintain the heart's ability to contract and to produce an adequate cardiac output. When this happens, the raised intracellular calcium concentrations cause cardiac hypertrophy.

So what does all this have to do with the substance now called calcineurin? Calcineurin is a calcium-regulated phosphatase that initiates cardiac hypertrophy when it is expressed in an active form. Calcineurin is activated by prolonged increases in basal concentrations of calcium. This suggests that calcineurin may play a pivotal role in the link between calcium and its effects on causing the heart to become hypertrophied.

This recent description of the role of calcineurin would be nothing more than an aficionado's nuance about how the heart works were it not for the fact that if calcineurin is the final end point that causes cardiac hypertrophy in those with hereditary cardiomyopathies, there just might be something that can turn it off. Both cyclosporin and a substance known as FK506 inhibit calcineurin. Animal models with hypertrophic cardiomyopathies have been successfully treated, but human trials are barely under way. It will be interesting to see whether either one of these "off-the-shelf" pharmaceuticals is capable of making a big muscle smaller.

Since I know nothing more about calcineurin, this commentary closes with the question: Do cold hands mean a warm heart? Well, apparently the old adage does have a scientific basis. Investigators in Salt Lake City examined hand temperature (taken topically on the fingernail of the middle finger), and compared this temperature to core body temperature in 219 individuals (divided into roughly equal numbers of men and women). Women had a mean core temperature of 98.6°F (SD, 0.8), whereas the mean core temperature for men was 97.4°F (SD, 0.8). The mean hand temperature for women was 87.2°F (SD, 6.7) compared with men, whose hand temperature was 90.0°F (SD, 5.5). These differences are all significant, statistically.

To rephrase this, women are more likely to have cold hands, and at the same time, to have warmer hearts. Thus, the adage, "cold hands, warm heart" is based on real differences in temperature. Actually, this makes some sense. Chances are that a good bit of Adam's core heat was removed when the Maker took his rib to create Eve. This phenomenon may also explain why some men get cold feet when it's time to get serious about a warm heart.

J.A. Stockman III, M.D.

Myocardial Bridging in Children With Hypertrophic Cardiomyopathy: A Risk Factor for Sudden Death
Yetman AT, McCrindle BW, MacDonald C, et al (Univ of Toronto)
N Engl J Med 339:1201-1209, 1998   12–20

Introduction.—The possibility that ischemia can lead to sudden death in children with hypertrophic cardiomyopathy has been suspected based on of the presence of ST-segment depression immediately before ventricular fibrillation on ambulatory monitoring, on the documentation of a higher incidence of perfusion defects on thallium scans in patients with a history of serious cardiac events, and on findings of transmural myocardial infarction at postmortem examination. Children with a diagnosis of hypertrophic cardiomyopathy who had cardiac catheterization and angiography were reviewed to determine the prevalence and clinical significance of myocardial bridging of the left anterior descending coronary artery.

Methods.—To determine whether myocardial bridging was present, angiograms from 36 children with hypertrophic cardiomyopathy were reviewed. An assessment was made of the characteristics of systolic narrowing of the left anterior descending coronary artery caused by myocardial bridging and the duration of residual diastolic compression. Clinical data were also reviewed.

Results.—In 10 (28%) of the children, myocardial bridging was present. For a mean of 50±17% of diastole, compression of the left anterior descending coronary artery persisted. Children with bridging had more chest pain than those without bridging (60% vs 19%); more cardiac arrest with subsequent resuscitation (50% vs 4%); and more ventricular tachycardia (80% vs 8%). Patients without bridging had an increase in systolic blood pressure with exercise (43 ± 31 mm Hg), whereas those without bridging had a decrease in systolic blood pressure with exercise (17 ± 27 mm Hg). Greater ST-segment depression with exercise was seen in children with bridging than in those without bridging, as was a shorter duration of exercise. Patients with bridging had a greater degree of dispersion of the QT interval, corrected for heart rate on the electrocardiogram, than those without bridging. Among patients with bridging, the estimate of the proportion of patients who had not died or had cardiac arrest with subsequent resuscitation, 5 years after the diagnosis of hypertrophic cardiomyopathy, was 67%, in comparison to 84% among those without bridging (Fig 3).

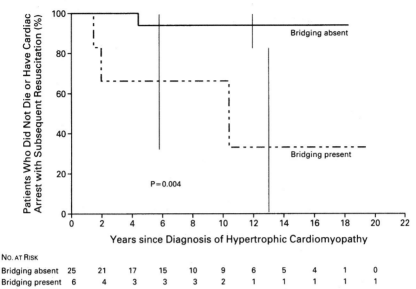

NO. AT RISK

Bridging absent	25	21	17	15	10	9	6	5	4	1	0
Bridging present	6	4	3	3	3	2	1	1	1	1	1

FIGURE 3.—Kaplan-Meier estimates of the proportions of patients who did not die or have cardiac arrest with subsequent resuscitation from the time of diagnosis of hypertrophic cardiomyopathy, according to the presence or absence of myocardial bridging. Five patients who had an event at presentation that led to the diagnosis of hypertrophic cardiomyopathy have been excluded (4 with bridging and 1 without bridging). *Vertical lines*, 95% confidence intervals. *P* value calculated with the log-rank test. (Reprinted by permission of *The New England Journal of Medicine*, from Yetman AT, McCrindle BW, MacDonald C, et al: Myocardial bridging in children with hypertrophic cardiomyopathy: A risk factor for sudden death. *N Engl J Med* 339:1201-1209. Copyright 1998, Massachusetts Medical Society. All rights reserved.)

Conclusion.—In children with hypertrophic cardiomyopathy, myocardial bridging is associated with a poor outcome and with myocardial ischemia.

▶ This article reminds us that some segments of our coronary arteries may be buried within the myocardium of the outer wall of the heart. Coronary arteries are supposed to be draped around the outer heart wall, not within the heart wall, except as they terminally branch and end. The term "myocardial bridging" refers to this phenomenon. In individuals with myocardial bridging, as the heart contracts in systole, the "bridged" coronary arteries are compressed and blood flow either slows or stops. If you happen to be a child with hypertrophic cardiomyopathy and if you also have myocardial bridging of your left coronary artery, you are at high risk of sudden death. The precise role of myocardial bridging, ischemia, and sudden death in patients with hypertrophic cardiomyopathy is controversial, since coronary profusion normally occurs during diastole. Systolic compression would normally be expected to have little or no effect on coronary blood flow. What we see in this article, however, is that affected patients have a distinct lag in blood flow during diastole in coronary arteries that have been compressed during systole. They never fill their coronary arteries the way they should. The practical implication of these data is that one might consider surgery for patients who have hypertrophic cardiomyopathy and who are at unusual risk for sudden death because of myocardial bridging. The surgery involved would require the unroofing of a myocardial bridge. There are data to suggest a beneficial effect of this surgical procedure, although the number of patients so operated upon has been small. Prior to this report, the actual mechanism of sudden death in hypertrophic cardiomyopathy was somewhat unclear. Most children with this disease have a low incidence of ventricular arrhythmias. It may well be that the combination of myocardial bridging and hypertrophic cardiomyopathy in a subset of children is what proves to be the lethal double whammy. Needless to say, now that this article has appeared, we may very well see more angiograms being performed as part of the evaluation of hypertrophic cardiomyopathy in children.

This is the last commentary in the Heart and Blood Vessels chapter, so as we often do, we will close with a "whodunit." Your training comes in handy one day while at a local bookstore, one of the types that is part of a large national chain. While perusing the aisles, you come to stand next to a young, middle-aged adult woman who suddenly complains of dizziness and passes out before your eyes. As you provide assistance, you notice that this woman is wearing a medical alert bracelet. The bracelet says that she has an implantable cardioverter-defibrillator. You look around, and realize that you are only about 2 feet from the exit pathway of the store. What maneuver do you perform to save this patient's life?

You should grab the patient and drag her away from the store's exit. This happened to a recently described adult who, while standing in a bookstore, received a shock from his implanted defibrillator. As it turns out, he was standing just 2 feet from an electronic anti-theft–surveillance device that was built into the casework surrounding the exit of a bookstore. A number of electromagnetic devices can trigger such defibrillators. Slot machines, remote-control devices for toys, and electronic anti-theft–surveillance equipment have all been reported to cause discharge of implantable defibrillators. Such discharges can cause a heart to stop. Fortunately, the defibrillators will trigger again to restart a heart, but only after symptoms such as syncope have occurred.[1]

There are approximately 400,000 anti-theft–surveillance devices now in use. Acoustomagnetic electronic surveillance systems produce a variety of interactions with pacemakers including asynchronous pacing, tachycardia, inhibition of the pacemaker, and system-induced pacing. Patients with implantable defibrillators rarely get into trouble with such surveillance devices unless they dawdle around them. The same holds true for patients with pacemakers. Patients with pacemakers, particularly those who are dependent on them, should take care to minimize their contact with acoustomagnetic systems by passing quickly through anti-theft detection gates in stores.[2]

J.A. Stockman III, M.D.

References

1. Santucci PA, Haw J, Trohman RG, et al: Interference with an implantable defibrillator by an electonic antitheft-surveillance device. *N Engl J Med* 339:1371-1374, 1998.
2. McIvor ME, Sridhar S: Interaction between cardiac pacemakers and anti-shoplifting security systems. *N Engl J Med* 339:1394-1395, 1998.

13 The Blood

False-Positive HIV-1 Test Results in a Low-risk Screening Setting of Voluntary Blood Donation
Kleinman S, for the Retrovirus Epidemiology Donor Study (Westat Inc, Rockville, Md)
JAMA 280:1080-1085, 1998   13-1

Introduction.—The detection of antibodies to HIV-1 results in a diagnosis of HIV-1. Testing involves a screening enzyme immunoassay and the Western blot assay. The Western blot assay has required the detection of bands of 3 specific HIV-1 gene products, including a core (Gag) protein (p24), an envelope (Env) glycoprotein (gp41 or gp120/160), and a polymerase protein (p31; endonuclease). In 1993, the criterion for requiring p31 reactivity was dropped, and since then, low-risk individuals have been falsely classified as HIV-1 infected. A large blood donation database was reviewed to investigate the prevalence of false positive HIV-1 Western blots.

Methods.—More than 5 million allogeneic and autologous blood donors donated blood in a 4-year period, and of those, 421 donors tested positive for HIV-1 by Western blot. These individuals also had HIV-1 RNA polymerase chain reaction (PCR) testing and follow-up HIV-1 serology.

Results.—Thirty-nine of 421 donors (9.3%) met the criteria of possible false positivity because they lacked reactivity to p31. PCR proved that 20 (51.3%) were not infected with HIV-1. The false positive prevalence was 0.0004% of all donors and 4.8% of Western blot-positive donors.

Conclusion.—The combination of enzyme immunoassay and Western blot testing in blood donor and other HIV-1 screening programs may cause a false diagnosis of HIV-1 infection. Counseling should be given to those who test positive with a Western blot but lack the p31 band, as there is uncertainty about the conclusion that they may be HIV infected. Further testing should be conducted on these individuals with RNA PCR and HIV serologic analysis.

▶ My goodness, the story around HIV screening detection has become quite complicated. Fifteen years ago, when screening for HIV became possible with the use of a method to detect antibodies to HIV-1, we knew that the initial screening detection method, an enzyme immunoassay, would sometimes have false positive results. We thought the problem was solved when a 2-stage process—beginning with a screening enzyme immunoassay and followed by a supplementary test to confirm the specificity of the result—became routine. The supplementary test was the HIV-1 Western blot assay. It soon became clear that even with this 2-stage diagnostic process, some who did not have HIV infection were being misdiagnosed as having this deadly infection. Because of concerns about possible false positive reactions, the Food and Drug Administration (FDA) recommended that those who tested positive with the 2-stage process also be specifically examined for detection of several HIV-1 gene products. The FDA made the noose much tighter in terms of minimizing the number of false positives.

The rub with such approaches is that one will possibly sacrifice sensitivity for specificity. For this reason, a few years ago, the FDA backed off of the requirement for what is known as p31 testing for those who were thought to be HIV infected. The result is what we see in this report, namely, that about 5% of individuals who are antibody positive when donating blood in the United States (thought to be low-risk for HIV infection) will be incorrectly characterized as being HIV infected by current technologies. The misclassification of even a single HIV-uninfected person as being infected will have disastrous consequences for that individual as well as for the individual's family. On the other hand, 19 out of 20 who have been through the whole route of confirmatory screening will, in fact, be HIV infected. The issue is whether misdiagnosing 1 in 20 is a legitimate price to pay for picking up everyone who is able to be detected by current methodologies. You will have to be the judge.

You can see a lot more about HIV infection in the Infectious Disease and Immunology chapter. When we speak of blood products and risks of infection, please recognize that the health professionals at greatest risk these days are phlebotomists. Do you know how many blood specimens a year the average phlebotomist obtains? The typical phlebotomist at the Mayo Clinic can answer this query for you. The Rochester, Minnesota facility employs approximately 200 such individuals. The average phlebotomist takes 10,000 specimens per year.[1] Concern about needle-stick injuries at Mayo led to the introduction of additional safety training and equipment, such as one-handed recapping boxes. This resulted in a fall in the rate of needle-stick injuries from 1.5/10,000 venipunctures to 0.2/10,000. Imagine drawing blood thousands of times a year and having a risk of just 1 needle-stick injury once every 5 years! Not bad for such a sticky career.

J.A. Stockman III, M.D.

Reference

1. Stacey M: Phlebotomy. *Mayo Clinic Proc* 73:611-615, 1998.

Detection of a Novel DNA Virus (TTV) in Blood Donors and Blood Products

Simmonds P, Davidson F, Lycett C, et al (Univ of Edinburgh, Scotland; Edinburgh and South East Scotland Blood Transfusion Service, Scotland; Royal Infirmary of Edinburgh, Scotland)

Lancet 352:191-195, 1998   13–2

Introduction.—The search for infectious viral agents responsible for residual post-transfusion non-A, non-B hepatitis that is not caused by hepatitis C virus has revealed a novel virus, a transfusion-transmitted virus (TTV). This newly discovered DNA virus has been implicated as a cause of post-transfusion hepatitis. The frequency of TTV viremia in blood donors in Scotland was assessed to determine the extent to which TTV contaminates clotting factors VIII and IX. The possible etiologic role of TTV in cryptogenic fulminant hepatic failure (FHF) was also studied.

Methods.—The plasma of blood donors and patients with FHF along with blood products (clotting-factors VIII and IX concentrates), underwent DNA extraction. TTV was detected by polymerase chain reaction (PCR) using primers from a conserved region in the TTV genome.

Results.—Nineteen of 1000 (1.9%) nonremunerated regular blood donors had TTV viremia. Infection was observed more frequently in older blood donors (mean age, 53 years) than in donors infected with hepatitis C virus and other parenterally-transmitted viruses. Ten (56%) of 18 batches of factor VIII and IX concentrates manufactured from like nonremunerated donors and 7 (44%) of 16 batches of commercially available products were contaminated with TTV. Solvent and detergent treatment had little effect on the detection of TTV in factors VIII and IX by PCR; these virucidal agents seemed to inactivate TTV infectivity. Four (19%) of 21 patients with FHF had TTV infection. In 3 patients, TTV infection was detected at the disease onset and was thus not excluded from being the cause of the disease. The TTV infection was detected more frequently in

TABLE 2.—TTV Infection in Hemophilic Patients

Severity	Treatment Before 1986*	Proportion TTV Positive
Haemophilia A		
Mild	Y	1/9 *(11%)*
Moderate	Y	3/18 *(17%)*
Severe	Y	13/32 *(41%)*
Haemophilia B		
Mild	Y	1/9 *(11%)*
Moderate/severe	Y	4/7 *(57%)*
von Willebrand	Y	1/9 *(11%)*
Total	Y	23/84 *(27%)*
Haemophilia A	N	1/19 *(0-5%)*

*Y = treated with non-virally inactivated clotting factor concentrates; N = treatment with virally inactivated concentrates only.

(Courtesy of Simmonds P, Davidson F, Lycett C, et al: Detection of a novel DNA virus [TTV] in blood donors and blood products. *Lancet* 352[9123]:191-195, 1998. Copyright by The Lancet Ltd., 1998.)

patients with hemophilia who were treated with nonvirally inactivated concentrates than in blood donors (Table 2).

Conclusion.—The TTV viremia is common in the blood-donor population. Transmission of TTV by transfusion of blood components may have already happened extensively. At present, there is an urgent need for clinical assessment of infected donors and recipients of blood and blood products and determination of the etiologic role of TTV in hepatic and extrahepatic disease.

▶ Just what the world needs, another transfusion associated viral disease. First there was hepatitis A. Then there was hepatitis B. Following that came non-A, non-B hepatitis. Most of the latter was recategorized into a newly identified virus some years back called hepatitis C virus. Then there was hepatitis D (delta virus), seen in association with hepatitis B. Even more recently described is the hepatitis G virus (HGV/GBV-C), which although widespread, is not a cause of serious illness. Lastly, in 1997, a new transfusion-related virus was described in a patient with post-transfusion non-A, -B, -C, -D, or -G hepatitis. Lacking a name for this virus, it has been assigned the title "TTV" (transfusion-transmitted virus).

The abstracted article shows us that TTV is reasonably common (2% of all regular blood donors have PCR-demonstrable TTV in their blood). The high frequency of TTV infection in hemophiliac patients indicates that TTV is likely to be transmitted by treatment with blood and blood component products. Hemophilia factor concentrates that are heat-treated, however, are TTV PCR negative. Factor concentrates that are solvent or detergent-produced do contain TTV PCR-detectable virus.

Now that we know that there is 1 more TTV, the issue to be pursued is whether this causes significant illness. The ability of TTV to cause posttransfusion hepatitis has been documented by a description of the association of TTV viremia, and transaminase increases post transfusion. Transaminase levels increase 6 to 9 weeks posttransfusion in blood product recipients.

The above is the bad news. The good news is that other investigations have recently shown that the TTV virus rarely, if at all, causes chronic liver disease. In a study of some 72 patients with chronic liver disease of ill-defined origin, the prevalence of TTV DNA in affected individuals was no different than the population at-large.[1]

There is very little written about TTV in children. We don't know for sure that it might not cause significant liver disease in those who become infected. It is also clear that TTV can be transmitted by other means than a transfusion, because most children who are TTV-positive have never received transfusions. We also don't know if maternal TTV infection can cause problems in a baby. Stay tuned to the litany of the alphabet soup of transfusion-related viruses. Chances are fairly good that TTV will be assigned a more conventional letter name. Maybe we should call it "Z" with fingers crossed that it will be the very last hepatitis virus. Lots of luck.

J.A. Stockman III, M.D.

Reference

1. Naoumov NV, Petrova EP, Thomas MG, et al: Presence of newly described human DNA virus (TTV) in patients with liver disease. *Lancet* 352:195-197, 1998.

Effect of Consumption of Food Cooked in Iron Pots on Iron Status and Growth of Young Children: A Randomised Trial
Adish AA, Esrey SA, Gyorkos TW, et al (McGill Univ, Quebec; Jimma Inst of Health Sciences, Ethiopia; UNICEF, New York; et al)
Lancet 353:712-716, 1999   13–3

Introduction.—About 50% of children and women and about 25% of men are affected by iron deficiency anemia in less-developed countries. A consequence of anemia is slow growth. Many countries seek a cost-effective and convenient control strategy since the effects of anemia on health and economic welfare can be severe. When cheaper and lighter aluminum pots became available, the use of iron pots, which were used routinely in many developing countries, was abandoned. It is known that iron pots can leach iron into foods; however, their role in the control of iron deficiency anemia has not been studied. The effect on iron deficiency of the introduction of iron pots into households in Ethiopia was studied.

Methods.—There were 407 Ethiopian children, one per household, included in the study to determine the effects of iron or aluminum cooking pots. The households were randomly assigned to receive an iron pot or an aluminum pot. To minimize the differences between the 2 groups, except for iron acquired by children through foods cooked in iron pots, the mothers were given elemental iron supplements of 60 mg daily for 3 months if they were given an aluminum pot. Intention-to-treat was the basis of analysis. Change in children's hemoglobin concentration, weight, or length over the study period were the main outcome measures. A laboratory study of total and available iron in traditional Ethiopian foods cooked in iron, aluminum, and clay pots was also conducted.

Results.—In the iron-pot group, the change in hemoglobin concentration was greater than in the aluminum-pot group with a mean difference of 1.3 g/dL between groups. In weight gain, the mean difference to 12 months between groups was 0.1 kg, and in length gain to 12 months, the mean difference was 0.6 cm. In foods cooked in iron pots, total and available iron was greatest, except for available iron in legumes, for which there was no difference among types of pots.

Conclusion.—Lower rates of anemia and better growth were found in Ethiopian children fed food from iron pots than in children whose food was cooked in aluminum pots. A useful method to prevent iron deficiency anemia may be the provision of iron cooking pots for households in less-developed countries.

▶ This is one neat little report. Imagine diminishing or eliminating dietary iron deficiency anemia by putting an iron pot in every kitchen. But wasn't it

Shakespeare who said, "Double, double toil and trouble; fire burn, and cauldron bubble"? Might there be some problems such as iron overload as an associated risk with the use of iron pots? Apparently not.

Given the fact that worldwide, iron deficiency is the single most common nutrient deficiency, and also a deficiency with us here in the United States, wouldn't it make sense to alter our cooking techniques with a low-cost, sustainable strategy that would improve iron intake to whole families and communities? This actually sounds reasonable since alternative methods to prevent iron deficiency, including food fortification, have not been very effective in certain parts of the world. In 1998, UNICEF, the World Health Organization, and the International Nutritional Anemia Consultative Group published guidelines for iron supplementation in children aged 6 to 24 months. They recommended 18 months of daily supplementation with iron and folic acid for babies of normal birth weight (22 months if birth weight was low).[1] It has turned out that this aim is unrealistic for most young children in developing countries. Similarly, food fortification is at an extremely rudimentary stage in poor countries. In this context, perhaps cooking in iron pots should be thought about as a remedy and systemically evaluated as an alternative strategy.

So what does this have to do with life here in the United States? Do we need an iron pot in every kitchen if we have two cars in every garage? Even as a wealthy nation, we still have 3% of our children with iron deficiency. Several times that percent of our teenagers have iron deficiency. Why not cook with iron skillets? The likelihood of producing iron overload seems remote.

There is a set of iron skillets and pots in our kitchen at home, hand-me-downs from my mother's kitchen. They are used on a regular basis although they no longer fry bacon and eggs every morning as they once did 50 years ago. The only problem with iron pots and pans is that they can and do rust if you don't dry them off or oil them lightly after each use. Actually, iron oxide (rust) is better absorbed than even elemental iron from the pans, so rust is not a nutritional deterrent.

...let Shakespeare's cauldron bubble.

J.A. Stockman III, M.D.

Reference

1. Staltzfus RJ, Dreyfuss ML: Guidelines for the use of iron supplements to prevent and treat iron deficiency anemia. INACG, WHO, UNICEF. Washington, DC, International Life Sciences Institute (ILSI), July 1998.

Unexplained Refractory Iron-deficiency Anemia Associated With *Helicobacter pylori* Gastric Infection in Children: Further Clinical Evidence
Barabino A, Dufour C, Marino CE, et al (G. Gaslini Inst, Genoa, Italy; Ospedali Galliera, Genoa, Italy)
J Pediatr Gastroenterol Nutr 28:116-119, 1999   13–4

Background.—Most cases of *Helicobacter pylori* infection in children are associated with recurrent abdominal pain, gastric dyspepsia, or duodenal ulcer. These authors described 4 children who had iron-deficiency anemia associated with *H. pylori* gastric infection.

> *Case Reports.*—The 4 children ranged in age from 4 years to 13 years 7 months; 3 were boys and 1 was a girl. All patients had iron-deficiency anemia (hemoglobin levels of 8.2 to 10.6 g/dL), all had normal iron absorption test results, but none responded to iron supplementation and/or packed red cell transfusion. Immunoglobulin G antibody titers to *H. pylori* were measured by enzyme-linked immunosorbent assay, and all 4 patients had greatly elevated titers (between 48% and 71%; normal, less than 15%). *H. pylori* was confirmed by histologic analysis in all 4 patients; 2 had gastrointestinal symptoms, and 2 did not.
>
> Each patient underwent a course of drug therapy (amoxicillin, bismuth, tinidazole, ranitidine, and/or omeprazole) ranging from 15 days to 1 month 15 days to eradicate *H. pylori* infection. Immediately after the infection was eradicated, hematologic profiles and iron stores were as low as they had been before treatment. However, iron supplementation for a period of from 3 weeks to 3 months improved hematologic and iron profiles in all patients. Patients remained normal, with no anemia and no evidence of *H. pylori* infection, at their last follow-up visit 11 months to 3 years after their profiles normalized.

Conclusion.—None of these children with iron-deficiency anemia responded to iron supplementation until the *H. pylori* infection was eradicated. This strongly suggests a causal role for this microorganism in these patients. Yet eradication of *H. pylori* was not enough because iron metabolism did not normalize until supplemental iron was again added to the diet. This suggests that, as the bacteria died, the iron stores were also lost and were not available for hemopoiesis. Thus, clinicians should consider *H. pylori* infection (whether symptomatic or not) in children who have unexplained iron-deficiency anemia that does not respond to iron supplementation or packed red blood cell transfusion.

▶ Iron-eating bacteria. Amazing! Who would have thought that a bacterium such as *H. pylori* would interfere with iron metabolism in such a way as to not only cause iron deficiency via gastrointestinal bleeding, but also to cause medicinal iron to be ineffective as part of the treatment of the iron deficiency caused by the gastrointestinal bleeding. Indeed, that's exactly what *H. pylori* does.

It is well known that microorganisms rely on a host's iron in order to grow. *H. pylori*, which can cause gastritis and duodenal ulcers, acquires its iron from human lactoferrin. There are laboratory studies showing that human lactoferrin does support *H. pylori* growth in the laboratory at very high levels. We also see from this report that among young patients with gastritis secondary to *H. pylori* infection, the organism sequesters iron for its own metabolism. Giving iron orally cannot override this problem.

Most of us have not thought about *H. pylori* as being a parasite but, indeed, it is. It sneaks into us and stays. It consumes our bodily iron for its own purposes. It causes an iron refractory, iron deficient anemia. The only way to adequately correct the hematologic problem is to stamp out the bug first and then treat with iron.

If there is a message in all this, it is that the next time you see a child with iron deficiency who fails to respond to oral iron therapy (assuming that the iron was properly given), you may want to think about *H. pylori* infection as a potential reason why this problem is occurring. *H. pylori* infection is relatively easy to treat with antibiotics and with bismuth. Giving iron without treating the underlying cause of the anemia helps the offending organism but doesn't do much for the host.

Antibiotics first, iron second.

Lastly, do not forget that things other than blood can cause black stool. The bismuth used to treat *H. pylori* infection can do this as well. The usual suspects when it comes to black bowel movements are as follows: melena, iron preparations, bismuth, lead salts, licorice, charcoal, coal, and dirt. Eating unusually large amounts of Oreo cookies can also cause black stools, a malady that goes by the term "Hydroxy fecalis." Lastly, please recognize that ingestion of as little as 250 mg of vitamin C can cause what otherwise would have been a guaiac-positive stool to be a negative one. A properly done guaiac test requires being off vitamin C for 72 hours before a stool sample is obtained.

J.A. Stockman III, M.D.

High Absorption of Fortification Iron From Current Infant Formulas
Hertrampf E, Olivares M, Pizarro F, et al (Universidad de Chile, Santiago)
J Pediatr Gastroenterol Nutr 27:425-430, 1998   13–5

Introduction.—Infant formulas are designed to meet nutritional needs of infants when breast milk is not possible. Little is known about the estimates of absorption of fortification iron from cow's milk and infant formulas. Modifications that could affect iron absorption have been performed on formulas during recent decades. Iron bioavailability from milk-based formulas was measured.

Methods.—Measurements were taken of the bioavailability of isotopically labeled iron (^{55}Fe and ^{50}Fe) from several infant formulas adminis-

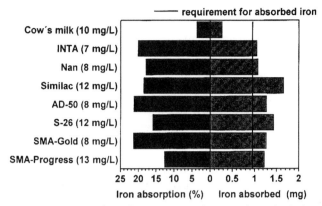

FIGURE 1.—Geometric means of iron absorption (%), and amount of iron absorbed in consumption of 750 mL of each of the different milks studied. Formulas are: 1 developed by the Institute of Nutrition and Food Technology, University of Chile, Santiago; NAN, Nestlé-Chile, Santiago, Chile; Similac and AD-40; Ross Laboratories, Columbus, OH; and S-26, SMA-Gold, SMA-Progress, Wyeth-Ayerst International, USA. (Courtesy of Hertrampf E, Olivares M, Pizarro F, et al: High absorption of fortification iron from current infant formulas. *J Pediatr Gastroenterol Nutr* 27:425-430, 1998.)

tered to contraceptive-using women between the ages of 30 and 50. A powdered, whole cow's milk was compared to 6 infant formulas and 1 follow-on formula. The results were normalized to an absorption of 40% from a reference dose of iron.

Results.—Infant formulas had consistently higher iron bioavailability (19%) than the unmodified cow's milk (4%). There was intermediate iron absorption of the follow-on formula (13%). Assuming a consumption of 750 mL/day of formula, formulas with 8 mg/L iron and 1 with 7 mg/L supply approximately 1 mg of absorbed iron (Fig 1). The iron needs of most infants are covered by infant formulas during their period of greatest vulnerability. The absorption of approximately twice the infant iron requirements would occur with formulas containing 12 mg/L iron.

Conclusion.—High iron bioavailability is found with current infant formulas, which is an appealing argument for lowering the level of iron fortification in infant formulas. The iron needs of term infants during their first year of life would be provided by formulas containing 7 to 8 mg/L of iron.

▶ Worldwide, iron deficiency remains a significant problem. Here in the United States, the prevalence of iron deficiency anemia has declined from about 9% to under 3% in the less-than-24-month–old population, all within the last 15 to 20 years. The reason why this article is important is that it tells us that there has been a change over time in the amount of iron that is absorbed from current infant formulas. Now, some 19% of iron, on average, is absorbed, compared with the 4% to 10% from previously reported series of infants. This means that we may not need as much iron in formulas as is currently recommended by the American Academy of Pediatrics. The Academy suggests that 12 mg/L of iron is the appropriate target for infant formulas. Virtually all fortified formulas in the United States contain this amount of iron. The math would tell us, however, that formulas with 7 to 8 mg/L would be more than adequate to cover the amount of required iron. There are data showing that formulas with as little as 4 mg/L of iron (formulas available overseas) prevent iron deficiency in the first 2 years of life. No one has shown, however, that using a 12 mg/L iron-enriched formula does any harm. Thus, there will be a great deal of debate and anguish, and perhaps some argument, about whether we should lower our recommendations when it comes to iron supplementation.

We are learning more and more about how iron is absorbed and what regulates this absorption. It would appear that iron transport across cellular membranes, gut and elsewhere, is regulated by a particular gene known as *DCT1/Nramp2*. The identification of this gene and other members of the related gene family may help address a number of unanswered questions about iron deficiency and the nonhematologic manifestations of iron deficiency. Iron deficiency has been linked to defects in psychomotor and cognitive function, impaired exercise tolerance and work performance, impaired intestinal absorption of a variety of substances, including decreased absorption of fats and vitamin A and increased absorption of lead, and finally to impaired white-cell function and immunity. The gene involved with iron transport, if defective for any reason, could affect cell cycles, mitochondrial protein processing, susceptibility to infection, and brain function. Some have even suggested that a defect in this gene may be the cause of what we occasionally see clinically, iron deficiency anemia unresponsive to iron therapy. If you want to read more about what regulates iron movement in the body, the genes involved, and the potential relationship with cognitive abnormalities in the presence of iron deficiency, see the superb commentary of Gallagher and Ehrenkranz.[1]

J.A. Stockman III, M.D.

Reference

1. Gallagher PG, Ehrenkranz RA: Understanding iron absorption and metabolism. *J Pediatr Gastroenterol Nutr* 27:610-613, 1998.

Prenatal Diagnosis of Fetal RhD Status by Molecular Analysis of Maternal Plasma

Lo YMD, Hjelm NM, Fidler C, et al (Chinese Univ of Hong Kong, China; John Radcliffe Hosp, Oxford, England)
N Engl J Med 339:1734-1738, 1998
13–6

Background.—The Rh blood group system is involved in hemolytic disease of the newborn. In cases where the mother is RhD-negative and the father is heterozygous, there is a 50% chance that the child will be RhD-positive. Several groups have analyzed the possibility of determining fetal RhD status from fetal cells isolated from the maternal circulation.

TABLE 1.—Results of RhD Genotyping of Fetuses of RhD-negative
Women With the Use of the RhD PCR Assay*

Trimester of Pregnancy	RhD-Positive Fetus†	RhD-Negative Fetus†
	No. of Positive Fetuses on PCR Testing/Total No. of Fetuses (%)	
First	7/9 (78)	0/3
Second	22/22 (100)	0/8
Third	8/8 (100)	0/7

*The RhD PCR assay used plasma samples from the women.
†The RhD status was determined by serologic analysis of cord-blood samples in the case of samples obtained during the first or third trimester and by PCR testing of amniotic fluid in the case of samples obtained during the second trimester.
(Reprinted with permission of *The New England Journal of Medicine*, from Lo YMD, Hjelm NM, Fidler C, et al: Prenatal diagnosis of fetal RhD status by molecular analysis of maternal plasma. *N Engl J Med* 339:1734-1738. Copyright 1998, Massachusetts Medical Society. All rights reserved.)

The feasibility of fetal RhD genotyping from fetal DNA extracted from maternal plasma samples was investigated.

Methods.—Blood samples were collected from 57 women with singleton pregnancies, who were patients at the John Radcliffe hospital. Of these 57 women, 12 were in the first trimester, 30 in the second trimester, and 15 in the third trimester of pregnancy. Ten were primigravidas. A sample of cord blood was collected after delivery. DNA was extracted from plasma samples and amniotic fluid, and real-time fluorogenic polymerase chain reaction (PCR) analysis was performed with a combined thermal cycler and fluorescence detector with the ability to monitor the progress of individual PCR reactions optically.

Results.—Among the 57 pregnancies, 39 fetuses were RhD-positive and 18 were RhD-negative (Table 1). Results of maternal plasma analysis were completely concordant with the results of amniotic fluid analysis in samples from women in the second or third trimester of pregnancy. Among the maternal samples collected in the first trimester, 2 yielded false-negative results, and the results in the other 10 were concordant with serologic analysis.

Conclusions.—Noninvasive fetal RhD genotyping can be performed rapidly and accurately with fetal DNA extracted from maternal plasma beginning in the second trimester of pregnancy. This method could potentially be used for the diagnosis of many disorders involving single genes.

▶ Rh disease is still with us. We must be as aggressive as ever at making sure that an Rh-negative woman does not become Rh sensitized. Currently, unless the father of a child is known to be RhD-negative, all Rh-negative women must receive Rh$_0$(D) immune globulin at 28 weeks of pregnancy, after abortion or threatened abortion, after amniocentesis or chorionic villus sampling, and after any other invasive intrauterine procedure. All of this would be unnecessary if one could be certain that a baby in utero were Rh-negative. The rub is when a mother is Rh-negative and a father is Rh-positive. There is a 50-50 chance that the father is actually heterozygous for the RhD antigen (slightly more than 50% of people are). In cases in which the father is heterozygous for the RhD gene and the mother is Rh-negative, there is a 50% chance that the unborn baby will be RhD-positive and a 50% chance that he or she will be negative. Determining the prenatal RhD status of such fetuses is helpful because if a baby is Rh-negative, no further testing or therapeutic maneuvers are needed. If the fetus is Rh-positive, immune globulin is given at 28 weeks, etc., and various studies are done to determine whether fetal hemolysis might be present during pregnancy.

The importance of the article abstracted is impossible to underestimate. Prior to this report, the only way of determining fetal RhD status was either by taking a sample of amniotic fluid or by obtaining a chorionic villus biopsy and testing for Rh status by PCR. Both of these techniques are invasive. Both techniques can cause leakage of fetal cells into the maternal circulation, with sensitization of the mother, albeit with a reduced incidence with the use of $Rh_0(D)$ immune globulin. The way around this is to see if one can detect evidence of fetal genetic material in the maternal circulation that would give a clue to its Rh status. We learn that it is possible to detect RhD messenger RNA in maternal plasma, if it is present there. We also see that this can be done as early as the first trimester in most instances. By early in the second trimester, all Rh-positive fetuses can be detected with a simple blood test on the mother.

Maternal blood samplings are now being done with increasing frequency to diagnose genetic and other disorders of the fetus. It has been used to prenatally diagnose Down syndrome in the fetus. As our ability to do surveillance on a pregnant woman's blood evolves, it will likely be possible to detect many other fetal abnormalities with nothing more than a sample of venous blood, not from the placenta but from a mother's arm. An unborn baby has no secrets from its mother. A sample of maternal blood tells it all.

J.A. Stockman III, M.D.

Long-term Safety and Effectiveness of Iron-Chelation Therapy With Deferiprone for Thalassemia Major
Olivieri NF, Brittenham GM, McLaren CE, et al (Univ of Toronto; Columbia Univ College of Physicians and Surgeons, New York; Univ of California, Irvine; et al)
N Engl J Med 339:417-423, 1998   13–7

Background.—Deferiprone, an orally active iron-chelation agent, is being studied as a treatment for iron overload in patients with thalassemia major. Animal studies have shown that prolonged treatment is correlated with a decrease in the efficacy of deferiprone and exacerbation of hepatic fibrosis. Annual hepatic iron stores were determined by chemical analysis of liver biopsy specimens and/or magnetic susceptometry.

Methods.—Seventy-two biopsy specimens from 19 patients treated with deferiprone for more than 1 year were examined. Forty-eight liver biopsy

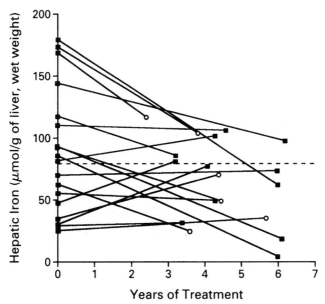

Years of Treatment

FIGURE 1.—Initial and final hepatic iron concentrations in 18 patients with thalassemia major treated with deferiprone. The *dashed line* indicates the value of 80 μmol of iron per gram of liver tissue, wet weight, above which there is an increased risk of cardiac disease and early death due to iron loading during long-term treatment with deferoxamine. *Squares*, concentrations determined by liver biopsy; *circles*, concentrations determined by magnetic susceptometry. (Reprinted by permission of *The New England Journal of Medicine*, from Olivieri NF, Brittenham GM, McLaren CE, et al: Long-term safety and effectiveness of iron-chelation therapy with deferiprone for thalassemia major. N Engl J Med 339:417-423. Copyright 1998, Massachusetts Medical Society. All rights reserved.)

specimens obtained from 20 patients treated with parenteral deferoxamine for more than 1 year were also assessed.

Findings.—Eighteen of the 19 patients given deferiprone received the drug continuously for a mean of 4.6 years. At final analysis, 7 of these patients had hepatic iron levels of at least 80 μmol/g of liver, wet weight. Fourteen of the 19 patients with multiple biopsies performed for more than 1 year could be evaluated for hepatic fibrosis progression. Twelve of the 20 deferoxamine-treated patients could be assessed for progression. Fibrosis had progressed in 5 deferiprone-treated patients, compared with none of the deferoxamine-treated patients. The estimated median time to progression of fibrosis was 3.2 years in the deferiprone-treated patients. After adjustment for initial hepatic iron concentration, the estimated odds of fibrosis progression increased by a factor of 5.8 with each additional year of deferiprone therapy (Fig 1).

Conclusions.—Deferiprone apparently does not sufficiently control body iron burden in patients with thalassemia. In addition, this agent may worsen hepatic fibrosis. Further research is warranted.

▶ Deferoxamine, the only drug proved effective in preventing iron overload in patients with thalassemia major, was introduced into clinical practice more than a quarter of a century ago. It has been documented to reduce liver iron concentration and can prevent the progression to cirrhosis. Treatment with deferoxamine, however, is not ideal. It must be administered as many as 6 days a week via a continuous subcutaneous infusion over a 12-hour period. Needless to say, such treatments are time consuming and uncomfortable. Most children don't like the therapy, and compliance becomes increasingly poor, particularly in the teenage years. Some children and adults treated with deferoxamine have serious side effects, including local skin reactions, hearing loss, neurotoxicity, renal damage, lung toxicity, growth retardation, and local infection. The cost of the drug and its administration are quite high.

Because subcutaneous deferoxamine therapy, in a sense, is so cruel, investigators have been looking for years for alternative oral iron-chelating agents. The only oral agent that has been investigated extensively is deferiprone. This drug is currently licensed in India for the treatment of iron overload, and several studies have suggested that negative iron balance can be achieved, although the long-term efficacy of deferiprone therapy in patients with thalassemia major has remained controversial. It too can cause serious side effects, including low granulocyte counts, arthritis, gastrointestinal tract disorders, and zinc deficiency.

In the abstracted article, Olivieri et al. suggest that long-term deferiprone therapy has a risk/benefit ratio that does not favor its use. Deferiprone itself may even cause hepatic fibrosis.

Despite the report of Olivieri et al., the case against deferiprone has not been totally made. The limited number of patients studied, the small size of the liver-biopsy specimens examined, and the differences between patients with worsening fibrosis and those without progression weaken the conclusions of this article. Because the drug is available and is licensed for use in some parts of the world, it would be important to follow data from India and elsewhere to determine just how safe and effective this agent is. Chances are that we will not see it licensed in this country any time soon, however.

Meanwhile, as the search for the ideal chelating agent continues, we should be doing everything possible to limit the amount of iron ingested by children with thalassemia major. Commercially available breads are iron-fortified, as are most breakfast cereals. The same is true of most prepackaged flours. These should be avoided, to a reasonable extent. Homemade pasta and breads made from natural flour that never see iron enrichment are great and may even block some iron absorption from other dietary sources. The best thing, however, is to drink tea with most meals. Substances in tea block the absorption of more than 90% of inorganic iron in the diet. Tea time is a good time anytime when it comes to thalassemia major.

J.A. Stockman III, M.D.

Pediatric Bone Marrow Cellularity: Are We Expecting Too Much?

Friebert SE, Shepardson LB, Shurin SB, et al (Case Western Reserve Univ, Cleveland, Ohio; Univ Hosps of Cleveland, Ohio)
J Pediatr Hematol Oncol 20:439-443, 1998   13–8

Introduction.—To diagnose hypocellular or hypercellular conditions, to monitor the course of disease, to determine optimal drug dosage, and to evaluate response to therapy, the assessment of bone marrow celullarity in the pediatric patient is useful. Loose evidence-based standards have shown that marrow cellularity is nearly 100% at birth and that it decreases by about 10% in each decade of life. A large retrospective review of pediatric bone marrow samples was conducted to determine whether cellularity assessments are correct when current methods of sample acquisition are used and to evaluate the effect of malignant and nonmalignant diagnoses on the marrow cellularity of a child.

Methods.—There were 448 bone marrow core biopsy or clot specimens, of which 45 were samples from healthy donors. The biopsies were taken from the posterior iliac crest of patients younger than 1 to 18 years, of whom 55% were male.

Results.—The entire sample had a mean cellularity of 65.4%. In boys and girls, cellularity was similar, but with age, it varied. In patients younger than 2 years, cellularity was highest (at 79.8%), declining in patients 2 to 4 years old (to 68.6%) and in patients 5 to 9 years old (to 59.1%) (Fig 1). In older patients, 10 to 14 years, it remained stable at 60.1% and in patients aged 15 to 18 years, it was 61.1%. In patients with an underlying nonhematomologic malignancy, mean cellularity was similar to that of healthy donors, but it was roughly 6% higher in patients with hematopoietic disorders, after adjusting for age and gender (Fig 2).

Conclusion.—Current techniques of marrow collection and standardized analysis show average cellularity during the first 2 decades of life to be lower than previously estimated. Until the age of 5 years, cellularity

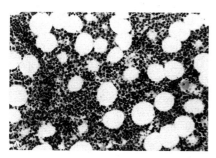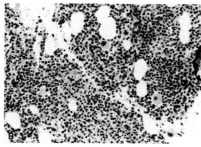

FIGURE 1.—**A,** bone marrow core biopsy with a cellularity of 60% (hematoxylin and eosin). **B,** bone marrow core biopsy with a cellularity of 80% (hematoxylin and eosin). (Courtesy of Friebert SE, Shepardson LB, Shurin SB, et al: Pediatric bone marrow cellularity: Are we expecting too much? *J Pediatr Hematol Oncol* 20:439-443, 1998.)

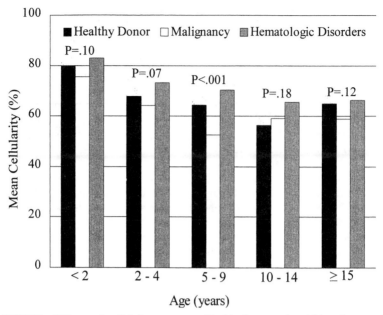

FIGURE 2.—Differences in cellularity among normal healthy donors, patients with nonhematopoietic malignancies, and patients with nonmalignant hematologic disorders, stratified according to age. (Courtesy of Friebert SE, Shepardson LB, Shurin SB, et al: Pediatric bone marrow cellularity: Are we expecting too much? *J Pediatr Hematol Oncol* 20:439-443, 1998.)

declined with age and was fairly constant thereafter. Differences according to diagnosis were relatively small, after adjusting for age.

▶ This article was selected merely because it represents the only study done in recent times that tells us what the normal bone marrow cellularity is during childhood. Most of us learned that newborns had packed marrows and that elderly adults had relatively hypocellular marrows. In general, this is true, albeit with significant variation among individual patients. The importance of the study reported is that it collected data using a gold standard method to determine marrow cellularity. This is a bone marrow biopsy, performed on the posterior iliac crest, using a marrow biopsy needle (the Jamshidi needle). Prior to this report, the only existing data related largely to the old-fashioned needle aspiration technique of trying to determine marrow cellularity by looking at blood smears, rather than looking at fixed biopsy specimen materials. Chances are that you will not be spending a lot of time trying to figure out whether a particular patient has a cellular or hypocellular marrow. This is best left to the hematologists, oncologists, and hematopathologists. It is nice to know, however, what they are talking about when they report back bone marrow cellularity. The information provided in this article will help you in that regard.

J.A. Stockman III, M.D.

Postsplenectomy Course in Homozygous Sickle Cell Disease

Wright JG, Hambleton IR, Thomas PW, et al (Univ of the West Indies, Kingston, Jamaica)
J Pediatr 134:304-309, 1999   13–9

Background.—In patients with sickle cell disease, does removing the spleen do more harm than good? These authors followed 130 patients with sickle cell disease who were treated by splenectomy to determine whether they were at increased risk of serious complications.

Methods.—The 130 patients (64 males and 66 females) underwent splenectomy for chronic hypersplenism (CHS) (n = 84; median age, 5.9 years) or acute splenic sequestration (n = 46; median age, 2.3 years). Age- and sex-matched control patients had sickle cell disease but did not undergo splenectomy. The frequencies of bacteremia and death were compared between groups throughout follow-up (median follow-up, 8.5 years in the patients with acute splenic sequestration and 7.4 years in their control patients, 6.5 years in the patients with CHS and 7.2 years in their control patients). Additionally, 90 patient-control pairs were followed for 5 years after splenectomy to determine the frequency of painful crisis, acute chest syndrome, and febrile episodes.

Findings.—In the group as a whole, mortality did not differ significantly between the patients (6 patients with CHS died, 3 patients with acute splenic sequestration died) and the control patients (12 died). The groups also did not differ in the frequency of bacteremias (4 patients with CHS, 6 patients with acute splenic sequestration, and 12 control patients). Within the 90 patient-control pairs, both painful crises (odds ratio [OR], 1.47) and acute chest syndrome (OR, 1.88) were significantly more common in the patients who underwent splenectomy. Furthermore, acute chest syndrome was significantly more common among the patients with acute splenic sequestration (OR, 3.38) than among those with CHS. The incidence of febrile episodes did not differ between groups.

Conclusion.—Splenectomy was not associated with an increased frequency of bacteremias or death in these patients with sickle cell disease. Thus, this procedure should not be deferred in appropriate patients because of concern about increased serious morbidity or mortality.

▶ Russell E. Ware, M.D., Ph.D., Department of Pediatric Hematology-Oncology, Duke University Medical Center, Durham, NC, comments:

The spleen has long been a source of medical mystery. Hippocrates thought the spleen contained "black bile," whereas Galen suggested that it purified "humors" from the blood.[1] We now recognize that the spleen performs several critical functions including filtration of opsonized bacteria and production of antibody responses. Asplenic patients are highly susceptible to overwhelming sepsis, particularly with encapsulated bacteria such as *Streptococcus pneumoniae* or *Hemophilus influenzae*, so the spleen is preserved whenever possible.

But removal of the spleen is sometimes necessary. The spleen performs quality control on circulating erythrocytes by requiring deformation through the narrow Cords of Billroth. This function is usually reserved for senescent erythrocytes but can include younger erythrocytes that are misshapen because of intrinsic defects (e.g., membrane abnormalities, hemoglobinopathies, enzyme deficiencies) or extrinsic forces (e.g., antibody coating, mechanical shearing). In these settings, the spleen can enlarge and become burdensome, and splenectomy is beneficial.

For children with sickle cell disease, the spleen can be life saving or life threatening, depending upon the circumstance. Hypoxia and sickling within the spleen usually lead to its demise with eventual involution. Occasionally, the spleen enlarges rapidly and traps circulating blood cells (acute sequestration). If the child recovers, the spleen may remain large and cause CHS. We previously advocated splenectomy for these patients, while recognizing the possibility of an increased risk of infection.[2] The article by Wright et al. abstracted here provides clarity for this dilemma by describing 130 children with sickle cell disease who underwent splenectomy over a 22-year period. Compared with control patients, splenectomized children were no more likely to go on to bacteremia or death. Perhaps one mystery involving the spleen has been solved. Once the spleen is functionally dead in patients with sickle cell disease, it provides no clear benefit. If the spleen enlarges and causes sequestration or CHS, clinicians should strongly consider elective splenectomy, coupled with pneumococcal vaccination and penicillin prophylaxis, as a reasonable therapeutic option.

R.E. Ware, M.D., Ph.D.

References

1. Rosse WF: The spleen as a filter (editorial). *N Engl J Med* 317:704-706, 1987.
2. Kinney TR, Ware RE, Schultz WH, et al: Long-term management of splenic sequestration in children with sickle cell disease. *J Pediatr* 117:194-199, 1990.

Beneficial Effect of Intravenous Dexamethasone in Children With Mild to Moderately Severe Acute Chest Syndrome Complicating Sickle Cell Disease
Bernini JC, Rogers ZR, Sandler ES, et al (Univ of Texas, Dallas; Children's Med Ctr, Dallas)
Blood 92:3082-3089, 1998   13–10

Introduction.—One of the most frequent complications requiring hospitalization is acute chest syndrome, which is characterized by fever, cough, chest pain, dyspnea, and new pulmonary infiltrates. A previous study found that high-dose intravenous methylprednisolone shortened the duration of hospitalization and reduced opioid requirements in children with painful events. It was hypothesized that corticosteroids might reduce the severity of acute chest syndrome since the pathophysiologies of acute chest syndrome and vaso-occlusive crisis are similar. To assess the efficacy of intravenous dexamethasone in children with mild or moderately severe acute chest syndrome, a randomized, double-blind placebo-controlled study was conducted.

Methods.—Forty-three children with a median age of 6.7 years who had sickle cell disease and acute chest syndrome were randomized to receive intravenous dexamethasone at 0.3 mg/kg or placebo every 12 hours in 4 doses. The 2 groups had similar demographic, clinical, and laboratory characteristics.

Results.—In the dexamethasone-treated group, mean hospital stay was shorter (47 vs 80 hours). Clinical deterioration was prevented, and the need for blood transfusions was reduced with dexamethasone therapy. The dexamethasone-treated patients had significantly reduced mean duration of oxygen and analgesic therapy, number of opioid doses, and duration of fever. Of the 7 patients readmitted within 72 hours, 6 were in the dexamethasone group. One of them had respiratory complications. There were no side effects clearly related to dexamethasone. The only variables that appeared to predict response to dexamethasone were gender and previous episodes of acute chest syndrome.

Conclusion.—In children with sickle cell disease hospitalized with mild to moderately severe acute chest syndrome, intravenous dexamethasone had a beneficial effect. Further study of this therapy is necessary.

▶ This report demonstrating the beneficial effects of steroids when used as part of the management of acute chest syndrome in patients with sickle cell disease comes from the same group in Dallas that has shown similarly unique benefits from steroids used as part of the management of painful crisis (vaso-occlusive crisis). This is the first report of the use of steroids in patients with sickle cell disease and acute chest syndrome, and the conclusions are to be respected. In fact, although this is a relatively small study, many centers have begun including steroids as part of the management of this potentially fatal complication of sickle cell disease. When hospital stays are cut in half, who can complain?

Please note that the authors chose to use dexamethasone as their steroid of choice. Griffin et al. studied the role of methylprednisolone (15 mg/kg) in patients with sickle cell disease and painful crises.[1] The duration of pain relief and hospital stay were significantly reduced in the steroid group. However, an excessive number of patients randomized to methylprednisolone were readmitted because of recurrence of pain. Concerns about administering such high doses of methylprednisolone and a possible rebound effect suggested the use of a lower dose of a longer-acting steroid such as dexamethasone in the study abstracted above. In fact, the dexamethasone dose and schedule used were comparable to those previously employed in infants and children with bacterial meningitis and croup.

Until alternative data are produced, it would seem wise to take a tip from these authors and use dexamethasone as part of the management of acute chest syndrome. It will be a while before we know if there is a long-term benefit in terms of preventing the permanent lung damage so common in these patients. But it seems only logical to think that such sequelae will be less in treated children. Also, please do not ask why dexamethasone works.

It is an antiinflammatory agent. It inhibits the production of cytokines and alters arachidonic acid metabolism. There is also evidence that steroids can prevent pulmonary fat embolism, fat embolism being a cause of acute chest syndrome.

Before leaving the topic of pain and sickle cell disease, consider this: the next time you see a child with sickle cell disease who complains of a toothache, do not think that the child may simply have a dental abscess. In a recent case-control study adjusting for oral hygiene, 49% of patients with sickle cell disease, compared with just 8% of control subjects, had had maxillary or mandibular toothache pain in the previous 12 months. The significant majority of sickle cell disease patients with such pain demonstrate no dental pathology, whereas not a single control subject had pain in the absence of such pathology.[2] A toothache isn't always what it seems, especially if you have a hemoglobinopathy.

And while we're on the topic of hemoglobinopathies, the fifth survivor of homozygous α-thalassemia was recently described. Recall that babies affected with alpha thalassemia die in utero. Without any alpha chains, you cannot form either fetal or adult hemoglobin. However, current technologies involving cordocentesis and intrauterine transfusion can now keep such babies alive. If they survive the intrauterine period, of course, they will be transfusion-dependent for the rest of their lives. However, with early bone marrow transplantation, it is now possible to save the lives of some of these babies. Alpha thalassemia syndromes are quite common, even in the United States, particularly in those of Asian ancestry. As other experimental therapies (in utero stem-cell transplantation or gene replacement therapy) become more available, maybe we will see more than just five survivors of this interesting disorder.[3]

J.A. Stockman III, M.D.

References

1. Griffin TC, MacIntire D, Buchanan GR: High dose intravenous methylprednisolone for pain in children and adolescents with sickle cell disease. *N Engl J Med* 330:733, 1994.
2. Toothache in sickle cell disease (editorial). *Br Dent J* 185:90-92, 1998.
3. Ng CHL, Cheung KL, Lee CH, et al: Is homozygous α-thalassaemia a lethal condition in the 1990s? *Acta Paediatr* 87:1197-1199, 1998.

The Costs of Children With Sickle Cell Anemia: Preparing for Managed Care

Bilenker JH, Weller WE, Shaffer TJ, et al (Johns Hopkins Univ, Baltimore, Md)
J Pediatr Hematol Oncol 20:528-533, 1998   13–11

Background.—Caring for children with chronic illness is expensive, and employer-sponsored insurance and Medicaid programs are increasingly moving these families into managed care arrangements. But how will chronically ill children fare under managed care? These authors identified some of the financial issues associated with the care of children with sickle cell anemia that must be faced to ensure that these children receive an optimum level of care.

Methods.—The authors analyzed 2 claims databases to identify all children 18 years old or less who were not institutionalized and for whom a medical insurance claim was filed in fiscal year 1992 (Federal Employees Health Benefits Program, or FEP) or fiscal year 1993 (Washington State Medicaid Program, or WSMP). Expenditures for children with sickle cell anemia were determined and compared with those of children without this diagnosis.

Findings.—The WSMP database included 56 children with sickle cell anemia. In this database, total expenditures for a child with sickle cell anemia averaged $8221, or almost 9 times more than the average expenditure of $938 for children without sickle cell anemia (Table 1). Most of the higher costs of care for children with sickle cell anemia were related to inpatient expenditures ($5894 vs $304 for children without sickle cell anemia; a 19-fold difference). Most of the children (55 of 56) had expenditures of less than $20,000, and 1 child's expenditures were as low as $142; however, 1 child had expenditures of more than $177,000. As for average physician payments, those for children with sickle cell anemia were 4.5 times greater than those for children without sickle cell anemia, and per capital payments averaged $887 (10.8% of the mean total expenditure for a patient with sickle cell anemia). Many different types of physicians (pediatricians, general practitioners, others) provided care for children with sickle cell anemia, and no one type of provider accounted for the majority of care. The FEP database included 100 children with sickle cell anemia. In this database, total expenditures for a child with sickle cell anemia averaged $11,686, or 10.4 times higher than the average expenditures for children without sickle cell anemia. Similar to the WSMP database, most of the higher costs of care for children with sickle cell anemia were related to inpatient expenditures, which averaged 18.8 times higher in the children with sickle cell anemia. Expenditures in these 100 children ranged from $40 to $166,574, but most (89%) had total expenditures less than $20,000.

TABLE 1.—Medicaid Expenditures for Children With Sickle Cell Anemia Compared to All Children by Type of Service

	Total Average Payment Per Child	Type of Service				
		Inpatient	Outpatient	Physician Payments	Prescription Medications	Miscellaneous
Children with SCA	8,221.0	5,894.0	893.0	887.0	266.0	281.0
All children	939.0	304.0	99.0	199.0	59.0	278.0
Ratio*	8.8	19.4	9.0	4.5	4.5	1.0

*Represents row 1 divided by row 2.
Abbreviation: SCA, sickle cell anemia.
(Courtesy of Bilenker JH, Weller WE, Shaffer TJ, et al: The costs of children with sickle cell anemia: Preparing for managed care. *J Pediatr Hematol Oncol* 20:528-533, 1998.)

Conclusions.—In managed care plans, providers assume the financial risks for a patient's health outcomes in exchange for a per-member-per-month fee. Unless appropriate risk adjustment systems are in place to account for the greatly increased costs for children with sickle cell anemia, their access to care and even the quality of that care may suffer. The standards of care most vulnerable under capitation would seem to be newborn screening, access to specific procedures and specialty providers, access to facilities, and comprehensive education for families.

▶ This report is all about risk adjustment. Risk adjustment is not possible unless one knows the extent of a particular risk. Children with sickle cell disease, or with any other chronic disease, are behind the eight-ball in a managed care environment that fails to provide appropriate risk adjustment. We see that it "costs" an average of slightly in excess of $8000 per year to care for a patient with sickle cell disease. This is approximately 9 times the national expenditure for the average child. The actual expenditures in this series ranged from a low of $40 to $177,014 per year. In an era of capitated managed care, those who care for patients with sickle cell disease are themselves at risk because of the extraordinary variation in cost associated with what these children require. One way of limiting risk is reinsurance. An example of this is stop-loss insurance, where plans or providers are responsible for the cost of care up to a predetermined dollar threshold, such as $5000. Once this figure is reached, the reinsurer becomes responsible for cost. The reinsurer is paid a premium for accepting this risk.

The science of risk adjustment in pediatrics is still somewhat in its primitive phase. The National Association of Children's Hospitals and Related Institutions (NACHRI) has done all of us a great service by defining (to the extent possible) which diagnoses carry a need for such a risk adjustment. It is important for us to become familiar with the concept of risk adjustment so that we have the tools to provide the very best care for those with a variety of chronic diseases, just one of which is sickle cell anemia.

J.A. Stockman III, M.D.

Preliminary Report: rhG-CSF May Reduce the Incidence of Neonatal Sepsis in Prolonged Preeclampsia-associated Neutropenia
Kocherlakota P, La Gamma EF (State Univ at Stony Brook, NY)
Pediatrics 102:1107–1111, 1998   13–12

Introduction.—A major cause of premature delivery is pre-eclampsia, which is associated with neutropenia in up to 57% of newborns. It was previously shown that recombinant human granulocyte colony-stimulating factor (rhG-CSF) increased the neutrophil count in pre-eclampsia–associated neutropenia, increased the absolute neutrophil count within 48 hours, and improved survival in septic-neutropenic neonates. The incidence of bacterial sepsis in this at-risk group may be reduced by prophylactic therapy with this cytokine. The dose of rhG-CSF required to raise the

absolute neutrophil count in pre-eclampsia–associated neutropenic neonates, who had an absolute neutrophil count below 1500/mm³ for more
than 3 consecutive days after birth was determined.

Methods.—There were 15 ventilated neonates with pre-eclampsia–associated neutropenia for 3 or more consecutive days in the postnatal week.
Ten neonates received an intravenous infusion of rhG-CSF at 10 µg/kg per
day for 3 days and 5 received 5 µg/kg per day for 3 days. These patients
were compared to 13 case-matched control neonates. The neutrophilic
responses and incidence of neonatal sepsis in the next 28 postnatal days
were measured.

Results.—In the 10 µg/kg per day, the absolute neutrophil count increased by twofold in 24 hours, by fourfold in 72 hours, and 14-fold by the
seventh day (Fig 1). In the 5 µg/kg per day, there was a 20-fold increase at
72 hours and a fivefold increase at 7 days. In the control group, only a

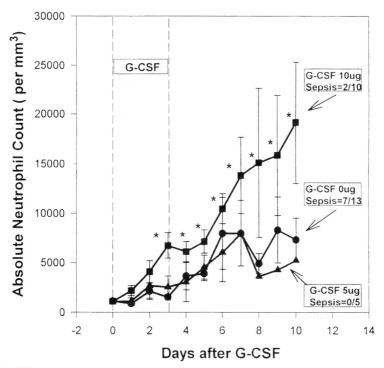

FIGURE 1.—Neutrophil response after the rhG-CSF treatment with preeclampsia-associated neonatal
neutropenia. Changes in the absolute neutrophil count throughout time for each of the 3 treatment groups
are indicated. The numbers in the labeled boxes indicate the number of patients who went on to be
diagnosed with infection after the first 3 days of the rhG-CSF or conventional treatments; the denominator
is the total number of patients in each group. The period during which the 3 daily morning doses of
rhG-CSF (none for control patients) were given is indicated by the vertical dotted lines. *$P < .05$ versus
baseline for all absolute neutrophil count values after the third day of therapy for the 10-µg group only
(analysis of variance followed by Dunnet's multirange testing). Other time points were not statistically
significant from baseline in either the 5-µg or the no-drug control group. Differences between groups are
not significant at any timepoint in a 2-way analysis of variance (time vs treatment). (Reproduced with
permission of *Pediatrics*, from Kocherlakota P, La Gamma EF: Preliminary report: rhG-CSF may reduce
the incidence of neonatal sepsis in prolonged preeclampsia-associated neutropenia. *Pediatrics* 102:1107-
1111, 1998.)

fourfold increase was seen at 7 days. The control group had a 54% incidence of sepsis while the rhG-CSF–treated group had a 13% incidence of sepsis.

Conclusion.—When compared with conventional therapy, 4hG-CSF increases the absolute neutrophil count significantly (at 10 µg/kg per day × 3 days) and reduces the incidence of neonatal sepsis in critically ill, ventilated neonates with prolonged pre-eclampsia–associated neutropenia.

▶ Dr. Joyce M. Koenig, assistant professor of Pediatrics, University of Florida College of Medicine, comments:

The variety of hyporegenerative neutropenia that occurs in neonates delivered after maternal pregnancy-induced hypertension was once thought to be a transient phenomenon without associated problems. However, mounting evidence suggests that this neutropenia results in an increased risk of late-onset sepsis.[1-4] Drs. Kocherlakota and La Gamma provide preliminary results showing that the administration of rhG-CSF to these patient can increase circulating neutrophil counts and reduce the incidence of nosocomial sepsis.

While these results are encouraging, the prophylactic use of rhG-CSF in neutropenic neonates born to hypertensive mothers should be approached cautiously. A clearer comparison will require greater numbers of patients and control subjects prospectively treated in a blinded fashion. In addition, Schibler et al.[5] recently observed, in a double-blind trial, that administration of rhG-CSF to neutropenic infants with suspected sepsis failed to elevate their absolute neutrophil count above those of the placebo group, and moreover, failed to improve their clinical outcome. Calhoun et al.[6] have observed G-CSF receptors on nonhematopoietic tissues of human fetuses, suggesting that administration of rhG-CSF to neonates might have effects other than the predicted hematopoietic action. Thus, recommendations for the use of rhG-CSF for treating neutropenia in neonates born to hypertensive mothers must await the results of larger clinical trials.

J.M. Koenig, M.D.

References

1. Gray PH, Rodwell RL: Neonatal neutropenia associated with maternal hypertension poses a risk for nosocomial infection. *Eur J Pediatr* 158:71-73, 1999.
2. Doron MW, Makhlouf RA, Katz VL, et al: Increased incidence of sepsis at birth in neutropenic infants of mothers with preeclampsia. *J Pediatr* 125:452-458, 1994.
3. Cadnapaphornchai M, Faix RG: Increased nosocomial infection in neutropenic low birth weight (2000 grams or less) infants of hypertensive mothers. *J Pediatr* 121:956-961, 1992.
4. Koenig JM, Christensen RD: Incidence, neutrophil kinetics, and natural history of neonatal neutropenia associated with maternal hypertension. *N Engl J Med* 321:557-562, 1989.
5. Schibler KR, Osborne KA, Leung LY, et al: A randomized, placebo-controlled trial of granulocyte colony-stimulating factor administration to newborn infants with neutropenia and clinical signs of early-onset sepsis. *Pediatrics* 102:6-13, 1998.
6. Calhoun DA, Donnelly WH Jr, Du Y, et al: Distribution of granulocyte colony-stimulating factor (G-CSF) and G-CSF–receptor mRNA and protein in the human fetus. *Pediatr Res* 46:333-338, 1999.

A Randomized, Placebo-controlled Trial of Granulocyte Colony-stimulating Factor Administration to Newborn Infants With Neutropenia and Clinical Signs of Early-Onset Sepsis

Schibler KR, Osborne KA, Leung LY, et al (Univ of Utah, Salt Lake City)
Pediatrics 102:6-13, 1998   13–13

Introduction.—The reduced host defense status of neonates is caused by multiple factors, including quantitative and qualitative neutrophil defects. Granulocyte colony-stimulating factor (G-CSF) stimulates neutrophil precursor proliferation, causes enhanced phagocytosis, and is the physiologic regulator of emergency neutrophil production and function. The study determined whether recombinant human G-CSF administration increased bone marrow stored and precursor neutrophils, whether it accelerated production of neutrophils, and whether it was safe in newborn infants with neutropenia and clinical signs of early-onset sepsis.

Methods.—The study included 20 infants with neutropenia and clinical signs of early-onset sepsis who were randomized in the first 3 days of life to receive G-CSF at 10 µg/kg per day or placebo for 3 days. Cultures were obtained from all infants, and antibiotics initiated. Measurements were made of circulating absolute neutrophils, immature-to-total neutrophil ratio (I/T ratio), bone marrow neutrophil storage pool, neutrophil proliferative pool, and plasma G-CSF concentrations.

Results.—By day 2, circulating absolute neutrophil counts increased in both G-CSF and placebo groups. In both groups, the I/T neutrophil ratio decreased. During the study period, no significant differences were noted in the absolute neutrophil counts or I/T ratio between the 2 groups. At study entry or on day 2, no differences were observed bone marrow neutrophil storage pool and neutrophil proliferative pool between the 2 groups. No differences were also noted in the secondary outcome measures, including severity of illness, morbidity, and mortality between the 2 groups.

Conclusion.—Circulating absolute neutrophil count, bone marrow neutrophil storage pool or neutrophil proliferative pool did not increase with administration of recombinant human G-CSF to infants with neutropenia and clinical signs of early-onset sepsis when compared to placebo. In severity of illness, morbidity, or mortality, no differences were seen between those who received placebo and those receiving G-CSF. There were no adverse effects of administration of G-CSF.

▶ Dr. Edmund F. La Gamma, professor of Pediatrics and chief, Division of Newborn Medicine & The Regional Neonatal Network of Westchester Medical Center's Children's Hospital, New York Medical College, Valhalla, comments:

Bacterial sepsis accounts for about 45% of deaths after 2 weeks postnatal age in the extremely low birth weight (ELBW) neonate (e.g., < 800 g at birth).[1] The hope of improved survival and a reduced occurrence of infection remains alive through the potential for augmenting neutrophil function with cytokines, such as G-CSF. Three recent reports address this problem but differ markedly with enrollment criteria for sepsis and neutropenia (Manroe criteria or an absolute neutrophil count <2000 or <1500 × 24 hours cells/mm³).[2-4] The overall severity of illness in each study paralleled the extent of the reduction in the ANC as did the authors' interpretation of the drug's presumed benefits. Unfortunately, none of these or previous studies are powered sufficiently to enable a conclusive recommendation to be made to a practicing clinician regarding its appropriate application. Nevertheless, based upon this and other evidence in adults, a therapeutic window of opportunity for use of G-CSF in neonates appears to lie in the proper selection of the highest acuity patients; particularly, if they are neutropenic and show clear systemic signs of sepsis. At present, systemic sepsis plus neutropenia defined as less than 1500 (or < 1000 cells/mm³, perhaps for 12-24 hours) based upon a vast oncology/transplant experience is prudent since compelling evidence does not yet exist proving efficacy in non-neutropenic patients at any age. The randomized trial by Schibler et al. was well intended but had weak criteria for sepsis that were based primarily on white cell counts and "risks" of infection, resulting in too many unconvincing "infected" neonates. They then used an infusion concentration of G-CSF much less than 15 µg/mL, which is likely to affect the proteins stability and thus to reduce its efficacy. The nonrandomized reports by Barak et al.[2] and by Kocherlakota and La Gamma[1,3] used more traditional clinical signs of systemic sepsis, including hypotension and metabolic acidosis, which may have resulted in selection of higher-acuity subjects. Both of these teams of investigators interpreted their data to advocate for continued experimentation. Barak illustrated a decrease in the neutrophil proliferative pool and an increase in the neutrophil storage pool after the fifth day of treatment. Schibler began therapy after an I/T ratio exceeded 0.25 and reported no change in neutrophil proliferative pool but a decrease in the neutrophil storage pool. One can interpret these findings positively as consistent with observations in adult lineage response and release schedules. Importantly, failure of a marrow response was associated with high mortality. Perhaps, most notable at the evolutionary stage of this intervention, is that none of these authors identified any adverse events attributable to the use of G-CSF. Each of them concluded that multicenter trials (currently in progress) are needed to establish a properly powered evaluation of the potential usefulness of G-CSF intervention in septic neonates. Therapy with G-CSF before then should be considered experimental (i.e., unproven).

E.F. La Gamma, M.D.

References

1. Kocherlakota P, La Gamma EF, Ahmad M, et al: Neonatal sepsis—an unsolved problem, in Morstyn G, Dexter TM, Foote M (eds): *Filgrastim in Clinical Practice* ed 2. New York, Marcel Dekker, 1998, pp 469-490.
2. Barak Y, Leibovitz E, Mogilner B, et al: The in vivo effect of recombinant human granulocyte-colony stimulating factor in neutropenic neonates with sepsis. *Eur J Pediatr* 156:643-646, 1997.

3. Kocherlakota P, La Gamma EF: Human granulocyte colony-stimulating factor may improve outcome attributable to neonatal sepsis complicated by neutropenia. *Pediatrics* 100(1):e6, 1997.
4. Schibler KR, Osborne KA, Leung LY, et al: A randomized, placebo-controlled trial of granulocyte colony-stimulating factor administration to newborn infants with neutropenia and clinical signs of early-onset sepsis. *Pediatrics* 102:6-13, 1998.

Is Bone Marrow Aspiration Needed in Acute Childhood Idiopathic Thrombocytopenic Purpura to Rule Out Leukemia?

Calpin C, Dick P, Poon A, et al (Univ of Toronto)
Arch Pediatr Adolesc Med 152:345-347, 1998   13–14

Background.—Bone marrow aspiration (BMA) is commonly done in children with acute idiopathic thrombocytopenic purpura (ITP) to exclude leukemia. However, this procedure is uncomfortable and costly. The prevalence of leukemia in a series of BMA samples obtained to confirm the provisional diagnosis of ITP in children was investigated to determine whether this procedure is necessary.

Methods and Findings.—Data on all 484 BMAs performed in children, aged 6 months to 18 years, with "typical" contemporaneous hematologic features of ITP between 1984 and 1996 at 1 center were analyzed retrospectively. None of the BMA studies revealed leukemia in the 332 children with typical hematologic features of ITP. The risk of missing the diagnosis of leukemia was less than 1% in this population.

Conclusions.—Routine BMA appears to be unnecessary in children with typical signs and symptoms of acute ITP. In this series, the yield of BMA for leukemia was low.

▶ One more study that tells us a bone marrow examination is not necessary in patients who look like, smell like, and otherwise act like they have childhood ITP. If a patient has a history consistent with ITP, a physical examination that shows no hepatosplenomegaly or unusual adenopathy, and the blood counts are perfectly normal other than a low platelet count (including a good look at the peripheral blood smear), you can put away the BMA tray. You will not miss a case of acute leukemia.

We don't need any more evidence that a BMA is unnecessary for the majority of children being evaluated for ITP. The data are perfectly clear. Enough is enough.

J.A. Stockman III, M.D.

Reticulated Platelet Counts in the Diagnosis of Acute Immune Thrombocytopenic Purpura

Saxon BR, Blanchette VS, Butchart S, et al (The Hosp for Sick Children, Toronto)
J Pediatr Hematol Oncol 20:44-48, 1998
13–15

Background.—For most children with acute immune thrombocytopenic purpura (ITP), the condition is diagnosed by invasive bone marrow aspiration. These authors described a noninvasive method of diagnosing ITP, by counting reticulated platelets (RPs).

Methods.—RPs are young platelets (high RNA content) whose production increases as platelet production increases. Because increased platelet production is associated with ITP, RP counts should also be higher in patients with ITP. To test this hypothesis, the authors compared RP counts from 15 patients with acute ITP (3- to 14-year-olds), 20 patients with acute lymphoblastic leukemia (6 months to 13 years old), 10 patients with aplasia (4 months to 14 years old), and 27 healthy control subjects (2.5 to 17 years old). All subjects provided venous blood samples, which were mixed with edetic acid, labeled with a platelet-specific monoclonal antibody, incubated with thiazole orange, and analyzed by flow cytometry. The thiazole orange fluorescence histogram was set at a standard gate to capture 1.3% ± 0.5% of the lyophilized platelet control subjects.

Findings.—Mean RP counts were significantly higher in the patients with acute ITP (RPs were 32.9% ± 10.2% of all platelets) than in the patients with acute lymphoblastic leukemia (6.6% ± 3.1%), the patients with aplasia (3.4% ± 2.0%), and the healthy control subjects (7.9% ± 2.9%) (Fig 1). RP counts did not differ significantly among the latter 3 groups.

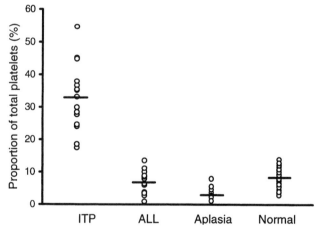

FIGURE 1.—Reticulated platelet counts for each diagnostic group, shown as percentage of total platelets. *Horizontal lines* indicate means. *Abbreviations: ITP*, immune thrombocytopenic purpura; *ALL*, acute lymphoblastic leukemia. (Courtesy of Saxon BR, Blanchette VS, Butchart S, et al: Reticulated platelet counts in the diagnosis of acute immune thrombocytopenic purpura. *J Pediatr Hematol Oncol* 20:44-48, 1998.)

Conclusion.—The whole-blood cytometric analysis of RP counts is a highly sensitive and specific means of diagnosing acute ITP in children. This method clearly differentiates between acute ITP and aplastic anemia that presents with thrombocytopenia in that RP counts in the latter condition are not significantly elevated. Further research is needed to determine whether RP measurements could make a difference in the diagnosis of thrombocytopenias that are difficult to distinguish, such as post–bone marrow transplantation thrombocytopenia and platelet destruction or bone marrow suppression of various causes (for example, drugs).

▶ If you are still a nonbeliever when it comes to the data that tell you you no longer need to do a bone marrow aspiration as part of the evaluation of ITP, the data from this report should help convince you otherwise. Not only is a bone marrow aspiration not necessary, but there is a perfectly good noninvasive test that can tell you whether a thrombocytopenia is caused by bone marrow failure or by increased platelet turnover, and does so with a reasonable degree of reliability. The test is an RP count, similar in concept to a red cell reticulocyte count.

RP counts seem to discriminate extremely well between acute ITP and thrombocytopenias of other types. If the results of this report hold up, we now have a relatively simple way to cleanly distinguish ITP as a cause of thrombocytopenia from leukemia or aplastic anemia. The only rub is that most hospital laboratories will not have the sophisticated equipment necessary to perform this test. However, there are enough centers around with flow cytometry that, hopefully, you will be able to get this study done by sending some blood off.

J.A. Stockman III, M.D.

Treatment of Childhood Acute Immune Thrombocytopenic Purpura With Anti-D Immune Globulin or Pooled Immune Globulin
Tarantino MD, Madden RM, Fennewald DL, et al (Univ of Louisville, Ky; Kosair Children's Hosp, Louisville, Ky)
J Pediatr 134:21-26, 1999   13–16

Background.—The optimal treatment for acute immune thrombocytopenic purpura (ITP) is unclear. The efficacy of anti-D immunoglobulin (anti-D) or pooled IgG immune globulin (IVIG) in the initial treatment of children with ITP was investigated.

Methods.—The records of 33 children with acute ITP diagnosed between 1995 and 1997 were reviewed. All had received either 45 to 50 µg/kg of anti-D or 0.8 to 1 g/kg of IVIG.

Findings.—Time to a platelet count of 20×10^9/L or higher was a mean of 1.54 days in the IVIG group and 1.26 days in the anti-D group. Time to a platelet count of 40×10^9/L or greater was a mean of 1.77 days in the IVIG and 1.49 days in the anti-D groups. Children receiving IVIG were hospitalized for 2.1 days, and those given anti-D, 1.9 days. Net hemoglo-

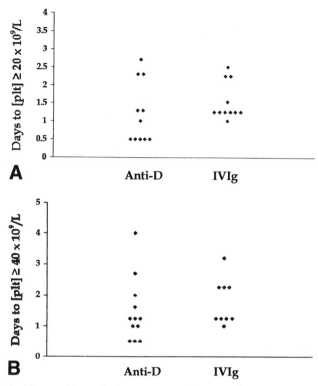

FIGURE 1.—Time to achieve a platelet concentration of $\geq 20 \times 10^9$/L (**A**) and 40×10^9/L (**B**) after treatment with either anti-D (n = 11) or IVIg (n = 11). Data included in this graph were obtained from patients who had an initial platelet count $<20 \times 10^9$/L and a platelet count measured ≤ 24 hours from the start of treatment (**A**) and approximately daily until the platelet count was $\geq 40 \times 10^9$/L (**B**). *Abbreviation: plt*, platelet count. (Courtesy of Tarantino MD, Madden RM, Fennewald DL, et al: Treatment of childhood acute immune thrombocytopenic purpura with anti-D immune globulin or pooled immune globulin. *J Pediatr* 134:21-26, 1999.)

bin concentration declined after IVIG and anti-D therapy by 9.1 and 4.5 g/L, respectively. None of the patients needed intervention for hemolysis (Fig 1).

Conclusions.—Anti-D and IVIG appear to be equally effective in the treatment of acute ITP in children. Randomized, controlled trials are now needed to definitively establish the role of anti-D in this setting.

▶ This is one of several studies summarized in this year's YEAR BOOK dealing with the management childhood acute ITP. In the report by Tarantino et al., we see that anti-D immune globulin generally is as effective as IVIG in raising the platelet count of affected children. The concept of using anti-D in the treatment of acute ITP in children has been around now for over a decade. The thought behind such an offbeat therapy comes from the theory that anti-A and anti-B antibodies, present in low amounts in IVIG preparations, caused a small degree of hemolysis in patients with blood types A, B, or AB, and this hemolysis facilitated blockade of Fc receptors within the spleen. With such a blockade, antibody-coated platelets would not be as easily removed by the spleen and the platelet count would rise. Indeed, anti-D via such a mechanism does raise the platelet count in Rh-positive individuals with ITP, although we now know that the anti-A and anti-B antibodies present in IVIG are not the reason why IVIG itself is effective.[1] The advantages of anti-D over IVIG are pretty obvious. The side effects of the former are almost negligible (a mild drop in hemoglobin is the worst that is seen). As importantly, the cost of anti-D globulin is a fraction (about one twentieth) of the cost of a standard treatment cycle of IVIG.

The real issue is whether any therapy is needed for most children with ITP. In fact, the overwhelming majority of children with ITP do well with virtually any treatment, including no treatment. The trick is to identify those who might get into trouble early. That is not as easily determined as one might think as we see in the article which follows.

J.A. Stockman III, M.D.

Reference

1. Sturgill MG, Nagabandi SR, Drachtman RA, et al: The effect of ABO and Rh blood type on the response to intravenous immunoglobulin (IVIG) in children with immune thrombocytopenic purpura (ITP). *J Pediatr Hematol Oncol* 19:523-525, 1997.

Major Hemorrhage in Children With Idiopathic Thrombocytopenic Purpura: Immediate Response to Therapy and Long-term Outcome
Medeiros D, Buchanan GR (Univ of Texas, Dallas; Children's Med Ctr of Dallas)
J Pediatr 133:334-339, 1998   13–17

Background.—Though idiopathic or immune thrombocytopenic purpura (ITP) in childhood is usually benign, in some children the bleeding is moderate to severe. Children with ITP and major hemorrhage were studied to determine treatment response and long-term outcomes.

Methods.—The medical records of 332 children with ITP diagnosed at 1 center in the past 10 years were reviewed. Major hemorrhage was defined as intracranial hemorrhage, epistaxis necessitating cautery or nasal packing, gross hematuria, or other bleeding causing a decrease in hemoglobin concentration.

Findings.—Fifty-eight children (17%) had a total of 68 episodes of major hemorrhage. Fifty-six of these episodes were treated with corticosteroids, IV immunoglobulin (IVIG), or both. Platelet counts increased to 20,000/mm³ or more within 14 hours of seeking medical care after only 18% of evaluated events. Twenty-eight percent of the children with major hemorrhage continued to have platelet counts of less than 20,000/mm³ after 7 days. Twenty-seven of 49 children available for assessment had ITP

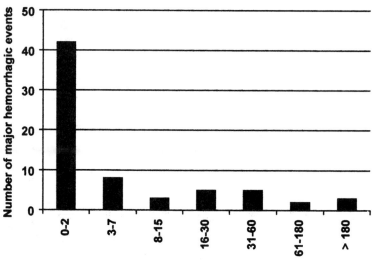

FIGURE 1.—Interval from initial diagnosis of idiopathic thrombocytopenic purpura to episode of major hemorrhage. (Courtesy of Medeiros D, Buchanan GR: Major hemorrhage in children with idiopathic thrombocytopenic purpura: Immediate response to therapy and long-term outcome. *J Pediatr* 133:334-339, 1998.)

resolution within 6 months. Twenty-one had chronic ITP, and 1 child died of sepsis (Figs 1 and 2).

Conclusions.—Seventeen percent of the children with ITP had major hemorrhage. Only a minority of these children had an immediate increase in platelet count after receiving IVIG, corticosteroids, or both. Further research is needed to establish optimal treatment for individual children.

▶ The consensus is that there remains no consensus regarding the management of ITP in children. Until there is a high-quality prospective study

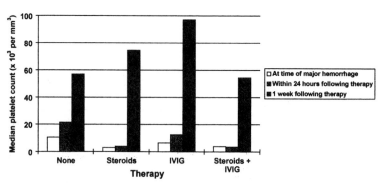

FIGURE 2.—Median platelet count before, within 24 hours, and 7 days after therapeutic intervention in 68 episodes of major hemorrhage. (Courtesy of Medeiros D, Buchanan GR: Major hemorrhage in children with idiopathic thrombocytopenic purpura: Immediate response to therapy and long-term outcome. *J Pediatr* 133:334-339, 1998.)

comparing the clinical course of untreated versus treated ITP, we are left to our own devices about how to manage these patients. Should we use steroids? Should we use IVIG? Should we use anti-D globulin? Should we do nothing except carefully observe? If a study were designed to examine various therapeutic approaches, what would be its end point? Would it be a determination of the rate of rise of the platelet count? As yet, it has not been determined that initial platelet count, or the change in initial platelet count accurately predicts the occurrence of clinically significant bleeding.

If you want to read more about new treatments for ITP, see the excellent editorial of Modak and Bussel.[1] You'll see that in addition to IV anti-D and dexamethasone, treatments in development for ITP include anti-CD40 ligand and thrombopoietin. Anti-CD40 ligand inhibits T-cell help to B cells and may have curative effects by decreasing autoantibody levels. Thrombopoietin levels in patients with ITP are normal, rather than increased; therefore, administration of thrombopoietin might be of some help to increase platelet production. Neither of these forms of therapy, of course, will be very helpful in the first day or two of the management of ITP, the period of greatest risk for serious bleeding.

One of the major problems in sorting out effective therapies is the relatively low frequency of serious complications of ITP. Some years ago, it was estimated that some 14,000 patients would have to enter a clinical trial to determine the benefits of one therapy versus another. That's a lot of patients to enroll. We will have to have a lot of patience to wait for the results of such a study.

J.A. Stockman III, M.D.

Reference

1. Modak SI, Bussel JB: Treatment of children with immune thrombocytopenia purpura: Are we closer to resolving the dilemma (editorial)? *J Pediatrics* 133:313-314, 1998.

Von Willebrand Factor–Cleaving Protease in Thrombotic Thrombocytopenic Purpura and the Hemolytic-Uremic Syndrome

Furlan M, Robles R, Galbusera M, et al (Univ Hosp, Bern, Switzerland; Mario Negri Inst for Pharmacological Research, Bergamo, Italy; Gen Hosp, Vienna; et al)
N Engl J Med 339:1578-1584, 1998
13–18

Background.—Plasma samples from patients with thrombotic thrombocytopenic purpura (TTP) and the hemolytic-uremic syndrome (HUS) contain unusually large forms of von Willebrand factor (VWF). The large multimers may result from a deficiency in the protease that cleaves VWF. These authors examined VWF-cleaving protease activity in patients with TTP or HUS.

Methods.—Blood samples were obtained from 30 patients with TTP (24 had nonfamilial TTP; 6 had the familial form), 23 patients with HUS (13 had nonfamilial HUS; 10 had the familial form), and 120 normal control subjects. Samples were assayed to determine the activity of the VWF-cleaving protease. Plasma samples were mixed and incubated with varying volumes (4:1, 1:1, and 1:5) of control plasma to identify any inhibitors of this protease.

Findings.—VWF-cleaving protease activity was normal in all the samples from controls. Moderate (4 patients) or severe (20 patients) deficiency in this protease was found in all 24 patients with nonfamilial TTP when it was measured during an acute episode. Mixing studies showed inhibition of protease activity in 20 patients (83%); 5 samples were assayed, and in all 5 immunoglobulin (Ig)G was identified. Plasma samples from the 6 patients with familial TTP revealed no VWF-cleaving protease activity at all, but mixing studies revealed no inhibitor. In contrast, VWF-cleaving protease activity was normal (11 patients) or only slightly decreased (2 patients) in the 13 patients with nonfamilial HUS when it was measured during an acute episode, and was normal in all 10 patients with familial HUS. Samples from 12 patients with HUS (5 familial; 7 nonfamilial) were studied to assess the degradation of VWF by the protease; in all 12 samples, protease activity was normal.

Conclusions.—VWF-cleaving protease was either completely absent or (typically) severely inhibited in patients with familial and nonfamilial forms of TTP. Samples from most patients with nonfamilial TTP indicated an inhibitor, which was determined to be IgG. Samples from the patients with the familial form, however, showed no inhibitors. Thus, the nonfamilial form appears to be caused by IgG inhibition of the VWF-cleaving protease, whereas a constitutional deficiency of this protease is present in patients with the familial form. VWF-cleaving protease activity was normal in the patients with HUS. These differences in protease activities may be useful in distinguishing patients who have TTP from those who have HUS.

▶ HUS is a fascinating disorder. It would appear that inhibitory antibodies against VWF-cleaving protease occur in patients with TTP, but not in youngsters with HUS. So what is the background on all of this and why is this information important? It was way back in 1924 that Dr. Eli Moschcowitz described the abrupt onset of petechiae and pallor, followed rapidly by paralysis, coma, and death, in a 16-year-old girl. The terminal arterioles and capillaries in this doomed teenager were occluded by hyaline thrombi, later determined to consist mostly of platelets without perivascular inflammation or endothelial desquamation. Moschcowitz had a theory, a wrong theory: he suspected a "powerful poison which had both agglutinative and hemolytic properties" as a cause of this frightening new disease, which we now know as TTP. Not much happened for the next 60 years until in the early 1980s, when unusually large multimers of VWF were found in the plasma of patients with chronic relapsing TTP. At that time, a report concluded that patients with recurring TTP had a defect in the processing of these unusually large multimers, which tended to become entangled within the structure of endothelial cells, causing adhesion of platelets in a massive manner following the vascular damage. Chronic relapsing TTP is an unusual disease. More common is the single, sometimes lethal, episode of this disorder. What Furlan et al., as well as Tsai and Lian,[1] tell us is that single episodes of TTP are characterized by absence of plasma VWF-cleaving protease activity during the acute episodes, but activity returning to normal on recovery. An IgG autoantibody against the components of the enzyme probably accounts for the lack of protease activity in most of these patients.

All this seems to make some sense, since before there was any inkling of the pathophysiologic process underlying TTP, the disease could be managed (or prevented in those patients who had relapses of the disease) by infusion of only a few units of fresh frozen plasma or cryoprecipitate. No one really knew what was being infused, but the patients got better. It turns out that these plasma products were replacing the missing VWF-cleaving protease that is absent from plasma in patients with chronic relapsing TTP. In patients with single episodes, lots of plasma has to be given, which usually means that plasmapheresis is the treatment of choice. The disappointment in all this is that the more we know about TTP, the less new knowledge we have about HUS. The latter remains a fascinating disorder of essentially unknown origin. Stay tuned for further information as we learn more about these thrombotic disorders.

J.A. Stockman III, M.D.

Reference

1. Tsai H-M, Lian EC-Y: Antibodies to von Willebrand factor-cleaving protease in acute thrombotic thrombocytopenic purpura. *N Engl J Med* 339:1585-1594, 1998.

Clinical Significance of Lupus Anticoagulants in Children
Male C, Lechner K, Eichinger S, et al (Univ of Vienna)
J Pediatr 134:199-205, 1999   13–19

Background.—In adults, antiphospholipid antibodies are associated with thrombosis and thrombocytopenia. Whether this association also exists in children, however, is unclear. These authors followed 95 children with lupus anticoagulants (LA) to determine the associated clinical manifestations and the time course of clinical and laboratory abnormalities.

Methods.—The subjects were 95 children (48 boys and 47 girls; median age, 5.3 years) with LA. Their clinical manifestations and laboratory test results at diagnosis were examined. Results of serial laboratory tests and clinical examinations were available for 83 patients over a median follow-up of 1.9 years (range, 5 weeks to 19.1 years). Clinical data of interest were recent symptoms, medication use, chronic bleeding, previous thrombosis, operations, and family history. Laboratory studies included activated partial thromboplastin time (APTT), prothrombin time, fibrinogen, clotting factor assays, factor II antigen assay, and a complete blood count. LA was diagnosed by a positive APTT, a positive plasma mixing study, and a positive phospholipid confirmation test.

TABLE 1.—Children With Presence of Lupus Anticoagulants Seen With Bleeding Symptoms

Patient No.	Clinical Presentation At Diagnosis				Laboratory Abnormalities (Apart From LA)		Duration of Bleeding	Follow-up Laboratory Abnormalities (At Final Examination)	Total Observation Time
	Sex	Age (y)	Associated Disease	Type of Bleeding	Clotting Factor (Activity)	Plt Count (G/L)			
1	F	4.1	Enteritis (adenovirus+)	Purpura	Factor II, 10%	Normal	7 d	LA−, FII normal (after 7 wk)	6.6 y
2	F	4.3	Upper respiratory tract infection (adenovirus+)	Bruising	Factor II, 9%; Factor IX, <1%; Factor XII, 46%	Normal	14 d	APTT+, mix+, confirm −; Factors II, IX, and XII normal (after 2 wk)	4.5 y
3	M	4.7	Enteritis (adenovirus+)	Melena	Factor II, 18%	Normal	6 d	LA+, Factor II normal (after 2 wk)	2 wk
4	M	8.2	Enteritis (adenovirus+)	Bruising	Factor II, 5%	Normal	5 d	LA−, Factor II normal (after 4 wk)	1.7 y
5	M	2.3	Enteritis (adenovirus+)	Hemorrhagic diarrhea	Factor II, 16%; Factor, XII 33%	125	3 d	LA−, Factor II normal (after 2 wk)	6.3 y
6	F	12.7	Chorea	Bruising	Normal	77	1.8 y +	APTT+, mix−, confirm −, Plt 64	1.8 y
7	F	13.6	None	Epistaxis	Normal	136	<1 d	LA− (after 18 wk), Plt 174	13 mo
8	M	2.8	None	Bruising	Normal	Normal	<1 d	LA−	21.6 y
9	M	4.6	Pneumonia	Posttraumatic bleeding	Normal	Normal	<1 d	LA− (after 10 wk)	6.4 y

Note: Lupus anticoagulant was diagnosed based on a positive activated partial thromboplastin time, a positive plasma mixing study, and a positive phospholipid confirmation test.

Abbreviations: LA, lupus anticoagulant; *Plt,* platelets; −, negative; +, positive/abnormal; *mix,* plasma mixing study; *confirm,* phospholipid confirmation test; *APTT,* activated partial thromboplastin time.

(Courtesy of Male C, Lechner K, Eichinger S, et al: Clinical significance of lupus anticoagulants in children. *J Pediatr* 134:199-205, 1999.)

Findings.—At diagnosis, most of the patients (80 of 95, or 84%) had no symptoms, and LA was diagnosed incidentally. In fact, only 9 of the patients (10%) were seen with a bleeding disorder (Table 1). Five of these 9 patients had transient severe hypoprothrombinemia that developed after adenovirus infection, and 3 had mild-to-moderate thrombocytopenia. Other laboratory abnormalities at diagnosis included thrombosis in 5 patients (5%). Of the 80 patients who were free of symptoms at diagnosis, none had subsequent bleeding, thrombotic complications, or autoimmune disease. Follow-up of 83 patients indicated normal APTT values in 48 (58%). Although 32 patients (38%) still had elevated APTT, they did not fulfill all the criteria for LA. As for the remaining 3 patients, they had persistent positive LA, anticardiolipin, and antinuclear antibodies 1.4, 2.8, and 7.5 years, respectively, after diagnosis. All 3 of these patients had presented with thrombosis, and 1 experienced recurrent thrombosis.

Conclusion.—In most of these children with LA, clinical complications did not develop, and the increase in LA was transient. Ten percent of the children with LA experienced moderate bleeding at presentation, typically in association with hypoprothrombinemia or thrombocytopenia. Five percent of the children with LA experienced thrombosis at presentation, typically children more than 10 years old (80%) and girls (80%), and thrombosis was strongly associated with persistent elevations in LA levels.

▶ Dr. Donna DiMichele, assistant professor of Pediatrics, Weill Medical College of Cornell University, and director, Regional Comprehensive Hemophilia Diagnostic & Treatment Center, New York Presbyterian Hospital, New York, comments:

The authors should be commended for their significant contribution to the pediatric hemostasis literature. Although retrospective, this 30-year review of the diagnosis, presentation, and long-term surveillance of LA in children is the most comprehensive to date and provides an excellent reference for pediatric hematologists. This type of study is made possible by the continued existence of academic centers of excellence that can: (1) serve as noncompeting referral centers for patients with hemostatic disorders and (2) perform consistent laboratory testing that is also investigative in nature and does not merely fulfill minimal criteria for diagnosis and clinical patient management because of reimbursement constraints. For these reasons, such a study is becoming progressively more difficult to perform in United States academic centers.

This review yields the following important and, in general, reassuring information about LA in children: (1) 84% are clinically asymptomatic and their condition is most frequently diagnosed through routine preoperative screening; (2) 96% (including all with asymptomatic or hemorrhagic presentations) are self-resolving but over a period that remains ill-defined; (3) associated hemorrhagic symptoms are infrequent (10%), mild, and most often accompanied—although not necessarily predicted—by transient hypoprothrombinemia or moderate thrombocytopenia; (4) they are rarely (1%) associated with systemic lupus erythematosus in the general pediatric population, in contrast to a reported high frequency among previously studied cohorts with this disease; and (5) although unusually associated with thromboembolic disease at presentation (5%), this symptom in the older child and adolescent (especially if female) may define a subgroup with "true disease" in whom the LA is persistent and associated with other "autoimmune" laboratory parameters, and for whom the recurrent risk of thrombosis may necessitate long-term anticoagulation.

The clinical significance of associated thrombotic risk factors in this subset of patients was not addressed in this review. This question is among several that can only be answered by a well-designed multicenter, prospective study of the natural history of LA in children.

D.M. DiMichele, M.D.

High Risk of Cerebral-Vein Thrombosis in Carriers of a Prothrombin-Gene Mutation and in Users of Oral Contraceptives
Martinelli I, Sacchi E, Landi G, et al (Univ of Milan, Italy)
N Engl J Med 338:1793-1797, 1998   13–20

Background.—A recently discovered mutation in the prothrombin gene (G20210A) has been identified as a common cause of deep-vein thrombosis of the lower extremity. The role of this mutation in causing cerebral-vein thrombosis, however, is not known. This study evaluated the risk of cerebral-vein thrombosis associated with this prothrombin gene mutation, both alone and in combination with other risk factors for cerebral-vein thrombosis.

Methods.—The participants were 40 patients with idiopathic cerebral-vein thrombosis (9 men and 31 women; median age, 31 years), 80 subjects with deep-vein thrombosis of the lower extremity (18 men and 62 women; median age, 30 years), and 120 healthy control subjects (27 men and 93 women; median age, 32 years). Subjects were matched to control subjects by age, sex, geographic origin, and level of education. Each participant provided a blood sample, and DNA was analyzed for the G20210A prothrombin gene mutation and the G1691A factor V mutation (another established genetic risk factor for deep-vein thrombosis). Other nongenetic risk factors for venous thrombosis, including the use of oral contraceptives, surgery or immobilization, or pregnancy, were also included in statistical analyses to determine their associations with cerebral-vein thrombosis.

Findings.—The prevalence of the G20210A prothrombin gene mutation was similar in patients with cerebral-vein thrombosis (8 of 40, or 20%) and in subjects with deep-vein thrombosis of the lower extremity (14 of 80, or 18%). This gene mutation was significantly more prevalent in patients and in subjects compared with control subjects (3 of 120, or 3%). Prevalences of the factor V mutation were similar: 6 of 40 patients (15%), 15 of 80 subjects (19%), and only 3 of 120 control subjects (3%). Oral contraceptive use was significantly higher in the female patients (96%) and in the female subjects (61%) compared with female control subjects (32%). All 3 of these factors were significantly associated with the risk of cerebral-vein thrombosis (Table 2), with odds ratios of 7.8 (for the factor

TABLE 2.—Risk of Cerebral-Vein Thrombosis in the Presence of Genetic Coagulation Defects and Nongenetic Risk Factors*

Risk Factor	Odds Ratio (95% Confidence Interval)
Genetic coagulation defects	
G20210A prothrombin-gene mutation	10.2 (2.3-31.0)
G1691A factor V mutation	7.8 (1.8-34.1)
Other risk factors for thrombosis	
Surgery, trauma, or immobilization	—
Pregnancy or postpartum state	—
Oral-contraceptive use†	22.1 (5.9-84.2)

*Patients with cerebral vein thrombosis were compared with healthy controls.
†The odds ratio was calculated for women without other risk factors for thrombosis.
(Reprinted by permission of *The New England Journal of Medicine*, from Martinelli I, Sacchi E, Landi G, et al: High risk of cerebral-vein thrombosis in carriers of a prothrombin-gene mutation and in users of oral contraceptives. N Engl J Med 338:1793-1797. Copyright 1998, Massachusetts Medical Society. All rights reserved.)

V mutation), 10.2 (for the G20210A mutation), and 22.1 for oral contraceptive use. The risk of cerebral-vein thrombosis was even greater for women using oral contraceptives who also had the prothrombin gene mutation (odds ratio, 149).

Conclusions.—As is the case with deep-vein thrombosis of the lower extremities, a G20210A mutation in the prothrombin gene and a factor V mutation are independent risk factors for the development of cerebral-vein thrombosis. Furthermore, oral contraceptive use was an independent predictor of cerebral-vein thrombosis, and oral contraceptive use in combination with the G20210A greatly increased the risk of cerebral-vein thrombosis. Nonetheless, indiscriminate screening of oral contraceptive users for this gene mutation would not be cost-effective. Furthermore, the withholding of oral contraceptives in women with no symptoms must be balanced by the increased risk of venous thromboembolism associated with pregnancy itself. For women who have symptoms and who have the gene mutation, oral contraceptives should be discontinued.

▶ There are lots of reasons why venous thromboses develop in children and adults. Protein C, protein S, and antithrombin deficiencies can do this. A G1691A mutation in the factor V gene, commonly known as factor V Leiden, does this as well. "The recent discovery of a transition from guanine to adenine at position 20210 in the sequence of the 3′ untranslated region of the prothrombin gene has widened the spectrum of inherited" causes of thromboses. Next to the mutation in the factor V gene, this prothrombin-gene mutation is now recognized to be the most common genetic reason for deep-vein thrombosis of the lower extremities. Certain other conditions, such as the use of oral contraceptives and the nephrotic syndrome are also associated with this tendency toward overclotting. Finally, acquired abnormalities such as the presence of antiphospholipid antibodies are also associated with an increased risk of venous thrombosis.

The report abstracted tells us about the relationship between the G20210A mutation and the problem of idiopathic cerebral-vein thrombosis.

Apparently, having this mutation in the prothrombin gene increases one's risk of cerebral-vein thrombosis by some 10-fold. The patients in this series in whom a cerebral-vein thrombosis developed had a wide range of symptoms, including headache, focal neurologic deficits, dysphasia, seizures, and impaired consciousness. So what does all this mean to you, the practicing pediatrician? The findings reported raise two questions. One is whether screening for the prothrombin-gene mutation would be appropriate in adolescents and young women before oral contraceptives are prescribed. The other question is whether withholding oral contraceptives from carriers of the prothrombin-gene mutation would be worthwhile. "Indiscriminate screening for the prothrombin-gene mutation would probably not be useful cerebral-vein thrombosis" is a relatively rare condition. The incidence of cerebral-vein thrombosis is not precisely known but is likely to be lower than the incidence of approximately 1 per 1000 persons per year reported for deep-vein thrombosis. Thus, screening would not be cost-effective, even though the risk of deep-vein thrombosis in oral contraceptive users who have the factor V mutation is greater than the risk in those who have only one of these risk factors.

With respect to the second question, the withholding of one of the most effective methods of contraception, pregnancy in and of itself increases the risk of venous thromboembolism. Therefore, one can reasonably recommend that carriers of the prothrombin-gene mutation who have had an episode of thrombosis should discontinue the use of oral contraceptives but that symptom-free carriers should not.

There is a great deal of controversy among adolescent care providers about the pros and cons, clottingwise, of oral contraceptives. Some are now screening for the most common inherited clotting abnormality that predisposes to deep-vein thrombosis, factor V Leiden, before writing a prescription for an oral contraceptive, particularly if a patient is in a population at greater risk of this (northern European white ancestry). Whether screening for factor V Leiden is appropriate and whether screening for the prothrombin-gene mutation is appropriate will remain controversial until someone does a serious cost-effective analysis on this topic.

J.A. Stockman III, M.D.

Prevalence of the Factor V Leiden Mutation in Children and Neonates With Thromboembolic Disease
Hagstrom JN, Walter J, Bluebond-Langner R, et al (Univ of Pennsylvania, Philadelphia; The Children's Hosp of Philadelphia)
J Pediatr 133:777-781, 1998   13–21

Introduction.—Thromboembolic disease is increasingly being recognized in children and neonates. In adults, one risk factor for deep vein thrombosis is resistance to active protein C; others are surgery, malignancy, oral contraceptives, disorders of the hemostatic system, antithrombin II deficiency, protein S deficiency, plasminogen deficiency, dysfibrino-

TABLE 3.—Prevalence of Factor V Leiden in Neonates and Children With Thrombosis

	Neonates		Children		Total	
	N	FVL	N	FVL	N	FVL
Venous	7	0	25	4 (16%)*	32	4 (13%)
DVT/PE	3	0	20	4 (20%)*	23	4 (17%)*
Sinus thrombosis	4	0	5	0	9	0
Arterial	26	6 (23%)*	27	2 (7%)	53	8 (15%)*
CNS	22	6 (27%)*	25	2 (8%)	47	8 (17%)*
Systemic	4	0	2	0	6	0
Total	33	6 (18%)*	52	6 (12%)	85	12 (14%)*

(Courtesy of Hagstrom JN, Walter J, Bluebond-Langner R, et al: Prevalence of the factor V Leiden mutation in children and neonates with thromboembolic disease. *J Pediatr* 133:777-781, 1998.)

genemia, and the anti-phospholipid antibody syndrome. A mutation in the coagulation factor V gene (factor V Leiden) has been found to be the basis for the activated protein C resistance. The association of the factor V Leiden mutation with arterial and venous thromboembolic disease in children and neonates was investigated through a retrospective chart review.

Methods.—The clinical records of 33 neonates and 52 children with thromboembolic disease were retrospectively analyzed. DNA analysis was used to screen for the factor V Leiden mutation, and also allowed for identifying patients as normal, heterozygous, or homozygous.

Results.—Of 85 patients, 12 were heterozygous for factor V Leiden (14.1%), and none were homozygous (Table 3). Eight of 47 patients who had arterial central nervous system events were positive for the factor V Leiden mutation (17%), including 6 of 22 neonates (27%). Four of 32 patients with a venous thrombosis were factor V Leiden positive (12.5%). Protein C deficiency was not seen in any of the patients. Protein S deficiency was seen in 3.5%. Antithrombin II deficiency was seen in 1.2% of patients. Anti-phospholipid antibodies were seen in 16.5% of patients.

Conclusion.—The factor V Leiden mutation plays a role in the development of arterial and venous thrombotic events in neonates and children.

▶ Each of the last several years, the YEAR BOOK OF PEDIATRICS has updated its audience on factor V Leiden-related issues. It was in 1993 that the first reports began to appear related to resistance to the action of activated protein C. This phenomenon was found to be present in about 40% of patients with otherwise-unexplained venous thromboses. Subsequently it was learned that the problem is caused by inheritance of a mutation in coagulation factor V gene that renders the protein less readily susceptible to inactivation by activated protein C. Heterozygotes for this mutation have a 7-fold increase in the risk for venous thrombosis. Those who are homozygous have an 80-fold increase in risk. This disorder would be an otherwise-obscure entity were it not for the fact that in the general population, the prevalence of the factor V Leiden mutation (the heterozygote) is 3% to 6%. In adults, factor V Leiden is the single most common identifiable defect in patients with venous thromboses of the legs. In this study from Philadelphia, we see that being a heterozygote for factor V Leiden is an extremely common cause of both arterial and venous thromboses in both newborns and older children.

As noted in prior commentaries in earlier YEAR BOOKS, factor V Leiden is particularly common in those of Scandinavian ancestry and is relatively uncommon in African Americans, with intermediate prevalence in those of other ethnic groups. The following table consists of data from the U.S. Census Bureau, and shows how diverse the great melting pot of America is when it comes to our composition, by country of origin, for the U.S. population.

Group	Population (in Millions)
1. German	57.9
2. Irish	38.7
3. English	32.7
4. African American	23.8
5. Italian	14.7
6. Mexican	11.6
7. French	10.3
8. Polish	9.4
9. Dutch	6.2
10. Jewish*	6.0
11. Scotch-Irish	5.6
12. Scottish	5.4
13. Swedish	4.7
14. Norwegian	3.9
15. Russian	3.0
16. French Canadian	2.2
17. Welsh	2.0
Spanish	2.0
Puerto Rican	2.0
20. Slovak	1.9
21. Danish	1.6
Hungarian	1.6
23. Chinese	1.5
Filipino	1.5
American Indians	1.5
26. Czech	1.3
27. Portuguese	1.2
28. Greek	1.1
29. Swiss	1.0
Japanese	1.0

*About 80% of American Jews trace their ancestry to Germany, Poland, and Russia.

None of the above would be important except that we are seeing more and more venous thromboses in kids. The reason is that central venous catheters are being used more frequently, and the morbidity associated with central venous catheter-related deep venous thromboses is substantial.[1] The next time you run into a youngster with such problems, at least think about the possibility of factor V Leiden-related difficulties.

J.A. Stockman III, M.D.

Reference

1. Massicotte MP, Dix D, Monagle P, et al: Central venous catheter related thrombosis in children: Analysis of the Canadian registry of venous thromboembolic complications. *J Pediatr* 133:770-776, 1998.

Increased Risk for Fetal Loss in Carriers of the Factor V Leiden Mutation

Meinardi JR, Middeldorp S, de Kam PJ, et al (Univ Hosp Groningen, The Netherlands; Academic Med Ctr, Amsterdam; Univ Hosp Maastricht, The Netherlands)

Ann Intern Med 130:736-739, 1999   13–22

Background.—Carriers of the factor V Leiden mutation probably have an increased risk for fetal loss because of placental thrombosis. However, previous research has not consistently demonstrated this risk.

Methods.—In a retrospective study, a cohort of 228 factor V Leiden mutation carriers and 121 noncarrier relatives seen at 3 university hospitals were studied. All had been pregnant at least once.

Findings.—Fetal loss occurred in 31.6% of the mutation carriers and in 22.3% of the noncarriers. Miscarriage occurred in 29.4% and 17.4%, respectively, and stillbirth in 5.7% and 5%, respectively. Ten percent of carriers and 4% of noncarriers had recurrent fetal loss. Compared with noncarriers, mutation carriers had an adjusted odds ratio of 2.12 for fetal loss, 2.08 for miscarriage, and 1.6 for stillbirth. The risks for fetal loss and stillbirth were greater in homozygous carriers than in heterozygous carriers (Table).

Conclusion.—Factor V Leiden mutation carriers are at greater risk for fetal loss, especially miscarriage, than noncarriers. The risk for recurrence of fetal loss is also increased in carriers compared with noncarriers, and that for fetal loss and stillbirth is increased in homozygous carriers compared with heterozygous carriers.

▶ Here is another report showing that those who are carriers of the factor V Leiden mutation do, indeed, have a much higher than expected risk of miscarriage. In this series, almost 1 in 3 pregnant carriers had a pregnancy resulting in a stillbirth. These are higher numbers than had been previously reported, but the data do seem believable. Should an otherwise normal pregnancy end in a stillbirth, the mother must be evaluated for a hypercoagulable syndrome so that the next time she becomes pregnant, that pregnancy can be managed appropriately, including management with the use of anticoagulants early on.

On a slightly different, but related, topic, there is a lot going on these days in terms of new understandings of antithrombotic agents. Generally, these are categorized into 2 classes: anticoagulants and antiplatelet agents. It is in the former category that so much new knowledge is being developed. Anticoagulants inhibit thrombin generation and fibrin formation. The established long-standing antithrombotic anticoagulants, heparin and coumarin,

TABLE.—Fetal Loss in Women With the Factor V Leiden Mutation and Their Noncarrier Relatives

Variable	Carriers	Noncarriers	Odds Ratio (95% CI)*	P Value
Women, *n*	228	121		
Women with fetal loss, *n* (%)	72 (31.6)	27 (22.3)	2.01 (1.07-3.75)	0.03
Women with miscarriage, *n* (%)	67 (29.4)	21 (17.4)	2.70 (1.39-5.25)	0.003
Women with stillbirth, *n* (%)	13 (5.7)	6 (5.0)	1.29 (0.45-3.69)	>0.2
Pregnancies, *n*	654	352		
Pregnancies ending in fetal loss, *n* (%)†	107 (16.4)	32 (9.1)	2.12 (1.35-3.33)	<0.001
In heterozygous carriers	98 (15.0)	32 (9.1)	2.02 (1.34-3.05)	<0.001
In homozygous carriers	9 (23.7)	32 (9.1)	4.07 (1.66-9.95)	<0.001
In homozygous compared with heterozygous carriers			2.01 (0.94-4.32)	0.07
Pregnancies ending in miscarriage, *n* (%)	88 (13.5)	26 (7.4)	2.08 (1.33-3.25)	0.001
In heterozygous carriers	82 (13.3)	26 (7.4)	2.03 (1.29-3.20)	0.002
In homozygous carriers	6 (15.8)	26 (7.4)	2.93 (1.52-5.77)	0.001
In homozygous compared with heterozygous carriers			1.46 (0.80-2.66)	>0.2
Pregnancies ending in stillbirth, *n* (%)	19 (2.9)	6 (1.7)	1.60 (0.58-4.43)	>0.2
In heterozygous carriers	16 (2.6)	6 (1.7)	1.39 (0.49-3.96)	>0.2
In homozygous carriers	3 (7.9)	6 (1.7)	6.36 (1.04-38.93)	0.045
In homozygous compared with heterozygous carriers			4.85 (0.82-25.58)	0.08

*Odds ratios, adjusted for age and number of pregnancies, were estimated by random-effects modeling to compare pregnancies.
†Terminated and ectopic pregnancies excluded.
(Courtesy of Meinardi JR, Middeldorp S, de Kam PJ, et al: Increased risk for fetal loss in carriers of the factor V Leiden mutation. *Ann Intern Med* 130:736-739, 1999.)

are effective but have fairly significant limitations. The development of new antithrombotic agents has been stimulated by clinical needs and by advances in biotechnology that have made it possible to produce drugs that target specific steps in thrombogenesis.

The pharmacokinetic and biophysical limitations of heparin can be overcome by these new classes of anticoagulants. Of the latter, low–molecular weight heparin and direct inhibitors of thrombin have been evaluated clinically. Although coumarins require careful laboratory monitoring because of concerns about safety, orally active direct inhibitors of thrombin and factor Xa may replace coumarins altogether. The new glycoprotein IIb/IIIa antagonists have shown clear benefits and have already become important antithrombotic agents for various conditions. The latter antagonists are antiplatelet agents that are more effective and controllable than aspirin. If you want to read more about what's new and what's on the horizon when it comes to antithrombotic agents, see the superb review of Hirsh et al.[1]

This is the last entry in the Blood chapter, so we will close with a quiz: You are a medical missionary and are about to head off to the jungles of South America for the next year. The rub is that you have recently developed chronic atrial fibrillation and you must take warfarin (Coumadin). There will be no way that you can reach a laboratory to have periodic coagulation testing done. The question is; What test can you perform that will act as a surrogate for formal coagulation testing to determine whether you are properly anticoagulated?

You can do what a 45-year-old technician, on long-term anticoagulation with a Coumadin product because of chronic atrial fibrillation, did when he started a new job in China. Because he was uncertain about the facilities for monitoring anticoagulation there, he designed a procedure based on the idea that anticoagulated blood runs further over an obliquely placed glass slide than non-anticoagulated blood and that the lengths of the blood trail would correspond to the degree of anticoagulation. This fellow took a glass slide (40 cm × 5 cm × 8 mm), and cleaned it with aftershave. After piercing one of his fingertips with a lancet, he positioned 1 drop of blood at the upper end of the glass slide on a flat surface without kneading the pierced finger. He made certain that the diameter of the blood drop was consistently between 6 and 8 mm, or the puncture was repeated. Immediately after placing the drop, he tilted the slide to 65.5 degrees. This angle was achieved by folding a rectangular sheet of paper twice and putting this wedge against a wall. The glass slide was pushed up the wedge as quickly as possible. The blood drop started to run down the slide and as soon as it stopped, after approximately 1 minute later, he measured the length of the blood trail with a ruler. By repeatedly testing the accuracy of the method, he found that optimal anticoagulation, in comparison with formal laboratory testing, was achieved if the blood trail length was 25 ± 2 cm. If the blood trail length was less than 23 cm, he increased his Coumadin by a small amount for the next 3 days. He did this test every 3 days throughout his 5-month stay in China without complications. To ensure a constant temperature during the testing, he did the test at a temperature of 20°C to 22°C, heating his room when he was in cold parts of China and doing the test early in the morning in hot areas.

If you think the above is so much fooey, it is not.[2] Indeed, the accuracy of this method was verified in 10 anticoagulated patients in which, instead of a paper wedge, a wooden frame was created to achieve reproducible correct angles. It was found that the correlation between formal clotting test values and the blood trail lengths was significant at an R value of -0.882.

What can beat a simple, cheap, quick, and reproducible test? Wouldn't it be interesting if this test could be used not just to measure anticoagulation effects, but to determine if coagulation defects actually exist?

J.A. Stockman III, M.D.

References

1. Hirsh J, Weitz JI: New antithrombotic agents. *Lancet* 353:1431-1436, 1999.
2. Finsterer J, Stollperger C, Janko O: Homemade anticoagulation monitor. *Lancet* 352:962, 1998.

14 Oncology

Myopathic Changes As a Paraneoplastic Sign in Childhood Acute Lymphoblastic Leukemia
Shuper A, Gilai AN, Stark B, et al (Tel Aviv Univ, Israel; Alyn Children's Hosp, Jerusalem, Israel)
Clin Pediatr (Phila) 37:565-568, 1998   14–1

Background.—Muscular disorders are very unusual paraneoplastic phenomena in children. The report of a girl in whom myopathy was the initial symptom of acute lymphoblastic leukemia (ALL) is presented.

Case Report.—Girl, first evaluated 2 months after birth because of enlarged occipital lymph nodes. The only physical abnormalities were generalized lymphadenopathy and an enlarged spleen and liver. Hemoglobin was 8.9 g/dL. Red blood cell indices and morphology and leukocytosis were normal. Three weeks later, the white blood count increased further, and the differential count shifted mildly to the left. Bone marrow aspiration showed myeloid hyperplasia with a few myeloblasts. An interim diagnosis of juvenile chronic myeloid leukemia was made, but the absence of fetal erythropoiesis and thrombocytopenia prompted the case to be classified as undetermined myeloproliferative state, and close observation was planned. During the next few months, the liver and spleen regressed partially, and the white blood cell count normalized. The patient had normal development until aged 5 years, when she began to have gait difficulties. She soon became unable to ambulate independently and was confined to a wheelchair. Neurologic assessment revealed marked weakness of all pelvic girdle muscles. An extensive evaluation yielded normal findings. However, needle electromyography showed small motor unit potentials and large turns and amplitude (T/A) values, suggesting that a decreased number of muscle fibers were participating in voluntary movements. Apparently, some myopathic changes had occurred without affecting conduction along motor or sensory fibers or the synaptic junction. The parents refused muscle biopsy. About 3 months after the onset of these symptoms, the patient was found to have severe thrombocytopenia. Bone marrow aspiration, which had been normal previously, was now compatible with early B

CD10-positive ALL. Treatment, on the basis of the INS-89 proto-col, resulted in hematologic remission and complete resolution of the child's neurologic signs. Two and a half years later, neurologic findings were normal except for a mild reduction in deep tendon reflexes resulting from chemotherapy.

Conclusions.—Muscle disorders may be the first sign of a wide range of lymphoproliferative disorders. The paraneoplastic myopathy present in the child described is presumed to be an autoimmune phenomenon, which may occur in adults as well as children, probably more often in persons with myelodysplastic syndromes.

▶ Most who deal with children are unfamiliar with "paraneoplastic signs." The reason why is straightforward. Paraneoplastic phenomena generally occur in adults with malignancy. Specifically, they are signs or symptoms that appear unrelated to a malignancy, but in fact are frequently the herald for a cancer, leukemia, or lymphoma. An unexplained high calcium, watery diarrhea, polymyositis, dermatomyositis, unexplained high hemoglobins, hy-pertension, precocious puberty, and opsoclonus/myoclonus syndrome are all examples of paraneoplastic signs associated with childhood malignancies.

In the case of this 5-year-old girl, she presented with a very aggressive myopathy as a prelude to a later diagnosis of ALL. Her neurologic findings were consistent with the Eaton-Lambert syndrome, a myasthenia-like dis-order that has been sporadically reported in association with acute lymphatic leukemia and with neuroblastoma in children.[1,2]

One of the tricks that we teach residents at morning report when an ill-defined case is presented is to outline broad categories of differential diagnoses rather than specific ones. For example, one would always place on a differential diagnosis of an ill-defined sign or symptom the possibility of an obscure infectious disease or the possibility of an immunologic/rheumatic disorder, and one should also include the possibility of a malignancy. Once one at least thinks of the possibility of a malignancy, one then can begin to weigh what unusual or rare possibilities might be the etiology of a particular patient's problem. It is not a stretch to think that a child with an ill-defined muscular skeletal problem might have a malignancy such as ALL.

Please see the articles that follow, which remind us of something that we should always be aware of; namely, a child with a limp that is otherwise unexplained could easily have an acute leukemia.

J.A. Stockman III, M.D.

References

1. de Graaf JH, Tamminga RYJ, Kamps WA: Paraneoplastic manifestations in chil-dren. *Eur J Pediatr* 153:784-791, 1994.
2. Shor NF: Nervous system dysfunction in children with paraneoplastic syndrome. *J Child Neurol* 7:253-258, 1992.

The Limping Child: A Manifestation of Acute Leukemia

Tuten HR, Gabos PG, Kumar SJ, et al (Alfred I duPont Inst, Wilmington, Del)
J Pediatr Orthop 18:625-629, 1998   14–2

Background.—Clinicians often evaluate children for a limp with no clear history of injury. Common causes of atraumatic limp are a septic joint, acute osteomyelitis, transient synovitis, Lyme disease, and juvenile rheumatoid arthritis. Atraumatic limp can also be a manifestation of acute leukemia. One series was reviewed.

Patients and Findings.—Nine children brought to 1 center for a limp with no history of trauma between 1990 and 1996 were subsequently diagnosed as having leukemia. These children comprised 11.6% of the total number of children diagnosed with leukemia at that center and in that period. The 6 boys and 3 girls were aged from 15 months to 13 years. None had an underlying chronic medical condition. However, recent illness was common, including otitis media and upper respiratory infections. A case review revealed certain clinical and laboratory features that helped establish the diagnosis. Every child had an irritable hip or knee, with the hip being the site of pain in 78%. Seventy-eight percent of the children were febrile at the initial assessment. All children had anemia and neutropenia. Lymphadenopathy and hepatosplenomegaly were also common findings. Thrombocytopenia, often profound, occurred in 6 patients. White blood cell counts were often normal or only slightly diminished but were increased markedly in 3 children. Seven children had a marked leukocytosis. Seven had blast cells present on the peripheral blood smear, indicating that their absence does not exclude the diagnosis of leukemia. The erythrocyte sedimentation rate (ESR) obtained in 4 patients, was increased in all. A C-reactive protein was obtained in 1 patient and was increased. Bone marrow biopsy verified the diagnosis in all the children (Table 1).

Conclusions.—The presence of antalgic gait with pain of variable intensity and duration, an irritable hip or knee, a mild-to-moderate increase in body temperature, lymphadenopathy, hepatosplenomegaly, increased ESR, thrombocytopenia, anemia, reduced neutrophils, elevated lymphocytes, or blast cells on the peripheral blood smear should alert clinicians to the possibility of acute leukemia in children with atraumatic limping. Bone marrow biopsy confirms the diagnosis.

▶ It's easy to see how a child who presents with hip pain, fever, and an elevated ESR might be thought to have a rheumatologic or infectious disorder, when in fact, a malignancy is present. In this series, the majority of patients had hip pain (78%), and the majority also had fever. Fortunately, the diagnosis was not missed in any patient because the CBC in all showed anemia and neutropenia. Even though leukemic cells were not present in the peripheral smear, no reasonable person would have skipped doing a bone marrow, which in every case easily made the diagnosis.

TABLE 1.—Clinical and Laboratory Findings for the 9 Patients

Case	Age	Race	Sex	Duration of Symptom (Weeks)	Limp	Night Pain	Joint Pain	Bone Pain	Location of Pain	Temperature (degC)	Concurrent Infection	Other Physical Findings	X-ray Findings	Bone Scan
1	15 mo	White	M	14	Right	No	Right hip	No	—	39	Diarrhea, otitis, URI	Bruising, petechiae	None	Positive
2	24 mo	White	M	8	Left	No	Left hip	Yes	Radiates to knee	35.5	No	Pallor, adenopathy, splenomegaly	None taken	Not done
3	27 mo	Black	M	1	Left	No	Left hip	No	—	37.6	No	Adenopathy	Osteopenia	Negative
4	37 mo	White	F	1	Left	No	Left hip	No	—	38.5	No	Hepatosplenomegaly	None	Positive
5	4 yr	White	F	2	Left	No	Left hip	No	Radiates to knee	37.6	No	Meningitis, hepatomegaly, adenopathy	None	Not done
6	5 yr	White	M	4	Right	Yes	Right hip	No	Radiates to thigh	36.5	URI, diarrhea	—	None	Positive
7	8 yr	White	M	2	Bilat.	Yes	Bilat. hips	Yes	Radiates to thighs	38	Otitis media, sepsis	Pallor, bruising, hepatospleno-megaly	None	Negative
8	9 yr	Black	F	9	Bilat.	No	No	Yes	Tibias	38	No	—	None taken	Not done
9	13 yr	White	M	6	Right	No	Right knee	No	Radiates to hip	37.7	No	Pallor, weight loss	None taken	Not done

Abbreviation: URI, upper respiratory infection.
(Courtesy of Tuten HR, Gabos PG, Kumar SJ, et al: The limping child: A manifestation of acute leukemia. *J Pediatr Orthop* 18[5]:625-629, 1998.)

Between 10% and 15% of children in the institution that was the origin of this report had hip pain and limp as the presenting sign of their leukemia. This statistic should remind us that in addition to a long list of potential causes of hip pain (a list that includes septic joint, acute osteomyelitis, transient synovitis, Lyme disease, juvenile rheumatoid arthritis, etc.), we must remember that leukemia should be considered. For more on the topic of leukemia masquerading as joint symptoms, see Abstract 14–3.

J.A. Stockman III, M.D.

Malignancies in Children Who Initially Present With Rheumatic Complaints

Cabral DA, Tucker LB (Univ of British Columbia, Vancouver; Tufts Univ, Boston)
J Pediatr 134:53-57, 1999   14–3

Introduction.—Rheumatic complaints are common among patients with malignancy. In pediatrics, rheumatic presentations of malignancies are infrequently reported. The presence of musculoskeletal pain, joint swelling, or limp may suggest chronic arthritis. Persistent fever, constitutional symptoms, or evidence of multisystem disease may suggest systemic arthritis, systemic lupus erythematosus, or vasculitis. Early diagnosis and treatment can help in successful therapy for childhood malignancy. Diagnosis of malignancy should be considered earlier among patients referred to the pediatric rheumatologist.

TABLE 1.—Provisional Referring Rheumatic Diagnoses and Final Diagnoses in 29 Children Ultimately Diagnosed With Malignancy

Diagnosis	n	%
Referring diagnosis		
JRA	12	41
Nonspecific connective tissue disease	4	14
Discitis (?JRA)	3	10
Juvenile spondyloarthropathy	3	10
SLE	2	7
Kawasaki disease	2	7
MCTD	1	3
Lyme disease	1	3
Juvenile dermatomyositis	1	3
Final diagnosis		
Leukemia	13	45
Neuroblastoma	6	21
Lymphoma	3	10
Ewing's sarcoma	3	10
Mixopapillary ependymoma	1	3
Epithelioma	1	3
Thalamic glioma	1	3
Sarcoma	1	3
JRA	2	7

(Courtesy of Cabral DA, Tucker LB: Malignancies in children who initially present with rheumatic complaints. *J Pediatr* 134:53-57, 1999.)

TABLE 3.—Frequency of Clinical Features in 29 Children With
Malignancy Initially Presenting to a Rheumatologist

Clinical Features	n	%
Features typical of many rheumatic disorders		
Musculoskeletal pains	24	82
Fever	16	54
Fatigue	15	50
Weight loss	13	42
Hepatomegaly	8	29
Arthritis	7	25
Abnormal gait	6	21
Lymphadenopathy	5	18
Splenomegaly	4	14
Rash	3	11
Features atypical of most rheumatic disorders		
Night sweats	4	14
Ecchymoses or bruising	4	14
Abnormal neurologic signs	3	10
Abnormal masses	2	7
Ptosis	1	3
Urinary incontinence	1	3

(Courtesy of Cabral DA, Tucker LB: Malignancies in children who initially present with rheumatic complaints. *J Pediatr* 134:53-57, 1999.)

Methods.—Twenty-nine children, ages 1 to 15.5 years, with malignancy referred to pediatric rheumatology centers were retrospectively reviewed.

Results.—On referral, the suspected diagnoses were: juvenile rheumatoid arthritis, discitis, nonspecific connective tissue disease, systemic lupus erythematosus, spondyloarthropathy, Kawasaki disease, mixed connective tissue disease, Lyme disease, and dermatomyositis (Table 1). Among the final diagnoses were: leukemia, neuroblastoma, lymphoma, Ewing's sarcoma, ependymoma, thalamic glioma, epithelioma, and sarcoma. Features of many rheumatic disorders were found among patients, including musculoskeletal pains (82%), fever (54%), fatigue (50%), weight loss (42%), hepatomegaly (29%), and arthritis (25%) (Table 3). There were also features suggestive of malignancy, including nonarticular bone pain (68%), abnormal initial investigations (68%), clinical features atypical of

TABLE 4.—Frequency of Worrisome Clinical Features or Initial Findings
Suggestive of Malignancy in 29 Children Presenting to a Rheumatologist

Worrisome Clinical Features	n	%
Nonarticular bone pain	20	69
Back pain as a principle presenting feature	9	31
Bone tenderness	8	28
Severe constitutional symptoms	9	31
Clinical features atypical of rheumatic disease	14	49
Abnormal initial findings	19	66

(Courtesy of Cabral DA, Tucker LB: Malignancies in children who initially present with rheumatic complaints. *J Pediatr* 134:53-57, 1999.)

most rheumatic disease (48%), severe constitutional symptoms (32%), back pain as a major presenting feature (32), and bone tenderness (29%) (Table 4). Night sweats, ecchymoses and bruising, abnormal neurologic signs, abnormal masses, and ptosis were among the atypical features. Tests that showed abnormal findings on initial investigations were complete blood count/smear, discordant erythrocyte sedimentation rate and platelet count, elevated lactate dehydrogenase level, plain skeletal x-ray films, bone scan, and abdominal ultrasound. In 40% of patients, findings of investigations before referral to the rheumatology clinic were not recognized as abnormal.

Conclusion.—The pediatric rheumatologist would see patients with a diverse group of malignancies, other than leukemia. Typical features of childhood rheumatic disorders should be familiar to pediatric care providers. In the presence of any atypical or discordant clinical features, rheumatic diagnoses should be re-evaluated.

▶ Balu H. Athreya, M.D., Pediatric Rheumatology, Alfred I. duPont Hospital for Children, Wilmington, Del, comments:

Juvenile rheumatoid arthritis (JRA)—in the process of being renamed juvenile idiopathic arthritis—is a clinical exclusion diagnosis. The exclusion process never stops. I have known children who carried a diagnosis of JRA for up to 6 months before a diagnosis of leukemia or neuroblastoma. One child developed inflammatory bowel disease 12 years after the diagnosis of JRA!

There are 3 major categories of JRA—systemic, pauci articular, and the polyarticular. Pediatricians are well aware of the fact that systemic features, such as fever, lymphadenopathy, and hepatosplenomegaly, can occur in both the systemic type of JRA and leukemia. What is not well-known is that malignancy must be considered in the differential diagnosis of polyarticular and pauci articular varieties of JRA also. It is also important to recognize that solid tumors appearing with musculoskeletal symptoms and positive antinuclear antibody does not necessarily mean a rheumatic disorder is present.

The authors have convincingly pointed out the importance of thinking about malignancies in children with rheumatic complaints. As an average, we see 2 or 3 referred patients a year in our pediatric rheumatology clinic because of rheumatic symptoms or for evaluation of positive antinuclear antibody who happen to have a malignancy. Based on personal experience and data from this article, I suggest the following table of differential diagnosis for children presenting with rheumatologic signs and symptoms who in fact have other problems:

• Systemic: Acute lymphatic leukemia
Acute monocytic leukemia
Acute eosinophilic leukemia
Neuroblastoma
Paraneoplastic syndrome (positive ANA)

- Polyarticular: Acute lymphatic leukemia
                   Acute monocytic leukemia
                   Hodgkin's lymphoma
                   Lymphomatoid granulomatosis (with its new names)
- Monarticular: Pigmented villonodular synovitis
                   Synovial chondromatosis
                   Hemangioma
                   Lymphangioma

One point in the history needs further emphasis. The characteristics of pain associated with leukemia are different from the pain of rheumatic diseases, particularly JRA. Children with JRA are stiff, but rarely complain about pain. But the pain in malignancy is out of proportion to the amount of swelling around the joint. Often the pain in leukemia is worse at night. Also, as the authors point out the tenderness is over the bones around the joint and also over other bones, such as the tibia and the sternum.

In this era of cost containment, the authors make an extremely important point: You do not need fancy and expensive studies to arrive at the diagnosis. Rely on physical examination; perform simple laboratory tests; and more important, look at those results carefully. The answer may be staring at you!

B.H. Athreya, M.D.

Clinical Significance of Minimal Residual Disease in Childhood Acute Lymphoblastic Leukemia
Cavé H, for the European Organization for Research and Treatment of Cancer–Childhood Leukemia Cooperative Group (Hôpital Robert Debré, Paris; et al)
N Engl J Med 339:591-598, 1998   14–4

Background.—The clinical implications of residual disease detection after treatment of acute lymphoblastic leukemia (ALL) are not clear. The predictive value of the presence or absence of detectable residual disease at several time points in the first 6 months after complete remission of childhood ALL were investigated.

Methods.—One hundred seventy-eight of 246 patients treated with a uniform chemotherapy protocol were monitored for residual disease with 1 or more clone-specific probes. Junctional sequences of T cell–receptor or immunoglobulin gene rearrangements were used, and residual disease was quantified by a competitive polymerase chain reaction (PCR) assay.

Findings.—At each time point studied, the presence or absence and level of residual disease were correlated significantly with the risk of early relapse. Patients at high risk for relapse after the completion of induction therapy or at a later time were identified by PCR measures. In a multivariate analysis including immunophenotype, age, risk group, and white cell count at diagnosis, the presence or absence and level of residual disease was the strongest independent prognostic factor (Fig 1).

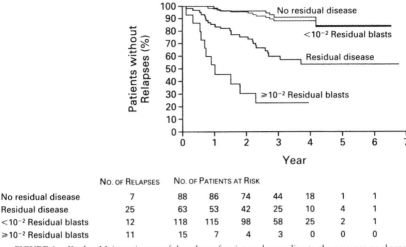

FIGURE 1.—Kaplan-Meier estimates of the relapse-free interval according to the presence or absence and level of residual disease in patients with a first complete remission of ALL at the end of induction therapy. *P* < .001 for the comparison between patients with residual disease and those without residual disease and for the comparison between patients with ≥10^{-2} residual blasts and those with <10^{-2} residual blasts. Nine of the 15 patients with a high level of residual disease (≥10^{-2} blasts) died, as compared with only 4 of the 118 with a lower level of residual disease (<10^{-2} blasts). The number of patients shown below the graph are the numbers at standard or very high risk for whom bone marrow samples were available. In 18 patients, residual disease was detected but was not quantified. (Reprinted by permission of *The New England Journal of Medicine*, from Cavé H, for the European Organization for Research and Treatment of Cancer-Childhood Leukemia Cooperative Group: Clinical significance of minimal residual disease in childhood acute lymphoblastic leukemia. *N Engl J Med* 339:591-598. Copyright 1998, Massachusetts Medical Society. All rights reserved.)

Conclusions.—Residual disease after induction of remission of ALL is a powerful prognostic indicator. The presence of residual disease as seen by PCR can identify patients at risk for relapse and should be considered when making decisions about alternative therapy.

▶ Times have certainly changed. When this editor was a fellow in training in hematology (not really all that long ago), the only commonly used prognostic features related to children with ALL were age and the total white count. The younger you were (under 1 year of age) and the older you were (over 10), the poorer the prognosis. A white count at presentation greater than 50,000 was a bad sign. One could also tell whether the leukemia was T cell in origin, and that was a bad prognostic feature. A little while later, various chromosomal translocations were identified, which when present, carried an increased risk of treatment failure. Better than even some of these prognostic features is the current description of the PCR assay. With PCR technology, one can pick out leukemic cells in blood or bone marrow samples. One can then find those children who are responding more slowly than others even if the child is in a "technical" remission (less than 5% lymphoblasts in the bone marrow).

The fact that high-risk children do better with more aggressive therapies is also noted in the article which follows. If there is any lesson in all this, it is that the microscope has been relegated to an increasingly minor position as far as telling us who is or who is not in a true remission. PCR is pushing it aside. Only when the leukemic cell burden rises to a figure of 10^{11} to 10^{12} does the microscope tell us there is disease. Death usually occurs when there are approximately 10^{13} leukemic cells. With chemotherapy, remission occurs and disease can no longer be identified with a microscope when the cell number falls to fewer than 10^{10}. The "remission" achieved is actually only a somewhat arbitrary point toward the end of a continuum of leukemic cell number and destruction. Only when no cells are left is a true cure seen. PCR helps us know when this is more likely to happen. It has a sensitivity in detecting malignant cells down to the level of 10^{-4} to 10^{-5}.

There are a number of hematologists/oncologists who are already proposing to increase the intensity of treatment in patients with persistently high levels of minimum residual disease (PCR-positive patients) who are technically in remission. Whether this will lead to additional benefits remains to be seen, but undoubtedly more will be learned about the biology of leukemia as this problem is more aggressively approached.

To read more on this topic, see the superb editorial of Alec Morley.[1]

J.A. Stockman III, M.D.

Reference

1. Morley A: Quantifying leukemia. *N Engl J Med* 339:627-629, 1998.

Augmented Post-induction Therapy for Children With High-Risk Acute Lymphoblastic Leukemia and a Slow Response to Initial Therapy

Nachman JB, Sather HN, Sensel MG, et al (Univ of Chicago; Univ of Southern California, Los Angeles; Children's Cancer Group, Arcadia, Calif; et al)
N Engl J Med 338:1663-1671, 1998   14–5

Background.—In children with high-risk acute lymphoblastic leukemia (ALL), a slow response to initial chemotherapy is associated with a poor outcome, despite intensive treatment. The efficacy of augmented postinduction therapy in such patients was investigated.

Methods.—Three hundred eleven children with newly diagnosed ALL were enrolled in the randomized trial between 1991 and 1995. The children were aged 1 to 9 years with white cell counts of at least 50,000/mm³ or 10 years or older, had a slow response to initial treatment, and entered remission at the end of induction chemotherapy. One hundred fifty-six patients received standard therapy, and 155, augmented treatment.

Findings.—Five-year outcomes were significantly better in the augmented treatment group than in the standard therapy group. Event-free survival was 75% and 55%, respectively, and overall survival, 78.4% and 66.7%, respectively. The difference between treatments was most marked

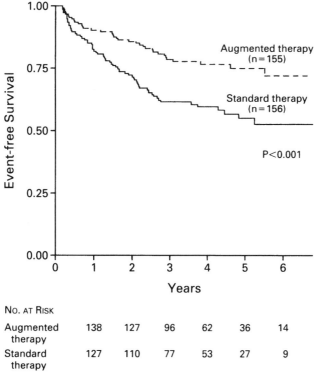

FIGURE 1.—Event-free survival during 5 years of follow-up in patients with ALL, according to the type of post-induction chemotherapy. *Dashed line*, augmented therapy; *straight line*, standard therapy. (Reprinted by permission of *The New England Journal of Medicine*, from Nachman JB, Sather HN, Sensel MG, et al: Augmented post-induction therapy for children with high-risk acute lymphoblastic leukemia and a slow response to initial therapy. *N Engl J Med* 338:1663-1671. Copyright 1998, Massachusetts Medical Society. All right reserved.)

among children aged 1 to 9 years all of whom had white cell counts of at least 50,000/mm³. In the entire cohort, risk factors for an adverse event included a white cell count of 200,000/mm³ or greater, nonwhite and nonblack race, and the presence of a t(9;22) translocation. The toxic effects of augmented treatment were substantial but could be managed (Figs 1 and 2).

Conclusions.—Most children with high-risk ALL and a slow response to initial treatment will have excellent outcomes with augmented postinduction chemotherapy. The extent of cytoreduction seen after 1 to 2 weeks of induction chemotherapy is a useful indicator of the susceptibility of leukemic cells to chemotherapeutic agents.

▶ Here is another article showing us that those who respond slowly to initial therapy with childhood leukemia may need more aggressive therapy. In addition to high white count, these investigators found that race other than black or white, and the presence of specific chromosomal translocation

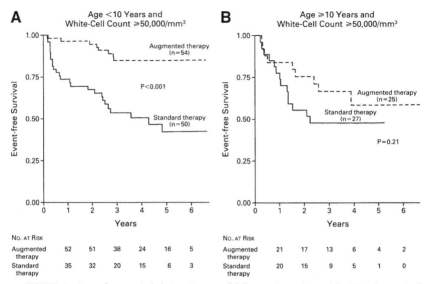

A Age <10 Years and White-Cell Count ≥50,000/mm³

B Age ≥10 Years and White-Cell Count ≥50,000/mm³

FIGURE 2.—Event-free survival during 5 years of follow-up in patients with ALL who received standard therapy or augmented therapy, according to age and white-cell count at diagnosis. **A**, children aged < 10 years; **B**, children aged ≥ 10 years. (Reprinted by permission of *The New England Journal of Medicine*, from Nachman JB, Sather HN, Sensel MG, et al: Augmented post-induction therapy for children with high-risk acute lymphoblastic leukemia and a slow response to initial therapy. *N Engl J Med* 338:1663-1671. Copyright 1998, Massachusetts Medical Society. All right reserved.)

[t(9;22)] are potential indications for more than just routine therapy. Please note that aggressiveness in the treatment of childhood leukemia does not come without a price. We see in this study that the toxic effects of augmented therapy are considerable, although in most instances manageable. What we don't know is whether more aggressive therapy will carry with it late sequelae. Late sequelae of treatment of ALL occurs in a small, but real number of survivors of the disease. Cranial irradiation has been implicated in the development of brain tumors (generally occurring about 10 years later), neuropsychological deficits, and endocrinopathy that can lead to short stature, obesity, precocious puberty, and osteoporosis. Many children with profound growth retardation caused by cranial irradiation or intensive chemotherapy receive growth hormone therapy after completing antileukemic therapy. An adequate final height can be achieved in most cases with replacement therapy. This therapy fortunately apparently does not increase the risk of leukemia relapse. Acute myeloid leukemia may develop in some patients after treatment for ALL, particularly in patients who have received intensive treatment with etoposide and teniposide. The latency period here is relatively short, approximately 3 years. The long-term survival rate of patients with ALL who develop AML is abysmal. The 1 other side effect of chemotherapy for ALL is cardiomyopathy if anthracyclines have been used at high dose.

If there is good news in the ALL data, it is that the incidence of cancer birth defects is not increased among offspring of adult survivors of childhood ALL.

To read more on the topic of potential future therapies for childhood ALL, see the excellent review on this topic by Pui and Evans.[1]

J.A. Stockman III, M.D.

Reference

1. Pui C-H, Evans WE: Acute lymphoblastic leukemia. *N Engl J Med* 339:605-614, 1998.

Residual Disease Detection Using Fluorescent Polymerase Chain Reaction at 20 Weeks of Therapy Predicts Clinical Outcome in Childhood Acute Lymphoblastic Leukemia
Evans PAS, Short MA, Owen RG, et al (Gen Infirmary at Leeds, England; St James's Hosp, Leeds, England)
J Clin Oncol 16:3616-3627, 1998   14–6

Background.—Although 95% of pediatric patients with acute lymphoblastic leukemia (ALL) will achieve remission, 25% will relapse. Currently, identification of these patients (so more aggressive or novel therapies can be appropriately targeted) is difficult, and an independent prognostic marker would be clinically useful. The predictive value of residual disease detection at 20 weeks of therapy using a simple system was analyzed in 42 patients with ALL.

Study Design.—The study group consisted of 42 pediatric precursor-B ALL patients with standard-risk clinical features. These patients were treated according to the Medical Research Council UKALL X or XI protocols. Patients were evaluated with a combination of fluorescent consensus framework I and framework III immunoglobulin heavy-chain polymerase chain reactions (PCRs). Clonal rearrangements detected at presentation were reevaluated at week 20 of therapy.

Findings.—Of the 42 pediatric patients with ALL in this series, 35 had a clonal population detected at presentation. Of these 35, 30 were reanalyzed at week 20 of therapy. Nine of the 30 still had a detectable clonal rearrangement. Of these 9, 8 (89%) relapsed with a median disease-free survival of 27.5 months. Of the remaining 21 patients without a detectable clonal rearrangement at 20 weeks, only 6 (21%) have relapsed. The sensitivity of this method was 57% and the specificity 89%.

Conclusions.—It is possible to detect pediatric ALL patients with a high risk of relapse by using fluorescent immunoglobulin H PCR at week 20 of therapy. This simple, specific, and reliable test would permit those patients with a poor prognosis to be identified early so that alternative treatments could be initiated.

▶ Peter G. Steinherz, M.D., Department of Pediatrics, Memorial Sloan-Kettering Cancer Center, New York, comments:

We can achieve a 97% remission rate and a close to 80% long-term disease-free survival in children with ALL. Yet we have no idea if, to cure leukemia, we need to eradicate every last one of the 10^{12-13} leukemic cells present at diagnosis or if a reduction below a certain unknown critical level is sufficient. After a mere 2 log reduction in leukemic cell mass, remission, with no clinically detectable signs of disease, is attained. Close to 10^{10} subclinical leukemic cells remain and presumably gradually disappear with further therapy.

Detection of persistent residual disease or early warning of increasing subclinical leukemic burden heralding an impending relapse would be important if change of therapy at that point could alter the otherwise dismal prognosis. Microscopic morphology can demonstrate only more than 5% immature cells. Even then, it frequently cannot distinguish regenerating normal young cells from leukemic ones until a second evaluation is performed sometime later. Cytogenetic abnormality, when present, is more specific, but not much more sensitive since usually only 20 metaphases are analyzed. When a probe is available to a previously known chromosomal abnormality, fluorescent in situ hybridization (FISH) can scan 500+ cells, increasing sensitivity. PCR-based qualitative and quantitative methods have been developed to detect clonal rearrangement of the immunoglobulin or T-cell receptor gene in the leukemic cell. The limit of detection with these techniques is 10^{-3} to 10^{-6}, but at a considerable cost in time and effort required for the complex methodology. Unfortunately, even with the most sensitive and specific assay, there are patients who are positive and do not relapse and those who are negative and will subsequently reoccur. The fusion transcripts detected by PCR, while derived from leukemic cells, may not be leukemogenic. These "footprints" of leukemic cells have been seen in long-term survivors thought to be cured of their disease. The same mixed lineage leukemia fusion transcript associated with t(4;11) and poor prognosis infant leukemia has also been detected in normal fetal livers and marrow of infants without leukemia.[1] To further complicate matters, clonal evaluation can occur after diagnosis with new rearrangement in the cells at relapse that will not be detected by the original probe.

Whatever method one chooses to follow patients, the faster the leukemic cells disappear and the lower the detectable level of residual disease at any one time point, the better the prognosis.[2,3] The longer it takes between the initiation of therapy and measurement of the residual disease, the fewer patients found positive, but with more certainty of impending relapse.[4] Residual disease after more intensive therapy is worse than after inadequate treatment.[2]

The study by Evans et al. has several limitations. It confirms previous observations and may be a less complex technique, but even in the small, single institution study only 71% of the initial group could be evaluated at week 20.[3,4] This time point, plus the additional time for results to become evaluable, is probably too late for the initiation of successful change in therapy. Eight of the 9 positive patients relapsed fairly quickly. Unfortunately, 29% of the negative patients also had an adverse event. One wonders how useful the technique would be with a more effective therapy when less residual disease would be present. On the described regimen overall results were very poor by current standards. The disease-free survival of this group of mostly standard risk patients was 47% starting from week 20 of treatment, when it should have been at least 70% from time of diagnosis.

P.G. Steinherz, M.D.

References

1. Uckun FM, Herman-Hatten K, Crotty ML, et al: Clinical significance of MLL-4F4 fusion transcripts expression in the absence of a cytogenetically detectable t(4;11) (q2;q23) chromosomal translocation. *Blood* 92:810-821, 1998.
2. Steinherz PG, Gaynon P, Trigg M, et al: Cytoreduction and prognosis in childhood acute lymphoblastic leukemia. *J Clin Oncol* 14:2403-2406, 1996.
3. Roberts WM, Estrov Z, Ouspenskaia MV, et al: Measurement of residual leukemia during remission in childhood acute lymphoblastic leukemia. *N Engl J Med* 336:317-323, 1997.
4. Cave H, Van der Werff Ten Bosch J, Suciu S, et al: Clinical significance of minimal residual disease in childhood acute lymphoblastic leukemia. *N Engl J Med* 339:591-598, 1998.

Late Relapsing Childhood Lymphoblastic Leukemia

Vora A, Frost L, Goodeve A, et al (Royal Hallamshire Hosp, Sheffield, England; Greenwich Districht Gen Hosp, London; CTSU, Oxford, England)
Blood 92:2334-2337, 1998   14–7

Introduction.—Relapse of lymphoblastic leukemia usually occurs immediately after stopping treatment, and children who have been in remission for 10 years have been considered to be cured. In rare instances, however, relapse occurs even after 10 years, and it has been difficult to determine whether the patients had a true recurrence of the original clone or a second or secondary leukemia. The presence of an identical clone-specific molecular signature in lymphoblasts at diagnosis and its recurrence can now be documented. Children whose leukemia had been in remission for 10 or more years before relapse were studied to determine whether they had true recurrences or second malignancies.

Methods.—The study included 1134 of 2746 children, aged from 10 to 24 years, with lymphoblastic leukemia who survived 10 years or more, and of those, 12 (about 1%) had subsequently relapsed. DNA extracted from archived marrow smears was subjected to polymerase chain reaction analysis for the presence of an identical Ig heavy chain or T-cell receptor gene rearrangement at initial diagnosis and subsequent relapse to determine whether the relapse was a true recurrence rather than a second or secondary leukemia.

Results.—In all patients, relapse blast cells were shown to express the common lymphoblastic leukemia antigen, as well as an identical clonal Ig heavy chain or T-cell receptor gene rearrangement. To induce a second complete remission in all patients, a further program of therapy was successful. Four of the patients had a second relapse after 12 to 27 months.

At a follow-up of 12 to 108 months (median, 52) from relapse, the remaining 8 are in a continuing second complete remission.

Conclusion.—The possibility of relapse of childhood lymphoblastic leukemia after 10 years in remission still persists, although it appears to be small (about 1%). The study raises questions about how blasts can survive for so long in a quiescent state and when one can confidently declare a cure.

▶ Some things in life are unfair. Some things in life are very unfair. Included in the latter is the reemergence of leukemia after a 10-year period of dormancy. This specifically relates to acute lymphoblastic leukemia (ALL) during childhood. While recurrence of this malignancy after 10 years of remission is an uncommon phenomenon (only around 1% of patients relapse that far out), it still occurs.

For some time, it had been felt that a late relapse of childhood leukemia represented a new, second malignancy, rather than a "true" relapse. This is not the case, however. A relapse of the original leukemia can now be documented by establishing a pattern of genetic molecular findings in the lymphoblasts at recurrence and at diagnosis. If the same "signature" is found in the gene pattern, one can be confident that one is talking about the same disease having reemerged, albeit after many, many years.

Why malignant cells can sit dormant for long periods of time remains a mystery. The mechanism responsible for this dormancy is likely to involve either an ability of the clone of malignant cells to remain out of cell cycle (technically termed "G_0") for long periods, or the ability of host immune surveillance to keep a residual leukemia in check for a long period, but without eradicating it. Most feel that a breech in immune surveillance is the more likely cause of why some quiescent leukemias reemerge.

If there is any good news in such a sad occurrence, it is the relative ease with which these relapse leukemias can be reinduced and easily maintained in a second remission. Without question, all the stops should be pulled out in an attempt to salvage a patient who has had a recurrence of ALL after many years of remission. A patient with this "Rumpelstiltskin" type of leukemia still has a shot at a cure and should be afforded every opportunity to live a normal life span.

J.A. Stockman III, M.D.

Bone Marrow Transplantation for Children Less Than 2 Years of Age With Acute Myelogenous Leukemia or Myelodysplastic Syndrome
Woolfrey AE, Gooley TA, Sievers EL, et al (Fred Hutchinson Cancer Research Ctr, Seattle; Univ of Washington, Seattle)
Blood 92:3546-3556, 1998   14–8

Introduction.—In the primary therapy for children with acute myelogenous leukemia and myelodysplastic syndrome, allogeneic bone marrow transplantation plays an important role. Young children may have a different outcome regarding marrow transplantation, tolerance of high-dose therapy, and risks for long-term sequelae. Infants younger than 2 years of age transplanted for acute myelogenous leukemia or myelodysplastic syndrome were evaluated.

Methods.—There were 40 infants younger than 2 years of age who received bone marrow transplants in a 21-year period for the treatment of acute myelogenous leukemia or myelodysplastic syndrome. Among the 34 acute myelogenous leukemia patients, 13 were in first remission, 9 were in untreated first relapse or second remission, and 12 were in refractory relapse. These infants were treated with cyclophosphamide with total body irradiation or busulfan. The prophylaxis for graft-versus-host disease (GVHD) was methotrexate, methotrexate plus cyclosporine, or cyclosporine plus prednisone.

Results.—In the group with acute myelogenous leukemia, the rate of severe regimen-related toxicity was 10% and the transplant-related mortality rate was 10%. In 39% of allogeneic patients, acute GVHD occurred. In 40% of patients, chronic GVHD occurred. Relapse occurred in 23 patients with acute myelogenous leukemia and 1 patient with myelodysplastic syndrome and was the cause of death for 19 patients. For patients transplanted in first remission, the 2-year probability of relapse was 46%; for those untreated in first relapse or second remission, the 2-year probability of relapse was 67%; and for those transplanted in relapse, the 2-year probability of relapse was 92%. Second marrow transplants were given to 1 patient with myelodysplastic syndrome and 8 patients with acute myelogenous leukemia for the treatment of relapse; of these, 5 survive disease free at more than 1.5 years. For patients transplanted in first remission, the 5-year probability of survival was 54% and disease-free survival was 38%. For those patients transplanted in untreated first relapse or second remission, the 5-year survival rate was 33%, and for disease-free survival, it was 22%. None of the patients transplanted with refractory relapse survived disease free. Phase of disease at transplantation and pretransplant diagnosis of extramedullary disease were significantly associated with outcome. Growth failure and hormonal deficiencies were the long-term sequelae for all survivors. Neurologic development for all survivors was appropriate for age and survival performance was a median of 100%.

Conclusion.—Compared with older children, infants with acute myelogenous leukemia have similar outcome after bone marrow transplant, which should be performed in first remission whenever possible. For the majority of infants with myelodysplastic syndrome, allogeneic bone marrow transplant provides effective therapy.

▶ This report shows us that children, especially young children, are certainly not little adults. About the time this report was appearing, another showed up in *The New England Journal of Medicine* comparing chemotherapy with bone marrow transplant as part of the management of acute myeloid leukemia in first remission in adults.[1] The adult study was unequivocal. Regular old high-dose chemotherapy produced somewhat better overall survival than autologous bone marrow transplantation.

So what is different about young patients? Why do they do better with bone marrow transplantation for the treatment of acute myeloid leukemia in first remission? It would appear that in young patients, one can escalate postremission therapy provided autologous or allogeneic hematopoietic stem cells are transplanted. In children, the probabilities of survival and disease-free survival are 54% and 38%, respectively, for patients transplanted in first remission and only 33% and 22%, respectively, for untreated first relapse or second remission.

At one time it had been thought that infants would not tolerate the rigors of high-dose chemotherapy and bone marrow transplantation. Time has proven this belief to be untrue. Little people are extremely resilient and bounce back much better than adults. They tend to take everything you throw at them and still survive.

One quick comment about a renewed role for arsenic: Arsenic trioxide is now being employed as part of the management of refractory acute promyelocytic leukemia (APL), and other leukemias as well. Arsenicals were the first class of agents reported to induce responses in chronic myelogenous leukemia, but with the advent of modern chemotherapy, they fell into disfavor. The outcome of APL was dramatically altered with the addition of transretinoic acid to anthracycline-based chemotherapy in recent years. Cure rates in APL have increased from 30% to above 50%. The problem is what happens to patients who relapse. In such circumstances, arsenic compounds may prove to be very helpful. In one small study, 100% of relapse patients achieved a complete remission with the use of IV arsenic trioxide. The only side effects noted were arrhythmias, epigastric pain, skin rashes, and high blood sugar levels.[2]

Arsenic is a curious heavy metal. Too much of it will kill you. Just enough of it may save a life!

J.A. Stockman III, M.D.

References

1. Cassileth PA, Harrington DP, Appelbaum FR, et al: Chemotherapy compared with autologous or allogeneic bone marrow transplantation in the management of acute myeloid leukemia in first remission. *N Engl J Med* 339:1649-1656, 1998.
2. Arsenic trioxide studies in refractory acute promyelocytic leukemia (APL) and other leukemias (editorial). *Leukemia Insights* 3:1, 1998.

Outcomes Among 562 Recipients of Placental-Blood Transplants From Unrelated Donors

Rubinstein P, Carrier C, Scaradavou A, et al (New York Blood Ctr; Duke Univ, Durham, NC; Mount Sinai Med Ctr, New York; et al)
N Engl J Med 339:1565-1577, 1998   14–9

Background.—Transplantation of hematopoietic stem and progenitor cells from placental blood from unrelated donors can restore the function of bone marrow and sustain hematopoietic recovery. A program for banking, characterizing, and distributing placental blood for transplantation was described.

Methods.—The program served 562 recipients between 1992 and 1998. Placental blood was stored under liquid nitrogen and given to patients based on HLA type and leukocyte content. All recipients received prophylaxis against graft-versus-host disease (GVHD) according to the routine practice of each center.

Findings.—Cumulative engraftment rates, according to actuarial analysis, were 81% by day 42 for neutrophils and 85% by day 180 for platelets. Speed of myeloid engraftment was correlated mainly with the leukocyte content of the graft. Transplantation-related events were associated with the patient's underlying disease and age, the number of leukocytes in the graft, the degree of HLA disparity, and the transplantation center. The main predictors of outcomes after engraftment were age, HLA disparity, and center. Severe acute GVHD developed in 23% of the patients and chronic GVHD in 25%. In patients with leukemia, relapse rates were 9% in the first 100 days, 17% in the first 6 months, and 26% by 1 year. Relapse rates were associated with GVHD severity, type of leukemia, and disease stage.

Conclusions.—Stored placental blood is a useful source of hematopoietic stem cells for patients without a related histocompatible donor. Greater accessibility and methods to accelerate engraftment and reduce early morbidity would enhance the efficacy of this source. Adequate international standards that permit worldwide cooperation among placental-blood banks are needed.

▶ It's pretty obvious that some of the products of conception, such as the placenta and the cord with its blood, might be eventually found to have some use other than as a reason to have trash containers in delivery rooms. Before placental-blood transplantation became popularized in the last few years, almost all patients who needed a transplant of hematopoietic stem cells got them from a related donor. Sometimes stem cells were harvested from the patient him-/herself prior to being bombarded with chemotherapy, using the stem cells as a salvage procedure. The latter approach to stem cell replacement potentially carried the risk that the stem cells themselves might carry the malignancy back into a patient, depending on the nature of the original problem. Placental-blood transplantation seems to obviate so many problems that it has quickly become the procedure of choice in anyone who does not seem to have a related donor match. One of the theoretical benefits of a placental blood transplantation is that the graft itself might produce a low level graft versus malignancy effect that might not be seen with a totally compatible bone marrow. In the article abstracted, the investigators found no increase in the frequency of lymphoma, despite the absence of graft versus host disease, suggesting that it may be possible to achieve a graft versus lymphoma effect without an associated GVHD. Please be aware that worldwide the most common genetic disease for which hematopoietic stem cell transplantation has been used is beta thalassemia major. Such transplantation is being employed increasingly also in the United States for the treatment of patients with severe sickle cell anemia if a histocompatible donor is unavailable. Curiously, when used as part of the treatment of hemoglobinopathies, it is not absolutely necessary to completely replace the patient's own blood cell precursors for clinical benefit to be achieved. In other words, you can transplant placental blood without the extremely rigorous preparations that are used to treat malignancies. One of the reasons why placental blood is so advantageous for this purpose relates to the fact that there is a greater tolerance of it in ethnic groups in whom it is difficult to find histocompatible donors if one were to use the traditional bone marrow transplantation sources. As long as folks keep having babies, there should be a fairly ample supply of placental blood for transplantation purposes. Given the fact that random cord blood engrafts so well, companies that went into business to store a baby's own placental blood for possible later use have begun to fall on hard times.

J.A. Stockman III, M.D.

Congenital Abnormalities in Children With Acute Leukemia: A Report From the Children's Cancer Group
Mertens AC, Wen W, Davies SM, et al (Univ of Minnesota, Minneapolis; Univ of Southern California, Los Angeles; Fred Hutchinson Cancer Research Ctr, Seattle)
J Pediatr 133:617-623, 1998   14–10

Introduction.—The etiology in the case of most patients with childhood leukemia remains unknown. Specific chromosome abnormalities may be associated with certain cancers in infants and children. There is an increased risk for the development of leukemia among patients with genetic syndromes such as Down syndrome, neurofibromatosis, Fanconi's anemia, and ataxia telangiectasia. The risk of leukemia associated with selected congenital and genetic abnormalities was evaluated. Siblings of patients with leukemia were evaluated for possible familial genetic defects.

Methods.—There were 2117 patients diagnosed with acute lymphoblastic leukemia and 605 with acute myelogenous leukemia. A modified random digit dialing method was used to compare patients with matched regional population control subjects. A telephone interview with the biological mother was conducted to collect data on congenital abnormalities in index children and their siblings.

Results.—Patients with acute myelogenous leukemia had more birth defects than the control subjects, with significant increases in multiple birthmarks, Down syndrome, mental retardation, and congenital heart defects. No significant differences in the number of reported congenital abnormalities were seen between siblings of patients and siblings of control subjects. Children with acute lymphoblastic leukemia had more congenital abnormalities than the controls, with significant increases in multiple birthmarks, Down syndrome, congenital heart defects, and pancreas-digestive tract abnormalities.

Conclusion.—Children with Down syndrome, who are known to have an increased risk for leukemia, had many of the observed associations with congenital abnormalities. A genetic component to leukemia risk is suggested by the higher reported frequency of birthmarks among case patients.

▶ Parents and physicians alike have questioned whether there are congenital reasons why acute leukemias develop in children. For the average child who has the most common kind of leukemia—acute lymphoblastic leukemia—the jury is still out on this question. There is no question, however, when it comes to certain congenital abnormalities and their association with cancer, in general, in children. Aniridia and Wilms' tumor are linked, as is the Beckwith-Wiedemann syndrome with Wilms' tumor. Both disorders have had genes identified that are associated with tumor development.

Of course, there are other genetic syndromes—including Down syndrome, Fanconi's anemia, neurofibromatosis, and ataxia telangiectasia—that cause a child to have an increased risk for the development of leukemia. Even with these entities aside, children with acute lymphatic leukemia seem to have a higher chance of having certain congenital abnormalities in excess of their peers. These anomalies include birth marks, congenital heart defects, and pancreas–digestive tract abnormalities.

What the link is between genetic influences and leukemia risk remains a mystery in the case of most children with malignancy. Once we know more about such links, we will know a great deal more about what causes them and, potentially, a cure will be possible.

J.A. Stockman III, M.D.

A Prognostic Score for Advanced Hodgkin's Disease

Hasenclever D, for the International Prognostic Factors Project on Advanced Hodgkin's Disease (Univ of Leipzig, Germany; et al)
N Engl J Med 339:1506-1514, 1998   14–11

Objective.—Predicting the outcome of treatment for non-Hodgkin's lymphoma may identify patients who would benefit from reduced treatment and those who are unlikely to benefit from treatment. Freedom from

TABLE 2.—The Final Cox Regression Model

Factor	Log Hazard Ratio	P Value	Relative Risk
Serum albumin, <4 g/dl	0.40 ± 0.10	<0.001	1.49
Hemoglobin, <10.5 g/dl	0.30 ± 0.11	0.006	1.35
Male sex	0.30 ± 0.09	0.001	1.35
Stage IV disease	0.23 ± 0.09	0.011	1.26
Age, ≥45 yr	0.33 ± 0.10	0.001	1.39
White-cell count, ≥15,000/mm³	0.34 ± 0.11	0.001	1.41
Lymphocyte count, <600/mm³ or <8% of white-cell count	0.31 ± 0.10	0.002	1.38

Note: Hazard ratios and relative risks are for freedom from progression of disease in patients with the factors as compared with those without the factors. Plus–minus values are rate estimates ± SE (approximate 95% confidence intervals can be calculated as the rate estimates ±2 SE).

(Reprinted with permission of *The New England Journal of Medicine*, from Hasenclever D, for the International Prognostic Factors Project on Advanced Hodgkin's Disease: A prognostic score for advanced Hodgkin's disease. *N Engl J Med* 339:1506-1514. Copyright 1998, Massachusetts Medical Society. All rights reserved.)

progression was used to measure response to therapy in 5141 patients, aged 15 to 65 years, from 25 centers who were treated with combination chemotherapy, with or without radiation therapy, for advanced Hodgkin's disease.

Methods.—Patients outside the age range specified, patients receiving outmoded or palliative therapy, and patients whose outcome was unknown were excluded. Data from 4695 patients were analyzed. Patients received standard doxorubicin-containing regimens (more than 75% of patients) or MOPP or similar therapy (20%). Two percent of the patients underwent extensive radiotherapy, 5% received subtotal or total nodal

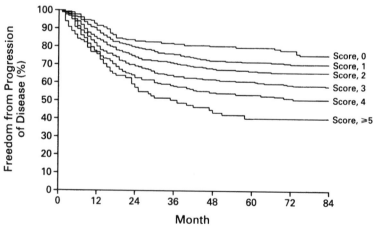

FIGURE 2.—Validation of the prognostic score in a group of 2,643 patients with incomplete data on albumin or lymphocyte values. Surrogate information was substituted for the missing data. The number and percentage of patients with each score were as follows: a score of 0, 196 patients (7%); 1, 671 (25%); 2, 809 (31%); 3, 578 (22%); 4, 292 (11%); and 5, 97 (4%). (Reprinted with permission of *The New England Journal of Medicine*, from Hasenclever D, for the International Prognostic Factors Project on Advanced Hodgkin's Disease: A prognostic score for advanced Hodgkin's disease. *N Engl J Med* 339:1506-1514. Copyright 1998, Massachusetts Medical Society. All rights reserved.)

irradiation, 33% received full or selected involved-field radiotherapy, and 60% received no irradiation.

Results.—Rates of freedom of progression and overall survival at 5 years were 66% and 78%, respectively. A 7-factor prognostic scoring system that predicted 5-year rates of freedom from progression of 45% to 80% (Table 2) was developed. This scoring system was also reproducibly predictive of overall survival, although there was no group of patients that could be identified as being at very high risk.

Conclusion.—The prognostic score may be useful for making specific therapeutic decisions for certain patients and for designing clinical trials, but it failed to help identify a specific group of patients at very high risk (Fig 2).

▶ As with most things, it is always helpful to know the score. The score in this case has to do with risk factors for determining the likelihood of a poor outcome in the treatment of Hodgkin's disease. Although this report focused largely on adults, more than 1300 study subjects were aged 15 to 24 years, and the prognostic scoring system certainly applies to this group as well.

Seven factors were identified as adverse prognostic features. Each one of them lowered by about 8% the likelihood that a patient would remain in remission. Although the factors are said to be independent of one another with respect to prognosis, several of the factors probably do relate to one another. For example, in patients with Hodgkin's disease a low albumin level is usually associated with leaky blood vessels, a result of elevations in inflammatory mediators that damage the capillary bed. A low hemoglobin value as a risk factor probably reflects the anemia of chronic disease/inflammation. A high white blood cell count and a low lymphocyte count probably reflect the same phenomenon. Nonetheless, there clearly were patients in this series who had one or more adverse risk factors without all of them being abnormal.

You may wonder why it is important in Hodgkin's disease to find out whether a person is likely or not likely to do well. Surely time will sort that out. The true reason for wanting to know who is at high risk has to do with the design of future therapy protocols. Should we be treating high-risk patients with higher-dose chemotherapy with or without stem-cell support? For patients with low-risk disease, might we not reduce the amount of aggressive therapy that we are now using? Clearly, patients with Hodgkin's disease are being cured at high rates these days. It's nice to see that patients with low risk scores have an 80% or better chance of living a normal life, a life that is free of risk of recurrence of their disease.

J.A. Stockman III, M.D.

Mass Screening for Neuroblastoma at 6 Months of Age: Difficult to Justify

Suita S, Tajiri T, Akazawa K, et al (Kyushu Univ, Fukuoka, Japan; Kumamoto Univ, Japan; Kagoshima Univ, Japan; et al)
J Pediatr Surg 33:1674-1678, 1998   14–12

Introduction.—A nationwide mass screening program for neuroblastoma has been conducted since 1985 for 6-month-old infants in Japan. Since then, the number of patients with neuroblastoma have increased and the number of those younger than 1 year of age with neuroblastoma have increased, but the number of advanced-stage neuroblastoma patients older than 1 year of age has not substantially changed. The effectiveness of this mass screening performed at 6 months of age was evaluated retrospectively, based on the available population data.

Methods.—A cohort of infants born from 1988 to 1992 was identified and compared to the cohort born during the pre–mass-screening period from 1980 to 1984. The cumulative incidence and mortality rates from neuroblastoma were determined in the screened infants and compared to the rates in the control cohort.

Results.—For screened children younger than 5, the cumulative incidence of neuroblastoma was 82 in 484,599; for unscreened children, it was 11 in 92,966. Findings at 6 months of age were negative in 14 of the 82 screened children. The cumulative mortality rates in children younger than 5 years did not differ between the screened and unscreened groups. Among the screened children, 6 of 7 patients who died were found to be negative at the 6-month screening, yet died of stage III or IV disease. The cumulative mortality rates from patients in both groups were not significantly different.

Conclusion.—The incidence and mortality from neuroblastoma were not reduced by Japan's mass screening for children less than 6 months of age. A favorable prognosis was found for the majority of the patients detected by mass screening. The prognosis of patients with unfavorable neuroblastoma, identified at over 1 year of age, was not improved by mass screening at 6 months of age.

▶ If the Japanese have thrown in the towel regarding screening for neuroblastoma at 6 months of age (or any time in the first year of life), so should everyone else. The Japanese started this ball rolling 15 years ago and the ball has bounced around creating controversy ever since. Neuroblastoma screening programs, based on the detection of catecholamine metabolite excretion in urine, were established in the hope of being able to diagnose this malignancy at an earlier age in order to improve outcomes. However, data published from early screening programs show that screening at 6 months of age may not meet this objective. In populations who have been screened in the first 6 months of life, an increased rate of localized neuroblastoma has been observed, but such screening has not led to a reduction in high-stage neuroblastoma cases in subsequent years of life. There is evidence that cases identified by biochemical screening may in fact have undergone spontaneous regression over the course of a year if they had been left undetected. By the way, most European countries that followed the lead of Japan in instituting screening programs for neuroblastoma have also thrown in the towel.[1] Some ideas which sound good at first just don't pan out. The trick is to know when to quit and cut one's losses. Mass screening for neuroblastoma never really caught on here in the US. Kudos to those who had some restraint.

J.A. Stockman III, M.D.

Reference

1. Craft AW, Parker L: Screening for neuroblastoma: 20 years and still no answer. *Eur J Cancer* 32:1540-1543, 1996.

Second Malignancies in Young Children With Primary Brain Tumors Following Treatment With Prolonged Postoperative Chemotherapy and Delayed Irradiation: A Pediatric Oncology Group Study
Duffner PK, and the Pediatric Oncology Group (State Univ of New York, Buffalo; et al)
Ann Neurol 44:313-316, 1998   14–13

Introduction.—Infants and very young children with malignant brain tumors have significantly worse survival rates than patients in any other age group. Infants tend to suffer irradiation-induced neurotoxicity, such as intellectual deterioration. Children younger than 3 years of age with malignant brain tumors were treated with prolonged postoperative chemotherapy to delay irradiation until they were better able to tolerate the effects on their central nervous system. Five of the 198 children developed second malignancies.

Methods.—A review was conducted of the 5 children who developed second malignancies. Four of the 5 children were younger than 2 years at diagnosis, with a cumulative risk at 8 years of 18.9%. Two children had received an initial diagnosis of choroid plexus carcinoma, 1 of ependymoma, 2 of ganglioglioma, and 1 of medulloblastoma.

Results.—The duration from diagnosis of the initial tumor to second malignancy was 33, 35, 57, 66, and 92 months. Lymphoproliferative disease occurred in 3 children younger than 2 years. Two children had myelodysplastic syndrome, both with monosomy 7 deletions, and 1 child had acute myelogenous leukemia after 24 to 26 cycles of chemotherapy, including 8 cycles of etoposide. Craniospinal irradiation was given to 2 of 3 children. Solid tumors occurred in 2 children, with 1 tumor developing at 5 years 6 months and the other at 2 years 11 months. After 26 cycles of chemotherapy and no irradiation, a sarcoma developed. After 12 cycles of chemotherapy and local craniospinal irradiation, a meningioma developed.

Conclusion.—Prolonged use of alkylating agents and etoposide with or without irradiation are potential causative factors for this high rate of secondary malignancies.

▶ Henry S. Friedman, M.D., professor of the Division of Pediatric Neuro-Oncology, Duke University Medical Center, Durham, NC, comments:

Treatment of patients with cancer, particularly young children, represents a balance of trying to achieve cure without doing unnecessary or excessive harm. Treatment of young children with brain tumors is a particular challenge because of the sensitivity of the developing central nervous system to both the damages produced by the tumor and the therapy used to treat it. This has led to a series of attempts to utilize chemotherapy to delay radiation and hopefully reduce long-term neurotoxicity. The Pediatric Oncology Group published the results of a trial utilizing therapy for children less than 3 years of age with brain tumors in 1993, detailing a survival higher than that of previously treated patients who received conventional surgery and radiotherapy. However, the use of chemotherapeutic agents, particularly alkylating agents, to produce secondary malignancies raised the concern by this group of investigators, even as the study started, that survivors might be prone to develop such tumors.

This article by Duffner et al., representing the efforts of the Pediatric Oncology Group, confirms this fear and indicates that 5 of 198 children treated on this protocol subsequently developed second malignancies. Three children developed hematopoietic malignancies, specifically myelodysplastic syndrome in 2 children and acute myelogenous leukemia in 1 child. Two children developed solid tumors, specifically a sarcoma and meningioma. This appears to be an acceptable complication, since the patient population treated has such a dismal prognosis when surgery and radiotherapy are used with exclusion of chemotherapy. Nevertheless, the refractory nature of these secondary malignancies (with the possible exception of meningioma) requires attempts to minimize use of particularly carcinogenic agents. Unfortunately, the topoisomerase I inhibitors and alkylating agents, which are known to be highly carcinogenic, are also the most active agents identified to date for the treatment of childhood brain tumors. For the present, use of chemotherapy in young children with brain tumors should be reserved for those children who have highly aggressive malignancies and who have no other meaningful therapeutic options.

H.S. Friedman, M.D.

Phase I Therapy Trials in Children With Cancer
Shah S, Weitman S, Langevin A-M, et al (Univ of Texas, San Antonio; McGill Univ, Montreal; St Jude Children's Research Hosp, Memphis, Tenn)
J Pediatr Hematol Oncol 20:431-438, 1998   14–14

Introduction.—The aims of phase I trials in patients with cancer are to examine the toxicity profile of promising new agents, to identify supportive measures to ameliorate drug toxicity, to note preliminary evidence of antitumor efficacy, and to determine a maximum tolerated dose of drug. Misconceptions may exist regarding phase I trials because of a lack of information. Overall response and toxicity rates, response rates of particular tumor types, drug doses at which responses occurred, and causes of death were determined.

Methods.—A review was conducted of peer-reviewed articles describing the results of single-agent phase I therapy trials in children younger than 21 years who had cancer. The review included 1606 patients with cancer in 56 single-agent pediatric phase I therapy trials during an 18-year period. Tumor-specific response data and doses of drugs that resulted in objective responses were recorded. Deaths that occurred because of drug toxicity, progressive disease, or complications of marrow aplasia, as well as drug doses that resulted in toxic death, were identified. The examination included temporal trends in response rates, toxicity, and number of patients entered in trials.

Results.—There were 1257 patients evaluated for response by tumor type, with an overall objective response rate of 7.9%. For patients with neuroblastoma, the response rate was highest (17.7%), followed by patients with acute myelogenous leukemia (11.6%). Response rates of less than 3% were found in patients with osteosarcoma and rhabdomyosarcoma. At 81% to 100% of the maximum tolerated dose, 60% of responses in patients with solid tumors occurred, although 42% of responses in patients with leukemia occurred at more than 100% of the maximum tolerated dose. In 7% of patients, death on study was noted. Death related to drug toxicity occurred in 0.7% of patients (Table 5). Death of 5.6% of participants occurred because of progressive disease. There was a trend of

TABLE 5.—Causes of Death in Pediatric Phase I Studies

Cause of Death	N	% Total Patients Entered	% of Total Deaths
Toxicity*	12	0.7	10.6
Progressive disease	90	5.6	79.9
Aplasia	11	0.7	9.7
Total	113	7.0	100

*Drugs and doses causing 11 of the 12 toxic deaths included carboplatin at 100% and 125%, 2'deoxycoformycin at 150%, 150%, and 200%, indicine at 150%, 150%, and 150%, IL-2 at 167% and 300%, and TNF at 100% of the maximum tolerated dose (*MTD*). Four patients died of acute liver toxicity. The mean dose causing a toxic death was 158% of the MTD.

(Courtesy of Shah S, Weitman S, Langevin A-M, et al: Phase I therapy trials in children with cancer. *J Pediatr Hematol Oncol* 20:431-438, 1998.)

TABLE 6.—Trends in Responses and Death Rates (1978 to 1996)

Years	Drugs	Trials	Patients Entered/ Evaluated	CR/PR Rate	DR	TD
1978-1984	8	8	313/293	5.5%	6.0	0.9
1985-1989	22	19	589/535	6.0	8.3	0.5
1990-1996	26	22	689/620	10.3	6.6	0.9

Abbreviations: CR, complete response; PR, partial response; DR, overall death rate; TD, toxic death rate.
(Courtesy of Shah S, Weitman S, Langevin A-M, et al: Phase I therapy trials in children with cancer. *J Pediatr Hematol Oncol* 20:431-438, 1998.)

increasing response rate, despite lessening trial size during the last 7 years of the study (Table 6).

Conclusion.—To determine the maximum tolerated dose, toxicity profile, and pharmacokinetics of new agents for use in children with cancer, phase I trials in children with cancer are a safe mechanism.

▶ You may wonder why parents would opt for entering their child with cancer in a phase I therapy trial. The intent of such a trial has one, and one only, specific objective: to evaluate the toxicity of a potentially promising new agent. In the process, other information about maximum lethal tolerated doses, pharmacologic profiling, and possible evidence of antitumor advocacy is collected. The goal in such a trial is not to find a magic bullet or cure. Miraculous outcomes virtually never happen. On the other hand, some patients (about 1 in 20) do experience some objective response, albeit not a cure. Stabilizing the clinical condition may be of help. On occasion, improvements in pain control and quality of life are obtained and are welcomed by both patient and parents. Although few patients in phase I therapy trials show significant benefit, equally few patients die as a result of the trial. The trick is to offer some benefit without producing untoward side effects that make the final days or months of the patient's life intolerable. If you ever have an opportunity to discuss pushing on with therapy at the phase I level with parents, please recognize that there is the possibility of some good in such therapy. Good not only for the patients, but for other patients who will follow. Without the critical information provided by phase I therapy trials, oncologists would have no knowledge of what the appropriate dosing of chemotherapy should be. Phase I therapy trials are not for everyone, but hopefully will be for enough patients that needed information can be obtained.

The Oncology chapter closes with a question. What malignancy is expected to double in incidence in the next 20 years? Clue: it is the same malignancy that killed Steve McQueen. It is mesothelioma. The risk of mesothelioma will be highest in those born between 1945 and 1950 because asbestos use in buildings, particularly in certain parts of the world such as Europe, peaked around 1970, when those born in 1950 started to work. The effects are only now beginning to be seen because mesotheliomas usually take 20 to 60 years to develop after exposure to asbestos. It can be expected that the prevalence of mesothelioma will peak around the year

2020 and then gradually decline, because asbestos use has been greatly reduced in the last 2 decades. In Europe, it is estimated that 1 in 150 of all men around age 50 will eventually die of mesotheliomas and the risk, of course, is much higher among those who have worked with asbestos.[1]

J.A. Stockman III, M.D.

Reference

1. Bonn D: Mesothelioma death may double within 20 years. *Lancet* 353:383, 1999.

15 Ophthalmology

Timing of Initial Screening Examinations for Retinopathy of Prematurity
Hutchinson AK, Saunders RA, O'Neil JW, et al (Med Univ of South Carolina, Charleston; Arizona Pediatric Eye Specialists, Mesa)
Arch Ophthalmol 116:608-612, 1998   15–1

Background.—The most appropriate time to begin screening examinations for retinopathy of prematurity (ROP) remains controversial. A retrospective analysis of premature infants was performed to determine whether a combination of chronological age and postconceptional age could be used to optimize the timing of screening.

Study Design.—The medical records of 326 eyes in 179 infants who underwent argon laser treatment for threshold ROP were reviewed. Birth weight, chronological age, and postconceptional age at treatment were entered into a database. This database was used to determine the most efficient method to diagnose the onset of ROP, requiring the smallest number of examinations to detect threshold ROP.

Findings.—The optimal ROP screening protocol based on the premature infant database, involved screening infants at 7 weeks of chronological age or 34 weeks of postconceptional age, whichever came first, but not before 5 weeks of chronological age. This protocol reliably detected the onset of threshold ROP while minimizing the number of unnecessary early examinations in this vulnerable population.

Conclusions.—The goals of an efficient screening program are to detect disease at the highest possible rate while minimizing the number of examinations that do not have an impact on care. The results of this study suggest that infants weighing no more than 1500 g or less at birth can be safely screened for ROP at 7 weeks of chronological age or 34 weeks of postconceptional age, whichever comes first, but not before 5 weeks of chronological age.

▶ It is not critically important for most pediatricians to know the best timing of initial screening examinations for ROP. It certainly doesn't hurt, however, to know when the neonatologist and the ophthalmologist should be keeping a careful eye out for the problem. Recently, the American Academy of Pediatrics, the American Association for Pediatric Ophthalmology and Strabismus, and the American Academy of Ophthalmology released a joint statement recommending that initial screening examinations for this disorder be performed between 4 and 6 weeks of chronological age or 31 and 30 weeks of postconceptional age. Although the concept of considering both chronological age and postconceptional age represents an advance over previous approaches, these guidelines lack some degree of specificity. For example, a conservative examiner might screen all infants at 4 weeks of chronological age regardless of postconceptional age, whereas a more liberal examiner could choose to screen infants at 33 weeks of postconceptional age regardless of chronological age. Although both regimens adhere to current recommendations, one can suspect that the more stringent protocol would result in many unnecessary examinations whereas the more liberal protocol might fail to diagnose the onset of early retinopathy of prematurity in a substantial number of infants.

Is there a middle ground? Apparently yes. Screening infants at 7 weeks of chronological age or 34 weeks of postconceptional age (whichever comes first), but not before 5 weeks of chronological age, seems to be the most reliable method to detect the onset of threshold retinopathy of prematurity while at the same time reducing the number of unnecessary early examinations. If there is a controversy about this topic going on in the nurseries that you are associated with, dig out this article and be proud that you know the insiders' information about what to do.

For another opinion on when to screen premature infants, see Abstract 15–2.

Finally, was your mama right when she said that reading too much would strain your eyes and cause you to need to start wearing glasses? The answer to this query comes from Singapore, where a careful study was done to determine the correlation between years of education and the probability of developing myopia. As it turns out, no fewer than 65% of university graduates in Singapore have myopia. This figure is quoted in a commentary in the *British Journal of Ophthalmology* that reviews evidence that the prevalence of myopia is closely associated with the number of years spent in full-time education.[1] The challenge for ophthalmologists is to figure out a way of preventing myopia without encouraging tiny tikes to drop out of preschool.

J.A. Stockman III, M.D.

Reference

1. Myopia in Singapore (editorial). *Br J Ophthalmol* 82:210-211, 1998.

Should Fewer Premature Infants Be Screened for Retinopathy of Prematurity in the Managed Care Era?
Wright K, Anderson ME, Walker E, et al (Univ of Tennessee, Knoxville)
Pediatrics 102:31-34, 1998   15–2

Introduction.—New screening guidelines for the timely detection of retinopathy of prematurity (ROP) in prematurely born infants have been recommended; these mandate screening for infants with birth weights of 1500 g or less or gestational ages of 28 weeks or less. Large infants are screened at the discretion of the attending pediatrician or neonatologist. Incidence figures for ROP derived from a comprehensive screening program based on the 1988 to 1996 American Academy of Pediatrics guidelines were reported to help reach a decision as to which infants to screen with a birth weight of more than 1500 g or a gestational age of more than 28 weeks so that the decision can be less discretionary and based more on evidence.

Methods.—In a 6-year period 707 infants were screened for ROP; the main outcome measure was maximum stage of ROP with respect to birth weight and gestational age.

Results.—In infants with gestational ages of 32 weeks or more or birth weights of 1500 g or more, no ROP of more than stage 1 was seen. Infants with gestational ages of 30 weeks or less or birth weights less than 1200 g made up the group that had threshold and stage 4 ROP.

Conclusion.—There would be 34.2% fewer infants who required screening if screening for ROP were limited to infants with birth weights of 1500 g or less compared with the previous recommendation of less than 1800 g, while missing no patients with ROP more than stage 1. However, several infants with more advanced retinopathy, including stage 4, could be missed if the gestational age cut-off was 28 weeks or less. The number of patients requiring screening could be reduced by 29.1% if criteria for screening for ROP were modified to include infants of gestational ages less than 32 weeks, compared with the previous recommendation of less than 35 weeks, without missing any patients with more than stage 1 of ROP. A savings of more than 1.5 million annually in the United States could be expected with a screening strategy of a birth weight of less than 1500 g or gestational age of less than 32 weeks, while missing no patients with stage 1 of ROP.

▶ Dr. Richard A. Saunders, Miles Professor of Ophthalmology, Medical University of South Carolina, comments:

The goals of an efficient screening program are to detect treatable disease at as high a rate as possible while simultaneously minimizing the number of examinations that yield normal findings or do not alter the course of clinical care. The large number of infants screened for ROP in the United States annually and the concentration of clinically important disease in infants of less than 1000 g birth weight and 28 weeks of gestational age appropriately raises questions about which infants should be screened in lower-risk categories. Although the authors correctly identify the cost savings associated with more restrictive protocols, elimination of unnecessary and potentially stressful examinations is also worthwhile because these may be hazardous to the infant. Recognized risks include external trauma, apnea or bradycardia (including cardiorespiratory arrest), adverse systemic effects of dilating eyedrops, and nosocomial infection. However, deciding exactly which examinations to eliminate is the crux of the problem. The approach taken by the authors is to reduce the number of infants eligible for screening. Equally important is deciding when to initiate and how frequently to perform ROP examinations in at-risk infants. In both instances, it seems that applying multiple criteria simultaneously yields more effective screening than using a single criterion alone.[1] This is the reason that the recently published screening guidelines from the American Academy of Pediatrics, the American Academy for Pediatric Ophthalmology and Strabismus, and the American Academy of Ophthalmology recommend the screening of all infants with birthweights of 1500 g or less *or* gestational ages of 28 weeks or less.[2]

On the basis of their retrospective study, the authors conclude that the use of the newly proposed gestational age cut-off of 28 weeks or less would have the "undesirable consequence of missing several cases of ROP more than stage 1," including 5 with stage 3 and 1 with stage 4. However, the real issue here is whether gestational age can be determined with sufficient accuracy to be used as the sole screening parameter at all. Furthermore, the authors' other conclusion that performance of screening ROP examinations in infants with birth weights greater than 1500 g is statistically unnecessary is also subject to question. In our database, 8 of 326 threshold eyes (2.5%) occurred in 4 infants (estimated gestational ages 30, 31, 31, and 34 weeks) with birth weights greater than 1500 g. Although the subject population was probably very different from the authors', this does emphasize the point that data from a single institution cannot necessarily be generalized to the population at large.

R.A. Saunders, M.D.

References

1. Hutchinson A, Saunders R, O'Neil J, et al: Timing of initial screening examinations for retinopathy of prematurity. *Arch Ophthalmol* 116:608-612, 1998.
2. Joint Statement of the American Academy of Pediatrics, the American Association for Pediatric Ophthalmology and Strabismus, and the American Academy of Ophthalmology: Screening examination of premature infants for retinopathy of prematurity. *Pediatrics* 100:273, 1997.

Geographical Variation in Anophthalmia and Microphthalmia in England, 1988-94
Dolk H, Busby A, Armstrong BG, et al (London School of Hygiene and Tropical Medicine)
BMJ 317:905-910, 1998   15–3

Background.—British press reports have described alleged clusters of anophthalmia and microphthalmia, and speculated that exposure to the fungicide Benomyl may have caused them. However, it was unclear whether the apparent clustering of these birth defects was real. This study assessed possible geographical variation and clustering of congenital anophthalmia and microphthalmia in England.

Methods.—All infants born with anophthalmia or microphthalmia from 1988 to 1994 were reported to a special registry. The analysis included a total of 444 cases, including 237 severe cases, 113 mild cases, and 94 cases of unknown severity. Twenty percent of cases in the severe subgroup were ascribed to a known etiology, e.g., a genetic syndrome. The prevalence of these abnormalities was determined by region and district, population density, and socioeconomic status. The study definition of clustering was a greater likelihood that the 3 nearest neighbors would be cases than expected by chance, or more cases within circles of fixed radius around a case than expected by chance.

Results.—During the period studied, anophthalmia or microphthalmia occurred with a prevalence of 1.0/10,000 births. Prevalence did not vary significantly on the regional or district level. Prevalence did vary by population density, with the lowest-density areas having relative risks of 1.79 overall and 2.37 for severe cases, compared with the highest-density areas. Socioeconomic deprivation did not appear to increase risk. Localized clustering did not appear.

Conclusions.—In contrast to British media reports, this study finds little evidence of geographic variation or localized clustering in the prevalence of anophthalmia or microphthalmia. These conditions are approximately twice as prevalent in rural areas, however. Further study is needed to confirm this finding and to assess risk factors for anophthalmia and microphthalmia.

▶ By way of background, microphthalmia describes a broad range of improperly developed, small eyes in newborn children. One end of the range is babies with complete absence of eyes, or anophthalmia. At the other end, cases are arbitrarily diagnosed because no clear cut border exists between mild microphthalmia and small normal eyes. Often the eye abnormality is part of a syndrome accompanied by other clinical features. Individual cases, however, may differ widely in their cause. Specific genetic factors, such as chromosomal abnormalities and inherited mutations in developmental genes, may form the underlying etiology. The disorder may also result from environmental influences on fetal development, such as exposure to certain infectious agents or teratogenic chemicals.

This report was selected for inclusion in the 2000 YEAR BOOK OF PEDIATRICS not so much because of the topic of anophthalmia and microphthalmia, which are important in and of themselves, but rather because it demonstrates how "clusters" of medical problems may be more visually apparent than reality apparent. Public concern was raised recently in England by the appearance of apparent clusters of anophthalmia and microphthalmia. The pesticide Benomyl produced by DuPont in Wilmington, Del., was the suspected cause of the alleged clustering. In response to a press campaign in Great Britain, the government established a research effort to determine whether the clustering was in fact real. Despite all the hoopla, it was not.

Clustering is a difficult concept to define precisely. It is important to distinguish a real cluster from the notion of a small individual cluster corresponding to an excess number of cases in one small area or around a suspected source of a problem. The fundamental problem when trying to assess the significance of a specific cluster is that the analysis almost always occurs after the fact—that is, some uncontrolled process recognizes the cluster as unusual, and then a subsequent statistical assessment is made. This is somewhat the opposite of the ideal for which statistical testing was designed—where a hypothesis is generated first and then subsequently tested on new data.

If you weren't aware of the most common cause of apparent, although not real, clustering, it is the well described "Texas sharp shooter" problem, in which a Texan fires randomly at a barn door and subsequently draws a bull's eye in the densest cluster of bullets. Even with a random, non-uniform, spacial pattern, it is sometimes possible to draw boundaries about apparent clusters in such a way that the density of observations in an area far exceeds one's expectation.

Please note that the Texas sharp shooter problem is very different from a Texas chain saw massacre. Body parts and chain saws should attract attention.

J.A. Stockman III, M.D.

Preseptal and Orbital Cellulitis in Childhood: A Changing Microbiologic Spectrum

Donahue SP, Schwartz G (Vanderbilt Univ, Nashville, Tenn)
Ophthalmology 105:1902-1906, 1998   15–4

Background.—The introduction of the *Haemophilus influenzae* type b (Hib) vaccine in 1985 dramatically decreased the incidence of haemophilus-associated diseases. Before the Hib vaccine, infection with *H. influenzae* was a significant cause of preseptal and orbital cellulitis. Fluid samples from children with preseptal or orbital cellulitis were examined to determine whether the microbiological spectrum changed since the introduction of the Hib vaccine.

Methods.—A retrospective review of medical records from 1986 to 1996 identified 70 children with preseptal cellulitis and 10 with orbital cellulitis. None of the patients had preseptal cellulitis caused by a chalazion. Data of interest included evidence of immunization with Hib vaccine and results of blood cultures, lumbar puncture, radiologic examination, and surgery.

Findings.—Of the children with preseptal cellulitis, 59 provided blood samples. Cultures were positive in only 6 of these samples (10%), and only 1 grew *H. influenzae*; the other 5 grew *Streptococcus* species. The sole culture that grew *H. influenzae* was from a child, aged 16 months, in 1987 who had not received the Hib vaccine. The immunization status was charted as "up to date" in more than half the patients, but clear documentation of Hib vaccination was noted in only 5 cases. Of the children with orbital cellulitis, 6 provided blood samples. Blood cultures were positive in only 1 of these samples, and grew alpha streptococcal species.

Six of these 10 children had orbital or subperiosteal abscesses, and surgical drainage was performed in 5 of them. Abscess fluid cultures were positive in all 5 samples; 3 grew streptococcal species and 2 grew *H. influenzae* and mixed *H. influenzae*/gram-positive cocci. The 2 children with *H. influenzae* infection were aged 5 and 12 years at the time of their infections, and the vaccine was probably not available when they were infants.

Conclusions.—The Hib vaccine has had a dramatic impact on the microbiology of preseptal and orbital cellulitis: Not since 1987 has there been a case of preseptal cellulitis associated with *H. influenzae* bacteremia at the authors' institution. In both preseptal and orbital cellulitis, streptococcal species are now the most common cause of the infection. These infections can typically be successfully treated with cephalosporins. Thus, whereas previously, *H. influenzae* infection in preseptal and orbital cellulitis required an aggressive approach to treatment, the different bacterial genus associated with these diseases today may warrant a more conservative approach.

▶ Another superb bacteriology study emanating from Vanderbilt. In this case, investigators reviewed the experiences pre- and post-introduction of the Hib vaccine as related to the bacterial causes of preseptal and orbital cellulitis in childhood. Indeed, the introduction of Hib vaccine has dramatically changed the scenery about the eye when it comes to infection. Numerous articles have commented on an overall reduction in the number of cases of hemophilus-associated meningitis, epiglottitis, buccal cellulitis, and otitis media. Data from the CDC currently suggest that as a result of this vaccine, there are now 7000 fewer cases of pediatric meningitis each year in the United States in comparison with the mid-1980s.[1]

The reason why the study from Vanderbilt is important relates to how we can now think about managing preseptal and orbital cellulitis. In the past, virtually everyone was managing these entities extremely aggressively, hospitalizing all children and treating them with intravenous antibiotics. Now we know that most infections are caused by *Strep* species. We also have superb imaging technologies that can precisely tell us the extent of the infection. We also now know that intramuscular ceftriaxone is extremely effective in the outpatient management in a number of pediatric infections. Thus it is prudent to reassess the standard treatment for both preseptal and orbital cellulitis in children. One can confidently say that intravenous antibiotics and lumbar puncture are not indicated for preseptal cellulitis in the absence of symptoms of bacteremia and meningitis. Orbital cellulitis obviously is a more risky disease, no matter what the organisms causing it. The authors of this article suggest that inpatient management with cefuroxime, 100 mg/kg per day intravenously in every 8 hour dosing is the appropriate parenteral coverage. They also suggest, alternatively, that outpatient management with intramuscular ceftriaxone could be adequate for mild cases if close follow-up can be assured. Older children with mild preseptal cellulitis can likely be treated with Augmentin (250 mg orally 4 times a day) and followed closely.

For more on the topic of how the introduction of the Hib type b immunization has changed the diseases children get and how we must take this into account, see the supplement that appeared in 1998 in the *Pediatric Infectious Disease Journal*. This supplement within volume 17 is entirely devoted to this topic.

While we're on the subject of things having to do with the orbits, how would you deal with the following? A 14-year-old boy is rushed to your office by his parents. The complaint is that he cannot see out of his left eye at all. The history indicates that he was wearing swimming goggles in a community pool when his goggles were struck by the elbow of a fellow swimmer. He noticed a slight pain at that time, but more importantly, he described a sudden blackout of vision in his right eye. As you examine this youngster, you see a slight bruise on his right brow. The right pupil fails to react to light. Fundus examination is normal, except that you seem to be unable to find the optic disc, which appears to be replaced by a black hole. When is a "black hole" not a black hole? What is going on here?

A black hole is not a black hole when it is, in fact, what is left after the optic nerve has been avulsed away from the retina. Although swimming is a relatively safe sport, and swimming goggles do reduce eye irritation and allow swimmers to see better, goggles can be a problem on rare occasions. Killer et al. reported the case of this 14-year-old boy who showed, on fundus examination performed 4 hours after an incident in the pool, that the optic disc had been avulsed and replaced by a cavity where the retinal fibers had retracted into the optic nerve sheath.[2] Other studies such as CT and MRI on such a patient had normal results, as has been reported previously in the literature. The mechanism that leads to avulsion of the optic disc when wearing swimming goggles is not fully understood. It is likely that when goggles were struck, the lower rim of the goggles pushed up against the eye, and the eyeball itself moved forward by a lever action, causing acute stretching of the optic nerve and leading to disruption of fibers and an avulsion of the optic nerve itself.

The lessons here are straightforward. Elbows and eye goggles in swimming pools don't mix. Also, not all black holes are in outer space. They can indeed represent a serious eye injury that leads to irreversible blindness.

J.A. Stockman III, M.D.

References

1. Schuchat A, Robinson K, Wenger JD, et al: Bacterial meningitis in the United States in 1995. Active Surveillance Team. *N Engl J Med* 337:970-976, 1997.
2. Killer HE, Blummer KB, Rust ON: Swimming goggle injury to the optic nerve. *Pediatr Ophthalmol Strabis* 36:92-93, 1999.

Therapy With a Purified Plasminogen Concentrate in an Infant With Ligneous Conjunctivitis and Homozygous Plasminogen Deficiency

Schott D, Dempfle C-E, Beck P, et al (Univ of Heidelberg, Mannheim, Germany; Hyland-Immuno Division of Baxter Healthcare, Heidelberg, Germany and Vienna; Univ of Tokushima, Japan; et al)

N Engl J Med 339:1679-1686, 1998   15–5

Introduction.—Ligneous conjunctivitis is a rare acute or chronic recurrent conjunctivitis characterized by conjunctival membranes that acquire a woodlike consistency from deposits of fibrin. It has been linked to severe plasminogen deficiency. This disease may be caused by a genetic defect with an autosomal recessive pattern of inheritance. A patient with homo-

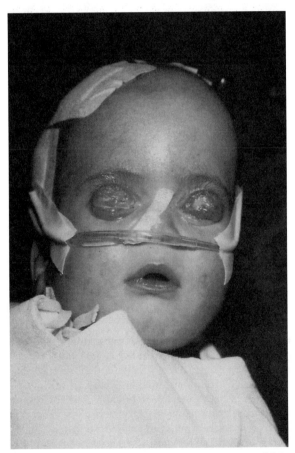

FIGURE 1.—Initial appearance of a child with homozygous plasminogen deficiency, showing the typical features of ligneous conjunctivitis. (Reprinted with permission of *The New England Journal of Medicine*, from Schott D, Dempfle C-E, Beck P, et al: Therapy with a purified plasminogen concentrate in an infant with ligneous conjunctivitis and homozygous plasminogen deficiency. *N Engl J Med* 339:1679-1686. Copyright 1998, Massachusetts Medical Society. All rights reserved.)

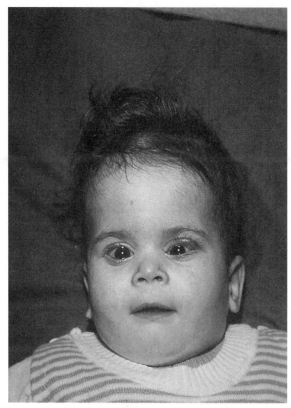

FIGURE 6.—Patient with homozygous plasminogen deficiency and ligneous conjunctivitis after 7 months of replacement therapy with lys-plasminogen. (Reprinted with permission of *The New England Journal of Medicine*, from Schott D, Dempfle C-E, Beck P, et al: Therapy with a purified plasminogen concentrate in an infant with ligneous conjunctivitis and homozygous plasminogen deficiency. *N Engl J Med* 339:1679-1686. Copyright 1998, Massachusetts Medical Society. All rights reserved.)

zygous plasminogen deficiency in whom ligneous conjunctivitis developed soon after birth is described.

> *Case Report.*—Newborn, second son of parents who were first cousins, had bilateral inflammation of the palpebral portion of the conjunctiva, with hypersecretion and formation of pseudomembranes detected 3 days after birth. At 2 weeks a thick, yellowish-white, fibrous, woody pseudomembranous layer of conjunctival proliferation developed and spread from the inner side of the upper and lower eyelids and completely closed both eyes (Fig 1). The pseudomembranes were removed several times, but regrew rapidly each time. Family studies revealed that the patient's parents and older brother had diminished levels of plasminogen antigen and activity, indicating heterozygous plasminogen deficiency. When the patient was 6 months old, a diagnosis of homozygous plasminogen

deficiency was proposed. Continuous IV infusion of 1000 casi-nolytic units of lys-plasminogen per 24 hours was administered. The patient's plasminogen level rose within 3 hours after treatment, and approached normal values within 24 hours. Within 3 days of the start of therapy the patient's symptoms were markedly improved, and findings subsequently became normal. At around 2 weeks the conjunctival pseudomembranes softened and were easily removed. Surgical specimens underwent histologic and genetic examination. Hematoxylin-eosin staining of parts of the conjunctival pseudomembranes showed fibrin-rich granulation tissue with a mixed neutrophil-rich perivascular infiltrate. Staining with an antibody specific for fibrin and fibrinogen showed diffuse fibrin deposits. Direct sequencing of fragments of exon 11 revealed a homozygous point mutation at position 1511 (G→T), leading to a stop codon (TAA) at position 460 (Glu460Stop). The catalytic domain of plasmin is eradicated by this mutation. The healthy brother and healthy parents of this patient were heterozygous for this mutation.

Conclusion.—Absence of plasmin activity caused formation of the fibrin-rich viscous or membranous material usually seen in patients with ligneous conjunctivitis. It is notable that no intravascular thromboembolic episodes occur in patients with ligneous conjunctivitis.

▶ This report was selected for inclusion in the YEAR BOOK OF PEDIATRICS because the editor had never heard of the entity "ligneous conjunctivitis." This form of acute or chronic recurrent conjunctivitis is quite unusual in that the conjunctival membranes acquire a woodlike consistency as a result of the deposition of fibrin into the conjunctiva. Worse yet, the cornea can be involved, and blindness results. Patients with ligneous conjunctivitis also have frequent and recurrent episodes of other types of upper airway infection, particularly nasopharyngitis and otitis media, along with lower respiratory tract findings that include tracheobronchial obstruction. Distant findings include vulvovaginitis and defective wound healing. The disease is now known to be due to a decrease in the fibrinolytic activity of blood.

Most of us tend to think of disorders associated with absence of the fibrinolytic system as causing intravascular thromboembolic phenomenon. We fail to remember that fibrinolytic activity is found (and is needed) in virtually all body fluids. It removes the small amounts of fibrin deposits that find their way into every part of the anatomy. In the eye, tears contain plasminogen activators released by the cornea. These ultimately result in the formation of plasmin, which rapidly clears fibrin from cornea and other eye tissues. Absent such plasmin, fibrin-rich viscous or membranous material accumulates, with the eventual development of ligneous conjunctivitis. An inflammatory reaction results in the woodlike appearance of dried out membranes in and about the eye. The same problem can occur in the airway and in the membranes about the vagina. Internal hydrocephalus has also been reported in patients with ligneous conjunctivitis, presumably as a result of obstruction of the natural flow of cerebrospinal fluid.

The baby reported above had a homozygous inactivating mutation of the plasminogen gene, resulting in severe plasminogen deficiency. Long-term plasminogen replacement in a very high dose normalized the findings in this baby (Fig 6).

Chances are that you may not run into a child with ligneous conjunctivitis. It is well worth knowing, however, about how the clotting system can cause signs and symptoms that are unrelated to blood problems. If you do see a child with eyelids as hard as Pinocchio's nose, remember that there is a therapy in the form of plasminogen.

Before we close this commentary on an unusual form of conjunctivitis, please recognize that a hurricane was responsible for one of the largest outbreaks of a common form of conjunctivitis. This was an outbreak of epidemic conjunctivitis in the U.S. Virgin Islands caused by enterovirus 70 (EV70) and CA24v. Following Hurricane Georges, some 1051 cases of acute hemorrhagic conjunctivitis were seen in 2 health department clinics and 1 emergency department of a hospital in St. Croix. Careful investigation by the Centers for Disease Control and Prevention estimated that this serious form of conjunctivitis developed in about 10% of all individuals in St. Croix following Hurricane Georges. The outbreak came almost immediately on the heels of the hurricane. Outbreaks of acute hemorrhagic conjunctivitis are characterized by high communicability, a shortened incubation period (1-2 days), and high secondary attack rates within households. Some outbreaks have been associated with rapid and efficient transmission, affecting more than 50% of persons in communities within a 1- to 2-month period. Spread of the virus most often occurs in areas where there is crowding and sharing of towels.[1]

If there is a lesson in all this, it is that when you're in the Islands during a hurricane, beware of beach towels. You may get more than a toweling-off from them.

J.A. Stockman III, M.D.

Reference

1. Acute hemorrhagic conjunctivitis: St. Croix, US Virgin Island, September-October 1998 (editorial). *MMWR* 47:899-900, 1998.

Ophthalmic Manifestations of Fibrous Dysplasia: A Disease of Children and Adults

Katz BJ, Nerad JA (Univ of Iowa, Iowa City)
Ophthalmology 105:2207-2215, 1998   15–6

Background.—In fibrous dysplasia, normal bone is replaced by immature bone and osteoid in a cellular fibrous matrix. Pain, swelling, and disfigurement throughout the skeleton can result from the fibroblastic expansion of affected bones. The etiology of fibrous dysplasia has not been defined. Malignant transformation is rare and often associated with previous irradiation. In about 20% of cases, craniofacial bones are involved. Most orbital lesions are monostotic, but frequently involve multiple skull bones and cross suture lines. Patients with fibrous dysplasia of orbital bones may seek treatment by an ophthalmologist because of facial deformities, loss of vision, or globe displacement, which may be the first clinical signs of the disease. Fibrous dysplasia is usually considered a disease of children and adolescents, but it can also occur in adults. The percentage of adults with ophthalmic complications of fibrous dysplasia was determined.

Methods.—In a retrospective study, 20 patients with fibrous dysplasia were investigated. Data were collected on patient demographics, major signs and symptoms, loss of vision, pattern of bone involvement, and radiographic appearance of fibrous dysplasia.

Results.—In contrast to populations previously reported, adults made up a significant percentage of these patients with ophthalmic complications of fibrous dysplasia. Of the 20 patients, 9 were younger than 18 years and 11 were 18 years old or older. The most common signs and symptoms were changes in facial contour and symmetry. Five patients had acute visual loss; 4 of these patients were adults. The most commonly affected facial bone was the maxilla. In most patients, monostotic lesions that crossed suture lines and involved multiple craniofacial bones were seen. CT results showed a characteristic pagetoid appearance with alternating areas of radiolucency and radiodensity in most of the lesions.

Discussion.—A diagnosis of fibrous dysplasia should not be ruled out on the basis of the age of the patient alone. Fibrous dysplasia of the orbital bones can cause significant dysfunction and disfigurement but is a treatable cause of blindness in both children and adults. In 1994, Bibby and Mc-Fadzean reported that 5 of 12 patients had progression of fibrous dysplasia beyond the teenage years. Also in 1994, Henderson reported that most patients with dysplasia of at least two cranial bones would probably have slow progressive disease indefinitely. The typical appearance of fibrous dysplasia on plain radiographs was originally described as a "ground glass" appearance. It can be difficult to differentiate fibrous dysplasia from meningioma because of their clinical and radiologic similarities. Both diseases involve slow, progressive globe displacement. Meningioma can induce a hyperostotic reaction in adjoining bone, making it resemble fibrous dysplasia on CT scans. The authors report that a pagetoid, heterogeneous appearance was seen in 12 of 13 CT scans of fibrous dysplasia, and in all cases, affected bones appeared "expanded" and had smooth, cortical boundaries. The hyperostosis of meningioma often shows a homogeneous thickening of bone with bone involvement often bowing into the temporalis fossa, and with some feathering of bone surfaces. There is also soft tissue involvement in meningioma, seen more easily on MRI, that is rarely seen in fibrous dysplasia.

▶ It's been some time since we have written of the topic of fibrous dysplasia in the YEAR BOOK OF PEDIATRICS. This report dealing with the eye manifestations of fibrous dysplasia overcomes the shortfall, since it not only updates us with respect to visual problems related to fibrous dysplasia, but also updates us on the overall topic. Even now, most cases of fibrous dysplasia remain of unknown cause. Polyostotic fibrous dysplasia in association with cutaneous pigmentation and endocrine dysfunction, the McCune-Albright syndrome, is one exception. The latter syndrome is known to be due to a mutation in the gene encoding a certain protein, the GTP-binding protein GNAS1. Bones of the face and cranium are fairly commonly involved with fibrous dysplasia and the lesions themselves usually tend to be single, but not always. While we have tended to think of fibrous dysplasia as affecting children, it certainly can affect adults, particularly if the problem has been quietly there all along, as is usually the case. When the bones in and about the eye are involved, as frequently does occur, visual impairment is the worry. In fact, visual impairment is the most common neurologic complication of fibrous dysplasia of the skull. It results from compression of the optic nerve. The rub is that the onset of the visual impairment may be so insidious that there is no time for surgical intervention, or that if intervention does take place, it's too late. Sometimes the visual loss is very precipitous and usually results from the fibrous dysplasia causing an ethmoid mucocele, or by its causing hemorrhage and/or an aneurysmal bone cyst.

This editor has been keeping a record of sorts of televisions news commentators' facial appearances. Try this yourself. News commentators generally tend to sit quite straight and look at the camera right on. It is easy under such circumstances to pick up any degree of facial asymmetry. You will find that asymmetry is much more common than you might expect and chances are very good that such asymmetry is due to mild degrees of fibrous dysplasia. An eyebrow a little higher than the other, the right side of the face being slightly smaller than the left side of the face, etc., seem to be much more prevalent than you might suspect. If you don't believe me about facial asymmetry in television personalities, take a good look at Barbara Walters. You'll see what I mean. Hugh Downs isn't all that perfect either.

J.A. Stockman III, M.D.

16 Dentistry and Otolaryngology

Halitosis in Children
Amir E, Shimonov R, Rosenberg M (Tel-Aviv Univ, Israel)
J Pediatr 134:338-343, 1999   16–1

Introduction.—A common complaint in the adult population is bad breath (halitosis). Usually it is due to microbial activity on the dorsal tongue between the teeth and periodontium. Chronic sinusitis, upper and lower respiratory tract conditions, various systemic diseases, and use of certain drugs have also been associated with bad breath. Few studies have addressed bad breath in children, and those that did examined children with upper respiratory tract infections. Bad-breath parameters and dental indexes were compared in a group of children with a primary family report of bad breath.

Methods.—During 3 appointments, 24 children, aged 5 to 14 years, were examined. Oral hygiene instructions were given after the second appointment. Odor judge scores (whole mouth, tongue, nose, and inter-dental areas), microbiologic tests (Oratest and BANA), and sulfide levels were the malodor-related parameters. The plaque index, the dental index, food impaction, bleeding, and tongue coating comprised the dental-related parameters. Analysis of variance, paired *t* tests, Pearson correlations, and multiple regression were used for statistical analyses.

Results.—Plaque index levels and Oratest were significantly associated with whole mouth odor. Tongue dorsum posterior odor was significantly associated with whole mouth malodor. Patients with interdental odor had significantly higher whole mouth malodor. Nasal malodor was significantly associated with tongue odor. Only at the second appointment were sulfide levels correlated with oral malodor levels.

Conclusion.—Oral malodor in children is related primarily to oral factors, as in adults. There were evident correlations between nasal and oral malodor, which suggested that a major role was played by postnasal drip.

▶ Halitosis is not something to sniff at. In kids, the smell of bad breath is related to both nasal and mouth odor. Its detection is readily obvious, in the nose of the beholder. The science of analyzing breath has moved along very,

very quickly. A whiff of a patient's breath can sometimes be enough to tell what is wrong. The fishy smell of compounds such as amines can indicate renal disorders. The sweet smell of acetone suggests diabetes. Scientists have recently developed a machine that can turn such detections into a science. Technology has been developed that can analyze a puff of breath for traces of gases that readily detect diabetes, renal failure, ulcers, and perhaps even malignancies.[1] The principles involved are the exact same principles used more than 20 to 30 years ago to identify trace gases in interstellar gas clouds. Kidney disease is detected by analyzing ammonia levels in breath. Stress levels can also be checked by tracking isoprene in breath. Preliminary data even suggest that breathalizers can detect hydrocarbons associated with bladder and prostate cancer.

Other scientists have capitalized on such breath analysis to develop an instrument known as the Haliometer, which measures one's degree of halitosis. The Haliometer is made by a company called Interscan Corporation here in the US. The Haliometer measures the amount of volatile sulfides in a patient's breath. The normal amount of volatile sulfides is less than 2 parts per billion.

As long as people have bad breath, you will see innovative ways to detect it, such as Haliometers, and even more innovative ways, perhaps curious ways, to treat it, such as Breathassure.

J.A. Stockman III, M.D.

Reference

1. Service RF: Breathalizer device sniffs for disease. *Science* 281:1431, 1998.

The Impact of WIC Dental Screenings and Referrals on Utilization of Dental Services Among Low-income Children

McCunniff MD, Damiano PC, Kanellis MJ, et al (Univ of Missouri–Kansas City; Univ of Iowa, Iowa City)
Pediatr Dent 20:181-187, 1998   16–2

Background.—The use of dental services has been associated with sex, race, income, and household size. The current cross-sectional study determined whether referrals from nondental health professionals affected the use of dental services by low-income populations.

Methods and Findings.—Three hundred nine mothers completed a self-administered, 32-item questionnaire to assess family oral health behaviors and dental service use. The mothers reported that a total of 27% of the children had been referred for dental care. In a bivariate analysis, a child having a dental visit was associated with a dental referral, child's age, mother's age, mother's perceived need for a dental visit for the child, household size, number of children in the household, and dental insurance for the child. However, logistic regression analysis demonstrated only age was a significant correlate.

Conclusions.—In this low-income population, the child's age was strongly associated with whether the child has seen a dentist. Additional research is needed to clarify the importance of referrals from nondental health professionals.

▶ It's interesting to see how recommendations vary for when children should be seen for their dental visits, particularly their first one. It's also interesting to see when children actually make those first visits. Many believe it is important to reach children at high risk for developing caries at a very young age. For example, the American Academy of Pediatric Dentistry recommends that a child's first visit to a dentist (for all children) should occur by the age of 1 year.[1] On the other hand, the Medicaid Early and Periodic Screening, Diagnosis and Treatment Program recommends screening and referral for dental care at an initial age of 3 years. It is fairly clear that children within the Medicaid population are at significantly greater risk of early dental problems. Take, for example, youngsters age 5 or younger covered under Medicaid. In this population, 2% of children consume 35% of all the resources spent on dental care within this age population.

This report gives us no clear indication about whether Women, Infant, and Children program (WIC) referrals actually result in an improvement in dental status. More time will be necessary to clarify the importance of WIC as a screening tool for this part of a child's health care. In all fairness, WIC cannot be responsible for solving all the ill health problems of children.

For more on WIC and the impact of a large-scale immunization initiative, see the report in the Infectious Diseases and Immunology chapter in this year's YEAR BOOK.

This year's YEAR BOOK is a bit shy on articles related to dentistry, so this commentary closes with a few fast facts about teeth and those who take care of teeth. First, data from the *World Almanac of the United States of America, 1996* tell us that dentists are not evenly distributed throughout the country. For example, there are more dentists per capita in the District of Columbia (at 122 per 100,000 population) than in any other city of the United States. Connecticut (80), New York (79), and Hawaii/New Jersey (78) are not far behind as states. On the other hand, Mississippi (38 per 100,000 population), New Mexico and Arkansas (41), and South Carolina, North Carolina, and Alabama (42) are the states with the fewest dentists.

Also, please recognize that breast-feeding can be associated with nursing caries. Weerheijm studied the characteristics and risk factors for caries in a group of Dutch children, breast-fed on demand over a prolonged period, whose mothers attended the meetings of the La Leche League.[2] On average, the children in this report were breast-fed until the age of 21.5 months. Some 15% of the children had caries by 28 months of age. The caries were due to a combination of having milk in the mouth on too many occasions during the day and having inadequate fluoride supplementation.

In western countries, please note that women who have had multiple pregnancies tend to lose their teeth more frequently as they age. Walker has observed that women of low socioeconomic status lose about 1 additional tooth per child, and women of high social status lose about 1 tooth for every

2 children by the time they reach middle to late middle age.[3] Why this is so is not clear, but presumably it has something to do with the effect of multiple pregnancies on calcium turnover and metabolism. One can presume that someone who has had a dozen or more pregnancies ought to be thinking about shopping around for dentures, sooner or later.

J.A. Stockman III, M.D.

References

1. American Academy of Pediatric Dentistry: Guidelines: Infant oral health care. *Pediatr Dent* 19:70, 1997.
2. Weerheijm S: Prolonged demand breast feeding and nursing caries. *Caries Res* 32:46-50, 1998.
3. Walker ARP: A tooth per child? *Lancet* 352:1386, 1998.

Effect of Treating Obstructive Sleep Apnea by Tonsillectomy and/or Adenoidectomy on Obesity in Children

Soultan Z, Wadowski S, Rao M, et al (State Univ of New York, Brooklyn)
Arch Pediatr Adolesc Med 153:33-37, 1999   16–3

Introduction.—Obese children with enlarged tonsils and/or adenoids can have obstructive sleep apnea, which may cause poor growth and failure to thrive. Known effects of obstructive sleep apnea in children are disturbed sleep and sleep deprivation with subsequent daytime hypersomnolence and decreased activities. Obesity may be caused by this decreased energy expenditure. This study determined whether treatment of obstructive sleep apnea by surgery improved sleep quality, decreased hypersomnolence, increased activity, and led to weight loss.

Methods.—There were 45 children with a mean age of 4.9 ± 2.4 years at operation who had tonsillectomy and/or adenoidectomy for obstructive sleep apnea. In this retrospective study, the children's weight and height changes after tonsillectomy and/or adenoidectomy were recorded, and the changes of the obese and morbidly obese patients were compared with those of the other patients.

Results.—At the time of surgery, there were 10 children who were morbidly obese, 7 who were obese, 3 who were underweight, and 25 who were of normal weight. Substantial weight gain occurred in 31 children, or 69%, including 10 of the 17 who were obese or morbidly obese. The score for weight from the entire group increased from 1.37 ± 2.49 to 2 ± 2.27. The height score increased from 0.03 ± 1.08 to 0.58 ± 0.94. In 28 patients, the body mass index, calculated as weight in kilograms divided by the square of the height in meters, increased.

Conclusion.—Increased gain in height, weight, and body mass index is associated with treating obstructive sleep apnea by tonsillectomy and/or adenoidectomy in most children, including the obese and morbidly obese.

▶ Taking out the tonsils and adenoids of obese children who have obstructive sleep apnea is treating the symptom without treating the cause. Please note that when a cause is so difficult to treat, as is true of obesity, sometimes it is better to treat the symptom, knowing that no cure has been effected. The rub is that these youngsters who no longer snore wind up gaining even more weight.

Obviously, you win some and lose some when you take out the tonsils of obese children.

J.A. Stockman III, M.D.

Assessment of Adenoidal Obstruction in Children: Clinical Signs Versus Roentgenographic Findings
Paradise JL, Bernard BS, Colborn DK, et al (Univ of Pittsburgh, Pa; Children's Hosp of Pittsburgh, Pa)
Pediatrics 101:979-986, 1998   16–4

Introduction.—A common childhood condition is chronic nasal obstruction attributable to large adenoids; however, few children with nasal obstruction complain about difficulty in nasal breathing. Mouth breathing

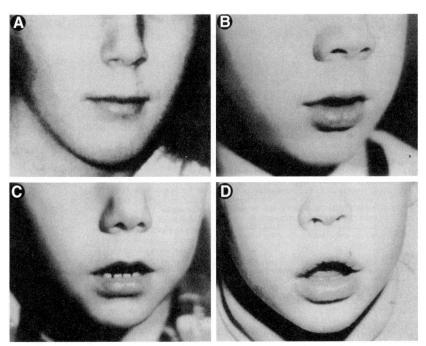

FIGURE 1.—Grades of mouth breathing: **A,** none; **B,** slight; **C,** moderate; and **D,** marked. (Reproduced by permission of *Pediatrics*, from Paradise JL, Bernard BS, Colborn DK, et al: Assessment of adenoidal obstruction in children: Clinical signs versus roentgenographic findings. *Pediatrics* 101:979-986, 1998.)

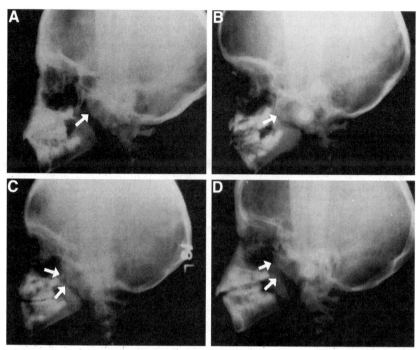

FIGURE 2.—In these lateral soft tissue roentgenograms, the anterior nasopharyngeal airway is defined as the space between the anterior border of the adenoid and the posterior wall of the maxillary antrum. The inferior nasopharyngeal airway is defined as the space between the inferior border of the adenoid and the superior border of the soft palate. The *arrows* point to the salient findings: A, normal-sized adenoid with ample anterior and inferior airways. B, markedly enlarged adenoid with narrowed anterior and inferior airways; C, large adenoid with ample anterior airway and narrowed inferior airway; and D, large adenoid with narrowed anterior airway and ample inferior airway. (Reproduced by permission of *Pediatrics*, from Paradise JL, Bernard BS, Colborn DK, et al: Assessment of adenoidal obstruction in children: Clinical signs versus roentgenographic findings. *Pediatrics* 101:979-986, 1998.)

and hyponasal speech have been the classic physical signs considered indicative of adenoidal nasal obstruction. A study was conducted to determine whether the presence and degree of adenoidal nasal obstruction in children can be assessed satisfactorily by simple clinical means and whether it correlates with roentgenographic assessments.

Methods.—A 4-point scale called the Nasal Obstruction Index, ranging from "none" to "marked," was used to rate the degree of children's mouth breathing (Fig 1) and speech hyponasality. Classifications of lateral soft tissue roentgenographs of the nasopharynx were based on assessment of adenoid size and of nasopharyngeal airway patency that showed either no obstruction, borderline obstruction, or obstruction (Fig 2). Levels of interobserver and intraobserver agreement concerning the classifications were also determined. Correlations in individual children between clinical rating and roentgenographic ratings of nasal/nasopharyngeal obstruction were determined. Using the roentgenographic ratings as the gold standard, the predictive values of clinical ratings were calculated.

Results.—There were 235 children measured for mouth breathing and 648 children measured for speech hyponasality; weighted κ values for interobserver agreement ranged from 0.84 to 0.91. There were 207 children assessed roentgenographically, and the value for interobserver agreement in assessing nasopharyngeal airway status was 0.92, whereas the intraobserver agreement for 191 children was 0.88. For concordance between Nasal Obstruction Index values and roentgenographic ratings in 1033 children, the Kendall's τ *b* value was 0.51. At the lower and upper extremes of 1.0 and ≥ 3.5, the nasal obstruction index values were highly predictive of concordant roentgenographic ratings.

Conclusion.—Standardized clinical ratings of the degree of children's mouth breathing and speech hyponasality can provide reliable and reasonably valid assessment of the presence and degree of adenoidal obstruction of the nasopharyngeal airway. At the extremes of either marked obstruction or no obstruction, these clinical assessments are particularly valid. To establish the presence of adenoidal obstruction, clinical assessment alone may be insufficient. When findings are unequivocally negative; however, clinical assessment can suffice to rule out adenoidal obstruction with a high degree of confidence.

▶ How many times a week in your office practice do you see children who are mouth breathers, who have funny voices and whose parent is concerned about enlarged adenoids? Some parent's complaints can be strong enough that you will need to confirm whether the adenoids are enlarged. There are very sophisticated ways to do this, including various rhinometric techniques for measuring nasal airflow, acoustical analysis of nasal respiratory sounds, acoustical measurement of nasal volume, simultaneous measurement of nasal and oral acoustical output in speech samples, and flexible fiberoptic endoscopy. All of these methods are beyond the reach of most primary care clinicians. Thus, in most instances, you are left with one option, the lateral soft tissue x-ray of the airway.

What Paradise et al. tell us is that, in many instances, you don't need an x-ray to inform you of what is going on. All you need to do is to look carefully at the child, and develop a skill in listening to children's voices so you can tell when hyponasal speech is present. The look involves seeing how much mouth breathing is happening. If you see no mouth breathing and you hear no hyponasal speech, you can be 100% certain there is not significant adenoidal obstruction. Contrarily, if there is obvious hyponasal speech and a wide open mouth, an x-ray is gilding the lilly. The child has big adenoids.

Read this article in detail. It is one of this past year's treasures from the literature. Paradise here on earth.

J.A. Stockman III, M.D.

A Comparison of Nebulized Budesonide, Intramuscular Dexamethasone, and Placebo for Moderately Severe Croup

Johnson DW, Jacobson S, Edney PC, et al (Univ of Calgary, Alta; Univ of Toronto; Astra Pharma, Mississauga, Ont)
N Engl J Med 339:498-503, 1998   16–5

Background.—Nebulized budesonide treatment reduces the symptoms of croup. However, the efficacy of budesonide compared with dexamethasone, the conventional treatment for croup, was analyzed.

Methods.—One hundred forty-four children with moderately severe croup were enrolled in a double-blind, randomized study. The children were given racepinephrine and a single dose of 4 mg of nebulized budesonide (group 1), 0.6 mg of IM dexamethasone per kilogram of body weight (group 2), or placebo (group 3). Assessments were performed before treatment and each hour for 5 hours after treatment.

Findings.—The hospitalization rates were 38% in group 1, 23% in group 2, and 71% in group 3. The children in the active treatment groups had greater improvement in croup scores than those receiving placebo. Children in group 2 had significantly greater improvement than those in group 1.

Conclusions.—Treatment with IM dexamethasone or nebulized budesonide improves moderately severe croup more rapidly than placebo. Dexamethasone was associated with the greatest improvement. Treatment with either active agent reduced the need for hospitalization.

▶ Croup is still with us. In children aged 1 to 2 years the annual incidence of croup is 60 per 1000. Hospitalization rates are reported to vary widely (1% to 30% of children with croup), but when hospitalization does occur, there is a real chance that a child will wind up getting intubated and require mechanical ventilation. It has been estimated that the annual cost of care for patients with croup in this country is about $60 million, two thirds of the cost being attributable to inpatient care. Thus anything that improves the outcome for the child with croup will yield significant financial benefits along with improvement in the morbidity associated with this problem.

Budesonide is a synthetic glucocorticoid with strong topical anti-inflammatory effects and low systemic activity. Nebulized budesonide is not approved for use in the United States. That is a shame because as the abstracted article shows, nebulized budesonide in this Canadian clinical trial was fairly effective. Even more effective was intramuscular dexamethasone, which, of course, is readily available.

The management of croup obviously begins with an assessment of the severity of airway obstruction. Oxygen is helpful if a child is cyanotic or otherwise appears hypoxemic. The use of humidified air, the mainstay of therapy, remains an option of unproved efficacy. A mist tent should be discouraged because most children in such tents are rendered virtually invisible, making ongoing observation extremely difficult. If humidified air is to be used, it should be given with a large-gauge gas-delivery tube (a "mist wand"). Many children with moderate-to-severe croup will benefit transiently from nebulized epinephrine (racemic epinephrine). The latter agent usually causes rapid clinical improvement within 30 minutes, but the effects are temporary, and in many patients, the degree of obstruction returns to pretreatment levels in less than 2 hours. The levo isomer of epinephrine has been shown to be as effective as the racemic form. The fact that children with croup who are ill enough to be seen by a pediatrician should receive glucocorticoids should come as no surprise, despite the debate that has raged in the last quarter century about the purported benefits of steroids. Most clinicians have long since been convinced of their efficacy. Here in the United States, the availability, ease of administration, and cost strongly favor oral or IM dexamethasone. As pointed out in an editorial on this topic, children who have been treated with nebulized epinephrine and dexamethasone may be sent home if clinical improvement is maintained for 2 to 3 hours after treatment.[1]

J.A. Stockman III, M.D.

Reference

1. Jaffe DM: The treatment of croup with glucocorticoids. *N Engl J Med* 339:553-554, 1998.

Controlled Trial of Universal Neonatal Screening for Early Identification of Permanent Childhood Hearing Impairment
Kennedy CR, for the Wessex Universal Neonatal Hearing Screening Trial Group (Southampton Gen Hosp, England)
Lancet 352:1957-1964, 1998   16–6

Introduction.—About 112 babies per 100,000 births can be affected by congenital bilateral permanent childhood hearing impairment of 40 dB or more relative to hearing threshold level. These children may greatly benefit from early management of hearing impairment, which would include such short- and long-term benefits as improved language, communication, mental health, and employment prospects. It was previously found that 2-stage neonatal screening with transient evolved otoacoustic emissions detection followed by automated auditory brain-stem response measurement was more than 99% specific. No previous studies have examined the incremental effect of such screening on the early diagnosis of permanent childhood hearing impairment. A controlled trial was conducted to investigate whether the addition of neonatal screening to the traditional health visitor distraction test, compared with the distraction test alone at 8 months, would increase detection and improve early management of babies with permanent childhood hearing impairment.

Methods.—There were 53,781 babies in the trial and of these, 25,609 were born during periods with neonatal screening. There were 1724 babies screened who had risk factors for permanent childhood hearing impairment, including a family history of hearing impairment, perinatal infec-

TABLE 2.—Neonatal Screening by Location and Risk Categories and Presence of Individual Risk Factors

Location and Risk Group*	Proportion of Screened Population (n=21 279)	
Postnatal wards		
Standard risk	84·5%	
High risk	5·1%	
Special/Intensive-care units >48 h		
Standard risk	6·5%	
High risk	3·0%	
Unclassified	0·9%	
Individual risk factors		
Family history of hearing impairment	6·6%	
Perinatal infection		
Suspected	3·8%	
Confirmed	0·5%	
Birthweight <1·5 kg	1·2%	
Anatomical deformity		
Craniofacial	0·5%	
Other		1·3%
Birth asphyxia		
Moderate	0·7%	
Severe	0·3%	
Chromosomal abnormality	0·2%	
Exchange transfusion		
Considered	0·3%	
Undertaken	0·02%	

*More than one risk factor was present in some babies.
(Courtesy of Kennedy CR, for the Wessex Universal Neonatal Hearing Screening Trial Group: Controlled trial of universal neonatal screening for early identification of permanent childhood hearing impairment. *Lancet* 352[9145]:1957-1964, 1998. Copyright by The Lancet Ltd.)

tion, an anatomical deformity, birth asphyxia, chromosomal abnormality, or exchange transfusion (Table 2). The screening periods lasted 4 to 6 months and were alternated with periods of no screening. A transient evoked otoacoustic emissions test was used to examine the babies, and those who failed had an automated auditory brain-stem response test on the same day. Babies with positive results were referred for audiologic assessment.

Results.—An 87% coverage of births was achieved with neonatal screening, with a false-alarm rate of 1.5%. There was an overall yield of 90 babies having bilateral permanent childhood hearing impairment of 40 dB or more relative to hearing threshold level per 100,000 target population. This was equivalent to 80% of the expected prevalence of the disorder in the population. During periods with neonatal screening, there were 71 more babies with moderate or severe permanent childhood hearing impairment per 100,000 target population who were referred before age 6 months than during periods without neonatal screening. There was a significantly lower rate of false negative results from neonatal screening than for the distraction test (4% vs 21%).

Conclusion.—For identifying permanent childhood hearing impairment early, neonatal screening is effective and may be particularly useful for babies with moderate and severe hearing impairment for whom early management may have the most benefit.

▶ Why shouldn't we be screening all babies for congenital deafness? It's more common than cystic fibrosis, galactosemia, or congenital hypothyroidism. In fact, in our country, moderate, severe, or profound hearing loss occurs in as many as 1 to 3 in 1000 live births. Should we miss it in the neonatal period, the consequences on speech development are profound. The impact on families is devastating. The cost to society over a lifetime can be huge.

All screening tests must be viewed in light of their sensitivity and specificity, positive predictive values, and negative predictive values. If the data from this report are to be believed, a very high percentage of babies will be detected with relatively few false positives. Such universal screening for hearing impairment in newborns is an ideal to be aimed at for all babies. If that ideal is too lofty a goal, then at least we should have programs aimed at screening all "high-risk" newborns. Certainly we should be looking at premature babies and babies who have had substantial prenatal or neonatal stresses including meningitis and intrauterine infection. Babies with a family history of deafness and babies with abnormalities of the ears, head, or neck, must be screened. Such high-risk babies account for as many as 50% of hearing-impaired children, so such limited screening would be a terribly good start, although still half of babies would be missed.

For more on the topic of the newborn with hearing loss and detecting hearing loss in the nursery, see the article that follows.

J.A. Stockman III, M.D.

The Newborn With Hearing Loss: Detection in the Nursery
Finitzo T, Albright K, O'Neal J (Univ of Texas, Dallas; Hearing Health Inst, Fort Worth, Tex; Texas Dept of Health, Austin)
Pediatrics 102:1452-1460, 1998   16–7

Introduction.—Children with hearing loss score higher on early language development if they receive early intervention. Detection of hearing loss in newborns is mandated in 20 states. If effective programs are to be implemented across the nation, there must be integration of pediatricians and other infant care providers into the detection process. Universal detection of hearing loss involves the birth admission screen, a follow-up and diagnostic component occurring 1 week to 3 months after discharge, and intervention services. The birth admission screen was examined by reviewing outcome measurements for newborns, and factors were evaluated that impacted the outcomes positively or negatively.

Methods.—There were 54,228 newborns screened. A physiologic test of auditory function was used for all newborns. They also had screening auditory brain-stem responses or transient evoked otoacoustic emissions. The newborns were screened in the newborn and intensive care nurseries before hospital discharge. Recordings were taken of the number of births screened, the number of newborns who passed the screen before discharge, the number of infants who returned for follow-up, and the number of newborns identified with hearing loss. A Birth Screening Performance Index was also calculated.

Results.—Of the newborns screened, 52,508 were screened before hospital discharge during their birth admission. Of these, 50,721 passed this screen. There were 1224 infants who returned for follow-up screen as outpatients. There were 113 newborns over a 3½-year span who failed the birth admission screening yet had hearing loss that was sensorineural in nature. There was an estimated incidence of hearing loss of 3.14/1000 infants.

Conclusion.—When audiology involvement, hospital support, and automated data and information management are present, screening in the nursery with low false positive rates can be achieved. Improvement is needed with follow-up measures. At-risk newborns may be assuredly connected to services with better tracking methods.

▶ Another report showing that hearing loss in newborn babies is common (3.14 affected babies per 1000 births). Another report showing us that we can screen for such hearing loss with either auditory brain-stem responses or transient evoked otoacoustic emissions without creating a lot of false positives.

Newborn hearing screening isn't without its problems. Even using the most advanced technology, were we to screen all babies, not just those at high risk or those who have visited an intensive care nursery, there would be some false positives. Some have shown that the false positives may indeed exceed the true positives in low-risk babies. That would make sense given the imperfect nature of the current screening tools. We have no knowledge of the potential impact of such false positives on parents or on the parent-child relationship. Anger, confusion, and frustration must occur for some in such circumstances.

Paradise provides us with a very useful commentary on this complex topic.[1] He reminds us that we urgently need a large randomized clinical trial of newborn screening to determine if the benefits outweigh the risks described above. The cost of such a trial would be high, but in fact these costs are minuscule in comparison with the first-year cost associated with putting into place a nationwide screening program that produces more problems than good.

As far as the 50% of deafness seen in babies that is attributable to genetic causes is concerned, the recent finding that mutations in a single gene (GJB2, encoding the connexin 26 molecule) causes childhood deafness in a large proportion of cases has revolutionized the field.[2] The reason why is that such forms of deafness can be detected with relatively straightforward gene screening programs. A molecular screen for a GJB2 mutation could turn out to be relatively inexpensive and certainly is not invasive. While not the only gene known to be involved with deafness, it does account for a substantive proportion of all the genetic causes of deafness.

J.A. Stockman III, M.D.

References

1. Paradise JL: Universal newborn hearing screening: Should we leap before we look? *Pediatrics* 103:670-672, 1999.
2. Cohn ES, Kelley PM, Fowler TW, et al: Clinical studies of families with hearing loss attributable to mutations in the connexin 26 gene (GJB2/DFNB1). *Pediatrics* 103:546-550, 1999.

Mutations in the Connexin 26 Gene (*GJB2*) Among Ashkenazi Jews With Nonsyndromic Recessive Deafness
Morell RJ, Kim HJ, Hood LJ, et al (NIH, Rockville, Md; Louisiana State Univ, New Orleans; Michigan State Univ, East Lansing; et al)
N Engl J Med 339:1500-1505, 1998   16–8

Introduction.—There are at least 20 genes that cause nonsyndromic recessive deafness if mutated. Mutations in the *GJB2* gene have recently been found to cause this form of deafness. This gene encodes a gap-junction protein, connexin 26, which is expressed in the inner ear. It may be important in maintaining endocochlear potential. More than 80% of nonsyndromic recessive deafness in Mediterranean Europeans is caused by inheritance of the 30delG mutant allele of *GJB2*. The contribution of mutations in *GJB2* to the prevalence of nonsyndromic recessive deafness was examined.

Methods.—Blood samples were obtained from members of 3 Ashkenazi Jewish families with nonsyndromic recessive deafness, Ashkenazi Jewish individuals seeking carrier testing for other conditions, and from members of other ethnic groups. Puretone audiometry, measurement of middle-ear immitance, and recordings of otoacoustic emissions were used to examine the hearing of persons who were heterozygous for mutations in *GJB2*.

Results.—Two frame-shift mutations in *GJB2* were detected in families with nonsyndromic recessive deafness: 167delT and 30delG. The prevalence of heterozygosity for 167delT, which is rare in the general population, was 4.03% in the Ashkenazi Jewish population; for 30delG, prevalence was 0.73. Genetic-linkage analysis revealed conservation of the haplotype for 167delG and existence of several haplotypes for 30delG. Audiologic evaluation of carriers of the mutant alleles who had normal hearing showed subtle differences in their otoacoustic emissions, indicating that the expression of mutations in *GJB2* may be semidominant.

Conclusion.—The 4.76% rate of carriers of mutations in *GJB2* is similar to that of other genes governing recessive diseases in the Ashkenazi Jewish population. Ashkenazi Jews may want to have their carrier status for mutations in the *GJB2* gene evaluated as part of genetic screening.

Blood samples should be examined for both the 167delT and 30delG mutant alleles.

▶ This report was selected for inclusion in the YEAR BOOK because it reminds us of how many deaf babies are born each year and what the causes of such deafness are. About 1 in 1000 children are born deaf, and of these, the vast majority (some 80%) are born with no associated clinical findings. Some half of all deafness of this type is genetic in origin. It has also been suggested that the genes causing deafness can cause progressive loss of hearing that only begins in adulthood. The gene involved (*GJB2*), is one that accounts for the most common cause of hereditary hearing loss. The *GJB2* gene is implicated in 50% of childhood deafness in some populations. This is particularly true within the Ashkenazi Jewish population.

Now we know that we can identify a fairly common gene causing deafness. The remaining issue is whether we should be screening individuals for the gene defect. As difficult as it was to find which gene caused deafness, it is even more difficult to decide what to do with the information now that we have it. This is made more complicated by the fact that the degree of hearing impairment in an affected fetus cannot be predicted on the basis of the degree of hearing impairment in another child in the family with the same gene mutation. There is much variation in the clinical presentation with identical genotypes. Even those who are homozygous for the mutation have been found to have hearing impairments ranging from mild to severe.

In the Ashkenazi Jewish population, the carrier rate for the *GJB2* gene is approximately 5%. This carrier rate is similar to that seen with other recessive diseases in the Ashkenazi Jewish population (Tay-Sachs disease, familial dysautonomia, and Gaucher's disease). The story with deafness is not as clean as with, say, Tay-Sachs disease regarding correlations of severity and gene mutations, but some couples may wish to opt for prenatal testing.

J.A. Stockman III, M.D.

Hearing Loss and Use of Personal Stereos in Young Adults With Antecedents of Otitis Media
Job A, Raynal M, Rondet P (Centre de Recherche du Service de Santé des Armées "Emile Pardé," La Tronche Cedex, France; Hôpital d'Instruction des Armées Percy, Clamart, France)
Lancet 353:35, 1999   16–9

Introduction.—Harmful effects of personal stereo use have been previously shown on hearing performances in young adults. Systematic medical assessments are given to men entering the army in France, and risk factors for deafness were assessed.

Methods.—There were 1208 men who had hearing status assessed by tonal automated audiometry. They were also interviewed about their hearing status and exposure to potential harmful sources of noise. Antecedents of childhood ear diseases were recorded, including history of repeated episodes of otitis media. A comparison was made between hearing thresholds of exposed and nonexposed groups.

Results.—In men who went to rock concerts and discos twice a month or more, the hearing threshold at 1.0 kHz was slightly increased in 38%. In 18% of men with noisy occupations, the hearing thresholds at 2 kHz and 4kHz were significantly increased. Personal stereos were the major factor influencing hearing. In 17% of men who used personal stereos for at least 1 hour per day, hearing thresholds were increased at all frequencies. The presence or absence of repeated episodes of otitis media in infancy or childhood greatly affected the harmful effect of stereo use. There were 114 men who had repeated otitis media episodes who were affected, whereas the men without previous otitis media were not affected by personal stereo use.

Conclusion.—In men with repeated episodes of otitis media in childhood, personal stereo use was shown to have clinically important effects. It is important to cure otitis in childhood. Personal stereo use is a risk factor for deafness in young people with a history of repeated episodes of otitis media.

▶ These investigators have hit upon a very interesting way of examining a captive audience in order to determine whether there is a potential relationship between hearing loss and the use of stereo headphones. Indeed there is. For Frenchmen who enter the military service as very young adults, routine hearing screening is performed. It turns out that young men who had previously attended rock concerts and discos 2 or more times a month experienced some degree of hearing loss. Additionally, those who had used personal stereos (the portable type with headphones), on average, had hearing losses of about 11 dB. That is not enough to get you out of the military, but it is enough to make you wonder whether these folks will wind up requiring hearing aids as they move through the latter stages of middle age. The problem is particularly difficult in individuals who have had prior episodes of otitis media.

Having repeated episodes of otitis media is a risk factor for hearing loss. Wearing headphones is a risk factor for hearing loss. Combining the two is even more of a risk factor. These days, a lot of runners wear earphones. That is even worse yet, a risk that destroys your hearing and your joints.

I have one final comment on hearing loss. See how you would answer the following question: Your triage nurse passes a query on to you that she cannot answer. A father called in with the following concern. For much of the father's life, he has been enamored with the hobby of model airplane flying. His 10-year-old son wants to get into the act as well. The father wants to know if there is a risk of hearing loss associated with the hobby. How would you answer? You answer should be *yes*. Model airplane flying as a hobby can affect hearing. Such airplanes generally use combustion engines which, if held at arm's length as one is working them, produce sound levels at about 112 dB. There is no question that such sound levels, even if intermittent, can cause prolonged hearing loss if exposure is frequent enough.

Please note that not all youngsters at risk for hearing loss experience this by playing with model airplanes. Even babies are theoretically at risk by having squeaky toys in their cribs. Were you aware that the average "squeaky toy" produces sounds that emanate at a level anywhere from 78 to 100 dB? 'Tis true.[1]

J.A. Stockman III, M.D.

Reference

1. Luxon LM: Toys and games: Poorly recognized hearing hazards. *BMJ* 316:1473, 1998.

Tympanostomy Tubes and Water Exposure: A Practical Model
Hebert RL II, King GE, Bent JP III (Med College of Georgia, Augusta)
Arch Otolaryngol Head Neck Surg 124:1118-1121, 1998   16–10

Introduction.—One of the most common otolaryngologic procedures performed today is myringotomy and tympanostomy tube placement. The most common complication is postoperative otorrhea, which some authorities attribute to water contamination of the middle ear via a patent tympanostomy tube. As a result, many physicians recommend ear plugs for swimming, diving, or even bathing as well as surface swimming in chlorinated pool or salt water only, no diving or deep swimming, and no exposure to soapy or contaminated water. Today, otolaryngologists differ widely in their recommendations of water precautions. This study determined whether, and under what conditions, water exposure causes middle ear contamination via a patent tympanostomy tube.

Methods.—An in vitro model of a human head containing an auricle, external auditory canal, middle ear, tympanic membrane with tympanostomy tube, eustachian tube, and mastoid cavity was developed. For detection of water entry, 2 electrodes connected to an external ohmmeter rested in the middle ear. Four types of water exposure were used to test the model: showering, bathing, hair rinsing, and swimming.

Results.—For showering, hair rinsing, or head submersion in 12.7 cm of clean tap water, no positive test results were obtained. However, with head submersion in soapy water, 10 of 97 tests were found positive, which was statistically different from clean water. Positive test results were found in 2 of 16 tests in a depth of 30 cm, in 3 of 18 tests in a depth of 45 cm, in 2 of 20 tests in a depth of 60 cm, and in 11 of 20 tests in a depth of 75 cm. At depths of more than 60 cm, there was a higher incidence of water entry into the middle ear. Between depths of 60 cm or less, no statistical difference was seen.

Conclusion.—Water entry into the middle ear is not promoted by showering, hair rinsing, or head submersion in clean tap water. Submersion in soapy water increased the probability of water contamination. The middle ear is infrequently affected by entry of pool water with head submersion; however, the incidence increases with deeper swimming at more than 60 cm. In patients with tympanostomy tubes, many of the frequently advised water precautions are unnecessary.

▶ How many times in the course of a month does a parent of a child with tympanostomy tubes ask you, "Can he get water in his ears?" The answer to this question has varied widely throughout the years ever since Dr. B.W. Armstrong introduced middle-ear ventilation tubes into our therapeutic armamentarium back in 1954. For the first 20 to 30 years, strict water precautions were the norm. Swimming was taboo. Only recently has the literature begun to focus on a more liberal approach that permits a number of activities, including swimming. Data, for example, suggest that swimming without earplugs carries no greater risk of ear drainage than swimming with earplugs in children with tubes.[1] Some have even suggested that children using ear protection actually have a higher incidence of otorrhea than children swimming without such protection.

This report continues to add information to our understanding of what constitutes a risk of otorrhea in children who have ear tubes. Exposure to clean tap water via head submersion, showering, or hair rinsing carries with it virtually no risk of getting fluid into the middle ear. However, if you go swimming well below the surface, there may be enough pressure to force water into the middle ear. Surface swimming is okay. While prophylactic use of otic antibiotic suspensions after water exposure theoretically helps prevent draining ears, this benefit has not been documented unequivocally. It is not recommended unless a patient has already developed problems.

If you think you've heard the last about tympanostomy tubes and water exposure, you must be ready to retire in the next few days. Dollars to donuts, there will be a new episode in the mini-series "Ear Tubes and Water" sometime in the very near future.

One last comment having to do with the ears. Were you aware that when driving along in a car, it is always best to leave a window slightly cracked or a sunroof slightly open? The reason why has to do with air bags. If you are in an accident in which the passenger compartment of an automobile were sealed tightly, you might develop a problem with your hearing. The cause is straightforward. When an airbag deploys, it produces a brief (<100 msec) intense (150-170 dB) pressure wave that propagates itself through the passenger compartment of the automobile. The actual magnitude of pressure produced relates to factors such as the vehicle size, the number of occupants, and the openness of the ventilation of the vehicle. Take, for example, the case of a 30-year-old man who was driving a station wagon at about 25 mph when the car went off the shoulder of the road. There was no collision, but the undercarriage of the station wagon struck an obstacle, deploying the driver's side airbag. At the moment of deployment, the driver was looking to his right and the airbag struck the left side of his face and head. Shortly thereafter, he noticed a hearing loss and tinnitus in his left ear. Audiometric thresholds showed profound hearing loss at low frequencies in his left ear. His right ear tested normal.[2]

Even without a direct strike to the ear, simple expansion of an airbag into a tightly closed space produces shock waves to the ears sufficient to cause temporary hearing loss and tinnitus. If you don't believe this phenomenon exists, ask the owner of a Volkswagen Beetle (the classic variety). That old "bug" was so tight that an owner sitting in the front seat would readily experience ear pain occasioned by compression of the air within the cabin when a car door was quickly slammed shut. Nothing loving about the love bug when it came to such a phenomenon.

J.A. Stockman III, M.D.

References

1. Becker GD, Eckderg TJ, Goldwater RR: Swimming and tympanostomy tubes: A prospective study. *Laryngoscope* 97:740-741, 1987.
2. Kramer MB, Shattuck TG, Charnock DR: Traumatic hearing loss following air-bag inflation. *N Engl J Med* 337:574-575, 1997.

Prevalence of Various Respiratory Viruses in the Middle Ear During Acute Otitis Media

Heikkinen T, Thint M, Chonmaitree T (Univ of Texas, Galveston)
N Engl J Med 340:260-264, 1999   16–11

Introduction.—The most common bacterial infection among children is acute otitis media, and it is the most frequent reason for outpatient antibiotic therapy. The annual costs of otitis media can exceed $3.5 billion in the United States. Respiratory viruses can have a crucial role in the etiology and pathogenesis of this disease. For major improvements in the management and prevention of otitis media, a better understanding of the effect of viruses and mechanisms of interactions between viruses and bacteria in otitis media is essential. Vaccines against viruses in the middle ear would have the greatest potential for reducing the frequency of otitis

TABLE 2.—Prevalence of Various Respiratory Viruses in the Middle Ear in Children With Acute Otitis Media

Virus	Viral Infection*	Virus in Middle-Ear Fluid
	No. of Cases (%)	
Respiratory syncytial virus	65	48 (74)†
Parainfluenza viruses	29	15 (52)‡
Influenzaviruses	24	10 (42)‡
Enteroviruses	27	3 (11)
Adenoviruses	23	1 (4)

*Viral infection was diagnosed by 1 or more methods: viral culture or antigen detection in the nasal-wash specimen, viral culture or antigen detection in the middle-ear fluid, or on the basis of an increase in viral titers by at least a factor of 4 from the time of acute illness to convalescence.
†P = .04 for the comparison with parainfluenza viruses and P≤.005 for the comparison with any of the other viral groups.
‡ P ≤ .01 for the comparison with enteroviruses or adenoviruses.
(Reprinted by permission of *The New England Journal of Medicine*, from Heikkinen T, Thint M, Chonmaitree T: Prevalence of various respiratory viruses in the middle ear during acute otitis media. *N Engl J Med* 340:260-264. Copyright 1999, Massachusetts Medical Society. All rights reserved.)

TABLE 3.—Specific Micro-organisms in the 43 Samples of Middle-ear Fluid That Contained Both Bacteria and Viruses

Bacterial Species	Respiratory Syncytial Virus (N=22)	Parainfluenza Viruses (N=10)	Influenzaviruses (N=8)	Enteroviruses (N=3)†
			No. of Cases (%)	
Streptococcus pneumoniae	8 (36)	1 (10)	8 (100)‡	1 (33)
Haemophilus influenzae	10 (45)	5 (50)	2 (25)	0
Moraxella catarrhalis	6 (27)	5 (50)	3 (38)	1 (33)

*More than 1 bacterial species was identified in samples from 8 ears.
†*Pseudomonas aeruginosa* was cultured in 2 ears with enteroviruses.
‡P = .003 for the comparison with respiratory syncytial virus, and P < .001 for the comparison with parainfluenza viruses (by Fisher's exact test).
(Reprinted by permission of *The New England Journal of Medicine*, from Heikkinen T, Thint M, Chonmaitree T: Prevalence of various respiratory viruses in the middle ear during acute otitis media. N Engl J Med 340:260-264. Copyright 1999, Massachusetts Medical Society. All rights reserved.)

media. The rates of middle-ear invasion by common respiratory viruses in children with acute otitis media and viral infection of the upper respiratory tract were determined.

Methods.—Four hundred fifty-six children, ages 2 months to 7 years, with acute otitis media were studied to determine the prevalence of various respiratory viruses in their middle-ear fluid. Middle-ear fluid specimens and nasal-wash specimens were obtained for viral and bacterial cultures and for the detection of viral antigens at enrollment and after 2 to 5 days of antibiotic therapy. Serologic studies of serum samples obtained during the acute illness and convalescence were conducted to assess the viral cause of the infections.

Results.—In 186 of the 456 children (41%), a specific viral cause of the respiratory tract infections was identified. In middle-ear fluid, respiratory syncytial virus was the most common virus identified. In 48 of the 65 children infected by this virus, it was detected in the middle-ear fluid (74%). Parainfluenza viruses (52%) and influenza viruses (42%) were also detected in the middle-ear fluid, as were enteroviruses (11%) and adenoviruses (4%) (Tables 2 and 3).

Conclusion.—During acute otitis media, respiratory syncytial virus is the principal virus invading the middle ear. The incidence of acute otitis media in children may be reduced by an effective vaccine against upper respiratory tract infections caused by respiratory syncytial virus.

▶ Stephen Berman, M.D., Children's Hospital, Denver, comments:

Improving our understanding of the pathogenesis of acute otitis media remains a vexing problem. Traditional thinking has cast the role of respiratory viruses as an indirect cause of acute otitis media by altering eustachian tube dysfunction. The inflammatory response caused by respiratory viral infections promotes aspiration of contaminated bacterial nasal pharyngeal secretions into the middle ear space. Bacterial infection within the middle ear is more likely when drainage and clearing mechanisms are impaired. The authors of this report challenge the validity of this pathogenesis model. The authors documented rates of middle ear and upper respiratory tract viral infections by determining the prevalence of respiratory viruses in both middle-ear fluid and nasal-wash specimens at the time of initial diagnosis of acute otitis media and after 2 to 5 days of antibiotic therapy. The findings suggest that certain viruses cause acute otitis media by directly invading the middle ear and producing inflammation. If respiratory virus infection causes acute otitis media only by altering eustachian function, one would expect that the frequency of acute otitis media associated with different viral respiratory pathogens would be similar. However, respiratory syncytial virus is more likely isolated from middle-ear fluid than other viruses, and acute otitis media is more likely to occur in children who experience respiratory syncytial virus.

Another interesting finding in this study was the association between bacterial pathogens and viral pathogens. *Streptococcus pneumoniae* was isolated more often in middle-ear fluid that also contained influenza viruses than in middle-ear fluid with other viral pathogens. The reason for this association is unclear. Perhaps, there is an interaction that predisposes to selective bacterial overgrowth of *S. pneumoniae* in the nasal pharyngeal space. There are important implications to this expanded pathogenesis model for acute otitis media. If respiratory viruses are active players in the pathogenesis of acute otitis media, it is possible that vaccines against respiratory syncytial virus and other viral pathogens will be more effective in preventing acute otitis media than bacterial vaccines. Pneumococcal vaccine in young children may have a transient impact on reducing episodes of acute otitis media, because non-vaccine serotypes may take over the ecological niches once held by the serotypes included in the vaccine.

The authors are commended for excellent detective work in unraveling the continuing mystery of the pathogenesis of acute otitis media. Unfortunately, this condition can still be considered otitis media with confusion.

S. Berman, M.D.

Otitis Media, the Caregiving Environment, and Language and Cognitive Outcomes at 2 Years
Roberts JE, Burchinal MR, Zeisel SA, et al (Frank Porter Graham Child Development Ctr, Chapel Hill, NC; Univ of North Carolina, Chapel Hill)
Pediatrics 102:346-354, 1998   16–12

Introduction.—It is still unknown whether otitis media with effusion (OME) causes delayed language development, despite the fact that several studies have shown an association. The mild-to-fluctuating hearing loss resulting from OME may make speech more difficult for a child to detect or to filter from background noise and may impair the child's processing of speech. Previous studies have not considered the child's caregiving environment. In a group of children whose history and development of

OME were prospectively monitored since infancy, a study was conducted of how children's OME history, hearing status, and caregiving environment during the first 2 years of life were related to the children's language and cognitive development at 2 years.

Methods.—The study included 86 African American infants aged between 6 and 12 months who attended group childcare centers. Serial ear examinations using otoscopy and tympanometry, serial hearing tests, 2 ratings of the child-rearing environment at home and in childcare, and language and cognitive outcomes were conducted between 6 and 24 months.

Results.—Between 6 and 24 months, 63% of children experienced either unilateral or bilateral OME, and 44% experienced reduced hearing sensitivity. Measures of language and cognitive skills were modestly correlated with the proportion of time with OME or with hearing loss; however, these relationships were no longer significant when the ratings of the home and childcare environments were also considered. Children with more hearing loss or otitis media effusion tended to live in less responsive caregiving environments. At 2 years, these environments were associated to a lower performance in vocabulary acquisition and expressive language.

Conclusion.—The quality of home and childcare environment was more strongly related to OME and hearing loss than to children's language and cognitive developments. This may be a result of the possibility that children in less-responsive caregiving environments experience conditions that make them more likely to experience OME. This may also be a result of the possibility that it is more difficult for caregivers to be responsive and stimulating with children with more OME.

▶ Roberts et al have challenged one of the sacred cows of pediatrics and have appeared to have made hamburger out of the old teaching that otitis media, sans other influencing factors, results in language and cognitive deficits in infants and toddlers. What these investigators have done is to attempt to carefully control for environmental influences that might seriously influence the likelihood that hearing loss secondary to OME would cause language delay. They pin most of the blame for delay in language skills on the quality of the home and childcare environment.

As one might suspect, this report and 1 previous from this same group in North Carolina has attracted quite a bit of reaction, some of it negative.[1] Whether the sacred cow should remain revered, or be led to slaughter remains to be seen. In the meantime, it seems wise to take OME extremely seriously. The same holds true for improving the quality of home and childcare environment. There are lots of causes for why children fail to develop their full potential.

J.A. Stockman III, M.D.

Reference

1. Roberts JE, Burchinal MR, Medley LP, et al: Otitis media, hearing sensitivity, and maternal responsiveness in relation to language during infancy. *J Pediatr* 126:481-489, 1995.

A Longitudinal Study of Otitis Media With Effusion Among 2- to 5-Year-Old African-American Children in Child Care

Zeisel SA, Roberts JE, Neebe EC, et al (Univ of North Carolina, Chapel Hill)
Pediatrics 103:15-19, 1999   16–13

Background.—These authors followed the natural history of otitis media with effusion (OME) in 2- to 5-year-old African American children attending community child care centers.

Methods.—The subjects were 86 African American children (40 boys and 46 girls) who were enrolled in a community child care center and who were developing normally. Subjects had been enrolled in a previous longitudinal study of OME, with a mean age at enrollment of 8.2 months. Beginning at 24 months of age and continuing through 60 months of age or until the child entered kindergarten, each child underwent biweekly assessments of middle ear status by pneumatic otoscopy and tympanometry (average number of ear examinations per child, 33).

Findings.—As the children became older, the prevalence of OME decreased. For children 24 to 30 months old, the mean proportion of examinations revealing bilateral OME was 12%; for children 54 to 60 months old, this figure dropped to 4%. Thirty-five children (41%) between 24 and 30 months of age (41%) had bilateral OME, whereas only 8 children (11%) between 54 and 60 months of age had bilateral OME. Conversely, the proportion of normal bilateral examination results increased with increasing age, from 77% for children 24 to 30 months of age to 88% for children 54 to 60 months of age. Episodes of bilateral OME lasting 4 months or longer were noted in 60 children before the age of 24 months; of these 60 children, only 8 had continuous episodes lasting this long after the age of 24 months.

Conclusion.—The incidence of OME decreased with increasing age in these children, as has been reported for other populations. Middle ear effusions are less prevalent after 2 years of age, even in children with previous episodes of OME lasting 4 months or longer.

Symptoms of Acute Otitis Media

Kontiokari T, Koivunen P, Niemelä M, et al (Univ of Oulu, Finland)
Pediatr Infect Dis J 17:676-679, 1998   16–14

Background.—Parents base their decision to seek medical care for a child with upper respiratory infection mainly on their assumption that the child's symptoms are related to acute otitis media (AOM). However, the symptoms of AOM are nonspecific. The sensitivity and specificity of parents' ability to predict AOM in their child, with each child serving as his or her own control, were studied.

Methods.—Eight hundred fifty-seven healthy children in daycare were followed up for 3 months. The symptoms of each child were compared during upper respiratory infections with and without AOM.

Findings.—One hundred thirty-eight children had upper respiratory infections with or without AOM during the study period. Earache was the symptom most strongly associated with AOM, although sore throat, night restlessness, and fever were also significantly correlated with AOM. In a logistic regression analysis, 71% of the patients were diagnosed correctly based on the symptoms of earache and night restlessness. The parents could predict the presence of AOM with a sensitivity of 71% and a specificity of 80%. Their positive and negative predictive values were 51% and 90%, respectively.

Conclusions.—Although symptoms are of limited value in distinguishing AOM from upper respiratory infection, parents can predict the presence of AOM somewhat reliably. More symptoms than previously reported seem associated with AOM.

▶ Chances are that even if you believe the findings of this report, you will not be prepared to put away your otoscope. To say this differently, just because parents can predict the presence of AOM with a sensitivity and specificity of 71% and 80%, this does not mean that a precise diagnosis by a skilled practitioner can be avoided.

One of our 3 daughters, Sam, had 1 episode after another of AOM in the first few years of life. She eventually needed pressure equalization tubes, indeed, on more than 1 occasion. Sam's parents knew when she had a new episode. Her brother and sister, who were only 4 years older, also could have easily made the diagnosis, so classic was her recurrent symptomatology. Still, we did what was right. She was seen every time she had symptoms, and somebody else wrote the prescription. Somebody else certainly put in the pressure equalization tubes. . . and yes, we were not *always* right. Every now and then Sam had a simple upper respiratory infection without middle ear problems, even though all of us swore that it was "her ears again."

J.A. Stockman III, M.D.

A Novel Use of Xylitol Sugar in Preventing Acute Otitis Media
Uhari M, Kontiokari T, Niemelä M (Univ of Oulu, Finland)
Pediatrics 102:879-884, 1998   16–15

Introduction.—Xylitol is a 5-carbon polyol with widespread use as a sweetening substitute for sucrose. It inhibits the growth of *Streptococcus mutans*, a bacteria causing dental caries. It also inhibits the growth of *Streptococcus pneumoniae*. Xylitol was evaluated for its effectiveness in preventing acute otitis media (AOM) in a randomized, controlled, double-blind trial.

Methods.—A total of 857 healthy children recruited from day care centers were randomized to 1 of 5 treatment groups: 165 were assigned to control syrup, 159 to xylitol syrup, 178 to control chewing gum, 179 to xylitol gum, and 176 to xylitol lozenges. The daily dose of xylitol ranged from 8.4 g in chewing gum to 10 g in syrup. Children were followed for occurrence of AOM.

Results.—Sixty-eight of the 165 children (41%) who received control syrup had at least 1 episode of AOM, compared with 46 of 159 children (29%) who received xylitol syrup. This was a 30% decrease in the incidence of AOM. The occurrence of AOM decreased by 40% in children who received xylitol chewing gum and 20% in children who received xylitol lozenges, compared with controls. There was a significantly lower incidence of AOM in children receiving xylitol gum or syrup. These children needed antimicrobials less often than controls. Xylitol was well tolerated in this cohort of day care children.

Conclusion.—Administration of xylitol sugar in gum or in syrup form was effective in preventing AOM and reducing the need for antimicrobials in young children.

▶ This 1 report, appearing in *Pediatrics*, probably received more attention than any other scientific report related to pediatrics in the year 1998. It qualifies as a potential recipient of the Academy Award of pediatrics, given the attention it has received.

Please note, however, that not all Academy awardees are deserving of honor, nor is this report, at least in this editor's opinion. It is very interesting. It provides new information, but the information it provides is fairly useless. Would anyone seriously think that to prevent AOM, one would put a child on a chronic prophylactic program of xylitol syrup or chewing gum? As an anti-infective, xylitol must be given several times a day. What parents are going to give their child a syrup or chewing gum several times a day? Given the fact that most AOM of a recurrent nature is in youngsters under the age of 2 years, who would allow such a young child to chew on gum?

Please note that xylitol is not totally without potential complications. It is largely unabsorbed in the gastrointestinal tract and frequently causes an osmotic diarrhea. It can also cause cramping abdominal pain. This problem has been described in the literature and is termed "chewing gum diarrhea."

There are only 2 potential therapeutic uses, as far as this editor knows, for chewing gum. The first we all know about and that is to relieve ear pain when ascending or descending in flight. The other is the observation that the chewing of gum can be very effective as part of the management of chronic rumination syndromes in teenage girls. Better to chew gum than ones cud. It is dubious whether a third use of gum (xylitol for preventing AOM) will be found to be realistic.

A few last remarks about chewing gum. First, there is indeed another benefit to chewing gum not mentioned above. If one chews a lot of gum, one can cause hypertrophy of one's masseter muscle. This produces the so-called masseteric look which teenagers in particular hold valuable these days. If you're not familiar with such a "look," it's also known as the "Brad Pitt look." The desired appearance is one in which the angle of the jaw has some prominence to it. For the more geriatric set in the YEAR BOOK audience who may not be familiar with Brad Pitt, Robert Redford is another good example of the masseteric look.

Finally, please also be aware that chewing a lot of gum is one of the most common reasons why one finds an elevated serum amylase in the absence of pancreatitis. Chewing gum exercises the parotid gland along with the masseter muscle, squeezing out the amylase enzyme.

J.A. Stockman III, M.D.

17 Endocrinology

Mortality in Patients With Congenital Adrenal Hyperplasia: A Cohort Study
Swerdlow AJ, Higgins CD, Brook CGD, et al (London School of Hygiene and Tropical Medicine; Middlesex Hosp, London; John Radcliffe Hosp, Oxford, England; et al)
J Pediatr 133:516-520, 1998   17–1

Background.—Congenital adrenal hyperplasia (CAH) is the most common adrenal disorder in children. It is caused by an inherited defect in 1 of 5 enzymes needed for cortisol biosynthesis, usually 21-hydroxylase or 11 β-hydroxylase. To date, no one has compared mortality in patients with CAH to that in the general population. The risk of death in a cohort of patients with CAH was reported.

Methods.—The cases of 333 children with CAH seen at several pediatric endocrinology departments in the United Kingdom since 1964 and monitored to mid-1996 were reviewed. Standardized mortality ratios were determined, and mortality in this cohort was compared with that in the general population after adjustment for sex, age, and calendar year.

Findings.—In the cohort of patients with CAH, all-cause mortality was 3 times higher than that expected. Mortality was significantly increased between 1 and 4 years of age, with a ratio of 18.3, but not at older ages. Mortality was increased in patients of Indian-subcontinent ethnicity, especially in girls. Most deaths appeared to be caused by adrenal crisis, frequently after infection.

Conclusion.—Although survival among patients with CAH has improved markedly since the introduction of steroid treatment, this disorder can still have fatal outcomes. Better communication with and education of parents with affected children, especially parents from immigrant ethnic minority groups, are needed.

▶ CAH is one of the disorders that is part of the standard teaching curriculum within pediatric residencies. None of us see it all that much, but we talk about it somewhat more because it is a disease that: (1) can be fatal and (2) should be able to be detected in most instances by neonatal screening.

The rub with neonatal screening is that in some patients, signs and symptoms of CAH will develop before the results of the neonatal screening are back. Also, sometimes specimens do get mixed up (don't they?). What the report abstracted here does is remind us that even if we do appropriately diagnose CAH in the newborn period (or later), there still remains some significant mortality. This does not, however, mean that the prognosis overall is not good. In fact, it is reassuringly good from these data.

With modern steroid replacement therapy, the problems seen with CAH, are likely to be related ones not specifically caused by the enzyme defect itself. For example, there are several reports of testicular and adrenal tumors that have developed in children with CAH as affected children age. It is possible that these patients were not treated with sufficient doses of steroids to suppress central stimulation of testicular or adrenal end organs. Also, in a few patients, various sarcomas have been reported to have developed. There is no explanation as to why this has occurred.

Please note that this report comes from Great Britain, where the highest mortality rate with CAH resides in patients of Indian ethnicity, particularly among girls. Excess deaths in this population appear to be caused by infections and are likely to be the result of an inadequate or delayed response to increasing steroid dosing during illness. Clearly, the parents of these kids did not receive the proper communication or did not understand it, which left the children vulnerable to adrenal insufficiency and death under stress.

The message is clear. Once one has made a diagnosis of CAH, one must be committed to a lifelong effort to be certain that families—particularly families of immigrant or minority status—clearly understand what the treatment of this disorder must be. Although the need for this understanding applies to many disorders, few are such that children will get into so much trouble so quickly should a parent fail to understand what needs to be done in certain circumstances.

Before leaving the topic of things related to adrenal glands, see if you can answer the following question. You volunteer your time in an AIDS clinic, providing care to teenagers and young adults. You notice that a number of patients who are HIV-infected have a "buffalo hump." Is this due to an adrenal overactivity? The answer is no. Recently, anecdotal reports of patients who developed a buffalo hump have appeared on the Internet. It has been noted that enlargement of the dorsocervical fat pad occurs after initiation of combination antiviral therapy that includes a protease inhibitor; this observation has led to the suggestion that the appearance of buffalo humps can be a consequence of such therapy in patients with AIDS.

The differential diagnosis of a buffalo hump is extremely limited. The etiologies can be counted on the fingers of a partially amputated hand. The causes are hypercortisolism (Cushing's syndrome) and protease inhibitor therapy. Few signs and symptoms have such a short list of causes.[1]

J.A. Stockman III, M.D.

Reference

1. Lo JC, Mulligan K, Tai VW, et al: "Buffalo hump" in men with HIV-1 infection. *Lancet* 351:867-870, 1998.

Childhood Hypoglycemia in an Urban Emergency Department: Epidemiology and a Diagnostic Approach to the Problem
Pershad J, Monroe K, Atchison J (Univ of Alabama, Birmingham)
Pediatr Emerg Care 14:268-271, 1998   17–2

Background.—Idiopathic ketotic hypoglycemia (IKH) is the most common cause of hypoglycemia in children aged 1 to 5 years. With appropriate treatment, the condition is benign. The epidemiology of IKH and a diagnostic approach are reported.

Methods and Findings.—Thirty-one patients were identified in a retrospective review of the medical records of patients seen in an emergency department between 1992 and 1995. The prevalence of hypoglycemia at this emergency department (ED) was 6.54 per 100,000 visits. In 18 (58%) patients, the diagnosis was IKH, for a prevalence of 3.9 per 100,000 ED visits. Patients with IKH were aged a mean of 27.7 months. The ratio of boys to girls was 2:1. Nine patients were black, 8 were white, and 1 was unavailable. Five children had weights below the 25th percentile. Fourteen

Hypoglycemia

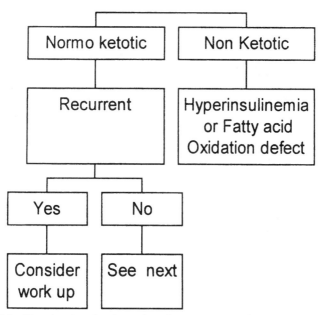

FIGURE 1.—Normoketotic and nonketotic hypoglycemia. (Courtesy of Pershad J, Monroe K, Atchison J: Childhood hypoglycemia in an urban emergency department: Epidemiology and a diagnostic approach to the problem. *Pediatr Emerg Care* 14[4]:268-271, 1998.)

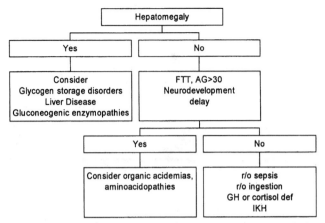

FIGURE 2.—First episode of "normoketotic" hypoglycemia. (Courtesy of Pershad J, Monroe K, Atchison J: Childhood hypoglycemia in an urban emergency department: Epidemiology and a diagnostic approach to the problem. *Pediatr Emerg Care* 14[4]:268-271, 1998.)

underwent hormone assessment, including insulin, growth hormone (GH), and cortisol. All had appropriately suppressed insulin levels and high cortisol levels. Thirteen of the 14 tested children had normal or high GH levels. The 4 children undergoing urine drug screens had negative findings. Although none of the children with IKH was febrile, 6 had sepsis workups, all of which were negative. In 15 of the 18 children tested, urine ketones were positive. The mean anion gap was 20. Eight children with IKH were discharged from the ED after their status normalized (Figs 1 and 2).

Conclusions.—The most common cause of hypoglycemia in children past infancy is IKH. Typically, affected children have been previously healthy, have normal growth and development, and are seen with a first episode of symptomatic fasting hypoglycemia and appropriate degree of ketonuria without hepatomegaly. Glucose administration usually relieves the symptoms. An extensive workup for endocrinopathy or inborn error of metabolism in such patients is not needed.

▶ The presentation of a youngster to an ED who has a low blood sugar is not that uncommon an occurrence. One sees that IKH is the most commonly identified cause of this problem. It is certainly the most common cause of hypoglycemia in childhood. It typically occurs in children aged between 1 and 5 years. It invariably resolves spontaneously by 8 to 9 years. Although technically this disorder is not considered to be pathologic, the hypoglycemic symptoms, when they occur, can be life threatening. The tip-off to the diagnosis is hypoglycemia resulting from fasting associated with ketosis and ketonuria. Affected patients do not have hepatomegaly or an anion gap. They respond rapidly to correction of their blood glucose levels.

All of us have been trained to recognize that unexplained hypoglycemia can be a manifestation of an endocrinopathy, an inherited inborn error of metabolism or a glycogen storage disease. The algorithm provided with this article should help you decide how far to go when first seeing a child who is observed with a low blood sugar. If episodes of hypoglycemia are recurrent or atypical, a workup for endocrinopathy, inborn errors of metabolism, and glycogen storage diseases should be considered. Other causes of low blood sugar should also be evaluated including GH deficiency and adrenal insufficiency. Never forget also that certain drugs are included in the differential diagnosis of hypoglycemia. Alcohol, salicylates, oral hypoglycemic agents, β-blockers, and β-2 agonists will cause this and can easily be picked up with routine drug screening

J.A. Stockman III, M.D.

Clinical Features of 52 Neonates With Hyperinsulinism
de Lonlay-Debeney P, Poggi-Travert F, Fournet J-C, et al (Hôpital des Enfants Malades, Paris; Université de Louvain, Brussels, Belgium; Ospedale Bambino Gesu, Rome)
N Engl J Med 340:1169-1175, 1999   17–3

Background.—Congenital hyperinsulinism can be caused either by diffuse abnormalities of pancreatic beta cells or by focal abnormalities involving adenomatous islet cell hyperplasia. Whereas a pancreas with diffuse involvement will likely require total or near-total pancreatectomy, focal hyperplasia can be treated with partial pancreatectomy to excise the abnormal area. These authors described the clinical manifestations and surgical outcomes in neonates with either diffuse or focal hyperinsulinism.

Methods.—The subjects were 52 neonates with hyperinsulinism who required surgery. Preoperatively, patients underwent transhepatic catheterization to locate the site(s) of insulin hypersecretion. Intraoperatively, tissues from the head, isthmus, body, and tail of the pancreas were examined histologically to confirm the extent of involvement. Thirty neonates had diffuse beta cell hyperfunction and underwent near-total pancreatectomy, whereas 22 neonates had focal hyperplasia and typically underwent partial pancreatectomy. All patients were monitored postoperatively by measurements of plasma glucose levels and glycosylated hemoglobin levels as well as by oral glucose tolerance tests.

Findings.—Clinical symptoms were similar between the patients with focal and diffuse hyperplasia. Focal hyperplasia has been associated with a loss of the maternal allele from chromosome 11p15 and a paternally inherited mutation of the sulfonylurea receptor type 1 gene. Mutations in the sulfonylurea receptor type 1 gene were found in 5 of the 22 patients with focal hyperplasia (Table 2). In these 22 patients, insulin hypersecretion was localized to the head of the pancreas in 9 patients, the isthmus in 3, the body in 8, and the tail in 2. Nineteen underwent partial pancreatectomy.

Postoperatively, all had normal postprandial plasma glucose concentrations, all were able to eat normally, and none required further surgery or

TABLE 2.—Location of Lesions as Determined by Pancreatic Venous Catheterization and Histologic Examination, Extent of Pancreatectomy, and Genetic Characteristics of the 22 Neonates With Focal Hyperinsulinism

Treatment and Patient No.	Age at Surgery	Location by Catheterization	Location by Histologic Examination	Extent of Pancreatic Resection	LOH in Lesion	Mutation of SUR1 Gene*
Partial pancreatectomy						
1	99 days	Head	Head	Head	NC	None
2	234 days	Body	Body	Body	Yes	None
3	117 days	Tail	Tail	Tail	Yes	R1421C†
4	91 days	Head	Head	Head	Yes	None
5	237 days	Body	Body	Body and tail	Yes	None
6	91 days	Body	Body	Body and tail	ND	None
7	73 days	Unknown	Body	Body and tail	ND	ND
8	142 days	Unknown	Body	Body and tail	Yes	None
9	27 mo	Head	Head	Head	ND	None
10	36 days	Body	Body	Body and tail	ND	del4138CGAC‡
11	139 days	Head	Head	Head	Yes	None
12	36 days	Isthmus	Isthmus	Isthmus and body	Yes	None
13	66 days	Body	Body	Body and tail	ND	ND
14	84 days	Isthmus	Isthmus	Isthmus and body	Yes	R842G§
15	58 days	Head	Head	Head	ND	ND
16	66 days	Head	Head	Head	Yes	None
17	69 days	Head	Head	Head	Yes	R1494W‖
18	44 days	Isthmus	Isthmus	Isthmus	Yes	None
19	99 days	Tail	Tail	Tail	Yes	ND
Near-total pancreatectomy						
20	88 days	ND	Body	Near-total	ND	ND
21	19 mo	ND	Head	Near-total	Yes	ND
22	20 mo	ND	Head	Near-total	Yes	R1494W‖

*Refers to heterozygous mutations in the NBF1 and NBF2 domains in peripheral blood lymphocytes from the patients and their fathers; other exons of the sulfonylurea receptor type 1 gene were not studied.
†R1421C was a missense mutation caused by a C→T transition at position 4261.
‡This mutation was a deletion of 4 nucleotides, CGAC, at positions 4138 to 4141 and the insertion of 3 nucleotides, GTG.
§This missense mutation was caused by a C→G transversion at position 2524.
‖This missense mutation was caused by a C→T substitution at position 44810.
Abbreviations: ND, not determined; LOH, loss of heterozygosity (loss of the maternal allele from chromosome 11p15 in the focal lesion); SUR1, sulfonylurea receptor type 1.
(Reprinted by permission of *The New England Journal of Medicine,* from de Lonlay-Debeney P, Poggi-Travert F, Fournet J-C, et al: Clinical features of 52 neonates with hyperinsulinism. *N Engl J Med* 340:1169-1175. Copyright 1999, Massachusetts Medical Society. All rights reserved.)

medical treatment (mean follow-up, 3.6 years). In no cases did hypogly-cemia, elevated glycosylated hemoglobin values, or glucose intolerance develop. Three of these 22 patients underwent near-total pancreatectomy, either because surgery was performed before pancreatic catheterization was available (1 patient) or partial pancreatectomy performed at another hospital did not resolve the hypoglycemia (2 patients). In the first patient, increasing hyperglycemia developed, and the patient had to be treated with insulin at 9 years of age; the latter 2 patients had hypoplastic lesions in the head of the pancreas that were resected, with subsequent resolution of hypoglycemia.

After near-total pancreatectomy in the 30 patients with diffuse hyper-insulinism, 13 had persistent hypoglycemia, diabetes mellitus type 1 de-veloped in 8, and hyperglycemia developed in 7 others. During the first year after surgery, plasma glucose concentrations normalized in only 2 of these 30 patients.

Conclusion.—Focal hyperinsulinism can be detected with preoperative pancreatic catheterization and intraoperative histologic examination. This disorder can be successfully treated with partial pancreatectomy, with little risk of the development of diabetes mellitus.

▶ Things have certainly changed since this editor was a resident in the early 1970s, when it comes to the management of newborns with persistent hyperglycemia caused by hyperinsulinism. In those days, the disease was inappropriately referred to as nesidioblastosis. Although diazoxide was avail-able and was used, it rarely controlled the insulin production and virtually all babies with hyperinsulinism and refractory hypoglycemia went to the oper-ating room and had a near-total pancreatectomy, with the consequent risk of the development of permanent diabetes mellitus.

What we see in this report is that slightly under half of babies do not require such vigorous approaches involving near-total pancreatectomy. The reason is that these babies have what is called adenomatous islet cell hyperplasia—also known as focal hyperinsulinism—rather than a diffuse hyperplasia of the beta cells of the pancreas. Focal hyperinsulinism is asso-ciated with the loss of a maternal allele from chromosome 11p15, leading to unbalanced expression of imprinted genes involving the control of cell growth. Somatic reduction to hemizygosity or homozygosity of a paternally inherited mutation of the gene for the sulfonylurea receptor type 1 leads to hyperinsulinism. The diffuse abnormalities causing hyperinsulinism repre-sent a heterogeneous disorder involving the gene encoding the sulfonylurea receptor, or the inward-rectifying potassium channel which can be caused by recessive or autosomal dominant disorders.

The rub with these 2 types of causes of hyperinsulinism and hypoglycemia in the newborn is that a surgeon cannot tell with the naked eye which is which. What needs to be done before the pancreas is operated on is to catheterize the pancreas and measure insulin levels from various parts of the organ. One should be able to tell whether the affected baby has a focal source for the hyperinsulinism or whether the pancreas is diffusely involved. In half the babies then, a subtotal pancreatectomy which corrects the problem with little or no risk of the subsequent development of diabetes mellitus can be successfully performed.

J.A. Stockman III, M.D.

Growth and Normal Puberty
Abbassi V (Georgetown Univ, Washington, DC)
Pediatrics 102:507-511, 1998   17–4

Objective.—The 2 most apparent signals of puberty are the pubertal growth spurt and the development of secondary sex characteristics. Pubertal growth begins with an acceleration phase, followed by a deceleration phase, then cessation of growth with epiphyseal closure. Previous

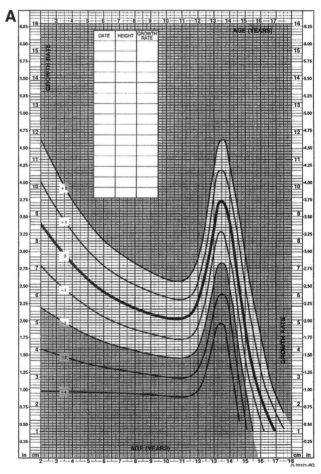

(Continued)

FIGURE 1 (cont.)

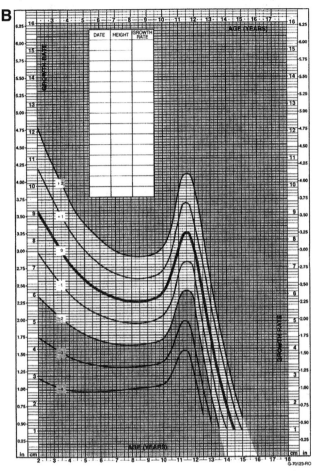

FIGURE 1.—Mean and SD height velocities in boys 2 to 18 years of age (A) and girls 2 to 15 years of age (B). Data from Tanner and Davies.[7] (Reproduced with permission of *Pediatrics*, from Abassi V: Growth and normal puberty. *Pediatrics* 102:507-511, 1998.)

studies of pubertal growth were reviewed to describe the growth characteristics of American children.

Methods.—The review included data from longitudinal growth studies from birth to maturity, longitudinal studies of growth during puberty, and cross-sectional studies. The reports were analyzed to describe the pubertal growth characteristics of age at take-off, the onset of growth acceleration; age at peak height velocity; peak height velocity; duration of puberty; and contribution of the pubertal growth spurt to final adult height.

Findings.—Age at take-off varied between the sexes, and within sex according to different variables. For children at an average growth rate, mean age at take-off was about 11 years for boys versus 9 years for girls.

Black girls were significantly more advanced in pubertal stage than white girls. Peak height velocity was 13.5 years for boys and 11.5 years for girls (Fig 1). Peak height velocity per year was 9.5 cm in boys and 8.3 cm in girls, with greatest peak height velocity for early-maturing children. Pubertal growth contributed 30 to 31 cm to height in boys, or 17% to 18% of final height; and 27.5 to 29 cm in girls, or 17% of final height. Pubertal height was not correlated with take-off height or adult height, but was negatively correlated with age at take-off. Age at take-off and at peak height velocity were significantly correlated with pubertal stage.

Conclusions.—The findings demonstrate the significant variation in pubertal growth characteristics by sex and other variables. For boys, mean age at take-off is 11 years and mean age at peak height velocity 13.5 years. For girls, these ages are 9 and 11.5 years, respectively. Clinical application of growth-velocity charts requires knowledge of the child's pubertal status and calculation of his or her growth velocity.

▶ You would think as we leave the 20th century, we would know how quickly children grow and when puberty begins. Nonetheless, it was only in the last couple of years that the National Center for Health Statistics provided data from cross-sectional growth studies to give us reasonably accurate information pertaining to pubertal age for boys and girls. The Center aggregated data from the Fels Research Institute studies, the Denver Child Research Council studies, the Harvard School of Public Health study, and the Guidance Study of the University of California at Berkeley. As expected, these showed that pubertal growth does begin earlier in girls (about two years) at about 9 years of age. Peak growth velocity in girls occurs at 11 years of age and 13 years of age in boys. This is at Tanner breast stage 2 to 3 for girls and Tanner testis stage 3 to 4 for boys. Girls generally stop growing at an average 14 years of age, but boys continue to stretch out until they are 17.

On a slightly different note, everyone knows the various Tanner stages of pubertal development, but few know about the Cooksey stages of pubertal development. Cooksey was the individual who defined the various patterns of pubertal voice development based on singing range and tessitura (most comfortable modal singing voice range).[1] Studies of the singing voices of boys during puberty confirm this classification to be valid and reliable. A comparison of the Cooksey classification of voice and the Tanner stage of 26 high school boys was recently undertaken.[2] It would appear that teenage boys' voices "break" late in puberty, not early. Maximum vocal changes occur somewhere between Tanner stage 3 and Tanner stage 4, and not toward the beginning of puberty as has been previously thought.

Someone once said: "When the training bra goes on, the trouble begins." For boys, one might say that "when the falsetto goes out and the baritone comes in, the trouble has really started."

Reading reports on childhood growth is a fascinating endeavor. Such reports are filled with terms such as "take-off growth," "acceleration," and "deceleration." Studies make this sound like rocket science when it is not. Most children do their own thing, in their own time, and in their own way.

They spurt when they want and they fizzle when they will. Knowing when all this happens may satisfy our morbid curiosity as care providers, but it doesn't change the reality of the inevitable happening when it chooses to happen.

J.A. Stockman III, M.D.

References

1. Cooksey JM, Becker RL, Wiseman R: A longitudinal investigation of selected vocal, physiologic, and acoustic factors associated with voice maturation in the junior high school male adolescent. *Proceedings of a Research Symposium on the Adolescent Voice*, vol 1. Buffalo, NY, State University of New York, Buffalo Press, 1984, pp 4-60.
2. Harries MLL, Walker JM, William DM, et al: Changes in the male voice at puberty. *Arch Dis Child* 77:445-447, 1997.

Birth Weight Influences the Initial Response to Growth Hormone Treatment in Growth Hormone–insufficient Children
Achermann JC, Hamdani K, Hindmarsh PC, et al (Middlesex Hosp, London)
Pediatrics 102:342-345, 1998   17–5

Introduction.—There is often a dramatic response in the first year a child undergoes growth hormone (GH) therapy. To program future development, there is the potential influence of fetal growth. Some adult diseases have been correlated with low birth weight. Children who have insufficient GH and who were born small for gestational age were shown to respond less well to GH treatment after 2 years than those who were born of appropriate birth weight. To investigate which factors most significantly influenced first-year growth response to GH treatment, data on birth weight SD scores for a population were used as 1 of the several variables in a group of children with pure isolated idiopathic GH insufficiency.

Methods.—Sixteen singleton white prepubertal children (11 boys and 5 girls) with isolated GH insufficiency were part of a longitudinal study of response to daily GH treatment of 15 to 26 IU/m²/week. During the 6 to 12 months before GH treatment and the 12 months after, change in height velocity SD scores was measured to reflect how responsive the children were to GH treatment. Age at treatment, birth weight SD score, peak GH response to insulin tolerance testing, midparental height SD score, and dose of GH administered were the potential influencing variables considered by regression analysis.

Results.—The mean birth weight SDS was −0.51. Birth weight SD score correlated positively with change in height velocity SD score. Peak GH correlated negatively with change in height velocity SD score. The influence of birth weight SD score on response to GH treatment was confirmed in stepwise linear regression analysis.

Conclusion.—In growth hormone–insufficient children, the continuum of birth weight influences initial response to GH treatment. Relative insensitivity in the GH or insulin-like growth factor axis may be the cause. Future studies should be conducted to determine the influence of birth weight on final height and the benefit of using higher doses of GH in these children.

Lack of Correlation Between Growth Hormone Provocative Test Results and Subsequent Growth Rates During Growth Hormone Therapy

Bell JJ, Dana K (Columbia Univ, New York; Genentech Inc, South San Francisco)

Pediatrics 102:518-520, 1998   17–6

Introduction.—Pituitary stimulation tests for diagnosis of growth hormone deficiency (GHD) do not necessarily reflect the actual growth hormone (GH) status of children with growth failure. On provocative testing, some slow-growing children without apparent GHD respond very well to GH treatment. Thus GHD appears to occur along a spectrum, from those with classic GHD—who do not produce or secrete GH—to those who have normal GH rates on testing but not enough for normal growth. This study examined the ability of pituitary stimulation tests to predict growth in response to recombinant GH therapy.

Methods.—The study included 24,843 children from the National Cooperative Growth Study database who had not received previous GH therapy. The peak GH level in response to pituitary stimulation was less than 10 µg/L in 57%, considered GHD; 10 µg/L or greater in 30%, considered a normal response; and unreported in 13%. These 3 groups were compared for their response to GH therapy. Responses were also studied in a group of 187 children who were healthy and growing normally, but were very short for age and sex.

Results.—All 3 groups of children showed a dramatic increase in growth rate during the first year of GH therapy, with means of 8.4 to 9.5 cm/yr. Thereafter, the growth rate decreased, stabilizing at 1.0 to 1.9 cm/yr greater than the baseline growth rate. Although growth rates in response to GH were significantly different between groups, there was substantial overlap. For the children with normal GH and normal growth, GH therapy increased growth rate by 7.7 to 9.2 cm/yr during the first year. Beyond 1 year, growth rates decreased to baseline or below.

Conclusions.—Pituitary stimulation testing cannot adequately diagnose the presence of GHD and cannot determine whether GH therapy is indicated for children with short stature. After an initial increase in growth rate, the response to GH therapy falls significantly in normally growing but short children. Thus GH therapy may not be of sustained benefit in these patients.

▶ If you have been puzzled about the value of GH testing, join the crowd. Now we see that the clinical presentation of a poorly growing child with low GH responses is often indistinguishable from that of a poorly growing child with adequate responses. Regardless of the peak GH response to testing, children will grow at a greater rate if they are treated with GH. This suggests that we should explore ways to diagnose GHD with more certainty than with the currently available tests. Another recent report has also indicated that abnormalities of GH secretion can be seen in children who have normal results on provocative GH tests, but who are growing slowly.[1]

The differences in GH secretion between slowly growing short children and normal children can be very subtle indeed. Neither provocative GH testing nor serial sampling is uniformly predictive of the response to GH in very short children. All this is exasperating. Thank goodness for our pediatric endocrine colleagues. They save the rest of us from pulling out our hair in trying to figure out what to do with these Danny De Vitos.

One final comment about growth and its measurement. Everyone knows that one gets shorter during the course of a day. The question is, can you get a reliable measurement at any time of the day by stretching the individual in question? The answer is, probably not, at least according to Fairbank.[2] It would appear that the well-known diurnal variation in height is mainly due to loss of fluid from the intervertebral discs rather than postural changes.[3]

J.A. Stockman III, M.D.

References

1. Diamond FB, Jorgensen EV, Root AW, et al: The role of serial sampling in the diagnosis of growth hormone deficiency. *Pediatrics* 102:521-524, 1998.
2. Fairbank J: Height measurements in stretching. *Lancet* 351:1212, 1998.
3. Botsford DJ, Esses SI, Oglivie-Harris DJ: In vivo diurnal variation in intervertebral disc volume and morphology. *Spine* 19:935-940, 1994.

Adult Height in Children With Growth Hormone Deficiency Who Are Treated With Biosynthetic Growth Hormone: The National Cooperative Growth Study Experience

August GP, Julius JR, Blethen SL (George Washington Univ, Washington, DC; Genentech Inc, South San Francisco)
Pediatrics 102:512-516, 1998   17–7

Background.—Few large studies have reported the adult height of children with growth hormone deficiency (GHD) treated with growth hormone (GH). Whether height gained in puberty by children with GHD treated with biosynthetic GH is comparable to that in otherwise healthy children with delayed bone ages was determined. In addition, whether the height SD score, which started to increase before puberty, continues to increase during puberty was examined.

Methods.—Four hundred eighty males and 194 females who had reached a chronological age of at least 20 or 18 years, respectively, or who had reached at least pubertal stage 4 and a chronological age of 16 or 14 years, respectively, comprised group 1. Group 2 was a subgroup of 153 males and 105 females who, in addition to the general criteria, had also attained a bone age of at least 16 or 14 years, respectively.

Findings.—In group 1, mean Tanner pubertal stage 2 was 14.1 years in the males and 12.6 years in the females. Bone age at this stage was 11.9 and 10.6 years, respectively, and the height SD score, −2.1 and −2.4, respectively. The total mean height gained in puberty was 22.4 cm in males and 17.4 cm in females. The percentage of adult height gained in puberty was 13.3% and 11.3%, respectively. Near-adult height SD score in males was −1.3 and in females, −1.6. The target adult height SD score was −0.4 and −0.5 in males and females, respectively. In group 2, these growth characteristics were similar in magnitude. In both groups, age at onset of Tanner stage 2 was negatively correlated with total height gained in puberty and the percentage of adult height gained.

Conclusions.—The growth characteristics of these study participants were similar to those observed in normal children and in previously reported smaller samples of children with GHD. Though the height SD score increased during puberty in these individuals, the target adult height SD score was not attained, which argues for early diagnosis and treatment of children with GHD.

▶ The more we learn about the effects of GH given as part of the treatment of GHD, the more we learn that we need to use it correctly. We need to strike while the iron is hot. The iron is hot not just during puberty, but for some period before puberty. If GH is administered shortly before or in conjunction with puberty, final adult height will fall somewhat short of what one might like for adult height. This is not because individuals with GHD do not grow as expected during puberty in comparison with their peers, when treated with GH, but rather that they have started off shorter to begin with. Catch-up is not to be expected.

In a time and era where every centimeter counts for success in life, for good and bad reasons, we should not be undertreating children with GHD. Although no children have ever died of being short, a few wish they had. The psychological disadvantages of being short, particularly in the teenage years, is not to be minimized. The authors are correct in their final conclusion: "If the final heights of children with GHD are to be optimized, then it is important that the diagnosis be made and treatment be initiated as early as possible to afford these children the opportunity to make up much of their height deficit before puberty."

For more on the topic of growth hormone and the treatment of short stature, see the report that follows (Abstract 17–8). One wishes that the writings on this subject were less complex, but that would be a neat trick given the intricacies of how humans operate. Einstein addressed this when he remarked: "Things should be made as simple as possible, but not any simpler." We can only go so far in making learning easy for ourselves.

J.A. Stockman III, M.D.

Effect of Growth Hormone Treatment on Adult Height of Children With Idiopathic Short Stature

Hintz RL, for the Genentech Collaborative Group (Stanford Univ, Calif; et al)
N Engl J Med 340:502-507, 1999   17–8

Introduction.—Results have been mixed for children treated with growth hormone (GH) for idiopathic short stature. Treatment can stimulate growth rate and SD scores for height. The effect of long-term GH therapy on adult height is unknown. The outcome of long-term GH therapy was assessed in 121 in children with idiopathic short stature.

Methods.—All children had an initial height below the third percentile, low growth rates, and maximal stimulated serum concentrations of GH of at least 10 µg/L. Patients were treated with GH at 0.3 mg/kg of body weight/week for 2 to 10 years. Eighty children reached adult height with a bone age of at least 16 years for boys and at least 14 years for girls and pubertal stage 4 or 5. The difference between predicted adult height before treatment and achieved adult height were compared with the corresponding difference in 3 groups of untreated normal or short-statured control subjects.

Results.—The mean SD score for height rose from −2.7 to −1.4 with GH treatment in the 80 patients who reached adult height (Fig 1). The mean differences between predicted adult height before treatment and achieved adult height were +5.0 cm and +5.9 cm for boys and girls, respectively. The difference among treated boys was 9.2 cm greater than the corresponding difference among untreated boys with initial SD scores of less than −2. The difference among treated girls was 5.7 cm greater than the difference among untreated girls. Few children achieved their mean midparental target height.

Conclusion.—Most patients with idiopathic short stature who were treated with GH therapy had a significant increase in growth rate. The decision to treat children with idiopathic short stature must weight the relative benefits, risks, and costs of treatment.

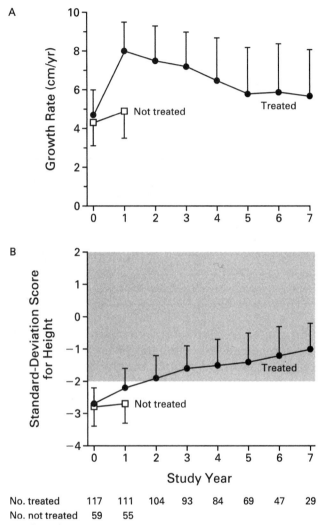

| No. treated | 117 | 111 | 104 | 93 | 84 | 69 | 47 | 29 |
| No. not treated | 59 | 55 | | | | | | |

FIGURE 1.—Effects of growth hormone treatment in children with idiopathic short stature. **A** shows the mean (± SD) growth rate anad **B** shows the mean (± SD) SD score for height. The value at time 0 is the growth rate for the preceding year or longer. The *numbers below the graphs* are the total numbers of children completing each year. Complete data for the pretreatment year were missing for 4 of the 121 children. Fifty-nine of the children were not treated in the first year, and their data are included both with the data for the untreated group and as part of the total data for the treated group. The shading in **B** represents the normal range for height. (Reprinted by permission of *The New England Journal of Medicine*, from Hintz RL, for the Genetech Collaborative Group: Effect of growth hormone treatment on adult height of children with idiopathic short stature. N Engl J Med 340:502-507. Copyright 1999, Massachusetts Medical Society. All rights reserved.)

Growth Hormone Treatment of Girls With Turner Syndrome: The National Cooperative Growth Study Experience

Plotnick L, Attie KM, Blethen SL, et al (The Johns Hopkins Univ, Baltimore, Md; Genentech Inc, South San Francisco)
Pediatrics 102:479-481, 1998   17–9

Background.—Biosynthetic growth hormone (GH) was approved recently for use in augmenting height in children with Turner syndrome (TS). The outcomes of GH treatment in girls with TS were analyzed.

Methods.—Data were obtained on 2798 girls with TS registered in a national database. Follow-up data on growth were available for 2475 patients, and data on adult height were available for 622.

Findings.—The mean age of girls with TS at database enrollment was 10.1 years. Mean GH treatment duration was 3.2 years. The mean height SD score increase was 0.8 compared with unaffected girls and 1.2 compared with TS standards. Growth rates increased from a mean 4 cm/yr before treatment to 7.5 cm/yr after 1 year of treatment. Treatment duration was the best predictor of change in height SD score. After 6 to 7 years of GH treatment, the cumulative change in mean height SD score was 2. The 622 girls for whom adult height data were available, who were older at GH initiation, achieved a height gain of 6.4 cm over pre-GH projected height after a mean 3.7 years of treatment. Their average adult height was 148.3 cm.

Conclusions.—Though GH treatment responses varied, such treatment was associated with very significant gains in growth and adult height in girls with TS. Treatment duration was the most important variable predicting adult height.

▶ Dr. Steven D. Chernausek, Division of Endocrinology, Children's Hospital Medical Center, Cincinnati, Ohio, comments:

Short stature and hypogonadism are dominant features of TS. Endocrinologists have attempted to improve adult height in patients with TS by giving anabolic steroids to stimulate growth and by delaying estrogen replacement to prolong the growth period. Though GH secretion is intact in TS, clinical studies using pharmacologic doses of GH show enhancement of statural growth and increase in final adult height. Such data ultimately led to approval of GH as a treatment for short stature due to TS in the United States and Europe, but controversy has remained as to the magnitude of the gain that results from treatment. Reports from clinical trials in the United States indicated an average gain of around 10 cm in final height, whereas others reported more modest gains and cautioned about unrealistic expectations of the treatment.[1,2] Because GH is expensive ($10,000-$30,000/yr) and involves daily injections for years, quantifying height gains is relevant to assessing the value of therapy. Plotnick et al. report the results from the National Cooperative Growth Study, which is a registry of patients receiving GH for a variety of conditions, including TS. Though not a formal clinical trial, it illustrates patterns of GH use and documents results achieved in large numbers of patients. The authors report an average gain of 6.4 cm in final height over that expected for patients with TS. Is a 2.5-inch gain worth it? How can we do better? Their study also shows that the treatment duration has a significant impact on the height gained. The patient group with final height data was older when they began GH (12.9 years), and therefore the relatively short treatment period probably limited their overall response. Initiating GH therapy at younger ages will give girls with TS more meaningful gains in adult height and also allow introduction of estrogen at ages more commensurate with the girls' peers.

S.D. Chernausek, M.D.

References

1. Rosenfeld RG, Attie KM, Frane J, et al: Growth hormone therapy of Turner syndrome: beneficial effect on adult height. *J Pediatr* 132:319-324, 1998.
2. Taback SP, Collu R, Deal CL, et al: Does growth-hormone supplementation affect adult height in Turner syndrome? *Lancet* 348:25-27, 1996.

Growth Hormone Treatment in Young Children With Down's Syndrome: Effects on Growth and Psychomotor Development

Annerén G, Tuvemo T, Carlsson-Skwirut C, et al (Uppsala Univ, Sweden; Karolinska Hosp, Stockholm; School of Life Science, Brisbane, Australia)
Arch Dis Child 80:334-338, 1999   17–10

Background.—The cardinal signs of Down syndrome are learning disability and short stature. Insulin-like growth factor I, regulated by growth hormone (GH) from about 6 months of age, may affect brain development. The long-term effects of GH therapy on linear growth and psychomotor development in young children with Down syndrome were investigated.

Methods and Findings.—Fifteen children with Down syndrome were treated with GH—initiated between 6 and 9 months of age—for 3 years. With treatment, mean height increased from -1.8 to -0.8 SD score (Swedish standard), compared with a decline from -1.7 to -2.2 SD score in an untreated control group. After GH therapy was stopped, growth velocity declined. Treatment had no effect on head growth, and no significant between-group differences in mental or gross motor development were noted. During GH treatment, low serum insulin-like growth factor I and insulin-like growth factor binding protein 3 levels normalized (Fig 1).

Conclusion.—GH therapy normalizes growth velocity in infants with Down's syndrome but does not affect head circumference or mental or gross motor development. When GH is stopped, growth velocity declines.

▶ After reading this report you may say, "Why would anyone want to do this study?" Children with Down syndrome are short and making them taller in

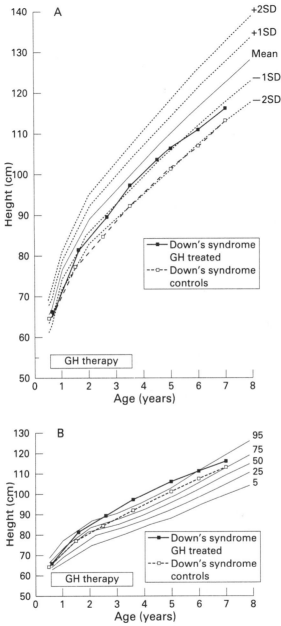

FIGURE 1.—Mean height of 12 boys and 3 girls with Down syndrome treated with GH for 3 years from the age of 6 to 9 months (mean, 7.4 months), compared with that of an untreated group of 6 boys and 9 girls with Down syndrome. **A,** the results are presented on the Swedish growth chart for normal boys. (From Annerén G, Tuvemo T, Carlsson-Skwirut C, et al: Growth hormone treatment in young children with Down's syndrome: Effects on growth and psychomotor development. *Arch Dis Child* 80:334-338, 1999. Courtesy of Karlberg P, Taranger J, Engström J, et al: Physical growth from birth to 16 years and longitudinal outcome of the study during the same period. *Acta Paediatr Suppl* 258:7-76, 1976.) **B,** the results are presented on the growth chart for boys with Down syndrome. (From Annerén G, Tuvemo T, Carlsson-Skwirut C, et al: Growth hormone treatment in young children with Down's syndrome: Effect on growth and psychomotor development. *Arch Dis Child* 80:334-338, 1999. Courtesy of Cronk C, Crocker AC, Peuschel SM, et al: Growth charts for children with Down syndrome: 1 month to 18 years of age. *Pediatrics* 81:102-110, 1988.)

no way is going to relieve them of a significant component of their disability or otherwise diminish whatever stigmatization occurs as the result of having Down syndrome. What is the sense in making a child with Down syndrome taller if it is just for the sake of adding a few inches?

The answer to this question is fairly complex, and, indeed, there may be a rationale for why this study needed to be done. For children with Down syndrome, their growth velocity reduces somewhere between 6 and 9 months and 3 years of age. Children with Down syndrome are usually of normal stature at birth. Between the second half of the first year of life and 3 years of age is also the period when the child with Down syndrome experiences a fall in intelligence. At 12 months of age the average IQ is about 70, but declines to 40 to 50, on average, at 36 months. During the period of decelerated linear growth and a falling IQ, the head circumference is also dropping off.

Thus, growth retardation in Down syndrome becomes pronounced during the period when lots of other things are going on and also during the period when GH normally starts to regulate overall growth. It was not unreasonable for these authors to speculate that there might be some link between what is going on with linear growth and with these other declining parameters. The conclusions are fairly obvious, though, in that although GH will make a child with Down syndrome grow, it does not cause the head to grow nor does it slow down the evolution of developmental lags, including intelligence.

If you care for children with Down syndrome, it is important for you to use the growth charts that are specific for children with this genetic defect. Simply plotting a child's growth with Down syndrome on a standard growth chart provides little useful information about how well that child is doing relative to peers with the same disorder. It is the latter comparison that is important, not the comparison with normal children. If you do not have a copy of the "Chart for Children with Down's Syndrome," see the classic article that appeared in *Pediatrics* in 1988.[1]

This is the last commentary in the Endocrinology chapter, so we'll close with a whodunit. As a pediatric endocrinologist, you occasionally have to cover the adult endocrinology services at your hospital. One weekend, you see a young man who has complaints of hot flashes and gynecomastia. He swears he is taking no medications or recreational drugs. He does not drink alcohol and has no risk factors for other types of liver disease. Physical examination shows bilateral gynecomastia. The penis and testes appear to be normal, as does the facial, axillary, and pubic hair. Liver, kidney, and thyroid functions are normal. Subnormal serum concentrations of testosterone, luteinizing hormone, and follicle-stimulating hormone are found. Serum estradiol concentrations are elevated. You suspect this individual is ingesting some estrogen-like substance. What is the substance?

There are lots of ways that you can unintentionally expose yourself to estrogens or estrogen-like substances in ointments, hair lotions, vaginal creams used by your sexual partners, or embalming cream. Indeed, embalmers are well-known to have an occupational risk of gynecomastia. The young man described above did not have any of these exposures. As it turns out, this fellow consumed large quantities of female urine provided to him at irregular intervals, though generally several times per week, by female sexual partners, at least 3 of whom were consuming estrogen-containing and progestogen-containing drugs, including estradiol, ethinyl estradiol, levonorgestrel, and dydrogesterone. Apparently this cocktail was enjoyed by the patient and the habit he had was continued for several years because he felt it subjectively improved his well-being.

Please note that drinking one's own urine is a traditional yogic practice. Specific data on the consequences of drinking urine are scarce, but the young man described above is the first reported to have partaken of large quantities of urine from members of the opposite sex and to have experienced gynecomastia as a consequence.[2]

Lastly, African American females aged 14 months to 43 years have been reported to have breast tissue and pubic hair development several months after starting the use of estrogen or placenta-containing hair products.[3] I have always wondered why we wasted placentas, but I would never have imagined that someone would want to put such products on her head!

J.A. Stockman III, M.D.

References

1. Cronk C, Crocker AC, Peuschel SM, et al: Growth charts for children with Down syndrome: 1 month to 18 years of age. *Pediatrics* 81:102-110, 1988.
2. Vierhapper H, Nowotny P: Gynecomastia and raised estradiol concentrations. *Lancet* 640:107-108, 1999.
3. Tiwary CM: Premature sexual development in children following the use of estrogen- or placenta-containing hair products. *Clin Pediatr* 37:733-740, 1998.

18 The Musculoskeletal System

The First Certifying Examination in Pediatric Rheumatology
Butzin D, Guerin R, Kredich D (American Board of Pediatrics, Chapel Hill, NC; Duke Univ, Durham, NC)
J Rheumatol 25:1187-1190, 1998   18–1

Background.—The first certifying examination in pediatric rheumatology was administered by the American Board of Pediatrics (ABP) in May 1992 to 94 candidates. This report describes the certifying examination process.

Process.—The ABP established a Sub-board of Pediatric Rheumatology that developed a detailed content outline for the examination. The 1992 examination consisted of 235 items with a 4½-hour time limit. To qualify to take this test, applicants were required to hold a current medical license and current certificate in pediatrics, to be recommended by a program director or chief of pediatrics, and to have the equivalent of 2 years of subspecialty fellowship training or 5 years of a combination of training and practice.

Results.—There were 94 examinees, and 80 passed this test. The total group average score was 76%. There was no significant difference between the average scores of those with and without formal training or between male and female examinees. The passing score was set at 1 standard deviation below the mean of the reference group, examinees with 2 or more years of fellowship training. The passing score was 70.5% correct. Eleven per cent of the passing candidates were international medical graduates. Most of the passing candidates were in their 40s (Fig 1).

Conclusions.—In 1992, 94 candidates sat for the first certifying examination in pediatric rheumatology. The overall pass rate was 85%. A recertification process will be offered beginning in 1999. The certifying examination was offered again in 1994 and 1996. The most recent examination was offered in November 1998. Requirements for future certifying examinations will include 3 years of full time fellowship training and verification of meaningful research.

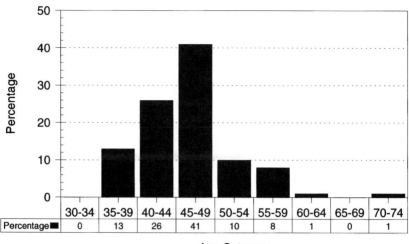

Percentage■	30-34	35-39	40-44	45-49	50-54	55-59	60-64	65-69	70-74
	0	13	26	41	10	8	1	0	1

Age Category

N = 80

FIGURE 1.—1992 Pediatric Rheumatology Certifying Examination. Age distribution of passing candidates. (Courtesy of Butzin D, Guerin R, Kredich D: The first certifying examination in pediatric rheumatology *J Rheumatol* 25:1187-1190, 1998.)

▶ Rheumatologic problems have been around a long time in pediatrics, and so have individuals who have been interested in these disorders. What haven't been around a long time, however, are board-certified pediatric rheumatologists. This is a relatively young subspecialty. The first subspecialists were certified only in 1992, when the first individuals identified themselves as experts in this area by applying for the first examination.

Many don't know how a "new" subspecialty comes about, at least with respect to board certification. It is actually not the ABP that starts the ball rolling in the creation of a new subspecialty. The impetus for this almost invariably comes from within the subspecialty itself. The board does not initiate the process but reacts to proposals from subspecialty professional societies. In considering the establishment of a new subspecialty certification program, the guiding principle is that children will be better served. The pediatric subspecialist is expected to serve as a teacher, a consultant, a researcher, and a provider of complex care but is not to supplant the general pediatrician in providing continuity of care. There must be evidence of a unique body of knowledge and a scientific basis for it. The application for certification in a subspecialty area by a professional society must include documentation of the numbers and distribution of specialists and the professional status of the field, training programs and curriculum, cost of training, and the effect of the new subspecialty on other disciplines. Subspecialty certification addresses these goals by establishing rigorous standards for subspecialty training, by verifying the knowledge base of candidates through a written examination, and by requiring periodic recertification. It was in 1992 that 94 candidates took the first certifying examination in pediatric rheumatology. Eighty passed. A second certifying examination was offered in 1994 and 1996, and a fourth examination was given in 1998. Currently, all applicants for examination must have had 3 years of full-time fellowship training after 3 years of residency in general pediatrics.

It is worthwhile every now and then to explain how a new subspecialty area comes about, at least with respect to physician certification. Recently two "new" subspecialty areas were approved: neurodevelopmental disabilities in childhood and developmental-behavioral pediatrics. Both of these subspecialty areas have faced an uphill battle in establishing themselves as creditable disciplines, since some care providers outside the community of pediatrics have thought that these disciplines were unnecessary. Thank goodness, advocacy on the part of children by those in the pediatric community and supporters elsewhere has seemed to swing the rhetoric toward acceptance of these disciplines as creditable and worthy of subspecialty certification.

J.A. Stockman III, M.D.

Clinical Criteria for Using Radiography for Children With Acute Knee Injuries
Cohen DM, Jasser JW, Kean JR, et al (Ohio State Univ, Columbus)
Pediatr Emerg Care 14:185-187, 1998   18–2

Background.—Acute knee injuries are common in children seen in the emergency department (ED), and radiographs are often obtained. However, knee fractures in this population are uncommon. Clinical criteria for selective radiography in children with injured knees were evaluated.

Methods.—The records of all children assessed radiographically for an isolated, acute knee injury in 1 ED during 1 year were analyzed. Exclusion criteria were injuries sustained more than 1 week earlier, injury isolated to superficial lacerations or abrasions, previous knee injury, and reassessment.

Findings.—Of the 254 patients in the study, 12 (4.7%) had a fracture. Inability to bear weight in the ED and inability to flex to 90° were associated with fracture. Point tenderness was not significantly correlated with fracture. Inability to bear weight combined with inability to flex to 90° would reduce the number of radiographs by 73%, with no fractures missed.

Conclusions.—The use of these clinical criteria to select children needing knee radiography may markedly decrease the number of unnecessary radiographs obtained in the ED. Point tenderness did not predict knee fracture well in this population.

▶ When was the last time you made a diagnosis of a broken knee? Probably never. The reason why is straightforward. Pain in the knee rarely is associated with a fracture. That, at least, is the situation in children. In adults, the rules are different. You will not miss a fracture in and about the knee if you do an x-ray on everyone who has knee pain, who is older than 55 years, who has tenderness at the head of the fibula, tenderness of the patella, an inability to flex the knee to 90°, or an inability to bear weight, both immediately after injury and in the ED. Any 1 of these in an adult is an indication for x-rays. These authors point out that no fractures would be missed if you ordered an x-ray in a child with knee pain if that child also had an inability to bear weight immediately after an injury or had difficulty flexing the knee to 90°. Clearly, radiography for knee injuries in children seems to be overused. It's not that children can't fracture their tibia, patella, or femur and experience knee pain, it's just that these are relatively uncommon circumstances as causes of knee pain. Following a few simple guidelines will allow you to make a diagnosis in those who do have a fracture without overusing x-rays in those who don't. Isn't it sweet?

Other things can also be a problem when you exercise. See if you can figure out the following. You practice pediatrics in Chicago. One busy morning you see 4 college-aged patients with the same signs and symptoms: chills, headache, myalgia, diarrhea, eye pain, and red eyes. They are all moderately ill. The only thing they have shared in common was that they had participated in a recent triathlon that took place in Springfield, Illinois. What do you suspect might have been going on? The Centers for Disease Control immediately knew what was going on. These patients, and 11% of everyone else who participated in the triathlon in downstate Illinois in mid-1998, came down with an acute febrile illness caused by a *Leptospira* infection. Leptospira infect a variety of domestic and wild animals. When these animals urinate, leptospira organisms find their way to damp soil, vegetation, mud, and fresh water ponds and lakes. No natural body of water can be expected to be totally free of leptospira.

Leptospirosis, the 842nd reason not to exercise.[1]

J.A. Stockman III, M.D.

Reference

1. Update: Leptospirosis and unexplained acute febrile illness among athletes participating in triathlons—Illinois and Wisconsin, 1998 (editorial). *MMWR* 47:673-676, 1998.

Effectiveness of Active Physical Training as Treatment for Long-standing Adductor-related Groin Pain in Athletes: Randomised Trial
Hölmich P, Uhrskou P, Ulnits L, et al (Amarger Univ, Denmark; Herlev Univ, Denmark; Glostrup Univ, Denmark; et al)
Lancet 353:439-443, 1999   18–3

Background.—Groin pain is a common problem for athletes in many sports. Although many disorders can cause groin pain, 1 of the most frequent causes is injury to the adductor muscle. Previous research has shown that exercises designed to strengthen a muscle might protect it from injury. These authors evaluated whether a physiotherapy (PT) program

Panel 1: **Elements of AT**

Module 1 (first 2 weeks)

1 Static adduction against soccer ball placed between feet when lying supine; each adduction 30 s, ten repetitions.
2 Static adduction against soccer ball placed between knees when lying supine; each adduction 30s, ten repetitions.
3 Abdominal sit-ups both in straightforward direction and in oblique direction; five series of ten repetitions.
4 Combined abdominal sit-up and hip flexion, starting from supine position and with soccer ball placed between knees (folding knife exercise); five series of ten repetitions.
5 Balance training on wobble board for 5 min.
6 One-foot exercises on sliding board, with parallel feet as well as with 90° angle between feet; five sets of 1 min continuous work with each leg, and in both positions.

Module II (from third week; module II was done twice at each training session)

1 Leg abduction and adduction exercises lying on side; five series of ten repetitions of each exercise.
2 Low-back extension exercises prone over end of couch; five series of ten repetitions.
3 One-leg weight-pulling abduction/adduction standing; five series of ten repetitions for each leg.
4 Abdominal sit-ups both in straightforward direction and in oblique direction; five series of ten repetitions.
5 One-leg coordination exercise flexing and extending knee and swinging arms in same rhythm (cross country skiing on one leg); five series of ten repetitions for each leg.
6 Training in sidewards motion on a "Fitter" (rocking base curved on top and bottom; user stands on platform that rolls laterally on tracks on top of rocking base) for 5 min.
7 Balance training on wobble board for 5 min.
8 Skating movements on sliding board; five times 1 min continuous work.

PANEL 1.—Elements of Active Training. (Courtesy of Hölmich P, Uhrskou P, Ulnits L, et al: Effectiveness of active physical training as treatment for long-standing adductor-related groin pain in athletes: Randomised trial. *Lancet* 353[9151]:439-443, 1999. Copyright by The Lancet, Ltd.)

that included active training (AT) for the adductor muscle would reduce pain in athletes with long-standing adductor-related groin pain.

Methods.—Sixty-eight male athletes had experienced sports-related groin pain for 2 or more months. None of men had inguinal or femoral hernia; prostatitis; urinary tract disease; vertebral pain; fracture of the pelvis or lower extremities; nerve entrapment of the ilioinguinal, genito-femoral, or lateral femoral cutaneous nerves; hip-joint disease; or bursitis of the hip or groin. All of the men experienced 2 or more of the following symptoms suggestive of adductor involvement: a characteristic symptom history (e.g., groin pain with coughing or sneezing), pain upon palpation of the symphysis joint, increased scintigraphic activity in the pubic bone,

Panel 2: Elements of PT

1 Laser treatment with a gallium aluminium arsen laser (Endolaser 465B; Enraf Nonius, Hvidovre, Denmark). All painful points of the adductor-tendon insertion at the pubic bone received treatment for 1 min, receiving 0·9 mJ per treated point. The probe was in contact with the skin at 90° angle.. The laser was fitted with an 830 nm (±0·5 nm) 30 mW, diode. Beam divergence was 4° and area of probe head was 2·5 mm².

2 Transverse friction massage for 10 min on painful area of adductor-tendon insertion into pubic bone.

3 Stretching of adductor muscles, hamstring muscles, and hip flexors. The contract-relax technique was used. The stretching was repeated three times and the duration of each stretch was 30 s.

4 Transcutaneous electrical nerve stimulation was given for 30 min at painful area. The apparatus used was a Biometer, Elpha 500, frequency 100 Hz and a pulse width of one and a maximum of 15 mA (100% effect).

PANEL 2.—Elements of Physiotherapy. (Courtesy of Hölmich P, Uhrskou P, Ulnits L, et al: Effectiveness of active physical training as treatment for long-standing adductor-related groin pain in athletes: Randomised trial. *Lancet* 353[9151]:439-443. Copyright 1999 by The Lancet, Ltd.)

and osteitis pubis around the symphysis joint. Subjects were randomly assigned to an AT program (n = 34) (Panel 1) or a PT program that did not involve AT (n = 34) (Panel 2). The AT program was targeted at improving strength and coordination of the muscles (especially the adductor) that act on the pelvis. Both programs were followed for 8 to 12 weeks, and participants were evaluated 4 months after the end of treatment to determine groin symptoms and current athletic involvement.

Findings.—Four months after the end of treatment, significantly more participants in the AT group had excellent outcomes (23 vs 4 participants) and were able to return to athletic participation without groin pain. Multiple regression analysis indicated that participants were much more likely to have unilateral rather than bilateral groin pain (odds ratio, 6.6 vs bilateral pain). After adjustment for unilateral groin pain in the model, men in the AT group were markedly less likely to experience pain (odds ratio, 12.7 vs PT group). Participants in the AT group also rated their improvement significantly better than men in the PT group rated theirs.

Conclusions.—An active training program to strengthen and improve coordination of the pelvic muscles (especially the adductor muscle) was effective in the treatment of long-standing adductor-related groin pain. Whether such an active training program could prevent adductor-related groin pain is worth investigation.

▶ There are no pediatricians who care for teenage athletes who have not recognized the problems associated with trying to figure out why one or another youngster engaged in sporting activities develops groin pain. In most cases, the pain is related to adductor muscle groups. The trick is to find a form of physical therapy that is effective without making the situation worse. What we learn from our colleagues in the Department of Orthopaedic Surgery at the Amarger University Hospital in Denmark is that one must be very precise about the type of physical therapy programs one chooses. For example, standard physical therapy programs, particularly those involving stretching exercises, only make the situation worse. On the other hand, physiotherapists experienced in active training programs aimed at coordination and strengthening of the muscles that stabilize the pelvis and hip joints, in particular the abductor muscles, will succeed more often than not. Obviously, the easiest way to treat a problem is to prevent it. Given the fact that athletes will be athletes, however, it's nice to know that there are forms of physical therapy that will work for common ailments like groin pain.

The preceding commentary ended with a whodunit, so this one, also on the topic of traumatic injuries, will as well. A 16-year-old boy comes into the emergency room with 24-hour history of pain in the right hip, causing him to limp. He is a known gymnast and recently has been exercising up to 4 hours a day in preparation for competition at the national level. He is taking no medications and denies taking anabolic steroids. His physical examination shows him to hold the hip in flexion. On extension, he is tender over the right hip. Abduction is normal, but there is slight pain on terminal flexion. He walks with a pronounced limp. Plain x-rays of the pelvis and hips have normal results. A CBC and sedimentation rate are also normal. A US of the hips is normal. Your diagnosis?

This patient exhibits what otherwise would be best termed the 843rd reason not to exercise. The patient described was a real one with a traumatic myositis of the psoas muscle. The diagnosis was made when a radioisotopic bone scan was performed to exclude bone abnormalities and possibly also aseptic arthritis. The scan showed normal uptake in the hips but revealed high uptake throughout the region of the right psoas muscle. A subsequent limited CT scan of the retroperitoneal space to exclude a psoas abscess showed enlargement of both psoas muscles, especially on the right. There was no evidence of abscess.[1]

"Psoas" not to hurt yourself, make gymnastics a visual sport; be an observer, rather than a participant.

J.A. Stockman III, M.D.

Reference

1. Stabler J: A case of traumatic myositis of the psoas in a gymnast. *Injury* 28:489-490, 1997.

Chronic Musculoskeletal Pain in Childhood
Song KM, Morton AA, Koch KD, et al (Children's Hosp and Med Ctr of Seattle, Wash; Texas Scottish Rite Hosp for Children, Dallas)
J Pediatr Orthop 18:576-581, 1998   18–4

Objective.—As many as 7% of school-age children have musculoskeletal pain that lasts longer than 3 months. No organic cause could be found in half of the children evaluated by these authors for chronic musculoskeletal or back pain. The Inappropriate Symptom Checklist (Fig 1) was evaluated to determine whether it could distinguish organic from inorganic pain in the pediatric population. Psychological profiles of children with organic and nonorganic pain were compared with each other and with those of pain-free children.

Methods.—Psychological profiles of 73 children, aged 8 to 16 years, with chronic pain or recurrent musculoskeletal pain of 6 weeks' or more

PLEASE CHECK ANY OF THE ITEMS THAT APPLY. IF NONE APPLY, LEAVE BLANK AND RETURN TO PSYCHOLOGY

INAPPROPRIATE SYMPTOM CHECKLIST

PATIENT'S NAME:_____ TSRHC ID #:_____

PHYSICIAN:_____ _____

NON-ORGANIC PHYSICAL SIGNS
1. Tenderness:
_____ Superficial-skin tender to light pinch over a wide area.
_____ Non-anatomic-deep tenderness over a wide area, not localized to an anatomic compartment or structure.
2. Simulation of Motion:
_____ Hip/knee/ankle (or other joint) pain with motion of the whole extremity which imitates motion of that specific joint.
3. Distraction:
A usual examination method is done and if positive the patient's position is changed and the exam repeated in a way that the patient will not recognize it. The best example is straight leg raising sitting vs. lying down, done sitting as if to look at the bottom of the foot.
4. Regional Findings:
_____ Non-anatomic sensory findings such as stocking anesthesia.
_____ Weakness of unusual nature such as giving way of many muscle groups that cannot be explained on a localized neurological basis,
5. Over-reaction (such as):
_____ Verbalization
_____ Facial expressions
_____ Unusual muscle tension
_____ Tremor
_____ Collapsing
_____ Sweating
6. Inappropriate Symptoms (include):
_____ Pain at the tip of the tail-bone
_____ Whole leg (or other extremity) painful
_____ Whole leg (or other extremity) numb
_____ Whole leg giving way
_____ 'In the past year have you had any spells with very little pain?' (No is a positive response for inappropriateness.)
7. Other:_____

FIGURE 1.—Inappropriate symptom checklist. (Courtesy of Song KM, Morton AA, Koch KD, et al: Chronic musculoskeletal pain in childhood. *J Pediatr Orthop* 18[5]:576-581, 1998.)

TABLE 1.—Medical Diagnosis of Organic Pain Group

Diagnosis	No.
JRA	12
Mixed connective tissue disease	3
Lupus	1
Psoriatic arthritis	2
Dermatomyositis	1
Lumbosacral plexitis	1
Legg-Perthes disease	4
Patellar dislocation	2
Spondylolysis	2
S/P posterior spinal fusion	2
Herniated nucleous pulposus	1
Wrist fracture	1
Osteochondritis dissecans	1
Shingles	2
Demyelinating motor and sensory neuropathy	1
Multiple hereditary exostosis	1
Total	37

(Courtesy of Song KM, Morton AA, Koch KD, et al: Chronic musculoskeletal pain in childhood. *J Pediatr Orthop* 18[5]:576-581, 1998.)

duration and of 14 control children (4 boys) were obtained. The Inappropriate Symptom Checklist was completed by each child's physician at the initial visit. Physicians rated their perceptions of each child's pain. There were 37 children (6 boys), aged 5 to 16 years, in the organic pain group and 36 (6 boys), aged 8 to 17 years, in the nonorganic pain group. The diagnoses are listed in Table 1.

Results.—The average Inappropriate Symptom Checklist score was 3, and two thirds of the nonorganic pain group had 2 or more checks. The average cost of evaluation was $4196, with an average hospital stay of 12 days. Seventy percent of the children incurred additional costs at other medical institutions. The organic pain group had an average Inappropriate Symptom Checklist score of 1.5. In 23 of 30 children with no inappropriate symptoms (76.7%), an organic cause was diagnosed. In 23 of 35 children with 2 or more inappropriate symptoms (65.7%), no organic cause was found. There were no differences in psychological values between groups, but significantly more children with nonorganic pain had relatives with chronic illnesses or pain.

Conclusion.—Among children with chronic pain, the Inappropriate Symptom Checklist was useful in separating those with an organic etiology from those with a nonorganic cause. Early psychological intervention is recommended for children with nonorganic pain to improve outcome.

▶ One of life's great challenges for the pediatrician is sorting out whether a child complaining of musculoskeletal pain has pain that is organic in origin or pain that is nonorganic in origin. As we see in this report, the differentiation in children is nowhere nearly as easy as in adults. The type of pain behavior that youngsters with nonorganic pain have more often than not does not assist us in clearly separating in a simple manner an organic diagnosis from a nonorganic diagnosis. This is one reason the cost of an evaluation runs so high in youngsters. In this report, such costs ran in excess of $4000 per case.

The value of this study from Texas is that it provides us with a checklist that sometimes will be helpful in distinguishing children who are likely to have a definable reason for their pain. Children without an identifiable cause should not be brushed off. They must not be classified as having psycho-somatic, hysterical, conversion, or somatization disorders, or hypochondri-asis with all the negative connotations associated with such diagnoses. Such terminology is best left on the chart since chronic pain, whether of organic or nonorganic cause, carries with it serious morbidity in childhood and screams out for proper management.

On a related topic, in the Newborn chapter, the subject of the illicit use of human recombinant erythropoietin by athletes was discussed (Abstract 1–7), as were the International Amateur Athletic Federation (IAAF) guide-lines which exclude any athlete with a hemoglobin concentration greater than 18.5 g/dL or a hematocrit value equal to or greater than 50% from competition on the basis of possible human erythropoietin use. But are such limits reasonable? Is there a variation between the type of athletic compe-tition and the normative range of hematologic values?

The answers are yes and yes. Yes, a hemoglobin of 18.5 and a hematocrit of 50% are reasonable ceilings in nonsmoking athletes. Such figures have been established as upper ranges of "normal," for example, for professional cyclists.[1] A recent study, however, finds that the normal range for hemoglo-bin and hematocrit in athletes very much depends on the type of athletic competition an individual is trained for. For example, power athletes (wres-tlers, etc.) tend to have lower hemoglobin and hematocrit values, averaging 14.9 g/dL and 43%, respectively. Endurance runners have hemoglobin levels that average 0.6 g/dL higher and hematocrit values 1% higher, respectively. The mean corpuscular hemoglobin concentration and volume are also sig-nificantly higher in endurance runners than in speed and power athletes. A 90th percentile for hemoglobin and hematocrit in endurance runners is 16.9 g/dL and 47%. If you see numbers higher than these, think about the possibility of doping.

J.A. Stockman III, M.D.

Reference

1. Saris WHM, Senden JMG, Brouns F: What is a normal-red cell mass for profes-sional cyclists? *Lancet* 352:1758, 1998.

Developmental Dysplasia of the Hip: A New Approach to Incidence
Bialik V, Bialik GM, Blazer S, et al (Rambam Med Ctr, Haifa, Israel; Technion-Israel Inst of Technology, Haifa)
Pediatrics 103:93-99, 1999   18–5

Background.—The incidence of developmental dysplasia of the hip (DDH) is unclear, mainly because criteria for defining a genuinely abnormal neonatal hip are ambiguous. An algorithm was developed to identify neonatal hips that, if untreated, would cause dysplasia to develop.

Methods.—Clinical and US assessment for DDH were done on 18,060 consecutive neonatal hips at 1 to 3 days of life. The study population did not include infants with skeletal deformities, neurologic or muscular disorders, or neural tube defects. Hips with any type of abnormality on US were examined again at 2 or 6 weeks, depending on the severity of the findings. Only hips with no improvement or deterioration of the initial abnormality were treated. The remainder were assessed periodically until the children were 12 months of age.

Findings.—Sonographic screening revealed 1001 deviations, for sonographic DDH incidence of 55.1 per 1000 hips. However, abnormalities persisted in only 90 hips, reducing the true incidence of DDH to 5 per 1000 hips. All other hips developed into normal hips. No additional instances of DDH were noted during follow-up.

Conclusion.—Two categories of neonatal hip abnormalities exist: one that eventually develops into a normal hip ("sonographic DDH") and one that deteriorates into a dysplastic hip, including full dislocation ("true DDH"). This classification system allows for a clear definition of DDH, enabling a more accurate determination of its incidence and more appropriate management.

▶ This report confirms what most have accepted, namely, that a high percentage of newborns with clinical and/or sonographic evidence of DDH will get better on their own. Indeed, it was Barlow himself who said that 88% of babies with a diagnosis of DDH would self-correct, no therapy being needed.[1] What is meritorious about the article abstracted is that it uses a combination of neonatal clinical examination and US to give us the "true" incidence of DDH, not only in the immediate newborn, but also in infants at several weeks of age. We find that about 5% of babies will have either positive results of a physical examination for DDH or positive US results shortly after birth. Of that figure, however, only about 10% remain abnormal at several weeks of age and require treatment. Based on this, the suggested incidence of DDH requiring treatment is only about 5 cases per 1000 newborns.

One of the true gurus of DDH—particularly with respect to much of the knowledge that we now have about the role of sonograms—is Dr. Ted Harcke from the Alfred I. duPont Institute in Wilmington, Delaware. In an editorial that accompanied the article abstracted, Dr. Harcke reminds us of 3 things. First he recalls for us the fact that regardless of how DDH is defined and its incidence calculated, the natural history of this condition is that most—overwhelmingly most—infants improve spontaneously with time and, therefore, would have required no treatment. Unfortunately, there are no up front findings that tell us which will and which will not ultimately respond on their own. Secondly, he reminds us that DDH is not a congenital problem and can actually show up *after* the newborn period; thus, the reason for the use of the current nomenclature rather than the original term, congenital dysplasia. Lastly, he recalls for us that sonography is extremely sensitive and will pick up lesions that are not detectable on clinical examination.

So if you are really uptight about the problem of missing DDH based solely on a clinical examination, sonography is your resource.[2]

By the time this commentary appears, we will likely have already seen the new American Academy of Pediatrics guidelines regarding DDH. These guidelines will clarify for you the role of sonography and the indications for initial treatment. If the prevalence of DDH requiring treatment turns out to be 5 cases per 1000 newborns, it will be very hard to justify a recommendation for routine sonographic detection screening in all newborns.

There is an art to medicine and to pediatrics in particular. The art of the physical examination should be the litmus test by which decisions are made about which baby has enough of a problem with DDH to require follow-up and, possibly, treatment. Please note that the treatment of DDH is not totally without its risks. Avascular necrosis post treatment is a known problem in a small, but real, subset of children.[3]

J.A. Stockman III, M.D.

References

1. Barlow TG: Early diagnosis and treatment of congenital dislocation of the hip. *J Bone Joint Surg* 44:292-301, 1962.
2. Harcke HT: Developmental dysplasia of the hip: A spectrum of abnormality. *Pediatrics* 103:152, 1999.
3. Segal LS, Boal DK, Borthwick L, et al: Avascular necrosis after treatment of DDH: The protective influence of the ossific nucleus. *J Pediatr Orthop* 19:177-184, 1999.

Inherited Risk Factors for Thrombophilia Among Children With Legg-Calvé-Perthes Disease
Arruda VR, Belangero WD, Ozelo MC, et al (State Univ of Campinas, Brazil; Univ of São Paulo, Brazil)
J Pediatr Orthop 19:84-87, 1999   18–6

Introduction.—Characterized by aseptic necrosis of the proximal femoral epiphysis, Legg-Calvé-Perthes disease is a self-limited pediatric hip disorder. The potential cause of this disease may be an impairment of the blood supply to the femoral head, probably from extrinsic compression of the vessels, as well as intravascular thrombosis. In up to 50% of patients who had a poor anticoagulant response of plasma to activated protein C, inherited thrombophilia was associated with a point mutation in the factor V Leiden. The most common inherited risk factors for hypercoagulability were investigated, including the mutation in the factor V gene, also known as factor V Leiden, the transition 20.210 G→A in the prothrombin gene, and also the homozygosity for the 677C→T transition in the methylene-tetrahydrofolate reductase gene.

Methods.—There were 61 children with Legg-Calvé-Perthes disease compared with 296 controls. Genomic DNA was obtained from the peripheral blood of the participants. A molecular diagnosis was performed.

Results.—In the patients with Legg-Calvé-Perthes, the prevalence of the factor V Leiden mutation was higher than in the controls (4.9 vs 0.7%). The prothrombin gene variant was not in any patient. When homozygosity for the methylenetetrahydrofolate reductase gene was determined, there was no difference between patients and controls (3.2% vs 2.6%).

Conclusion.—The only inherited risk factor associated with the development of Legg-Calvé-Perthes disease was the heterozygosity for factor V Leiden in this population. The risk for Legg-Calvé-Perthes disease was not increased by the prothrombin variant and the methylenetetrahydrofolate reductase gene, even though they were previously associated with vascular disease.

▶ This must be the year of the thrombophilia. Actually, it's probably the decade of the thrombophilia in as much as the topic of why children (and adults) clot too much was re-energized in the early 1990s with the description of the factor V Leiden mutation. Now we see that inherited thrombophilias are also a cause of common orthopedic problems, specifically Legg-Calvé-Perthes disease. The latter is what we also call idiopathic avascular necrosis of the femoral head.

The etiology of Legg-Calvé-Perthes disease has been unknown, although trauma, transient synovitis, venous congestion, hyperviscosity, coagulation abnormalities, and other mechanisms have been suggested. Recently, Glueck et al.[1] found evidence for inherited thrombophilia in approximately 75% of investigated patients suffering from this orthopedic difficulty. We see in the study from Brazil that heterozygosity for factor V Leiden was the only inherited risk factor associated with the development of Legg-Calvé-Perthes disease, albeit at a much lower rate of causality than earlier suggested.

The question of whether inherited thrombotic disorders are in fact *the* etiology of Legg-Calvé-Perthes disease remains open, particularly since a recent study from Austria examining 44 patients with this problem found only about 10% of cases could be ascribed to an inherited thrombophilia.[2] Not so controversial is the increased frequency of genetic thrombophilia in women with complications of pregnancy. You may wish to look at Abstract 1–3, which summarizes recent information demonstrating that women with serious obstetric complications have an increased incidence of mutations predisposing them to thrombosis and other inherited and acquired forms of excessive clotting.

While we're on the topic of things that cause hip and knee pain, please recognize that these represent signs and symptoms of a very old occupational hazard. A study of the skeletons stored beneath the crypt of St. Stephen's Monastery in Jerusalem has shown that almost all the monks buried there had arthritis of the knees.[3] The skeletons themselves are about 1500 years old. The assumption is that the knee damage was associated with frequent kneeling as the monks went through their daily pattern of worship. Is this the reason why present-day monks mostly stand during prayers?

J.A. Stockman III, M.D.

References

1. Glueck CA, Glueck HI, Greenfield D, et al: Protein C and protein S deficiency, thrombophilia, and hypofibrinolysis: Pathophysiologic causes of Legg-Perthes disease. *Pediatr Res* 35:383-388, 1994.
2. Gallistl S, Reitinger T, Linhart W, et al: The role of inherited thrombotic disorders and the etiology of Legg-Calvé-Perthes disease. *J Pediatr Orthopaed* 19:82-83, 1999.
3. Monks and arthritis (editorial). *The Sciences* 37:11, 1997.

Lyme Arthritis in Children: Clinical Epidemiology and Long-term Outcomes
Gerber MA, Zemel LS, Shapiro ED (Univ of Connecticut, Hartford; Yale Univ, New Haven, Conn)
Pediatrics 102:905-908, 1998   18–7

Introduction.—In areas of the country in which Lyme disease is endemic, the disease has become a relatively common cause of arthritis among children. There is a fear that in children who acquire Lyme disease with arthritic complications chronic, debilitating joint disease will develop despite appropriate antimicrobial therapy. Little is known about the long-term outcomes of children with Lyme arthritis who have not received appropriate antimicrobial therapy. To determine the clinical epidemiology of Lyme arthritis in children as well as their long-term outcomes, a long-term follow-up study was conducted.

Methods.—There were 90 children with a mean age of 8.3 years who were given a diagnosis of Lyme arthritis; 63% were boys. To obtain demographic, clinical, and follow-up data, medical records were reviewed and structured telephone interviews were conducted.

Results.—In 26% of the children, Lyme arthritis was preceded by early Lyme disease. However, appropriate antimicrobial therapy was given to only 35% of these children at that early stage. Arthritis of at least one knee was found in 90% of the children, whereas small joints were rarely involved (Table 1). There were 31 children who had arthrocentesis, and

TABLE 1.—Joints Affected in Children With Lyme Arthritis

Joint	No. (%)
Knee	81 (90)
Hip	13 (14)
Ankle	9 (10)
Wrist	8 (9)
Elbow	6 (7)
Others	6 (7)
Single joint	57 (63)
Multiple joints	33 (37)
Oligorticular (<4 joints)	90 (100)

(Reproduced by permission of *Pediatrics*, from Gerber MA, Zernel LS, Shapiro ED: Lyme arthritis in children: Clinical epidemiology and long-term outcomes. *Pediatrics* 102:905-908, 1998.)

their mean white blood cell count in the synovial fluid was 38,000 cells/mm³, with predominantly neutrophils (Fig 1). An erythrocyte sedimentation rate was determined for 79 children; the highest level for 77% of the children was more than 20 mm/hr, whereas for the rest it was more than 50 mm/hr. After the onset of symptoms, antimicrobial therapy was begun at 2 days to 5.5 years, with a median of 2 months. Antimicrobial therapy was not used at all for 5 of the children. A single episode of arthritis was reported by 51% of the children, whereas recurrent episodes of arthritis over a period of 1 week to 8 years was reported by 49% of the children. Chronic arthritis occurred in 2 children (2%); they had arthroscopic synovectomy. Ongoing musculoskeletal complaints that resulted in mild-to-moderate impairment in school or sports activities was found in 4 children at the follow-up, which was performed at a median of 7 years after the onset of the Lyme disease. None of these children had evidence of active arthritis.

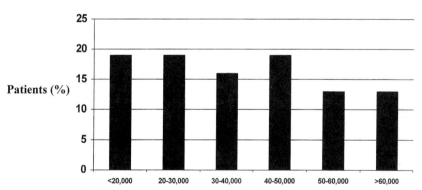

FIGURE 1.—White blood cell count in the synovial fluid of the 31 children who underwent arthrocentesis. (Reproduced by permission of *Pediatrics*, from Gerber MA, Zernel LS, Shapiro ED: Lyme arthritis in children: Clinical epidemiology and long-term outcomes. *Pediatrics* 102:905-908, 1998.)

Conclusion.—There is an excellent prognosis for children with Lyme arthritis who are treated with appropriate antimicrobial therapy.

▶ The more we learn about Lyme disease, the more we learn. In this case, we learn about both the presentation of Lyme arthritis and the long-term outcome of Lyme arthritis in children. Please note, however, that Lyme arthritis does not equal Lyme disease per se. This series consists of selected patients and is not population based. Thus, no comment can be made about the actual incidence of Lyme arthritis among children with Lyme disease, and the article makes no comment about the incidence of Lyme arthritis among children in the general population. In those children with Lyme disease in whom Lyme arthritis develops, we learn that single-joint disease is more common than multiple-joint (by a ratio of about 2:1). We also learn that "big" joints are more likely to be the joints involved, with the knee being the predominant one. Although the long-term outcome of children with Lyme arthritis appropriately treated with antimicrobial therapy is excellent, chronic arthritis is a real possibility in a subset of children.

Only a handful of studies have addressed the long-term outcomes in pediatric Lyme disease. Without antibiotic treatment, the possibility of late sequelae is real.[1] More recently, Salazar et al.[2] reported the results of a telephone follow-up of more than 5 dozen children with Lyme disease who received antibiotic treatment with penicillin, amoxicillin, tetracycline, or doxycycline. As long as 6 years after the acute illness, none of these children reported persistent arthritis, carditis, or neurologic disease. In a follow-up survey of the entire year-round population of Nantucket Island, Mass, there was no higher prevalence of musculoskeletal or neurologic symptoms, examination abnormalities, abnormal EKGs, or behavioral difficulties in children with a diagnosis of Lyme disease than in those with no history of the disease.[3] Abstract 18–8 provides details on this. The importance of the Nantucket study is that it is a report on long-term outcomes in patients with pediatric Lyme disease based on a whole population rather than on a clinical series of children presenting with only arthritis.

Although only a few pediatric patients with Lyme arthritis go on to have treatment-resistant chronic problems, those who do are indeed tough to treat. We now know that this may represent an autoimmune disease or an immune reaction to *Borrelia burgdorferi*, which upregulates a human protein known as leukocyte function–associated antigen 1 and starts a vicious cycle in which T cells continue to react to leukocyte function–associated antigen 1 even after the spirochete has been eliminated.[4]

Thank goodness for the Lyme vaccine. Even though we still don't know exactly who should receive it and for how many times, at least we have a crutch to lean on, knowing that there is something we can do to beat this tick-borne disease.

Chances are that Lyme disease is not as new as one might think. While this disease caused by *B. burgdorferi* was first reported in the United States not that long ago, the total number of cases seen in both the United States and Europe exceeds 12,000 each year. It was recently also described for the first time in Southeast Asia. A 45-year-old man living in Northern Taiwan was diagnosed in 1998. Investigators from the National Defense Medical Center (Taipei, Taiwan) have demonstrated that as many as 28% of rodents living in rural Taiwan are infected with *Borrelia* organisms.

The international team that tracks Lyme disease notes that even though this entity was initially identified only 20 years ago, it is so well-established throughout the northern hemisphere that it must be very old indeed. They also note that there is a wide degree of strain diversity that varies according to geography. Each strain is associated with a different pathologic and clinical presentation.[5]

J.A. Stockman III, M.D.

References

1. Szer IS, Taylor E, Steere AC: Long-term outcome of Lyme arthritis in children. *N Engl J Med* 325:159-163, 1991.
2. Salazar JC, Gerber MA, Goff CW: Long-term outcome of Lyme disease in children given early treatment. *J Pediatr* 122:591-593, 1993.
3. Wang TJ, Sangha O, Phillips CB, et al: Outcomes of children treated for Lyme disease. *J Rheumatol* 25:2249-2253, 1998.
4. Gross D: Treatment-resistant Lyme arthritis: An autoimmune disease? *Science* 271:703-706, 1998.
5. Moore P: Has Lyme disease crossed the Pacific Ocean? *Lancet* 351:963, 1998.

Emergency Department Presentations of Lyme Disease in Children
Bachman DT, Srivastava G (Univ of Vermont, Burlington; Univ of Texas, Houston)
Pediatr Emerg Care 14:356-361, 1998   18–8

Introduction.—The most commonly reported tick-borne disease is Lyme disease, with most cases occurring in the coastal Northeast, the Midwest, and the far West. A significant rate of misdiagnosis, partly caused by indiscriminate use of serologic tests, is accompanied by the current rise in the number of strictly defined cases of Lyme disease. It is not known how accurate practitioners of emergency medicine are in their recognition of Lyme disease. The clinical features of children with Lyme disease who came to an emergency department (ED) during a recent 3-year period were described.

Methods.—Pediatric patients who received a final diagnosis of Lyme disease during a 3-year period were included in a retrospective study of their demographic, historical, clinical, and laboratory data.

Results.—Subsequent to a visit to a pediatric ED, 29 children, ranging in age from 3 to 19 years, received a diagnosis of Lyme disease. Early localized disease with erythema migrans and varying degrees of systemic symptoms were seen in 4 patients. Early disseminated Lyme disease was seen in 10 patients with multiple erythema migrans, neurologic involvement, or carditis. Late Lyme disease with arthritis was identified in 15 patients. It was difficult to diagnose Lyme arthritis: 6 children were initially diagnosed with septic arthritis and 6 had arthrotomy. These patients

TABLE 3.—Stages of Lyme Disease and Recommendations for Testing and Treatment

Stage and Common Clinical Manifestations	Time of Onset Relative to Tickbite	Recommended Serologic Testing	Recommended Treatment*
Early localized disease Erythema migrans (EM) (may be accompanied by systemic systems)	7 to 14 days (range 3 to 28 days)	None if diagnosis certain (generally negative in early disease)	Age < 9 yr Amoxicillin 50 mg/kg/day divided tid × 21 days Age > 9 yr Doxycycline 100 mg bid × 21 days Alternative: Erythromycin 30-50 mg/kg/day divided qid × 21 days
Early disseminated disease Secondary EM Cranioneuropathy Aseptic meningitis Carditis, conduction delay Flu like illness without EM (rare)	2 to 12 wk	ELISA‡ (Western blot if equivocal) Treat based on clinical findings, exposure Consider repeat testing in 2 to 4 wk if initially negative	Secondary EM, cranioneuropathy†: As for erythema migrans Meningitis, carditis: Ceftriaxone 50-80 mg/kg/day single dose (max 2 g) × 14 to 21 days OR Penicillin G 200,000-400,000 units/kg/day (max 20 million units/day) divided q4th × 14 to 21 days
Late disease Arthritis Chronic CNS disease (rare)	6 wk to 2 years	ELISA (Western blot if equivocal) If negative Lyme disease unlikely	As for erythema migrans × 30 days Consider nonsteroidal anti-inflammatory Refractory arthritis, chronic CNS disease: As for meningitis

*Treatment may precipitate Jarisch-Herxheimer reaction.
†Corticosteroids not recommended for cranioneuropathy.
‡Enzyme-linked immunoabsorbent assay.
(Courtesy of Bachman DT, Srivastava G: Emergency department presentations of Lyme disease in children. *Pediatr Emerg Care* 14[5]:356-360, 1998.)

had marked elevations of the erythrocyte sedimentation rate and synovial fluid white blood cell counts, making it difficult to distinguish Lyme disease from septic arthritis. Lyme disease is a condition with distinct clinical stages and erythema migrans is the hallmark of early localized disease. Early disseminated disease symptoms include meningitis, cranial neuritis, multiple erythema migrans, and flu (Table 3).

Conclusion.—In children who are seen early in an ED, Lyme disease is a difficult, infrequent diagnosis. The predominant forms are early disseminated and late disease. In comparison with other ambulatory venues, the classic erythema migrans is uncommon in the ED. Lyme arthritis can be distinguished from septic arthritis if there is exposure in an endemic area. In the ED setting, underdiagnosis of Lyme disease may be more of a problem than overdiagnosis. Familiarity with Lyme disease's epidemiology and multiple manifestations is necessary for emergency medicine practitioners to make the diagnosis.

▶ The table accompanies this abstract (Table 3) should be of help to clinicians in sorting out the relative frequency of signs and symptoms of Lyme disease. Please note, though, that these cases presenting in the emergency room setting most likely represent a higher cohort of patients with less common and more severe forms of the disease. One can see that, in the emergency room, patients with Lyme disease present with erythema with migrans much less frequently than they present in the general pediatrician's office. Nonetheless, erythema migrans is the hallmark of early localized Lyme disease. Unfortunately, antibody testing is often negative and generally unnecessary at this stage, because the diagnosis can be established purely on a clinical basis. Treatment with oral antibiotics is all that is required. Treatment recommendations do vary with the stage of the disease, as noted in the table. Cranial nerve palsies, particularly involving cranial nerve VII, have become another hallmark of Lyme disease. The next time you see a patient with a Bell's palsy, at least think about the possibility of Lyme disease and draw appropriate titers. Now that we have a vaccine against Lyme disease, controversy has emerged about whom should receive it. Clearly this vaccine is not for everyone. It is intended only for those who are in endemic areas and who would otherwise be considered at high risk. Simply living in Lyme, Connecticut is not an indication for the vaccine, nor is living on Long Island. It takes more than locale to justify use of this somewhat expensive vaccine.

J.A. Stockman III, M.D.

Neurocognitive Abnormalities in Children After Classic Manifestations of Lyme Disease

Bloom BJ, Wyckoff PM, Meissner HC, et al (Tufts Univ, Boston; Tupper Research Institute, Boston; New England Medical Center, Boston; et al)
Pediatr Infect Dis J 17:189-196, 1998   18–9

Background.—Months to years after the classic manifestations of Lyme disease, affected adults may experience a subtle encephalopathy, characterized by memory impairment, irritability, and somnolence. Whether a similar disorder occurs in children is not known.

Methods.—Five children were seen in a Lyme disease clinic for assessment of neurocognitive symptoms that developed near infection onset or months after classic manifestations of Lyme disease. Detailed neuropsychologic testing was performed. The children were treated intravenously with ceftriaxone for 2 or 4 weeks and followed up for 2 to 7 years.

Findings.—The 5 patients exhibited behavioral changes, forgetfulness, and declining school performance concomitant with or months after erythema migrans, cranial neuropathy, or Lyme arthritis. The children also reported headache or fatigue, and 2 had a partial complex seizure disorder. All the children had immunoglobulin G antibody responses to *Borrelia burgdorferi* in serum and intrathecal immunoglobulin G antibody production to the spirochete. Two children had CSF pleocytoses. All children had normal intellectual functioning, but mild to moderate deficits in auditory or visual sequential processing were noted. The 4 children for whom follow-up information was available had gradual symptom improvement after therapy with ceftriaxone therapy.

Conclusions.—Neurocognitive symptoms may develop in children along with or after the classic manifestations of Lyme disease. Such symptoms may indicate an infectious or postinfectious encephalopathy associated with *B. burgdorferi* infection.

▶ Lyme disease is a tricky disease, especially when it comes to its neurologic manifestations. Following the acute manifestations of the disorder (erythema migrans and flu-like symptoms), acute neurologic abnormalities, including meningitis, encephalitis, cranial neuropathy, or radiculoneuritis may develop days to weeks later. Months to years later, intermittent episodes of arthritis or chronic neurologic abnormalities may develop, including encephalopathy, polyneuropathy, or, rarely, encephalomyelitis.

What we see in this report is that some patients may have only memory impairment with or without cerebrospinal fluid abnormalities, occurring many months to years after the classic manifestations of Lyme disease. The most common problem in diagnosis of this complication in both children and adults is to distinguish chronic Lyme encephalopathy from chronic fatigue syndrome, fibromyalgia, or somatoform disorders. This difficulty is compounded by the fact that a small percentage of patients may have these pain or fatigue syndromes in association with, or soon after, Lyme disease. Remember that an important clue to the diagnosis of fibromyalgia is widespread muscle and joint pain accompanied by tender points on examination, a relatively rare finding in Lyme disease. Chronic fatigue syndrome and fibromyalgia, even when they follow Lyme disease, seem not to respond in a sustained manner to antibiotic therapy.

If you see a child who has unusual or obscure neurologic symptoms, particularly those that, on neuropsychological testing, show abnormalities in auditory or visual sequential processing, think about the possibility that this could be due to prior Lyme disease. If serologic testing or other testing does suggest a prior infection, it would be wise to treat such children with a 1-month course of IV ceftriaxone if they have not previously received it.

J.A. Stockman III, M.D.

Outcomes of Children Treated for Lyme Disease
Wang TJ, Sangha O, Phillips CB, et al (Brigham and Women's Hosp, Boston; Children's Hosp Med Ctr, Boston)
J Rheumatol 25:2249-2253, 1998   18–10

Background.—Uncontrolled studies of antibiotic therapy for Lyme disease in children suggest that treatment outcomes are good, with little long-term morbidity. However, these studies have been based on case series and specialty clinic cohorts, which makes their results difficult to generalize. Outcomes of Lyme disease in children identified in a total population survey of an endemic island were analyzed in this study.

Methods and Findings.—The population-based, retrospective cohort study was conducted on an island off Massachusetts. Twenty-five children meeting the Centers for Disease Control case definition of previous Lyme disease were compared with 26 children with no history of Lyme disease. All affected children received antibiotics in the acute phase of illness. Mean duration since the initial manifestations of Lyme disease was 3.2 years. The prevalences of musculoskeletal and neurologic symptoms, abnormal findings on examination, abnormal EKG, and behavioral problems were no higher in children with previous Lyme disease than in those with no history of Lyme disease.

Conclusions.—This is the first controlled population-based study of the long-term outcomes of Lyme disease in children treated with appropriate antibiotic therapy. These children appeared to have no detectable long-term morbidity.

▶ As this report shows, the large majority of children with Lyme disease do just fine. We also know now that one of the reasons we are now saddled with this disease may be because of a vanishing breed of pigeon. It was recently noted that Lyme disease has its highest prevalence years in which oak trees lose their acorns (a phenomenon known as masting). At such times, the populations of mice tend to markedly increase. A major competitor of deer and mice for these bumper crops has been absent from the eastern deciduous forests of the United States for the better part of 100 years. It is the extinct passenger pigeon (*Ectopistes migratorius*). This bird is a nomadic wanderer that specializes on a diet of the super-abundant, but unpredictable, crops of mast. At one time here in the United States, carrier pigeon populations were estimated to be between 2 and 5 billion. They flew in enormous flocks, congregating wherever huge crops of acorns fell. The birds were so efficient at denuding the forest of nuts that many observers noted that native wildlife and feral hogs could not find sufficient food after a pigeon flock had passed through. Careful research of the illnesses found early in this century and in the last century have suggested that there was no Lyme disease. Is it possible that the presence of carrier pigeons controlled the population explosions of mice in mast years? Could the outbreaks of Lyme disease of the late 20th century have been a delayed consequence of the extinction of the carrier pigeon? The relationship of passenger pigeons to Lyme disease is not necessarily a story for the birds.[1]

J.A. Stockman III, M.D.

Reference

1. Blockstein DE: Lyme disease and the passenger pigeon. *Science* 279:1831, 1998.

Cutaneous Vasculitis in Children and Adults: Associated Diseases and Etiologic Factors in 303 Patients

Blanco R, Martínez-Taboada VM, Rodríguez-Valverde V, et al (Universidad de Cantabria, Santandar, Spain)
Medicine 77:403-418, 1998   18–11

Introduction.—Cutaneous vasculitis is characterized by nonspecific histopathologic findings and palpable purpura. It may be a primary disorder or a cutaneous manifestation of another entity, such as systemic necrotizing vasculitis, connective tissue disease, systemic bacterial infection, or malignancy, making it a diagnostic and therapeutic challenge. The disease associations and etiologic factors were assessed. The frequency of primary and secondary cutaneous vasculitis in different age groups were determined. Features that help to distinguish between the primary and secondary forms were determined.

Methods.—There were 172 adults and 131 children studied. The diagnosis was based on skin biopsy or the presence of typical nonthrombocytopenic palpable purpura. They were clinically classified as having primary cutaneous vasculitis, cutaneous vasculitis as a manifestation of systemic necrotizing vasculitis, or secondary cutaneous vasculitis. They had a complete blood count, Westergren erythrocyte sedimentation rate, biochemistry profile, urinalysis, and chest X-rays. Adults had an immunologic profile.

Results.—Primary cutaneous vasculitis was found in 130 of 131 children. This included Henoch-Schönlein purpura and hypersensitivity vasculitis. Only 120 of the 172 adults had primary vasculitis. It was a manifestation of systemic necrotizing vasculitis in 23 adults, such as

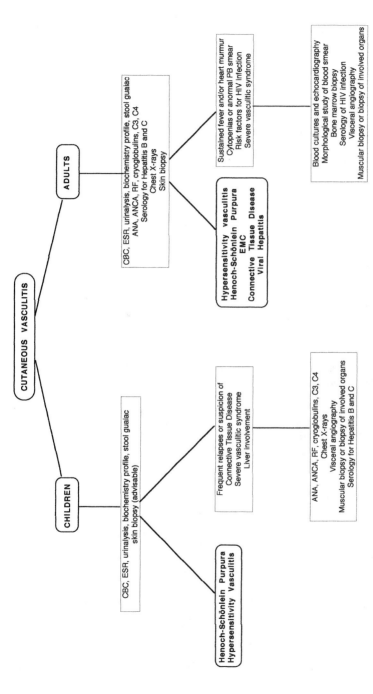

FIGURE 5.—Proposed work-up of patients presenting with cutaneous vasculitis. Children usually require a less extensive work-up than adults. *Abbreviations: ANA,* antinuclear antibodies; *ANCA,* antineutrophil cytoplasmic antibodies; *CBC,* complete blood count; *EMC,* essential mixed cryoglobulinemia; *ESR,* erythrocyte sedimentation rate; *HIV,* human immunodeficiency virus; *PB,* peripheral blood; *RF,* rheumatoid factor. (Courtesy of Blanco R, Martinez-Taboada VM, Rodriguez-Valverde V, et al: Cutaneous vasculitis in children and adults: Associated diseases and etiologic factors in 303 patients. *Medicine* 77[6]:403-418, 1998.)

Wegener granulomatosis, polyarteritis nodosa, and Churg-Strauss syndrome. It was secondary to other processes in 29 adults, including connective tissue disease or another autoimmune or rheumatoid disease (20), severe bacterial infections (5), especially bacterial endocarditis. For 4 patients, it was the presenting symptoms of an underlying malignancy. Clinical and laboratory data suggestive of the associated disorder were found in the patients who had cutaneous vasculitis as a manifestation of systemic necrotizing vasculitis or secondary to a connective tissue disease, severe bacterial infection, or malignancy. There was a benign clinical picture and outcome of primary cutaneous vasculitis in children and adults.

Conclusion.—A simple diagnostic work-up was suggested for children with cutaneous vasculitis (Fig 5). However, for adults, the diagnostic approach should be more cautious and the work-up more extensive. Of paramount importance for an adequate diagnosis and appropriate treatment is the early differentiation between primary cutaneous vasculitis, secondary cutaneous vasculitis, and cutaneous vasculitis presenting as symptoms of systemic necrotizing vasculitis, especially in adults.

▶ This report involves what is probably the largest combined series of adults and children with cutaneous vasculitis. Still, it is not large enough to tease out all the many varieties of vasculitis in children. Note, for example, that of 131 children with cutaneous vasculitis, 116 had Henoch-Schönlein purpura, leaving only hypersensitivity vasculitis and lupus to fill in the remainder of the causes of vasculitis. The spectrum of causes in a similar number of patients who are adults is quite a bit more diverse, because Henoch-Schönlein purpura is much less frequent. Do not forget the potential for polyarteritis nodosa, Wegener granulomatosis, rheumatoid arthritis, Sjögren syndrome, sarcoidosis, malignancies, and a variety of infections to also cause diffuse cutaneous vasculitis in children.

The next time you see a child with cutaneous vasculitis, if a diagnosis of Henoch-Schönlein purpura or hypersensitivity vasculitis does not jump out at you, follow the flow diagram and perhaps you will be more easily led to 1 of the less common, albeit very important, other causes of vasculitis in children.

Were you aware that the patron saint of lost souls (and objects), St. Anthony, may have suffered from peripheral vascular disease? The paintings of Mathis Gothardt-Neithardt, better known as Matthias Grünewald, show this. Grünewald is thought to have lived from around 1480 to 1524 and was one of the most celebrated painters of the so-called Rhenan School. His masterpiece is the Isenheim Altar, which can be seen in the Museum Unterlinden, Colmar, France. A fragment of this altar shows St. Anthony's Temptation. The history of this painting is quite interesting. Grünewald lodged for some time with St. Anthony's monastic order. Members of this order had the exclusive privilege of treating patients with the disease known as St. Anthony's fire, later identified as ergotism. For almost 100 years, several art historians have been aware that ergotism was shown in Grünewald's painting. Some of the monstrous creatures spinning around St. Anthony in his artwork show amputated fingers. If one looks at St. Anthony himself, one can easily decipher a bluish atrophy which is a classic sign of peripheral vascular disease, the first symptom of severe Raynaud's disease. Thus, Matthias Grünewald can be credited for the first indisputable pictorial representation of peripheral vascular disease, which in this case most likely relates to the use of ergots.

If you would like to see a superb reproduction of St. Anthony's fingers showing the Raynaud's phenomenon, see the report of Kahn.[1] St. Anthony is indeed the saint of lost souls. Chances are, however, that he was not 100% good at finding lost objects; he more likely than not lost a finger or two of his own to Raynaud's disease.

J.A. Stockman III, M.D.

Reference

1. Kahn M-F: St. Anthony's plague. *Lancet* 352:1478, 1998.

Juvenile Dermatomyositis at Diagnosis: Clinical Characteristics of 79 Children
Pachman LM, Hayford JR, Chung A, et al (Northwestern Univ Med School, Chicago; Ctrs for Disease Control and Prevention, Atlanta, Ga; Univ of Dallas, Tex; et al)
J Rheumatol 25:1198-1204, 1998   18–12

Background.—Juvenile dermatomyositis (JDM) is the most common idiopathic inflammatory myopathy of childhood. This study of a relatively large group of children with JDM examined presenting symptoms, demography, time of onset, and socioeconomic factors.

Study Design.—Seventy-nine patients with JDM under the age of 17 were recruited for this study from 1989 to 1992. A family interview was conducted and included information on onset, disease, demographics, patient's medical history, and household environment.

Findings.—All children had rash and proximal muscle weakness at diagnosis (Table 2). Other symptoms included muscle pain in 73%, fever in 65%, dysphagia in 44%, hoarseness in 37%, abdominal pain in 37%, arthritis in 35%, calcinosis in 23%, and melena in 13%. Muscle-derived enzyme levels were normal in 10%. An electromyogram was performed in 43 children, and 19% had normal results. Muscle biopsy was performed in 51 cases but was nondiagnostic in 20%. The median time from onset of disease to diagnosis differed significantly by racial group: 2 months for white children and 6.5 months for all minority children. The median time from onset of disease to treatment was 3 months for white children and 7.2 months for minority children. Calcinosis was associated with increased time between onset and diagnosis or therapy. In the 33 children with onset from June to September, rash was the first symptom in 83%. Therapy consisted of steroids in 91% and methotrexate in 10%.

Conclusions.—The study describes a series of 79 patients with JDM. At diagnosis, most children had rash, weakness, muscle pain, and fever.

TABLE 2.—Symptoms Present in 79 Children With
Newly Diagnosed JDM

Symptom	n (%)
Rash	79 (100)
Weakness	79 (100)
Muscle pain	58 (73)
Fever	51 (65)
Dysphagia	35 (44)
Hoarseness	34 (43)
Abdominal pain	29 (37)
Arthritis	28 (35)
Calcifications	18 (23)
Melena	10 (13)

(Courtesy of Pachman LM, Hayford JR, Chung A, et al: Juvenile dermatomyositis at diagnosis: Clinical characteristics of 79 children. *J Rheumatol* 25:1198-1204, 1998.)

Minority children experienced significant delays in diagnosis and treatment. Delayed diagnosis was associated with calcinosis.

▶ This may very well be the most important piece ever published in the pediatric literature in terms of the clinical description of dermatomyositis. The investigators pulled together a series of 79 children (an extraordinarily large number of children for such a relatively uncommon disorder) from a variety of institutions, pooling the data in a carefully constructed clinical protocol. In addition to muscle weakness, muscle pain and fever are the principal components at diagnosis. Some children will also complain of dysphagia, abdominal pain, hoarseness, or arthritis. Please use this article as your reference standard. You won't find a better clinical article on this topic.

J.A. Stockman III, M.D.

Fibrin D-Dimer As a Marker of Disease Activity in Systemic Onset Juvenile Rheumatoid Arthritis

Bloom BJ, Tucker LB, Miller LC, et al (Brown Univ, Providence, RI; Tufts Univ, Boston)
J Rheumatol 25:1620-1625, 1998   18–13

Introduction.—During active disease periods, children with systemic onset juvenile rheumatoid arthritis (JRA) often have hematologic abnormalities, such as anemia, leukocytosis, and thrombocytosis. In adults with rheumatoid arthritis, levels of d-dimer have been found to correlate with disease activity. Monoclonal antibodies specific for the d-dimer domain of products of the terminal steps of the fibrinolytic pathway can help detect fibrin degradation products (Fig 1). Other markers of disease activity in systemic lupus have been correlated with serial levels of d-dimer, which clinically responded to medications. The prevalence of coagulation abnormalities in patients with systemic JRA was studied, using d-dimer as a

FIBRINOGEN

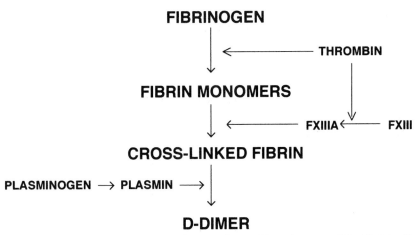

FIGURE 1.—The fibrinolytic pathway. In the terminal steps of this pathway, cross-linked fibrin is split into various products that contain dimers of the d-subunit of fibrin. In this study, an assay was employed to detect these subunits by use of monoclonal antibodies. (Courtesy of Bloom BJ, Tucker LB, Miller LC, et al: Fibrin d-dimer as a marker of disease activity in systemic onset juvenile rheumatoid arthritis. *J Rheumatol* 25:1620-1625, 1998.)

specific measure of fibrin degradation. It was also determined whether serial levels of d-dimer were related to response to medications and clinical events over time.

Methods.—The study included 24 patients with systemic JRA who had measurements taken of levels of d-dimer in addition to complete blood counts, erythrocyte sedimentation rate, maximum fever, duration of morning stiffness, and swollen joint count. In 11 patients, serial d-dimer levels were obtained. To determine any correlations between d-dimer and the other variables, linear regression analyses were done. To compare levels before and after treatment interventions, a student's paired *t* test was used. Concurrent clinical events, such as pericarditis, were compared against levels of d-dimer.

Results.—In 23 (96%) of 24 patients, elevated levels of d-dimer were found. When serial levels were analyzed, correlations between levels of d-dimer and fever and total leukocyte count, were found but not with other variables. In patients deemed to be clinical responders to immuno-modulatory agents, a significant reduction in levels both before and after treatment was noted. During the remainder of follow-up, elevated levels were indicative of severe disease. A benign disease course was indicated by lack of d-dimer.

Conclusion.—Coagulation abnormalities are more prevalent in children with systemic JRA than previously reported and are frequently found during periods of active disease, according to the use of a sensitive and specific marker for fibrinolysis known as d-dimer. Response to disease-modifying agents apparently parallels serial levels of d-dimer. The levels of d-dimer may predict outcome during a short follow-up period. Assessment of disease activity may be enhanced by fibrin d-dimer, a novel marker that when used in combination with known variables could help predict disease activity and response to medications in children with systemic onset.

▶ D-dimers appear to be almost always elevated in children with active systemic and/or arthritic disease. This should come as no surprise since elevated levels of d-dimer have now been described in adults with rheumatoid arthritis as well as other disorders associated with vasculitis, including systemic lupus and systemic sclerosis. In these adult disorders, d-dimer levels seem to correlate with disease activity and diminish in response to adequate therapy. Levels of d-dimers are not mere acute phase reactants like sed rates, which are known to poorly correlate with disease status in JRA.

A few fast facts about JRA. The prevalence of JRA has held steady in recent years and is estimated at 30,000 to 50,000 cases in the United States. JRA is more common in girls, with a female-to-male ratio of 3:2. There are 3 forms of JRA onset: systemic, which constitutes 11% to 20% of cases; polyarticular (5 or more joints), 17% to 40%; and pauciarticular, 40% to 72%. The peak age at onset of JRA remains between 2 and 4 years. One of the most serious complications of JRA is uveitis, which occurs in somewhere between 5% and 10% of cases. Unfortunately, up to 12% of children with uveitis associated with pauciarticular JRA will develop permanent blindness as a result of low-grade chronic intraocular inflammation. The vision-robbing consequences of low-grade uveitis occur extremely slowly, and typically over a period of 4 to 8 years. Most children who develop blindness are ironically those observed by ophthalmologists who opt to tolerate low-grade ocular inflammation, hoping to avoid the development of corticosteroid-induced ocular adverse effects, such as cataract and glaucoma.

To read more about JRA, including some of its long-term complications, particularly that of the associated uveitis, see the superb review of Nguygen and Foster.[1]

J.A. Stockman III, M.D.

Reference

1. Nguygen QD, Foster CS: Saving the vision of children with juvenile rheumatoid arthritis-associated uveitis. *JAMA* 280:1133-1134, 1998.

Autologous Haemopoietic Stem-Cell Transplantation in Four Patients With Refractory Juvenile Chronic Arthritis

Wulffraat N, van Royen A, Bierings M, et al (Univ Hosp for Children "Het Wilhelmina kinderziekenhuis," Utrecht, The Netherlands; Leiden Univ, The Netherlands)

Lancet 353:550-553, 1999   18–14

Background.—Autologous hematopoietic stem-cell transplantation (AHSCT) may be a feasible treatment for severe autoimmune disease refractory to conventional therapy. The cases of 4 children with severe forms of juvenile chronic arthritis (JCA) treated with AHSCT were reported.

Methods.—Three children with systemic JCA and 1 with polyarticular JCA were treated. Unprimed bone marrow was obtained 1 month before AHSCT, and T-cell depletion was performed with CD2 and CD3 antibodies. The preparative regimen consisted of antithymocyte globulin, 20 mg/kg; cyclophosphamide, 200 mg/kg; and low-dose total body irradiation, 4 Gy. Methotrexate and cyclosporine therapy were discontinued before AHSCT, and prednisone was tapered after 2 months. Drug-free follow-up ranged from 6 to 18 months.

Outcomes.—During follow-up, the children had a marked reduction in joint swelling, pain, and morning stiffness. Within 6 weeks, erythrocyte sedimentation rate and levels of C-reactive protein and hemoglobin were almost normal. Despite T-cell depletion, 3 children had a rapid immune reconstitution. In 2 patients, a limited varicella zoster virus eruption developed, necessitating aciclovir therapy.

Conclusion.—In these children with severe JCA resistant to conventional therapy, AHSCT induced disease remission and was well tolerated. Prolonged, prednisone-free growth catch-up and general well-being were documented. Longer follow-up is needed to determine whether these children have been completely cured of their disease.

▶ Who would have ever thought that we would be talking about AHSCT as part of the management of refractory JCA? Well, as we start the millennium, we, indeed, are now hearing about such approaches to serious autoimmune diseases such as rheumatoid arthritis. Indeed, AHSCT has been reported as a potential treatment for patients with a variety of severe autoimmune diseases including systemic sclerosis, multiple sclerosis, and systemic lupus erythematosus refractory to conventional treatment. What is done with this technique is to remove bone marrow about a month before the AHSCT. T cells are depleted from the bone marrow and, during this period, the patient receives antithymocyte globulin, cyclophosphamide, and low-dose total body irradiation. Methotrexate and cyclosporine, along with prednisone, are also part of this approach.

AHSCT for the management of severe JCA is not for the light of heart. It is also not for the fool-hearted. It obviously should not be rushed into, particularly as there are a number of new disease-modifying agents that are being studied in both adults and children. Two relatively new such agents are leflunomide and cyclooxygenase (COX)-2 inhibitors. The former is an immunomodulatory agent that inhibits de novo pyrimidine synthesis by selective inhibition of dihydroorotate dehydrogenase within T lymphocytes. There are excellent data that indicate that leflunomide effectively slows or stops the progression of arthritis in animals, and human data are also emerging.[1]

Lastly, COX-2 inhibitors have hit the millennium in full stride. In the past 100 years, aspirin has been the sort of mainstay as an analgesic, anti-inflammatory, and antithrombotic agent. However, by 1938 it was clear that aspirin did serious damage to the stomach. Nonsteroidal anti-inflammatory drugs developed since the 1960s also failed to achieve the goal of a "safer aspirin." The demonstration that inhibition of prostaglandin synthesis was central to both the therapeutic and toxic effects of aspirin and nonsteroidals appeared to establish the principle of no gain without pain with this approach to inflammation control. Is it possible that COX-2 inhibitors violate the principle of no pain, no gain? Might the "safe aspirin" be here at last? To read about COX-2 inhibitors, see the superb review by Hawkey.[2]

We close this chapter with a quiz question related to a common musculoskeletal disorder. What occupation can both worsen and improve the symptoms of a herniated disc? That occupation is stunt flying. Recently, a stunt pilot with a herniated L4-L5 disc was documented by MRI. He had sciatic pain and experienced serious worsening of this symptom when pulling out of a sharp dive, at which point his body was subjected to an estimated 5 Gs. The pilot empirically found that he could alleviate this pain by climbing to 10,000 feet and performing an outside loop, resulting in approximately −3 Gs of force on his body. These experiences were repeatedly demonstrated in the course of his professional flying, during which he performed aerobatics in high-performance fighter planes at military and civilian air shows.[3]

All of this makes some sense. In the supine position, in vivo lumbar intradisc pressure averages 50 kPa. In the standing position, these pressures double. They double again to 200 kPa in the sitting position. The pilot described above weighed 180 lbs. A reasonable estimate is that, at 1 G (normal gravity), approximately 120 lbs would be pressing on his lumbar spine in the erect position. At 5 Gs, this weight would increase 5-fold to 600 lbs, raising intradisc pressure, thus exacerbating any preexisting herniation. When he was doing his loops, however, the effect was as if he had a 360-lb traction weight placed on his spine, a weight easily capable of reducing an intradisc herniation.

The lesson here is straightforward. If you develop back pain, do a few loop-da-loops.

J.A. Stockman III, M.D.

References

1. Smolen JS, Kalden JR, Scott DL, et al: Efficacy and safety of leflunomide compared with placebo and sulphasalazine in active rheumatoid arthritis: A double-blind, randomised, multicentre trial. *Lancet* 353:259-266, 1999.
2. Hawkey CJ: COX-2 inhibitors. *Lancet* 353:307-314, 1999.
3. Choy DSJ: Positive and negative gravitational forces and herniated-disc sciatic pain. *N Engl J Med* 337:1396-1397, 1997.

19 Gastroenterology

Gastroesophageal Reflux in Preterm Infants: Norms for Extended Distal Esophageal pH Monitoring
Ng SC-Y, Quak S-H (Kandang Kerbau Women's and Children's Hosp, Singapore; Natl Univ of Singapore)
J Pediatr Gastroenterol Nutr 27:411-414, 1998   19–1

Background.—Gastroesophageal reflux disease is common in preterm infants and is typically diagnosed by extended distal esophageal pH monitoring. However, no reference data defining a normal extended distal esophageal pH in preterm infants have been published. These authors reported on the normal distal esophageal pH values found in preterm infants, and compared norms in this age group with those of other age groups.

Methods.—The subjects were 21 asymptomatic preterm infants (12 boys and 9 girls) with a mean birth weight of 1545 g and a mean postconceptional age of 30.7 weeks. Six of the infants had received xanthine derivatives for apnea of prematurity and 15 had not. None of the infants had any condition associated with reflux, and all were consuming 70% or more of their oral feedings (nursed in the prone position). At a mean of 14 days after birth, infants underwent extended distal esophageal pH monitoring for a mean of 20.58 hours, and characteristics of their reflux episodes were recorded.

Findings.—None of the measurements for infants who received xanthine derivatives were significantly different from those of infants who did not receive these drugs. Overall, the mean reflux index (percentage of total monitoring time during which the lower esophageal pH was less than 4 for 15 seconds or longer) was 0.7% ± 1.1% (Table 1). Infants experienced a mean of 7.6 ± 11.2 episodes of reflux each day, but only a fraction of the episodes (0.5 ± 1.1) lasted for more than 5 minutes. The longest episode of reflux that infants experienced averaged 4.2 ± 6.1 minutes. All of these data were similar to data reported for term infants, children, adolescents, and adults.

Conclusion.—The reported norms for extended distal esophageal pH monitoring reported here for preterm infants are similar to those in other populations. Establishment of reference values for preterm infants should help clinicians recognize and reduce the complications associated with gastroesophageal reflux disease in this population.

TABLE 1.—Esophageal pH Norms for Preterm Infants

pH Data	Mean ± SD Whole Group (n = 21)	With Xanthine (n = 6)	Without Xanthine (n = 15)
Total % time pH < 4 (RI)	0.7 ± 1.1	0.3 ± 0.2	1.16 ± 1.47
Total number reflux episodes per day	7.6 ± 11.2	3.8 ± 4.5	9.1 ± 12.8
Reflux episodes > 5 minutes per day	0.5 ± 1.1	0.2 ± 0.4	0.7 ± 1.2
Longest episode (min)	4.2 ± 6.1	1.3 ± 2.3	5.4 ± 6.8

Abbreviations: RI, reflux episode; *SD*, standard deviation.
(Courtesy of Ng SC-Y, Quak S-H: Gastroesophageal reflux in preterm infants: Norms for extended distal esophageal pH monitoring. *J Pediatr Gastroenterol Nutr* 27:411-414, 1998.)

▶ You know, if this report had appeared 25 years ago, it would have been titled "Normative Data for How Often and to What Extent Babies Burp." Babies don't burp now, they have gastroesophageal reflux, some babies to a greater extent, some babies to a lesser extent. With this new information, we know that the average normal infant refluxes 7.6 ± 11.2 times a day. We also see that babies born at 32 to 34 weeks tend to have more reflux episodes per day in comparison to those born earlier or later in pregnancy.

Life was a lot simpler when babies burped instead of refluxing. Life was also a lot simpler when there was no such thing as a grade 4 reflux. That was simply called a wet burp or upchuck. The topic of reflux is written about so much that it makes some of us adults want to upchuck.

While on the topic of reflux, an unusual opportunity presented itself a couple of years back when, during a manometric examination of an adult woman complaining of dysphagia, an earthquake occurred. The epicenter of this earthquake (in Umbria, Italy) was about 35 miles from where the esophageal study was being performed. The magnitude of the earthquake was 5.2 on the Richter scale. The woman in question was about halfway through the manometry when the seismic event struck. Sphincter pressure immediately dropped from 20 to 5 mm Hg. The study was repeated a few days later, and the esophageal pressure was found to be within the normal range (21 mm Hg).

Thus, it would appear that when your adrenalin is up, esophageal sphincter pressure drops. Earthquakes can do this. With this piece of trivia, you now know why those who experience earthquakes often have an opportunity to taste their breakfast, lunch, or supper, a second time.[1]

J.A. Stockman III, M.D.

Reference

1. Bassottti G, Fiorella S: Esophageal pressure during an earthquake. *Lancet* 351:806, 1998.

Heterogeneity of Diagnoses Presenting as Cyclic Vomiting

Li BUK, Murray RD, Heitlinger LA, et al (Ohio State Univ, Columbus; Columbus Children's Hosp, Ohio)
Pediatrics 102:583-587, 1998   19–2

Introduction.—The hallmark clinical feature of cyclic vomiting syndrome, in which no cause of the vomiting becomes apparent on testing, is a quantitatively high peak intensity of vomiting (4 or more times an hour) and low episode frequency (2 or fewer times per week). The etiology and pathogenesis of cyclic vomiting remain unknown. Possible causes of cyclic vomiting include migraine, epilepsy, disorders of metabolism, parent-child relationships, gastrointestinal dysmotility, autonomic dysfunction, hypothalamic dysfunction, and abnormal fatty acid oxidation. The diagnostic profile of children who have cyclic vomiting was established.

Methods.—Two hundred twenty-five children younger than 18 years who had at least 3 episodes of vomiting between which they were well throughout an 11-year period were studied. A combination of chart review and structured telephone interviews was conducted to determine the diagnosis of those who had a pattern of cyclic vomiting, as well as the results of diagnostic testing and responses to various treatments.

Results.—Idiopathic cyclic vomiting syndrome was the largest diagnostic category (88%). In those having complete cessation of episodes after therapy, extraintestinal disorders (7%) and gastrointestinal disorders (5%) were found to be the probable cause of vomiting (Table 2, A). Serious surgical disorders of the gastrointestinal system (malrotation), renal system (acute hydronephrosis), and CNS (neoplasm) were found in 12% of the children. Serious endocrine (Addison's disease) and metabolism disorders (disorder of fatty acid oxidation) were found in 2% of the children. Associated disorders, such as gastroesophageal reflux and chronic sinusitis were found among 41% of those with idiopathic cyclic vomiting syndrome; however, based on a partial response to therapy, these were then discarded as the main cause. There were 49% who had an identified disorder that most likely caused, or could have contributed to, the vomiting.

Conclusion.—Heterogeneous disorders that either cause or contribute to the vomiting can induce the cyclic pattern of vomiting. Systematic diagnostic testing to look for the underlying disorders is warranted, once the cyclic vomiting pattern is identified.

▶ So what is cyclic vomiting? Is it a variant of migraine? Or is it a manifestation of a seizure disorder, or possibly a disorder of metabolism? Is it, as recent studies suggest, merely a disorder of gastrointestinal motility, or is there something wrong with the brain, or is there a disturbance in fatty acid oxidation? Chances are, that in 1 or another patient, the cause of cyclic vomiting might be any of these, or several of these. Indeed, the diagnostic profile of cyclic vomiting is almost as long as your arm (see Table 2, A).

TABLE 2A.—Gastrointestinal and Extraintestinal Disorders That Cause Vomiting in Children With the Cyclic Vomiting Pattern

	Probable Cause	Associated Disorders
Gastrointestinal disorders		
Gastrointestinal inflammation		
GERD/esophagitis	4	34
Gastritis		5
Duodenitis	1	9
Gastrointestinal infections		
Giardiasis		1
Gastrospirillium		1
Entamoeba coli		1
Blastocystis hominis		1
Pinworms		1
Gastrointestinal motility		
Irritable bowel syndrome	1	5
Constipation		3
Gastrointestinal-surgical lesions		
Duplication cyst	1	
Malrotation*	3	2
Hirschsprung's disease*		1
SMA syndrome		1
Chronic appendicitis*	2	1
Adhesions	1	
Hepatobiliary and pancreatic		
Hepatitis		1
Choledochal cyst	1	
Cholelithiasis*	1	1
Gall bladder dyskinesia*		1
Pancreatitis		1
Extraintestinal disorders		
Otolaryngological		
Chronic sinusitis (3 cases)*	1	22
Pulmonary		
Asthma	1	1
Renal and gynecological		
Hydronephrosis 2° UPJ obstruction*		1
Hypercalciuria		1
Ovarian cyst		1
Nephrolithiasis	1	
Endocrine		
Diabetes mellitus type I		2
Metabolic		
VLCAD ± SCAD (heterozygote)	1	
Acute intermittent porphyria	1	
Suspected mitochondriopathies	2	
Neurological		
Epilepsy	1	
Brainstem glioma*	1	
Cerebellar medulloblastoma*	1	
Astrocytoma*	1	
Chiari malformation*		3
V-P shunt dysfunction*	1	2
Epilepsy	1	4
Psychological		
Depression, secondary gain		4
Total	27	115†

Abbreviations: GERD, gastroesophageal reflux disease; *SMA*, superior mesenteric artery; *UPJ*, ureteropelvic junction; *VLCAD*, very long chain acyl-CoA dehydrogenase deficiency; *SCAD*, short-chain acyl-CoA dehydrogenase deficiency.

(Reproduced by permission of *Pediatrics*, from Li BUK, Murray RD, Heitlinger LA, et al: Heterogeneity of diagnoses presenting as cyclic vomiting. *Pediatrics* 102:583-587, 1998.)

The next time you become involved with the care of a youngster with cyclic vomiting, step back for a minute and decide what will be a logical diagnostic approach based on that child's specific history and physical examination. If you get no clues other than the history of periodic vomiting, recognize that the tests with the highest yield are endoscopy, sinus films, and x-ray studies of the small bowel. Next in line would be studies that include blood glucose, electrolytes, liver and pancreatic enzymes, blood ammonia, lactic acid, urinary organic acids, serum carnitine, δ-aminolevulinic acid, and porphobilinogen. These are best done in conjunction with an actual episode of a cycle of vomiting. If all else fails, you may need to do a CT of the abdomen and a CT or MRI of the head.

You will have to decide whether these authors are correct in recommending an extensive evaluation for every child seen with cyclic vomiting. The yield will be about 50%. You will pick up some serious surgical disorders in a small, but real, number of children. Chances are very good that you will want to engage a pediatric gastroenterologist to help you sort through the multitude of diagnoses that can present as cyclic vomiting.

This commentary closes with a query having to do with things coming up from the stomach via rumination. Rumination as a symptom is rarely considered in the care of older children and adolescents, but as an eating disorder, rumination is commonly associated with failure to thrive in toddlers. The entity, also known as *merycism*, was first described in the 17th century when it was considered a somewhat sensual activity. Rumination refers to the voluntary regurgitation of partially digested food into the mouth, where it is subsequently rechewed and reswallowed or sometimes expectorated after chewing. Once thought to be a problem only of those with mental retardation, rumination has recently been identified as a not-so-infrequent problem in patients with bulimia. Curiously, it has also been described as a potentially normal variant of human behavior. So what is the latest in terms of nifty ways of treating rumination disorders? It's plain old chewing gum. Weakly et al. show the merits of this approach. Simply substituting a wad of gum for a wad of stomach contents often cures the problem.[1]

If you ever run into a youngster (or adult) who ruminates, tell them there is a way that they can double their pleasure, double their fun, with the "Wrigley effect." Chewing a stick of gum is far better than chewing one's cud like a cow.

J.A. Stockman III, M.D.

Reference

1. Weakly MM, Petti TA, Karwisch G: Case study: Chewing gum treatment of rumination in an adolescent with an eating disorder. *J Am Acad Child Adolesc Psychiatr* 36:1124-1127, 1997.

Transient Neonatal Cholestasis: Origin and Outcome

Jacquemin E, Lykavieris P, Chaoui N, et al (Hôpital de Bicêtre, Le Kremlin Bicêtre, France)

J Pediatr 133:563-567, 1998

19–3

Background.—Appropriate treatment for neonatal cholestasis relies on prompt identification of its specific cause. In many children, however, the cause cannot be detected, and cholestasis resolves spontaneously within a few months. One group of such patients was reported on.

Patients and Findings.—Ninety-two children first seen with neonatal cholestasis were included in the retrospective analysis. All children were followed until liver tests normalized. Eighty-one children had factors responsible for chronic or acute perinatal distress. The onset of jaundice occurred at a mean of 7 days. The mean duration was 3.5 months. Stools were initially discolored in 39 children, with color normalizing at a mean age of 1.7 months. Hepatomegaly was initially detected in 90 children, resolving at a mean of 13 months of age. Liver test results were normal by 1 year of age in 83 children. The mean age at normalization was 10 months. Liver histologic examination was performed in 70 children. Findings included moderate portal and lobular fibrosis, multinucleated giant hepatocytes, and hematopoietic foci. Follow-up liver biopsy specimens obtained from 15 children were normal or improved.

Conclusion.—In this large series of children, cholestasis of neonatal onset and unknown origin resolved spontaneously. Most such cases of transient neonatal cholestasis may be caused by a combination of several factors, including immaturity of bile secretion because of prematurity and perinatal insults, resulting in hepatic hypoxia or ischemia.

▶ This report teaches us an important lesson and that is that there are many causes of neonatal cholestasis, but when neonatal cholestasis is transient and goes away, it stays away. Unfortunately, neonatal cholestasis is frequently given the misnomer of neonatal hepatitis when, in fact, for most youngsters with transient neonatal cholestasis, there is virtually no evidence of an inflammatory or infectious process going on in the liver. The authors of this report suggest that neonatal cholestasis really results from a combination of factors including immaturity of bowel secretion potentially exacerbated by prematurity; chronic or acute oxygen deprivation of the liver as a result of intrauterine growth retardation, acute perinatal distress, or lung disease; liver damage caused by perinatal or postnatal sepsis; or a decrease in bile flow caused by delayed feeding, seen in children with necrotizing enterocolitis or in those receiving total parenteral nutrition.

Whatever the cause(s) of neonatal cholestasis, the diagnosis of transient neonatal cholestasis should not be made unless a thorough evaluation has been undertaken and the patient followed for a very long period. "All the usual suspects" should be evaluated and appropriate diagnoses excluded. Liver function studies and liver enzymes should be repeated 1 to 2 years after everything appears to have returned to normal. Only then can one say that this was truly an idiopathic case of neonatal cholestasis that was transient.

J.A. Stockman III, M.D.

A Defect in the Transport of Long-Chain Fatty Acids Associated With Acute Liver Failure

Al Odaib A, Shneider BL, Bennett MJ, et al (Yale Univ, New Haven, Conn; Univ of Texas, Dallas)
N Engl J Med 339:1752-1757, 1998   19–4

Introduction.—During periods of fasting, fatty-acid oxidation (FAO) has a major role in energy production. Fatty acids are mobilized from adipose tissue when body glucose is depleted and converted to ketone bodies, an alternative source of energy for peripheral tissue. Metabolic decompensation during fasting, hypoketotic hypoglycemia, and acute dysfunction of fatty acid–dependent tissues are common clinical features of disorders of FAO. Two boys had acute liver failure and were found to have a defect in the transport of long-chain fatty acids.

Methods.—One boy had hypoglycemia, hyperammonemia, and acute hepatic failure when he was 1 year old. He had 7 additional episodes of acute liver failure during the next 4 years. He had his most severe episode when he was 5, and after he had surgical reconstruction of the bile duct and liver transplantation, he was in good health. Another 5-year-old white boy had liver failure and mild encephalopathy. After he had a liver transplantation, he was in good health. Both patients had biochemical and histologic studies, as well as cell lines and enzyme assays.

Results.—One patient had a distinctive profile of the tissue homogenate that was characterized by low levels of myristic acid, palmitic acid, stearic acid, oleic acid, and linoleic acid with elevated levels of carnitine. Apparently he had a defect in the transport of long-chain fatty acids at the plasma-membrane level. Both patients had lower uptake of oleic acid in skin fibroblast. The length of the fatty acid tested correlated with the severity of the defect.

Conclusion.—The finding of a defect in fatty-acid uptake with severe clinical manifestations supports the view that active transport of long-chain fatty acids is required to maintain hepatic ketogenesis and energy supply during fasting for infants and young children. Further studies are necessary to better understand the underlying mechanisms of this disease.

▶ Estella M. Alonso, M.D., director of Hepatology and Liver Transplantation, Children's Memorial Hospital, and associate professor of Pediatrics, Northwestern University School of Medicine, Chicago, comments:

Acute liver failure is an uncommon, but important, problem in pediatrics. Approximately 50 children per year are considered for liver transplantation for this indication. Few of these children recover spontaneously, and the majority are never labeled with a specific (or satisfying) diagnosis. In fact, these children are probably affected by a variety of problems, including unknown viruses, and by a medley of metabolic disorders. Hepatologists and metabolism gurus are slowly navigating this chaos to try to define some of these diseases. This publication is an important contribution to that effort.

The history of the first patient included many clues pointing to an inborn error of FAO. Yet urine and plasma analyses, even during crisis, were unimpressive. Only extensive testing of this patient's cultured fibroblasts revealed this novel defect in fatty acid transport. The second patient presented with his first crisis at age 4, which is rather late, with most defects in FAO present in infancy. His screening metabolic work-up was quite nonspecific, and he took a short course toward liver transplantation. Most hepatologists, myself included, would not have bothered to harvest skin fibroblasts on this child. Someone did bother though, and both patients were found to have a pattern of impaired oxidation of long-chain fatty acids, which reversed when the fibroblast membranes were made permeable with digitonin. It is also important to note that the liver histology in these children was atypical for a FAO defect, which usually includes predominantly fatty change. Liver histology in these children revealed fibrosis, cellular disarray, and hepatocyte necrosis. The authors warn that children who have acute liver failure should still be evaluated for FAO defects, even if their liver histology is not typical.

So, what can we learn from this report? First, defects in fatty acid oxidation are probably responsible for an important fraction of acute liver failure in children. Second, our standard methods of screening for these defects are probably inadequate. Clinicians need to be more careful about looking for clues. Saving urine and serum before hypoglycemia is corrected may be the only opportunity to recognize hypoketotic hypoglycemia—the most important clue to this disorder. Third, a variety of patterns of liver injury may be associated with FAO defects. Therefore, should fibroblast studies investigate all children with non-viral, non-toxic acute liver failure? I think the jury is still out, but perhaps, with heightened awareness, we can become more effective in diagnosing FAO defects.

E.M. Alonso, M.D.

Relation Between Mutations of the Cystic Fibrosis Gene and Idiopathic Pancreatitis

Cohn JA, Friedman KJ, Noone PG, et al (Duke Univ, Durham, NC; Univ of North Carolina, Chapel Hill)
N Engl J Med 339:653-658, 1998 19–5

Introduction.—A potentially life-threatening disease, chronic pancreatitis is usually related to alcohol or it is idiopathic, but whether hereditary factors increase its likelihood is unknown. Cystic fibrosis is the most common inherited disease of the exocrine pancreas. Mutations of the cystic fibrosis transmembrane conductance regulator (CFTR) gene lead to dysfunction of the lung, sweat glands, vas deferens, and pancreas in cystic fibrosis. The gene may have a role in idiopathic chronic pancreatitis. Whether abnormal CFTR genotypes are predisposing factors for idiopathic pancreatitis was determined.

Methods.—Twenty-seven patients, with a mean age of 36 at diagnosis, had idiopathic pancreatitis. Testing of the DNA was conducted for 17 CFTR mutations and for the 5T allele in intron 8 of the CFTR gene. Associated with an inherited form of infertility in males, the 5T allele reduces the level of functional CFTR. If patients had 2 abnormal CFTR alleles, they were further tested for unrecognized cystic fibrosis-related lung disease. The nasal mucosa had measurements taken of baseline and CFTR-mediated ion transport.

Results.—At least 1 abnormal CFTR allele was found in 10 patients with idiopathic chronic pancreatitis (37%). There were 8 CFTR mutations detected, a prevalence ratio of 11:1. Both alleles were affected in 3 patients. Lung disease typical of cystic fibrosis, identified by sweat testing, spirometry, or base-line nasal potential-difference measurements, was not seen in these 3 patients. Abnormal nasal cyclic AMP-mediate chloride transport was seen in each.

Conclusion.—Mutations in the CFTR gene were strongly associated with pancreatitis in this group of patients referred for evaluation of idiopathic pancreatitis. The genotypes associated with male infertility resemble the abnormal CFTR genotypes.

▶ This article begins to fill in many of the blanks in our understanding of the relationship between CFTR gene abnormalities and the variable expression of states associated with these abnormalities, including cystic fibrosis. If there were a god involved with these various clinical expressions, that god's name would be Proteus, the Greek god from ancient mythology who could change himself from time to time at the drop of a hat in order to avoid capture. Indeed, the clinical manifestations of CFTR mutations are protean. Individuals with the cystic fibrosis gene mutation, which we now call the CFTR mutation, can have very little wrong with them, or a lot. Little is isolated obstructive azoospermia. At the other end of the spectrum is full-blown cystic fibrosis. Also included within the spectrum are congenital absence of the vas deferens, nasal polyposis, diffuse bronchiectasis, and, in adults, bronchopulmonary allergic aspergillosis. Each of these conditions has been associated with mutant CFTR genes, in the absence of clinical cystic fibrosis. Most of these disorders are not associated with elevated sweat chloride tests. As this abstract indicates, we now must add chronic pancreatitis to the list of clinical presentations of the CFTR mutation. There are lots of causes of chronic pancreatitis. It can be caused by a number of infectious agents. Alcohol consumption in excess can do this. The most common cause of the disease, however, is idiopathic (some 40% of cases). It is this idiopathic group of cases that is actually due to the inheritance of the CFTR gene. These findings are critically important, because it is entirely possible that having the CFTR gene should warn you that alcohol or certain drugs known to cause pancreatitis should be avoided.

The long and the short of this is straightforward. The next time you see a child with pancreatitis, a child for whom no etiology is apparent, think about getting a genotype done on that child to determine whether that child may have a CFTR (ΔF508 or otherwise) mutation.

J.A. Stockman III, M.D.

Coeliac Disease Hidden by Cryptogenic Hypertransaminasaemia

Volta U, De Franceschi L, Lari F, et al (Univ of Bologna, Italy)
Lancet 352:26-29, 1998   19–6

Introduction.—Previous studies have shown that many patients with untreated celiac disease have gluten-dependent liver involvement. An early biochemical sign of celiac disease free of gastrointestinal symptoms has been hypertransaminasemia of unknown, cryptogenic origin. Some cases of celiac disease may go unrecognized because diagnostic tests for celiac disease are not included among investigations for cryptogenic hypertransaminasemia. Patients with hypertransaminasemia were investigated to establish how many have celiac disease and to determine whether an unexplained increase in serum transaminases can be considered a high-risk condition for gluten-sensitive enteropathy.

Methods.—Fifty-five of 600 patients with liver disease due to raised serum transaminases had cryptogenic hypertransaminasemia after the exclusion of every known cause of liver disease. Indirect immunofluorescence was used to test these patients for immunoglobulin (Ig)A to endomysium and for IgA and IgG to gliadin.

Results.—Five patients tested positive for IgA to endomysium and IgG to gliadin. Four patients were positive for IgA to gliadin. Another patient who was not positive for antibodies to endomysium was positive for IgG to gliadin. Duodenal biopsy that showed a subtotal villous atrophy was found in the 6 antibody-positive patients, and this was consistent with celiac disease in the 5 patients with antibodies to endomysium. A normal small-intestine mucosa was found in the patient with only IgG to gliadin. Gastrointestinal symptoms were not seen in any of the 5 patients with celiac disease. Liver biopsy specimens taken from three of the five patients with flat mucosa showed a histologic picture of nonspecific reactive hepatitis. Within 6 months, transaminase concentrations reverted to normal in 4 patients with celiac disease who followed a strict gluten-free diet.

Conclusion.—Symptom-free celiac disease affects about 9% of patients with cryptogenic hypertransaminasemia. In these patients, consideration should be given to the performance of gluten-sensitive enteropathy and antibody screening for celiac disease by means of antibodies to endomysium and gliadin.

▶ How many of you have seen patients in your practice who are found to have an elevated liver transaminase level for which you could find no explanation? The next time you run into such an occurrence, think about the possibility that your patient may have celiac disease. In the series abstracted approximately 10% of adults with elevated enzyme levels of undetermined origin ultimately were shown to have celiac disease. The lesson is straightforward. The typical symptoms of celiac disease (diarrhea, flatulence, weight loss, and fatigue) may be as uncommon as they are common. Among the lesser known presentations of celiac disease, we must now consider also an elevation in liver enzymes levels. This can happen in the absence of any other sign or symptom of the disorder. This should not be too much of a surprise because biopsy-proven liver damage has been reported in most patients with untreated celiac disease who have other signs and symptoms of the problem.

This report is one of those little pearls that you run into every now and then in the literature. It links cryptogenic hypertransaminasemia to celiac disease. If such an association doesn't turn you on, it should. The elevations in serum transaminase levels in such circumstances are the tipoff to a disease that, if not treated (in this case with a gluten-free diet), could lead to a host of later consequences, including a greater risk of cancer (lymphoma in particular). The diagnosis of celiac disease can be easily suspected on the basis of a blood test (serum IgA/IgG to gliadin and IgA to endomysium). Such blood tests are highly predictive markers for celiac disease, which can then be confirmed by small-bowel biopsy.

J.A. Stockman III, M.D.

Role of Seroconversion in Confirming Cure of *Helicobacter pylori* Infection
Feldman M, Cryer B, Lee E, et al (Univ of Texas, Dallas; Dept of Veterans Affairs Med Ctr, Dallas, Tex)
JAMA 280:363-365, 1998   19–7

Introduction.—A growing trend exists for patients without ulcers to be tested for *Helicobacter pylori* infection. It is reasonable to want to determine effectiveness of antimicrobial treatment in patients who have recurrent symptoms. The sensitivity and specificity of *H. pylori* seroconversion in confirming cure of *H. pylori* infection was prospectively assessed.

Methods.—Twenty-three adults with active *H. pylori* infection with no history of peptic ulcer or chronic upper gastrointestinal tract symptoms had confirmation of infection by gastric biopsy and positive *H. pylori* serologic findings. All research subjects had a 14-day course of bismuth, tetracycline, and metronidazole. Serum samples were taken at baseline and at 1, 3, and about 18 months after completion of therapy to determine immunoglobulin (Ig)G serum antibodies to *H. pylori*. These data were compared with findings from serial gastric mucosal biopsy specimens. The *H. pylori* infection was considered cured when mucosal biopsy specimens from the gastric body and antrum no longer showed *H. pylori* organisms 18 months after therapy.

Results.—Fifteen (65%) of 23 research subjects were cured of gastritis and *H. pylori* infection, as determined by gastric biopsy. Mean antibody levels diminished from 92.5 U/mL at baseline to levels that were undetectable at final follow-up at 18 months. The remaining 8 (35%) research subjects were not cured and continued to experience persistent gastritis at 18 months. In these research subjects, the mean antibody level went from 130.6 U/mL at baseline to 89.7 U/mL at 18 months. The sensitivity and specificity of seroconversion (positive to negative test result) in determining cure of *H. pylori* infection were 60% and 100%, respectively.

Conclusion.—Cure of *H. pylori* infection led to elimination of gastritis and seroconversion in 60% of healthy research subjects. Seroconversion may be considered a reliable indicator of cure of *H. pylori* infection, however additional long-term studies are needed, particularly with the newer treatment regimens.

▶ *H. pylori* infections continue to puzzle us all. This article is 1 study performed in adults, but it is likely that its conclusions are applicable to children. In both children and adults, the question is frequently asked, is the patient cured, of their *H. pylori* infection. If there is a desire to confirm cure of *H. pylori* infection early after therapy, the process is not so easy. Urea breath testing or a gastric biopsy, obtained either endoscopically or nonendoscopically, are required, because *H. pylori* serum IgG antibody tests remain positive for many months after a cure. However, urea breath tests and gastric biopsy are time consuming and expensive, and biopsy is invasive. The longer the time from initial therapy, the more likely it is that serum IgG levels will fall. What we have not known, however, is how quickly IgG levels fall and what the sensitivity and specificity would be of paired-quantitative levels.

Comparing paired sera comparisons is difficult, if not impossible. Serum storage for prolonged periods is not practical. Many laboratories do not report quantitative antibody levels, but instead report results qualitatively as positive or negative. What the abstracted article tells us, however, is that one can do a single titer 18 months after completion of therapy, and if that titer is negative (a phenomenon known as reverse seroconversion), one can be 100% assured that the patient has been cured. On the other hand, a lingering titer does not necessarily mean the patient is still infected since some will still have positive titers in spite of negative biopsy specimens, a year and a half or more later. Although some 40% of subjects who are cured still have positive test results, those with negative results on IgG serologic testing clearly are cured.

To say all this differently, if a patient after initial treatment for *H. pylori* infection has recurrent symptoms, it is not necessary to do a repeat urea breath test or a gastric biopsy if that patient has a negative IgG antibody test. Your patient's symptoms are caused by something other than *H. pylori.*

Remember the term "reverse seroconversion." You will see it used more often for the diagnosis of a "cure" for diseases where antibody titers eventually fall to zero.

One final comment, this having to do with treatment of *H. pylori:* You're out of antibiotics. You're out of bismuth. You're in the middle of nowhere. How might you treat a *H. pylori* infection? The answer is, you might look around to see if anybody can give you a supply of mastic gum. Mastic is a resinous exudate contained in the stem and main leaves of *Pistacia lentiscus.* It is used as a food ingredient in the Mediterranean region. It is well known clinically that mastic gum is effective in the treatment of benign gastric ulcers and duodenal ulcers. One milligram per day for 2 weeks can cure peptic ulcers very rapidly, at least according to Huwez, Thirlwell, et al.[1]

Mastic gum is cheap and widely available, particularly in third-world countries. If your insurance plan doesn't pay for antibiotics, you might think about this alternative therapy.

J.A. Stockman III, M.D.

Reference

1. Huwez FU, Thirlwell D, Cockayne A, et al: Mastic gum kills *Helicobacter pylori* (letter). *N Engl J Med* 339:1946, 1998.

Helicobacter pylori Infection May Undergo Spontaneous Eradication in Children: A 2-Year Follow-up Study
Perri F, Pastore M, Clemente R, et al ("Casa Sollievo della Sofferenza" Hosp, San Giovanni Rotondo, Italy; Gasthuisberg Univ, Leuven, Belgium)
J Pediatr Gastroenterol Nutr 27:181-183, 1998   19–8

Introduction.—The most common chronic infection in humans may be *Helicobacter pylori* infection, which colonizes the stomach and is associated with gastritis, gastric and duodenal ulcer, and gastric cancer. Generally, this infection is acquired early in life and lasts several decades. It is unknown whether a spontaneous eradication of *H. pylori* can occur during childhood. It was determined whether *H. pylori* infection can be spontaneously eliminated in symptom-free, infected children.

Methods.—There were 304 children, ages 4.5 to 18.5 years, who were tested for *H. pylori* by means of C-urea breath test. This test was used because it is easy to perform, noninvasive, nonradioactive, and accurate, and can be repeated more times in the same person with no biologic hazard. The infected children were followed up every 6 months for as long as 2 years. Consumption of antibiotics was recorded among the children. A repeat C-urea breath test was given to children at each visit.

Results.—*H. pylori* infection was found in 85 children (27.9%). The follow-up study included 48 of the 85 infected children (56.4%). Negative results on C-urea breath tests were found in 8 (16.6%) of the infected children after 2 years. Antibiotics were given to 2 children for concomitant infections. At 6 months, one child was negative but then was found to be positive again at the next 6-month C-urea breath test. Persistent positive results were seen in 40 children, and of these 10 were given a short course of antibiotics.

Conclusion.—H. *pylori* infection may be a fluctuating disease with spontaneous eradication and possible recurrence, at least during childhood. The mechanisms underlying the complex relation between host and bacteria may act differently in children and adults.

▶ It's nice to know that H. *pylori* infection can go away on its own. Actually, that is not too surprising. Long before we even knew about H. *pylori* and how to treat it, we knew that children and adults with dyspepsia could, as often as not, have their symptoms go away on their own. Presumably, many of those latter individuals were patients who had H. *pylori* infection. This is not to say that we should not be treating patients who have documented H. *pylori* disease. A spontaneous regression rate within a 24-month period can only be expected in about 1 of 5 patients.

These data come at a time when we have also recently learned what the recurrence of infection with H. *pylori* is after adequate initial therapy. Kato et al.[1] tell us that reinfection with H. *pylori* is rare in children older than 5 years old once successful initial eradication has occurred. The actual reinfection rate is about 2.4% per patient-year. By the way, the latter data are from Japan, where the prevalence of H. *pylori* as detected by serum anti–H. *pylori* antibodies is approximately 20% among teenagers.

One final comment about H. *pylori* infection, and that is its relationship with gastric cancers. Thus far, we do not know too much about this relationship in children, but such an association certainly exists in adults; therefore, we should be worried about the potential in our pediatric-age population. The types of cancers seen in the stomach include carcinomas, lymphomas, and mucosa-associated lymphoid tissue lymphomas. What little information exists suggests that acquisition of H. *pylori* infection during childhood appears to be the critical risk factor for the later development of gastric cancers. In a superb study of the pathology of the stomach of patients with H. *pylori* infection, Jones et al.[2] have shown that the balance between gastric epithelial cell proliferation and programmed cell death (also known as apoptosis) is severely altered, favoring the development of malignancy.

To say all this differently, we don't want our kids to get infected with H. *pylori*, and if they do get infected, it is important to treat them adequately. Such treatment is associated with a low reinfection rate.

By the way, as far as treatment of ulcers is concerned, you may be seeing a resurgence of the use of milk, or at least calve's milk, for the management of peptic disease. While research is still at an early stage, laboratory studies suggest that bovine colostrum cuts the rate of gastric injury caused by nonsteroidal inflammatory drugs by as much as 60%. Colostrum from cows is sold over-the-counter as a health food supplement in most parts of this country.

Who would have ever thought that cow colostrum would be good for calves *and* humans?[3]

J.A. Stockman III, M.D.

References

1. Kato S, Abukawa D, Furuyama N, et al: *Helicobacter pylori* infection rates in children after eradication therapy. *J Pediatr Gastroenterol Nutr* 27:543-546, 1998.
2. Jones NL, Shannon PT, Coutz E, et al: Increase in proliferation and apoptosis of gastric epithelial cells early in the natural history of *Helicobacter pylori* infection. *Am J Pathol* 151:1695-1703, 1997.
3. Colostrum and gastric ulcers (editorial). *Gut* 44:653-658, 1999.

Pets Are Not a Risk Factor for *Helicobacter pylori* Infection in Young Children: Results of a Population-based Study in Southern Germany
Bode G, Rothenbacher D, Brenner H, et al (Univ of Ulm, Germany)
Pediatr Infect Dis J 17:909-912, 1998   19–9

Introduction.—Knowledge about the route of transmission of *Helicobacter pylori* infection remains incomplete. The infection is thought to be transmitted from person to person by the oral-fecal route or the oral-oral route. An important role in the transmission of the infection may be played by animals. Domestic feline and canine gastric tissue has revealed spiral organisms, and the stomachs of many animal species have their own highly evolved *Helicobacter* species. Generally, infection with *H. pylori* occurs during childhood. The relation of exposure to pets to the prevalence of *H. pylori* was assessed in children.

Methods.—There were 685 first-grade children included in the study. To determine active infection status, the C-urea breath test was used. Parents filled out a questionnaire to provide information about pets in the household, living conditions, and socioeconomic factors of the family. Gender was equally distributed, and most children were 6 years old. Parents had levels of education similar to the general adult population. There were 40.2% of children who had contact with pets, particularly rabbits (10.7%), cats (10.5%), and dogs (9.9%).

Results.—There was a 6.3% prevalence of infection. Contact with pets in general or a specific kind of animal was not associated with *H. pylori* infection, according to bivariate and multivariable analyses as evaluated by means of logistic regression. Pets were kept in the household for a mean of 49.9 months and varied from 31.1 months for guinea pigs and 73.0 months for dogs. None of the children with a dog in the household was infected.

Conclusion.—Among children in this population, pets in the household were not a risk factor for *H. pylori* infection.

▶ Thank goodness, Rover will be allowed to stay in the house. Apparently a kitty can as well, although cats remain on this editor's "good-for-nothing list"—prime candidates for an ample supply of material with which to string tennis rackets. Dogs seem to pose no risk at all.

Cats are well-established reservoirs for infections such as *Campylobacter jejuni* and *Salmonella* species, but as far as *H. pylori* is concerned, transmission from cats seems to be unimportant as a route of infection among children, although one recent report has described the isolation of *H. pylori* from cats.[1] Given the proclivity with which cats hack up their fur balls, one wonders if we might not see more in the way of transmission of this organism to kids from their pet Felix, if cats are ultimately shown to harbor this bug.

One additional comment regarding *H. pylori*, this having to do with the relationship between this infection and type 1 diabetes mellitus in children. In the early years of diabetes in children, the seroprevalence of *H. pylori* infection does not differ between patients with diabetes and control subjects. Subsequently, there is a much greater rate of acquisition of *H. pylori*, a phenomenon that has already been well described in adults and older patients with diabetes. It is at present impossible to establish whether the disease directly causes the increase by altering immunologic responses. *H. pylori* infection acquired in childhood and during adolescence could be one of the causes of chronic atrophic gastritis, which is frequently found in those who have long-standing diabetes mellitus.[2]

For more on the topic of *H. pylori* in pediatric patients and its diagnosis by serologic detection, see the superb editorial by Czinn.[3] You'll learn that commercially available serologic tests do not appear to have the necessary sensitivity or specificity to screen the large numbers of pediatric patients needed to determine who has and who does not have infection with *H. pylori*. This is not to say that a symptomatic patient who is seropositive should not be treated. On the other hand, seronegative patients cannot be presumed to be uninfected with *H. pylori*. Above all, there is insufficient evidence to say that all children with chronic abdominal pain should be empirically treated. That would be doing such patients a great disservice.

J.A. Stockman III, M.D.

References

1. Fox JG, Batchelder M, Marini R, et al: *Helicobacter pylori*–induced gastritis in the domestic cat. *Infect Immun* 63:2674-2681, 1995.
2. Salardi S, Cacciari E, Menegatti M, et al: *Helicobacter pylori* and type 1 diabetes mellitus in children. *J Pediatr Gastroenterol Nutr* 28:307-309, 1999.
3. Czinn SJ: Serodiagnosis of *Helicobacter pylori* in pediatric patients. *J Pediatr Gastroenterol Nutr* 28:157-161, 1999.

Extended Excretion of Rotavirus After Severe Diarrhoea in Young Children

Richardson S, Grimwood K, Gorrell R, et al (Royal Children's Hosp, Melbourne, Australia; Wellington School of Medicine, Wellington South, New Zealand)
Lancet 351:1844-1848, 1998   19–10

Introduction.—Rotaviruses are the primary cause of severe diarrhea in children. Duration of infection of rotavirus must be determined using highly sensitive techniques because human infection may be caused by the ingestion of only 1 plaque-forming unit. The duration of rotavirus excretion and fluctuations of antirotavirus immunoglobulin (Ig)A coproantibody were assessed in sequential fecal specimens collected from young children during the 100 days after hospital admission for severe rotavirus diarrhea.

Methods.—Fecal specimens were obtained daily for 14 days after hospital admission and weekly for a minimum of 100 days in 37 children who were hospitalized for severe rotavirus diarrhea. The 22 male and 15 female children were aged from 1 to 39 months. Stool specimens were screened for rotavirus by enzyme immunoassays and underwent analysis by reverse transcription–polymerase chain reaction. Enzyme immunoassays were used to estimate IgA coproantibodies.

Results.—Rotavirus excretion ranged from 4 to 57 days after onset of diarrhea. Excretion ceased within 10 days of hospital admission in 16 children (43%), between 10 and 21 days in 10 children (27%), and between 22 and 57 days in 11 children (30%) (Fig 1). The continued excretion of rotavirus was not correlated with age, symptom severity of symptoms during hospitalization, amount of virus excreted in initial disease stages, or serotype of the infecting rotavirus. Extended excretion of

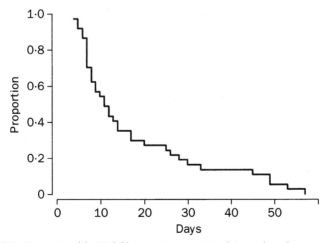

FIGURE 1.—Proportion of the 37 children excreting rotavirus relative to days after onset of rotavirus diarrhea. (Courtesy of Richardson S, Grimwood K, Gorrell R, et al: Extended excretion of rotavirus after severe diarrhoea in young children. *Lancet* 351[9119]:1844-1848, 1998. Copyright by The Lancet Ltd.)

rotavirus was significantly correlated with antirotavirus IgA coproanti-body boosts. Most boosts (68%) were related to rotavirus excretion, suggesting that the fluctuating coproantibody concentrations recorded during the surveillance period reflected an immune response to continuing replication of the rotavirus strain responsible for severe primary disease.

Conclusion.—About one third of young children with severe primary rotavirus infection may continue to excrete rotavirus particles for more than 21 days and up to 57 days after hospital admission. The intermittent excretion of rotaviruses for extended periods may make these young children reservoirs of infection. This phenomenon could contribute to the survival of human rotaviruses between epidemics.

▶ This article will get your attention. Before it appeared, most studies had suggested that fecal rotavirus shedding ceased within 10 days of the onset of symptoms in most children and within 20 days in almost all children. It was thought that extended excretion of this virus would only occur in immunocompromised children. Would that life be that easy. Continued excretion of rotaviruses for more than 21 days is common. In fact, virus excretion for close to 2 months should not be considered unusual if one uses as the gold standard virus detectable by polymerase chain reaction technology. You might say that such technology is too sensitive in picking up small quantities of the virus. Au contraire, human infection by rotavirus can be caused by the ingestion of a single plaque-forming unit of virus.

The implications of these findings are pretty straightforward. Once infants, toddlers, or children are infected with rotavirus, they are very able to infect others for a long period, setting the stage for not only epidemics of this diarrheal disease, but also persistence of the virus within communities between periods of epidemics. These findings also underscore the value of the rotavirus vaccine. Morbidity from rotavirus disease in the United States and the cost to our health care systems and society are substantial. The new FDA-rotavirus vaccine has been proved to be effective in preventing disease and decreasing the rate of hospitalization. This makes routine immunization with this vaccine potentially attractive. The rub, however, is the cost to the care provider of this vaccine, a cost that will be passed along. At the time of the announcement of the availability of this vaccine in August 1998, its manufacturer, Wyeth-Lederle, proposed a charge of $38.00 per vaccine dose. Add that to the additional expense for vaccine administration, and one can see that this vaccine could be only marginally cost effective from a societal standpoint. In fact, it could well be the least cost-effective vaccine used in the United States at that price. In the fall of 1998, the Public Policy Council representing the American Pediatric Society, the Association of Medical School Pediatric Department Chairs, and the Society for Pediatric Research went online with Wyeth to suggest that the vaccine price be lowered to no more than $20.00. They urged Wyeth to reduce the price of the vaccine to be certain as many children as possible could derive its benefits. Hopefully by the time this commentary is published, a lower-priced, and therefore more cost-effective vaccine has been made available and, hopefully, it is one that is not associated with a risk of intussusception.

This commentary shifts gears at this point to see how you would handle the following situation. You are brought a 7-week-old African American baby with a history of fever, emesis, and diarrhea. The temperature is 101.2°F. The fontanelle is flat and the rest of the examination is generally unremarkable, except that the child appears to be ill. Sepsis is suspected. The white blood cell count is 10,000/mm³ with 18% band forms, toxic granulations, and Döhle's bodies in neutrophils. Lumbar puncture, serum electrolytes, and chest x-rays had unremarkable results. You obtain blood, urine, and spinal fluid for culture and hospitalize the child after starting the administration of ceftriaxone. Within 48 hours, *Yersinia enterocolitica* is isolated from the blood. The patient's symptoms respond fairly quickly over a 3-day period, and an uneventful recovery occurs. The question is, How did this child develop this particular infection? The only clue you have is that this infant contracted the infection during a long Thanksgiving Day weekend.

If you put together the fact that this was an African American baby who became ill over Thanksgiving from an infectious agent that has its origins in enteric flora, you might have recognized that there was a possibility that this child, in one way or another, had been exposed to chitterlings. As it turns out, this baby's grandmother had prepared chitterlings on Thanksgiving Day for inclusion in the holiday dinner. She failed to wash her hands before preparing the baby's formula.

Consumption of chitterlings occurs principally over the Thanksgiving Day and New Year's Day holidays. A history of exposure to chitterlings should be investigated when potentially exposed infants are seen during the winter with enteric disease or signs of septicemia.[1] Pediatricians need to counsel about careful hand-washing for those who prepare entrails for human consumption.

J.A. Stockman III, M.D.

Reference

1. Bien JP: Anticipatory guidance and chitterlings. *J Pediatr* 133:712, 1998.

An Evidenced-based Clinical Pathway for Acute Appendicitis Decreases Hospital Duration and Cost
Warner BW, Kulick RM, Stoops MM, et al (Univ of Cincinnati, Ohio)
J Pediatr Surg 33:1371-1375, 1998   19–11

Background.—Clinical pathways are designed to reduce the overall costs associated with a particular diagnosis and to minimize variations in diagnosis and therapy between different practitioners, without negatively affecting patient outcomes. A clinical pathway for the most common surgical emergency in children was created and results are reported.

Methods.—The study included 2 groups of patients with acute appendicitis: 122 control patients (mean age, 11.5 years) who underwent surgery before the clinical pathway was in place and 120 patients (mean age, 11.2

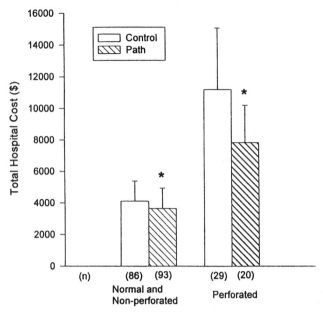

FIGURE 3.—Average total hospital cost (±SD) including home care for patients with either nonperforated or perforated appendicitis. Control patients were compared with pathway patients. *P < .05. (Courtesy of Warner BW, Kulick RM, Stoops MM, et al: An evidence-based clinical pathway for acute appendicitis decreases hospital duration and cost. *J Pediatr Surg* 33:1371-1375, 1998.)

years) whose condition was managed in accordance with an evidence-based clinical pathway. Two clinical pathways were created: 1 for a nonperforated appendix (symptoms between 24 and 48 hours, localized abdominal tenderness) and 1 for a perforated appendix. For pathway patients, intravenous access was established, and crystalloid fluids and antibiotics were administered preoperatively, but patients did not undergo radiologic or laboratory studies unless other conditions were suspected (eg, palpable mass, gallstones, etc). The nonperforated clinical pathway required the continuation of antibiotics for 1 additional dose, resumption of diet within 6 to 8 hours, and ambulation as early as possible. The perforated clinical pathway required the continuation of antibiotics for 7 days or more after surgery, a renal profile and determination of antibiotic levels on the first day after surgery, a complete blood count on the seventh day after surgery, and early consultation with home care services. Records were reviewed to compare demographic, clinical, and cost variables between the control group and the pathway patients.

Findings.—The control and pathway groups were similar in their rates of negative radiologic and laboratory tests (12.3% vs 9.2%, respectively) and in the incidence of perforation (26.2% vs 18.3%). However, emergency department management, hospital duration, and hospital costs differed significantly between the groups (Fig 3). Pathway patients received surgical consultation sooner (1.6 vs 2.5 hours), and they were more likely to be taken to the emergency room in less than 3 hours (38% vs 17%). For those with nonperforated appendicitis, significantly more pathway patients were discharged in 24 hours or less (67% vs 48%), and their hospital costs were lower ($1280 vs $4095). For those with a perforated appendix, pathway patients had a significantly shorter mean hospital stay (113 vs 185 hours) and lower mean hospital costs ($11,175 vs $7823).

Conclusions.—Use of the clinical pathway significantly improved response times in the emergency department and reduced hospital costs, without having a negative impact on diagnosis or therapy. The estimated annual savings for appendicitis under this pathway at the authors' institution is $164,800, about a 20% decrease compared with the control group's period.

▶ Nobody likes a cookbook, including this editor. It is difficult, nonetheless, to ignore any report that shows that with the use of a clinical pathway for diagnosis and treatment, cost is reduced and quality of care is improved. These are the precise findings from the Children's Hospital Medical Center in Cincinnati, Ohio. Recognizing that although significant differences may be detected in the white blood cell count determinations between patients with and without appendicitis, more often than not, there is substantial overlap. Thus a CBC is probably of limited usefulness. In Cincinnati, therefore, a white count and differential is not used in deciding which patients undergo appendectomy. It can serve as a baseline test in the follow-up in the postoperative period. In the same light, since an abnormal urinalysis may be seen in up to 50% of patients with acute appendicitis, this test can also be skipped. Similarly skipped is the abdominal radiograph. Only 1 in 10 patients with appendicitis show an appendicolith, and only 21% of patients will have any other abnormality on a plain film.

The consequence of not needing to do so many studies means that it is more likely that a busy surgical resident or attending physician will see a patient sooner than later since there is no waiting around for tests that will ultimately make little difference. This is probably one of the reasons why the patients in Cincinnati got out of the hospital faster, with lower hospital charges, if they were treated "on protocol." By the way, even if the appendix was perforated, the savings per patient per hospital stay amounted to $3350.

Acute appendicitis remains the most common reason for a child to be admitted to a pediatric surgical service. It also remains a diagnostic challenge. Part of the reason it is a diagnostic challenge relates to the many faces of the presentation of an acute appendix. Please see the article in the Genitourinary Tract chapter (Abstract 10–4), that warns us that a hot appendix can act like an "acute scrotum."

J.A. Stockman III, M.D.

Symptomatic Colonic Polyps in Childhood: Not So Benign

Hoffenberg EJ, Sauaia A, Maltzman T, et al (Univ of Colorado, Denver)
J Pediatr Gastroenterol Nutr 28:175-181, 1999   19–12

Introduction.—A common symptom of colonic polyps in children is lower gastrointestinal bleeding. Children can have multiple, rather than solitary, juvenile polyps, with up to 9% of children with juvenile polyps having 5 or more. Ten or more polyps is considered juvenile polyposis coli, and in these patients, there is an increased risk of adenocarcinoma of the colon. Colorectal cancer may be prevented in adulthood if children with juvenile polyposis coli can be identified early since it takes about 10 years for a polyp to develop into a malignancy. A series of children with colonic polyps was reviewed to compare the clinical features of those with juvenile polyposis coli and those without this problem, as well as to determine the prevalence of genetic alterations known to be common in colorectal tumorigenesis.

Methods.—There were 78 children, aged 0.4 to 18 years, with symptomatic colonic polyps and negative family history of polyps. The definition of juvenile polyposis coli was 10 or more juvenile polyps or any juvenile polyp in a relative of an index case of juvenile polyposis coli. Tests on polyps were conducted for *Ki-ras* mutations, p53 overexpression, and aneuploidy. All the children were evaluated for lower gastrointestinal

TABLE 2.—Clinical Data of 78 Children With Symptomatic Colonic Polyps

	JPC ($n = 9$)	Non-JPC ($n = 69$)	P
Symptom duration			
(mo median [range])	12 (1-24)	4 (0-18)	0.32
Reason for evaluation (%)*			
Rectal bleeding	8 (89)	68 (99)	0.22
Anemia	2 (22)	0 (0)	0.01
Abdominal Pain	1 (11)	4 (6)	0.39
Polyp characteristics			
Number (median (range)	14 (2-55)	1 (1->10)	0.001
Polyp type per patient (%)			0.001
Pedunculated	1 (11)	63 (91)	
Sessile	0	4 (6)	
Pedunculated and sessile	8 (89)	2 (3)	
Rectal prolapse of polyp (%)	0	16 (23)	0.19
Polyp with adenomatous			
change (%)	2 (22)	2 (3)	0.06
Polyp location (%)			0.001†
Anorectal	0	10 (14)	
Rectosigmoid	0	45 (65)	
Left-side	0	9 (13)	
Right-side	1 (11)	5 (7)	
Pancolonic	8 (89)	0	

*One child had both bleeding and anemia (JPC group), and 4 children had both bleeding and pain (1 in JPC, and 3 in non-JPC group).
†JPC versus non-JPC distribution of left-side, right-side, and pan-colonic polyps.
Abbreviation: JPC, juvenile polyposis coli.
(Courtesy of Hoffenberg EJ, Sauaia A, Maltzman T, et al: Symptomatic colonic polyps in childhood: Not so benign. *J Pediatr Gastroenterol Nutr* 28:175-181, 1999.)

bleeding. They were divided into those with juvenile polyposis coli and those without the problem.

Results.—Juvenile polyposis coli was found in 9 children (12%). Isolated juvenile polyps were found in 66 children (84%), and other types of polyps were found in 3 children (4%). The 9 children with juvenile polyposis coli were similar in age and symptom duration to the other children. However, they had more polyps and a greater likelihood of anemia, polyps with adenomatous change, and right-colon polyps (Table 2). In 3 of the 8 families with juvenile polyposis coli, polyps were identified in asymptomatic first-degree relatives. There was no identification of abnormalities in *Ki-ras*, p53, or aneuploidy.

Conclusion.—In children with symptomatic polyps, juvenile polyposis coli is common and is associated with right-colon polyps, anemia, and adenomas. Further study is needed to determine the risk of polyps and of colorectal cancer in relatives of individuals with juvenile polyposis coli.

▶ Rectal bleeding, sometimes profuse, is the herald sign of a colonic polyp in a child. In most cases, these turn out to be what are known as "juvenile" polyps, which have also been called hamartomatous retentive or inflammatory polyps. A child with unexplained rectal bleeding demands a colonoscopy not only to deal with the bleeding polyp itself but also to determine whether other polyps are present, which implies a polyposis syndrome. In contrast to isolated juvenile polyps, the polyposis syndromes (including Peutz-Jegher syndrome and juvenile polyposis coli disorder) are associated with an increased risk of colorectal cancer. The finding of 5 to 10 juvenile polyps is quite suggestive of juvenile polyposis coli, with 10 or more polyps being diagnostic. In such kids, the chance of developing adenocarcinoma of the colon runs as high as 30%. These cancers occur via transformation known as adenomatous change within an existing juvenile polyp. The average time for an adenomatous polyp to transform itself into a malignancy is about 10 years, so once a child is identified, regular surveillance via periodic colonoscopy is mandatory and will prevent colorectal cancer. Children with lots of recurrent polyps or too many polyps to remove should be considered candidates for colectomy.

Were you aware that gastrointestinal polyps could occur in places other than where you might think? For example, a 16-year-old was recently reported who had heartburn and mild dysphagia. The youngster had no history of vomiting or of gastrointestinal tract bleeding. An esophagogram showed evidence of a filling defect suggestive of a polyp, a diagnosis confirmed on endoscopy. As it turns out, at age 11, he had undergone an esophageal colonic interposition for an esophageal stricture secondary to caustic injury that had occurred some years earlier. The transverse colon with its middle colic artery was used for the interposition. The patient had no history suggestive of colonic polyp before this surgery, and there was no family history of colonic polyps or cancer.[1]

The next time you see a child with rectal bleeding, hopefully it will be from a fissure and not from a juvenile polyp. If it is due to a polyp, be aware that about 15% of such polyps are in association with a polyposis syndrome. The risk of malignancy in such situations is worrisomely high.

J.A. Stockman III, M.D.

Reference

1. Del Rosario MA, Croffie JM, Rescorla FJ, et al: Juvenile polyp in esophageal colon interposition. *J Pediatr Surg* 33:1418-1419, 1998.

Colonic Polyps: Experience of 236 Indian Children

Poddar U, Thapa BR, Vaiphei K, et al (Postgraduate Inst of Med Education and Research, Chandigarh, India)
Am J Gastroenterol 93:619-622, 1998   19–13

Background.—Juvenile polyps can be single or multiple and can be rectosigmoid or proximal to the sigmoid colon. Although juvenile polyps are thought to have little malignant potential, some studies have reported malignancies in patients with single juvenile polyps or with juvenile polyposis. These authors described the clinical characteristics and histologic findings of colonic polyps in children living in India and evaluated their malignant potential.

Methods.—The subjects were 236 children (male-female ratio, 3.5:1) 12 years old or younger (mean age, 6.12 years) who had colonic polyps. All patients were evaluated clinically and by colonoscopy. Polyps occurring singly (seen in 76% of patients) or in groupings of 2 to 5 (seen in 16.5% of patients) were removed during colonoscopy. The 17 patients with 5 or more polyps (that is, juvenile polyposis; 7% of patients) underwent serial colonoscopic polypectomies every 3 weeks until all polyps were removed. Patients who did not respond to colonoscopic polypectomy were treated by colectomy. Patients with juvenile polyposis were monitored by follow-up colonoscopy to ensure the completeness of polyps removal. Polyps were available for histologic examination from 152 patients (142 of whom had juvenile polyps).

TABLE 1.—Distribution of Polyps (Excluding Juvenile Polyposis)

Site	No. of Polyps (%)
Rectum	193 (72.0)
Sigmoid	52 (19.5)
Descending colon	10 (3.7)
Transverse colon	7 (2.5)
Ascending colon/cecum	5 (2.0)

TABLE 2.—Comparison Between Juvenile Polyps and Juvenile Polyposis

	Juvenile Polyps (n = 219)	Juvenile Polyposis (n = 17)	p Value
Age (yrs)	5.97 ± 2.62	7.68 ± 2.95	<0.05
Gender (M:F)	3.5:1	3.2:1	NS
Duration of symptoms (months)	12.24 ± 13.15	33.0 ± 27.0	<0.001
Rectal bleeding	99%	94%	NS
Polyps localized to rectosigmoid	90%	0%	<0.001
Adenomatous changes	5%	59%	<0.001
Polypectomy (session/child)	1.04 ± 0.20	4.76 ± 3.72	<0.001

(Reprinted by permission of the publisher, from Poddar U, Thapa BR, Vaiphei K, et al: Colonic polyps: Experience of 236 Indian children. *Am J Gastroenterol* 93:619-622. Copyright 1998 by Elsevier Science Inc.)

Findings.—The majority of polyps were solitary (76%), juvenile (93%), and located in the rectum (72%) or sigmoid colon (19.5%) (Table 1). Only 17 of the 152 polyps examined (11%) showed adenomatous changes, and these changes were significantly more common in patients with juvenile polyposis (59%) than in those with juvenile polyps (5%) (Table 2). Patients with juvenile polyposis were also significantly more likely to be older (7.68 vs 5.97 years) and have a longer duration of symptoms (33.0 vs 12.24 months). Polyps recurred in 10 of the 219 patients with juvenile polyps (5%). Of the 17 patients with juvenile polyposis, the colon was cleared in 8 patients (3 of whom required repeat polypectomy for recurrence), colectomy was required in 6 patients, and 3 patients were still undergoing serial polypectomies at the time of reporting.

Conclusion.—In most of these children, the polyps were solitary and rectosigmoid. Nonetheless, about 24% had multiple polyps (7% of whom had juvenile polyposis), and about 8% of the polyps were located proximally. Thus, all children with polyps should be examined by total colonoscopy. Juvenile polyposis has a higher neoplastic potential than juvenile polyps, and, thus, multiple polyps should be removed and their recurrence closely monitored by colonoscopy.

▶ The statistics about colonic polyps are pretty straightforward when it comes to children. If you are a pediatrician in general practice following somewhere between 1000 and 1300 children actively, whether you know it or not and whether the patient has or does not have symptoms, you will have about 10 to 13 children who have colonic polyps. Such polyps are among the most common causes of significant rectal bleeding. Most of the polyps are solitary and are located in the rectum or sigmoid colon.

Fortunately, juvenile polyps are benign. They are hamartomas. Thus far, only 5 cases of juvenile polyps have been described that have had adenomatous changes, and only 2 cases of colorectal malignancy evolving from juvenile polyps have been reported. This is not to say that juvenile polyposis is not a premalignant condition late in life. Most agree that, with time, there is a potential for the development of malignancy, but this most likely occurs at a significantly older age.

All juvenile polyps should be removed endoscopically to prevent rebleeding and also to prevent the later development of a malignancy. Fortunately, with current colonoscopy techniques, the procedure for dealing with them is very straightforward and relatively simple.

J.A. Stockman III, M.D.

Guideline for the Management of Pediatric Idiopathic Constipation and Soiling
Felt B, Wise CG, Olson A, et al (Univ of Michigan, Ann Arbor)
Arch Pediatr Adolesc Med 153:380-385, 1999   19–14

Background.—What is the best approach to the diagnosis and management of idiopathic constipation and soiling in children? These authors developed an evidence-based guideline for use by primary care physicians in approaching this problem.

Methods.—This multidisciplinary team of authors performed a MEDLINE search of publications from January 1975 through January 1998 to gather evidence regarding 3 primary questions: First, what is the best path to early, accurate diagnosis? Second, what are the best methods for adequate clean-out? Third, what are the best approaches for promoting patient and family compliance with management? The team identified 25 articles addressing these questions, then graded them according to strict criteria and created evidence tables for each of the 3 questions. They then developed the algorithm and clinical care guidelines by consultation and with consensus.

Findings.—The algorithm emphasizes the need for early identification of children with idiopathic constipation and soiling, the recognition of when they should be referred, and the importance of patient and family compliance. The first step is to rule out another disorder as the cause of the constipation and soiling. Once an idiopathic cause is confirmed, both the family and the patient should be educated about the physiologic basis of the condition and should understand that the condition is common and usually multifactorial. If impaction is present, disimpaction should be pursued with high-dose mineral oil, enemas, or a combination of enema, suppository, and oral laxative.

After full expulsion and as a next step for patients without impaction, the patient should enter a (minimum) 6-month maintenance phase to promote regular stool production and to prevent reimpaction. Maintenance therapy should include behavioral training, dietary changes, and oral medications such as mineral oil and senna syrup. After 6 months, patients should be weaned from laxatives, although maintenance therapy may be required for up to 24 months (with efforts to wean from laxatives at 6-month intervals). Recovery is defined as the production of 3 or more stools per week without soiling. For patients who fail to recover, physicians should consider the need to improve compliance, the need to revisit the differential diagnosis, or the need for further evaluation by a developmental behavioral pediatrician or a child psychiatrist.

Conclusion.—The algorithm and guideline presented were created based on evidence in the literature and can be used by primary care physicians to diagnose and manage children with idiopathic constipation and soiling.

▶ It's nice to know that we have a helping hand in the form of an algorithm to guide us in the management of a common pediatric problem: constipation and soiling. Algorithms are not for everyone, but sometimes cookbooks do help relieve us of the need to start from scratch every time we encounter similar types of problems. By the way, the guidelines from this report may also be found on the University of Michigan website (http://www.med .umich.edu/i/oca/practiceguidelines/).

While on the topic of helping hands, more than three quarter of children referred for chronic constipation were found in a referral center to have never had a digital rectal examination performed before the gastrointestinal referral.[1] In half of the cases, the children were subsequently found to have fecal impactions, implying that they had never received adequate "clean out" therapy before they showed up for their consultations. If you want to give a helping hand to these kids, put on a glove, do a digital rectal examination and start the treatment by diagnosing whether an impaction is present or not.

Please recognize that constipation can present itself in unusual ways. Take the case, for example, of an 11-year-old girl who came in with complaints of low back pain radiating down her legs. A diagnosis of sciatica was made, but the history suggested that she also had chronic constipation. After an MRI scan, it was clear that her lower abdomen was filled with feces (as a consequence of idiopathic megacolon). Hard feces filled the entire space between the sacrum and the pubic symphysis.

By the way, a good bowel movement (assisted by multiple enemas) relieved this child's sciatica. It must have been a grand opening.[2]

Lastly, my sister Patricia, a nurse, sent in a suggestion, via E-mail, for the treatment of chronic constipation that the readers of the YEAR BOOK might enjoy. She says that adults with this problem should prepare a cocktail of vodka, orange juice, and milk of magnesia. One might call this a "Phillip's screwdriver."

J.A. Stockman III, M.D.

References

1. Gold DM, Levine J, Weinstein TA, et al: Frequency of digital rectal examination in children with chronic constipation. *Arch Pediatr Adolesc Med* 153:377-379, 1999.
2. Frischhut B, Ojon M, Trobos S, et al: Sciatica as a manifestation of idiopathic megacolon: A previously undescribed causal relationship. *J Pediatr* 133:449, 1998.

Intolerance of Cow's Milk and Chronic Constipation in Children

Iacono G, Cavataio F, Montalto G, et al (Ospedale G di Cristina, Palermo, Italy; Università di Palmero, Italy)

N Engl J Med 339:1100-1104, 1998   19–15

Background.—A previous open study indicated that children with intolerance to cow's milk often have chronic constipation. Children with chronic constipation were evaluated in a double-blind crossover study to compare the effects of cow's milk and soy-based milk.

Methods.—The study included 65 children (29 boys and 36 girls, aged from 11 to 72 months) who had chronic constipation (1 bowel movement every 3 to 15 days) that was refractory to treatment with laxatives. All patients were consuming diets containing cow's milk (whole milk, dairy products, or commercial formulas) at study entry. Laboratory tests and a rectal biopsy were performed at baseline; 49 patients (75%) had anal fissures and perianal erythema or edema. Fifteen days after the baseline visit, patients were assigned to receive either cow's milk or soy milk for 14 days. After a 7-day washout period (diet was unrestricted) between treatment arms, patients were switched to the other type of milk for 14 days. Patients who had 8 or more bowel movements during a 14-day treatment arm were considered to have a response.

Findings.—During both treatment periods, none of the patients receiving cow's milk had a response. However, 44 of 65 patients (68%) receiving soy milk had a response, and their discomfort on defecation, erythema, and perianal edema resolved completely. After 1 month, the responders were challenged with cow's milk. Their constipation and discomfort on defecation returned with the cow's milk, and again disappeared with the soy milk. Furthermore, rectal biopsy was repeated in 20 responders 1 month after beginning the soy milk diet; 8 patients had normal histologic findings, and the other 12 patients showed significant improvement while off cow's milk. At baseline, symptoms suggestive of intolerance to milk (rhinitis, bronchospasm, dermatitis) were significantly more common in soy milk responders than nonresponders (11 of 44 patients [25%] vs 1 of 21 patients [5%]), as were hypersensitivities on immunologic testing (31 of 44 [71%] vs 4 of 21 [19%]). Responders were also significantly more likely to have had anal fissures and erythema or edema (40 of 44 [91%] vs 9 of 21 [43%] and biopsy evidence of rectal mucosa inflammation (26 of 44 [59%] vs 5 of 21 [24%]). Finally, after 8 to 12 months of drinking soy milk, cow's milk was reintroduced to 15 patients; all 15 developed constipation.

Conclusions.—In two thirds of these patients, the constipation was related to cow's milk. Children with anal fissures and erythema/edema and rectal mucosa inflammation were particularly likely to respond to a cow's milk-free diet, as were children with signs of milk intolerance or hypersensitivity. The improvement in histologic findings on rectal biopsy in 20 of the responders offers a mechanism for the constipation: In the patients with severe anal fissures, discomfort with defecation causes the child to retain feces in the rectum. This causes the stools to dehydrate and harden, thereby making the constipation worse.

▶ Another report providing convincing evidence that cow's milk is for calves and that the breast is best when it comes to humans. The popular teaching is that intolerance to cow's milk during early childhood results in chronic diarrhea, not constipation. Au contraire. Indeed, it would seem that intolerance to cow's milk is a very common cause of chronic constipation in children. The authors of this article suggest that cow's milk allergy with its resulting inflammation of the gastrointestinal tract produces irritative bowel movements resulting in anal fissures and that the latter ultimately cause chronic constipation via stool avoidance. This is an interesting weave that actually makes some sense.

Chronic constipation is a very common problem in children, and it's good to know that a fair percentage of it is caused by cow milk ingestion since this is readily preventable and easily treated. While on the topic of chronic constipation, recent information has emerged about Hirschsprung's disease. Data from a study in the United Kingdom suggest that we are doing too many rectal biopsies to make a diagnosis of Hirschsprung's disease.[1] In a retrospective review of 186 rectal biopsies from 141 children with chronic constipation, all of the 17 children with Hirschsprung's disease had the onset of their symptoms before 4 weeks of age. Not a single child who developed symptoms after 4 weeks of age was ultimately diagnosed as having Hirschsprung's disease. Please note that a very careful history was taken to be certain of when the first symptoms appeared in this British report. If the recommendations from this report had been followed, essentially all cases of Hirschsprung's disease would have been accurately diagnosed while at the same time some 60% of rectal biopsies that were negative would have been largely avoided.

This is the last entry in the Gastroenterology chapter, so we will close with a query. Do you know what *gut-lag* is? Gut-lag is the prosaic brother of jet-lag. Gut-lag (a.k.a., constipation) has now been described to commonly occur after long flights. It is equivalent of jet-lag of the bowel. Many travelers have apparently experienced this, but presumably because it is such a personal phenomenon, its existence has never made it into the literature—at least until recently.[2] It would appear that with gut-lag, a morning habit may continue to make its usually timely request, but at a more distant hour of the day, when the habit may not be accommodated. It would also appear that gut-lag subsides at about the same time jet-lag subsides. It is not amendable to melatonin therapy.

A betting person would say that much more will now appear in the literature about gut-lag. Is it worse flying against time zones in an easterly direction, or with them in a westerly direction? Stay tuned for answers to these pivotal questions in medicine. Whatever the answers show, it will be obvious that "east, west, home is best," as far as the potty is concerned.

J.A. Stockman III, M.D.

References

1. Ghosh A, Griffiths DM: Rectal biopsy in the investigation of constipation. *Arch Dis Child* 79:266-268, 1998.
2. Shuster S: Gut-lag: A silent dignity. *Lancet* 350:1488, 1997.

Subject Index

A

Abdominal
  discomfort as premenstrual symptom in adolescents, 229
  pain in juvenile dermatomyositis, 517
  symptoms in chronic fatigue syndrome, 179
  wall malformations and Down's syndrome, 151
Abuse
  physical, documentation of, 162
Academic
  performance
    declining, after classic manifestations of Lyme disease, 512
    expenditures per student and, 220
    sleep-disordered breathing and, 297
Accidental
  adolescent poisoning deaths, in U.S., 257
Acidosis
  Fanconi's renal tubular, due to ketogenic diet, 196
Acoustomagnetic
  electronic surveillance devices, interference with pacemakers, 352
Actinobacillus suis
  endocarditis due to, 340
Acyclovir
  for condyloma, 143
Addison's disease
  vomiting due to, cyclic, 527
Adductor
  -related groin pain in athletes, long-standing, active physical training as treatment for, 496
Adenoidal
  obstruction, clinical signs vs. roentgenographic findings, 449
Adenoidectomy
  for obstructive sleep apnea, and obesity, 448
Adenovirus
  infection after measles, mumps, and rubella vaccination, 56
  pertussis-like coughing due to, 75
Adolescent(s)
  alcohol use beliefs and behaviors among high school students, 233
  atherosclerosis in, prevalence and extent of, 322
  beach week as high school graduate rite of passage for, 225
  body composition development, in white females, 115

breast masses in girls, fine-needle aspiration of, 236
celiac disease in, gluten-free diet as nutritional risk factor in, 111
Chlamydia trachomatis screening for, home, in girls, 246
diabetes mellitus in, type 1, natural history of microalbuminuria in, 289
emergency department use by, in U.S., 227
fatigue in, chronic
  course and outcome, 178
  syndrome of, orthostatic intolerance in, 342
herpes zoster in, 45
homicide rates, in U.S., 255
hypercholesterolemia in, heterozygous familial, lovastatin for, 324
levonorgestrel use in, 250
medicine, 225
medroxyprogesterone acetate use in, depot, 250
Pap smear diagnoses in, 240
Pap smear screening in, routine, 252
poisoning deaths, in U.S., 257
pregnancy, and smoking, 310
premenstrual symptoms in, prevalence and severity, 229
psychiatrists, national distribution of, 185
rumination disorders in, chewing gum as treatment for, 529
sexual maturation in females with anorexia nervosa, self-assessment of, 235
sleep schedules and daytime functioning in, 231
vaginal infections in, evaluation without speculum, 243
Adrenal
  hyperplasia, congenital, mortality of, 471
African Americans
  in child care, otitis media with effusion in, 466
  chitterlings causing Yersinia enterocolitica infection in, in infant, 543
Age
  childbearing at early age as risk factor for infant homicide, 161
  distribution of pediatric practice, 182
  -related differences in clinical manifestations of congenital long QT syndrome, 346

Author Index

A

Abbassi V, 478
Achermann JC, 481
Adams MM, 215
Addis MF, 293
Adish AA, 359
Aeppli D, 313
Ainely-Walker PF, 138
Akazawa K, 424
Aker PD, 129
Albright K, 455
Allen AL, 142
Al Odaib A, 531
Amir E, 445
Andersen B, 246
Anderson AC, 171
Anderson ME, 432
Annerén G, 488
Aquino A, 149
Arditi M, 79
Armstrong BG, 434
Arruda VR, 504
Arvin AM, 54
Atala A, 275
Atchison J, 473
Attie KM, 487
Auerbach J, 223
August GP, 483
Avner JR, 90

B

Bachman DT, 509
Baghurst PA, 265
Baker MD, 90
Ballaban-Gil K, 196
Balon J, 129
Baorto E, 339
Barabino A, 361
Barnard M, 344
Barrow RE, 131
Barson WJ, 81
Bartholmey S, 106
Basson CT, 336
Bealer JF, 267
Beck P, 439
Belangero WD, 504
Belay ED, 116
Bell JJ, 482
Bell LM, 90
Bellini LM, 157
Benador N, 291
Bennett MJ, 531
Bennett RT, 277
Benson DW, 336

Bent JP III, 460
Berg-Kelly KS, 250
Berkowitz CD, 162
Bernard BS, 449
Bernini JC, 372
Bernstein GA, 259
Bhaskar B, 165
Bialik GM, 503
Bialik V, 503
Biederman J, 220
Bierings M, 521
Bilenker JH, 374
Birken CS, 181
Blake DR, 243
Blanchette VS, 382
Blanco R, 514
Blazer S, 503
Blethen SL, 483, 487
Bloom BJ, 512, 518
Bluebond-Langner R, 394
Bocian AB, 182
Bode G, 539
Bodensteiner JB, 198
Bogaerts H, 74
Boguniewicz M, 133
Bolte RG, 278
Bordley WC, 263
Boulet JR, 227
Braat DDM, 249
Bradley JS, 79
Brenner H, 539
Brenner RA, 160, 165
Bresee JS, 116
Brewer ED, 287
Brittenham GM, 366
Brook CGD, 471
Buchanan GR, 385
Buckley RH, 99
Burchinal MR, 464
Busby A, 434
Busse WW, 123
Butchart S, 382
Butterworth RJ, 208
Butzin D, 493

C

Cabral DA, 405
Callahan C, 196
Calpin J, 381
Carabin H, 92
Carlsson-Skwirut C, 488
Carr R, 26
Carrier C, 419
Carroll ME, 259
Carruth BR, 107

Carskadon MA, 231
Carta F, 293
Caserta MT, 48
Cavataio F, 552
Cavé H, 408
Chan DP, 201
Chaoui N, 530
Chatburn RL, 121
Chinchilli VM, 115
Chonmaitree T, 462
Christie JD, 157
Chung A, 517
Cisek LJ, 275
Cleckner-Smith CS, 229
Clemente R, 537
Cloyd JC, 187
Coelho P, 77
Cohen DM, 495
Cohn JA, 532
Colborn DK, 449
Cole CH, 20
Colton T, 20
Cook A, 103
Cook L, 76
Cortes D, 283
Corwin MJ, 164
Cox C, 271
Cromer BA, 250
Crowther ER, 129
Cryer B, 535
Culasso F, 318
Culnane M, 43
Curless RG, 200

D

Damiano PC, 446
Dana K, 482
Daneman D, 289
David TJ, 138
Davidkin I, 56
Davidson F, 357
Davidson PW, 271
Davies SM, 420
Davis GL, 60
Davis P, 126
Davy T, 71
Dean NW, 259
DeCamillo DM, 333
De Franceschi L, 534
de Kam PJ, 397
de Lonlay-Debeney P, 475
Dempfle C-E, 439
Dick P, 381
Dick PT, 71
Di Paolo FM, 318